DHA for Optimal Health

Special Issue Editor

Barbara Meyer

MDPI • Basel • Beijing • Wuhan • Barcelona • Belgrade

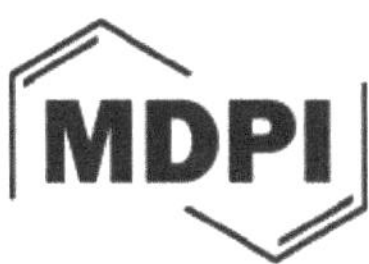

Special Issue Editor
Barbara Meyer
University of Wollongong
Australia

Editorial Office
MDPI
St. Alban-Anlage 66
Basel, Switzerland

This edition is a reprint of the Special Issue published online in the open access journal *Nutrients* (ISSN 2072-6643) from 2015–2016 (available at: http://www.mdpi.com/journal/nutrients/special issues/dha-brain-function).

For citation purposes, cite each article independently as indicated on the article page online and as indicated below:

Lastname, F.M.; Lastname, F.M. Article title. *Journal Name* **Year**, *Article number*, page range.

First Editon 2018

ISBN 978-3-03842-971-5 (Pbk)
ISBN 978-3-03842-972-2 (PDF)

Table of Contents

About the Special Issue Editor

Barbara Meyer, After studying biochemistry at Monash University in Australia, Barbara Meyer undertook her PhD at the Baker Medical Research Institute in Melbourne, Victoria. Barbara's first academic appointment was in the Department of Biomedical Science at the University of Wollongong in 1992 and she is now a Professor in the School of Medicine. Her current research is in the field of lipid and fatty acid metabolism; notably the role of omega-3 fatty acids in health and disease, including mental health and complicated pregnancies.

Preface to "DHA for Optimal Health"

The omega-3 long chain polyunsaturated fatty acids (n-3 LCPUFA) include eicosapentaenoic acid (EPA), docosapentaenoic acid (DPA) and docosahexaenoic acid (DHA) and this Special Issue is focussed on DHA for optimal health. It is well known that DHA is extremely important for neurological development, especially in the last trimester of pregnancy when the brain increases in size [1]. More recently it has been shown that increase in maternal plasma DHA concentration occurs very early in pregnancy, highlighting the importance of DHA at the critical time when the neural tube closure occurs [2].

There are other benefits of DHA, as evidenced by the publications in this Special Issue of DHA for Optimal Health.

Shi et al. [3] have shown that in cultured neurons isolated from mice that DHA combined with Lyciumbarbarum polysaccharide (LBP) protected neurons from oxygen-glucose deprivation/reperfusion injury. These results suggest that DHA and LPB are likely candidates for combined pharmacotherapy for ischemic stroke.

Walker et al. [4] showed that supplementation with n-3 LCPUFA (EPA and DHA) increased in blood cells and plasma fractions at the expense of various fatty acids and there is a dose response in all pools assessed. Specifically the n-3 LCPUFA displaced the following fatty acids in the various pools: linoleic acid (LA), gamma-linolenic acid (GLA), arachidonic acid (AA) and oleic acid (OA) in plasma PC; LA in plasma CE; OA in plasma TAG; AA and adrenic acid (AdrA) in erythrocytes; GLA in platelets, with no displacement of AA. This lack of displacement of AA in platelets is likely to be due to platelet function, whereby AA is used to produce eicosanoids involved in platelet aggregation. The differences in response to n-3 LCPUFA supplementation in these fatty acid pools could be of biological significance.

Abeywardena et al. [5] conducted a supplementation trial with stearidonic acid (SDA) compared to fish oil on anti-arrhythmic actions in rats. Supplementation with SDA resulted in increased EPA and DPA, but not DHA levels, which is similar to studies in humans [6]. However, DPA still had anti-arrhythmic effects, but not as great an effect as that of DHA. Hence, DHA has greater anti-arrhythmic effects than other n-3 PUFA.

Elsherbiny et al. [7] have shown that DHA supplementation maintains high DHA levels in the brains of pups even when they were weaned on DHA deficient diets. Another study has shown that when rats have been fed a restricted diet containing low levels of alpha-linolenic acid (ALA) at 0.8% and 0.2% of total fatty acids, their liver DHA reduced by 50% and 90% respectively, while their brain DHA was maintained when on the 0.8% ALA diet, and DHA levels only reduced by 40% at the extreme low dose of 0.2% ALA in the diet [8]. This study also showed that omega-6 docosapentaenoic acid (n-6 DPA) increased corresponding to the decrease in DHA [8], and it appears that n-6 DPA will take the place of DHA (during neurological development), until such time as DHA is restored in the diet [9]. Not only does this occur in rats, but there is evidence of this replacement in very early pregnancy in humans, as both n-6 DPA and DHA levels increase in maternal circulation in the first 45 days of pregnancy [2]. Moreover, in twin pregnancies (and this is even before the mother knows that she is having twins), the maternal plasma DHA concentrations double compared to singleton pregnancies and the maternal n-6 DPA concentrations triple over the first 45 days of pregnancy compared to singleton pregnancies [2].

Valenzuela et al. [10] conducted a randomised clinical trial assessing the efficacy of chia supplementation compared to control on being able to increase DHA levels in maternal blood and breastmilk samples. The chia intakes resulted in high ALA, commencing at 1.2 g per day and increasing to 9.5 g per day at delivery and 7.7 g per day at 6 months breastfeeding; corresponding to erythrocyte phospholipid levels of ALA from approximately 1% to 6% at delivery and 7% at 6 months breastfeeding. Erythrocyte EPA levels also increased from approximately 1% to 2.5% at delivery and 2% at 6 months breastfeeding. However, DHA levels did not increase and did not differ from baseline, delivery and 6 months breastfeeding. This lack of increase in DHA has been shown previously [11]. The LA levels decreased in breastmilk for the duration of the 6 month period. ALA levels were increased across the 6 months period of breastfeeding with a trend to decreased levels from 2 months to 5–6 months breastfeeding. There were no differences in EPA in breastmilk, but there was a significant increase in DHA levels in the first 3 months of breastmilk, and no significant differences in 4–6 months of breastfeeding. Due to the lack of DHA increase in erythrocytes and yet an increase in breastmilk DHA, the authors suggest that accretion of DHA in breastmilk is a highly regulated process [12].

A review by Minihane [13] has highlighted that, despite relatively limited evidence, the Apo E and FADS genotypes are emerging as being important on EPA and DHA status. Variant alleles of FADS are associated with lower DHA status and APOE4 carriers appear to have lower uptake of DHA in the brain as well as higher b-Oxidation of DHA than non-APOE4 carriers. Interestingly, APOE4 carriers have a 50% lower chance of reaching 90 years of age compared with non-APOE4 carriers [14].

Zheng et al. [15] showed that DHA ameliorates fructose induced triacylglyerol (TAG) accumulation in the liver by promoting B-oxidation of TAG in the liver and, therefore, less storage of TAG in the liver.

A meta-analysis of prospective cohort studies investigating the association of fish, n-3 LCPUA and incidence of elevated blood pressure by Yang et al. [16] showed that circulating n-3 CLPUFA was inversely associated with the incidence of elevated blood pressure with the summary risk ratio (SRR) of 0.67 (95% CI 0.55, 0.83) and DHA SRR of 0.64 (95% CI 0.45-0.88). This meta-analysis suggests that people with high levels of circulating n-3 LCPUFA (and especially DHA) have 43% (and 46% in the case of DHA) reduction in elevated blood pressure.

Nagayama et al. [17] showed that DHA, but not EPA suppressed the expression of monocyte chemotactic protein-1 (MCP-1) in arterial strips isolated from rats. They showed that DHA generated 4-hydroxy hexenal (4-HHE) which is an end product of n-3 CLPUFA which also suppressed MCP-1 expression. In contrast, DHA, EPA and 4-HHE stimulated MCP-1 expression in vascular smooth muscle cells. This apparent dual effect of n-3 LCPUFA on the regulation of MCP-1 expression warrants further investigation, but does highlight that DHA may be important in the pathogenesis of atherosclerosis.

DHA has been shown to have a beneficial effect on cognition throughout the lifespan which is explained in the review by Weiser et al. [18]. Van der Wurff et al. [19] showed that typically developing Dutch adolescents with high omega-3 index had improved cognition; specifically information processing and fewer errors due to increased attention. Lauritzen et al.'s [20] review on DHA effects on brain development and function, highlights the importance of DHA for optimal visual acuity development and the role of DHA in slowing cognitive decline, but also demonstrating beneficial effects of DHA through childhood and adult life.

Liu et al. [21] has shown that dietary DHA intake correlates with plasma erythrocyte and breastmilk levels of DHA in lactating women from various areas of China. The coastal areas have higher DHA intakes resulting in higher plasma, erythrocyte and breastmilk DHA levels. The opposite is true for inland areas of China. The median intake of DHA is 24 mg DHA per day (coastland), 14 mg DHA per day in Lakeland areas and only 9 mg DHA per day in inland areas of China. These results suggest that people who consume fish/seafood have higher DHA levels not only in their own circulation, but also in their breastmilk.

The Australian population is not meeting the recommended intakes for n-3 LCPUFA with only approximately 20% of the population meeting these recommended intakes [22]. Approximately 10% of women of childbearing age [22] are meeting the recommended intake of at least 200 mg DHA per day [23-29].

Ghasemifard et al. [30] compared a constant daily dose versus a once a week large 'spike' dose of n-3 LCPUFA in a rat based study. They showed that the large spike dose resulted in greater deposition of the n-3 LCPUFA in various tissues compared to the daily constant dose (when expressed as percent of total intake). This was due to less B-oxidation, and greater deposition rather than increased excretion of n-3 LCPUFA. This study suggests that a large dose of n-3 LCPUFA (from either supplements or the consumption of an oily fish meal once a week) may be better than daily smaller doses of n-3 LCPUFA in terms of increasing the n-3 LCPUFA status.

Fayet-Moore et al. [31] has developed four models, namely: (1) fish only; (2) fish, meat, eggs and enriched foods; (3) meat, eggs and enriched foods; and (4) enriched food only for vegetarian diets to meet the recommended intakes for n-3 LCPUFA. The easiest way to meet the recommended intakes for n-3 LCPUFA is through the consumption of fish and seafood. For vegetarians, there are other sources of n-3

LCPUFA and they include seaweed and algal oil supplements.

Barbara Meyer
Special Issue Editor

References

1. Makrides, M.; Gibson, R.A. Long-chain polyunsaturated fatty acid requirements during pregnancy and lactation. *Am. J. Clin. Nutr.* **2000**, *71*, 307S–311S.
2. Meyer, B.J.; Onyiaodike, C.C.; Brown, E.A.; Jordan, F.; Murray, H.; Nibbs, R.J.; Sattar, N.; Lyall, H.; Nelson, S.M.; Freeman, D.J. Maternal plasma dha levels increase prior to 29 days post-lh surge in women undergoing frozen embryo transfer: A prospective, observational study of human pregnancy. *J. Clin. Endocrinol. Metab.* **2016**, *101*, 1745–1753.
3. Shi, Z.; Wu, D.; Yao, J.P.; Yao, X.; Huang, Z.; Li, P.; Wan, J.B.; He, C.; Su, H. Protection against oxygen-glucose deprivation/reperfusion injury in cortical neurons by combining omega-3 polyunsaturated acid with lyciumbarbarum polysaccharide. *Nutrients* **2016**, *8*.
4. Walker, C.G.; West, A.L.; Browning, L.M.; Madden, J.; Gambell, J.M.; Jebb, S.A.; Calder, P.C. The pattern of fatty acids displaced by epa and dha following 12 months supplementation varies between blood cell and plasma fractions. *Nutrients* **2015**, *7*, 6281–6293.
5. Abeywardena, M.Y.; Adams, M.; Dallimore, J.; Kitessa, S.M. Rise in dpa following sda-rich dietary echium oil less effective in affording anti-arrhythmic actions compared to high dha levels achieved with fish oil in sprague-dawley rats. *Nutrients* **2016**, *8*.
6. James, M.J.; Ursin, V.M.; Cleland, L.G. Metabolism of stearidonic acid in human subjects: Comparison with the metabolism of other n-3 fatty acids. *Am. J. Clin. Nutr.* **2003**, *77*, 1140–1145.
7. Elsherbiny, M.E.; Goruk, S.; Monckton, E.A.; Richard, C.; Brun, M.; Emara, M.; Field, C.J.; Godbout, R. Long-term effect of docosahexaenoic acid feeding on lipid composition and brain fatty acid-binding protein expression in rats. *Nutrients* **2015**, *7*, 8802–8817.
8. Kim, H.-W.; Rao, J.S.; Rapoport, S.I.; Igarashi, M. Regulation of rat brain polyunsaturated fatty acid (pufa) metabolism during graded dietary n-3 pufa deprivation. *Prostaglandins Leukotrienes Essential Fatty Acids* **2011**, *85*, 361–368.
9. Kim, H.Y. Novel metabolism of docosahexaenoic acid in neural cells. *J. Biol. Chem.* **2007**, *282*, 18661–18665.
10. Valenzuela, R.; Bascunan, K.; Chamorro, R.; Barrera, C.; Sandoval, J.; Puigrredon, C.; Parraguez, G.; Orellana, P.; Gonzalez, V.; Valenzuela, A. Modification of docosahexaenoic acid composition of milk from nursing women who received alpha linolenic acid from chia oil during gestation and nursing. *Nutrients* **2015**, *7*, 6405–6424.
11. de Groot, R.H.; Hornstra, G.; van Houwelingen, A.C.; Roumen, F. Effect of alpha-linolenic acid supplementation during pregnancy on maternal and neonatal polyunsaturated fatty acid status and pregnancy outcome. *Am. J. Clin. Nutr.* **2004**, *79*, 251–260.
12. Das, U.N. Essential fatty acids: Biochemistry, physiology and pathology. *Biotechnol. J.* **2006**, *1*, 420–439.
13. Minihane, A.M. Impact of genotype on epa and dha status and responsiveness to increased intakes. *Nutrients* **2016**, *8*, 123.
14. Beekman, M.; Blanche, H.; Perola, M.; Hervonen, A.; Bezrukov, V.; Sikora, E.; Flachsbart, F.; Christiansen, L.; De Craen, A.J.; Kirkwood, T.B., et al. Genome-wide linkage analysis for human longevity: Genetics of healthy aging study. *Aging Cell* **2013**, *12*, 184–193.
15. Zheng, J.; Peng, C.; Ai, Y.; Wang, H.; Xiao, X.; Li, J. Docosahexaenoic acid ameliorates fructose-induced hepatic steatosis involving er stress response in primary mouse hepatocytes. *Nutrients* **2016**, *8*.
16. Yang, B.; Shi, M.Q.; Li, Z.H.; Yang, J.J.; Li, D. Fish, long-chain n-3 pufa and incidence of elevated blood pressure: A meta-analysis of prospective cohort studies. *Nutrients* **2016**, *8*.
17. Nagayama, K.; Morino, K.; Sekine, O.; Nakagawa, F.; Ishikado, A.; Iwasaki, H.; Okada, T.; Tawa, M.; Sato, D.; Imamura, T., et al. Duality of n-3 polyunsaturated fatty acids on mcp-1 expression in

vascular smooth muscle: A potential role of 4-hydroxy hexenal. *Nutrients* **2015**, *7*, 8112–8126.

18. Weiser, M.J.; Butt, C.M.; Mohajeri, M.H. Docosahexaenoic acid and cognition throughout the lifespan. *Nutrients* **2016**, *8*, 99.
19. van der Wurff, I.S.; von Schacky, C.; Berge, K.; Zeegers, M.P.; Kirschner, P.A.; de Groot, R.H. Association between blood omega-3 index and cognition in typically developing dutch adolescents. *Nutrients* **2016**, *8*.
20. Lauritzen, L.; Brambilla, P.; Mazzocchi, A.; Harslof, L.B.; Ciappolino, V.; Agostoni, C. Dha effects in brain development and function. *Nutrients* **2016**, *8*.
21. Liu, M.J.; Li, H.T.; Yu, L.X.; Xu, G.S.; Ge, H.; Wang, L.L.; Zhang, Y.L.; Zhou, Y.B.; Li, Y.; Bai, M.X., et al. A correlation study of dha dietary intake and plasma, erythrocyte and breast milk dha concentrations in lactating women from coastland, lakeland, and inland areas of china. *Nutrients* **2016**, *8*.
22. Meyer, B.J. Australians are not meeting the recommended intakes for omega-3 long chain polyunsaturated fatty acids: Results of an analysis from the 2011-2012 national nutrition and physical activity survey. *Nutrients* **2016**, *8*, 111.
23. EFSA Panel on Dietetic Products Nutrition and Allergies (NDA). Scientific opinion on dietary reference values for fats, including saturated fatty acids, polyunsaturated fatty acids, monounsaturated fatty acids, trans fatty acids, and cholesterol. *EFSA J.* **2010**, *8*, 1461.
24. AFFSA (France). Avis de l'agence francaise de securite sanitaire des ailments relatif a l'actualisation des apports nutritionels conseilles pour les acides gras. Available online: http://www.afssa.fr/cgi-bin/countdocs.cgi?Documens/NUT2006sa0359EN.pdf (accessed on 24 April 2018).
25. International Society for the Study of Fatty Acids and Lipids (ISSFAL). Available online: http://www.issfal.org/pufa-recommendations (accessed on 28 April 2018).
26. Koletzko, B.; Lien, E.; Agostoni, C.; Bohles, H.; Campoy, C.; Cetin, I.; Decsi, T.; Dudenhausen, J.W.; Dupont, C.; Forsyth, S.; et al. The roles of long-chain polyunsaturated fatty acids in pregnancy, lactation and infancy: Review of current knowledge and consensus statement. *J. Perinatal Med.* **2008**, *36*, 5–14.
27. D-A-C-H. Deutsche gesellschaft fur ernahrung, osterreichische gesellschaft fur ernahrung schweizerische gesellschaft fur ernahrungsforschung, schweizererische vereinigung fur ernahrung: Referenzwerte fur die nahrstoffzufuhr, umschau/braus verlag, frankfurt; 2008.
28. Superior Health Council of Belgium. Recommendations and Claims Made on Omega-3 Fatty Acids (shc7945). Available online: https://www.health.belgium.be/en/recommendations-and-claims-made-omega-3-fatty-acids-2004-shc-7945 (accessed on 3 May 2018),
29. March of Dimes. Omega-3 Fatty Acids during Pregnancy. Available online: https://www.marchofdimes.org/pregnancy/vitamins-and-other-nutrients-during-pregnancy.aspx (accessed on 30 April 2018),
30. Ghasemifard, S.; Hermon, K.; Turchini, G.M.; Sinclair, A.J. Metabolic fate (absorption, β-oxidation and deposition) of long-chain n-3 fatty acids is affected by sex and by the oil source (krill oil or fish oil) in the rat. *Br. J. Nutr.* **2015**, *114*, 684–692.
31. Fayet-Moore, F.; Baghurst, K.; Meyer, B.J. Four models including fish, seafood, red meat and enriched foods to achieve australian dietary recommendations for n-3 lcpufa for all life-stages. *Nutrients* **2015**, *7*, 8602–8614.

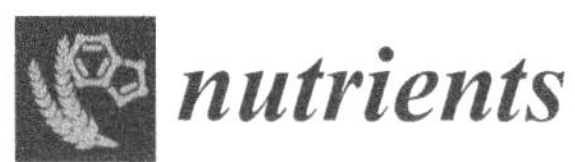 nutrients

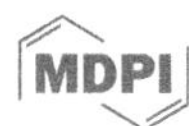

Article

What Is the Most Effective Way of Increasing the Bioavailability of Dietary Long Chain Omega-3 Fatty Acids—Daily *vs.* Weekly Administration of Fish Oil?

Samaneh Ghasemifard [1,†], Andrew J. Sinclair [1,†], Gunveen Kaur [2], Paul Lewandowski [1] and Giovanni M. Turchini [3,*]

[1] School of Medicine, Deakin University, Geelong 3220, Australia; E-Mails: sghasemi@deakin.edu.au (S.G.); andrew.sinclair@deakin.edu.au (A.J.S.); paul.lewandowski@deakin.edu.au (P.L.)

[2] Centre for Physical Activity and Nutrition Research (CPAN), School of Exercise and Nutrition Sciences, Deakin University, Burwood 3125, Australia; E-Mail: Gunveen.Kaur@deakin.edu.au

[3] School of Life and Environmental Sciences, Deakin University, Warrnambool 3280, Australia

* Author to whom correspondence should be addressed; E-Mail: giovanni.turchini@deakin.edu.au; Tel.: +61-3-55633312.

† These authors contributed equally to this work.

Received: 18 May 2015 / Accepted: 1 July 2015 / Published: 10 July 2015

Abstract: The recommendations on the intake of long chain omega-3 polyunsaturated fatty acids (*n*-3 LC-PUFA) vary from eating oily fish ("once to twice per week") to consuming specified daily amounts of eicosapentaenoic acid (EPA) and docosahexaenoic acid (DHA) ("250–500 mg per day"). It is not known if there is a difference in the uptake/bioavailability between regular daily consumption of supplements*vs.* consuming fish once or twice per week. In this study, the bioavailability of a daily dose of *n*-3 LC-PUFA (Constant treatment), representing supplements, *vs.* a large weekly dose of *n*-3 LC-PUFA (Spike treatment), representing consuming once or twice per week, was assessed. Six-week old healthy male Sprague-Dawley rats were fed either a Constant treatment, a Spike treatment or Control treatment (no *n*-3 LC-PUFA), for six weeks. The whole body, tissues and faeces were analysed for fatty acid content. The results showed that the major metabolic fate of the *n*-3 LC-PUFA (EPA+docosapentaenoic acid (DPA) + DHA) was towards catabolism (β-oxidation) accounting for over 70% of total dietary intake, whereas deposition accounted less than 25% of total dietary intake. It was found that significantly more *n*-3 LC-PUFA were β-oxidised when originating from the Constant treatment (84% of dose), compared with the Spike treatment (75% of dose). Conversely, it was found that significantly more *n*-3 LC-PUFA were deposited when originating from the Spike treatment (23% of dose), than from the Constant treatment (15% of dose). These unexpected findings show that a large dose of *n*-3 LC-PUFA once per week is more effective in increasing whole body *n*-3 LC-PUFA content in rats compared with a smaller dose delivered daily.

Keywords: bioavailability; EPA; DHA; DPA; metabolic fate; tissue deposition; frequency of intake

---

1. Introduction

A vast body of literature exists on the effect of long chain omega-3 polyunsaturated fatty acids (*n*-3 LC-PUFA) in the areas of infant development [1], cardiovascular disease, platelet aggregation [2], cancer [3], dementia, Alzheimer's disease, depression [4,5], and inflammation [6,7].

Recommendations for eicosapentaenoic acid (EPA; 20:5n-3) plus docosahexaenoic acid (DHA; 22:6n-3) intake have been put forth by several organizations globally, with ranges from 250 mg to 500 mg per day for adults with an additional 200 mg of DHA per day for pregnant and lactating women [8]. The recommendation for patients with coronary heart disease generally is 1 g EPA plus DHA per day, and for patients with high triglycerides the recommendations range from 1.2 to 4 g EPA plus DHA per day [8]. Some organisations, including the American Heart Association and Australian National Health and Medical Research Council, recommend foods (oily fish) once to twice per week [9], whereas others like the National Heart Foundation of Australia deal with nutrients daily based on daily intake (250–500 mg per day of EPA plus DHA) [10]. Accordingly, despite the actual quantity of recommended intake, it appears to be important to understand what feeding strategy, such as a constant daily dose or large doses fewer times per week, is more efficient to fulfil dietary requirements of EPA and DHA.

There are two human studies which have compared a constant daily dose of *n*-3 LC-PUFA *vs.* twice weekly doses of *n*-3 LC-PUFA [11,12]. Harris *et al.* [11] compared the bioavailability of EPA and DHA from twice weekly consumption of oily fish (3.40 g/week EPA + DHA) with daily fish-oil capsule supplementation (3.37 g/week EPA + DHA) in a 16 week study in 23 women; they found that there were no treatment differences in the EPA and DHA content of red blood cell membranes or plasma phospholipids. Browning *et al.* [12] compared the bioavailability of EPA and DHA from fish oil capsules (twice per week) with daily fish oil consumption. Male and female participants (n = 65) were given capsules (containing 6.54 g of EPA and DHA per week) either twice weekly or daily for one year. They found that there was no difference between treatments in the plasma phosphatidylcholine level of EPA and DHA, but that there were significantly higher levels of EPA and DHA in platelets and higher levels of EPA in mononuclear cells. Both studies used blood (plasma or red cell) levels of *n*-3 LC-PUFA as a proxy for bioavailability, which as discussed previously has significant limitations [13].

The aim of the present study was to compare the bioavailability and efficiency (as metabolic fate) of the same amount of dietary *n*-3 LC-PUFA administered either as a constant daily dose (Constant treatment)*vs.* a single weekly dose (Spike treatment). It was hypothesized that a single weekly dose of *n*-3 LC-PUFA would not be as bioavailable as a continuous daily dose of *n*-3 LC-PUFA.

2. Materials and Methods

2.1. Diet and Study Design

This study was performed following the Australian code for the care and use of animals for scientific purposes and approved by the Deakin University Animal Welfare Committee (G29-2012).

Forty eight 6-week old, sexually mature, healthy male Sprague-Dawley rats were purchased from Animal Resources Centre, Western Australia. Rats were housed in pairs (2 rats per cage; 24 cages in total) and acclimatised for a week on *ad libitum* normal chow diet. The 24 cages of rats were randomly divided into four groups of six cages each. One group (six cages) was sacrificed via CO_2 overdose at day 0 for the baseline data. The other three groups (six cages each) were randomly allocated to three different dietary treatments (feeding regimes), named "Control", "Constant" and "Spike". To achieve these three different dietary treatments, three specifically formulated diets were designed and manufactured to be iso-proteic, iso-lipidic (10% fat by weight, Speciality Feeds, Western Australia), and named: "No *n*-3 LC-PUFA diet", "Constant diet" and "Spike diet". The "No *n*-3 LC-PUFA diet" was formulated to contain no fish oil, and thus no *n*-3 LC-PUFA; the "Constant diet" was formulated to contain 0.7% of fish oil (mixed fish oils), and the "Spike diet" was formulated to contain a 4.9% of the same fish oil (a 7-fold higher level of *n*-3 LC-PUFA compared with the "Constant diet") (Table 1). Based on these three experimental diets, three different dietary treatments (feeding regimes) Control, Constant and Spike were implemented. In the "Control" treatment rats were fed only with the "No *n*-3 LC-PUFA diet", in the "Constant" treatment rats were fed only with the "Constant diet", and in the "Spike" treatment the rats were fed 6 days/week with the "No *n*-3 LC-PUFA diet", and one day per week with the "Spike diet". To ensure equal intake amongst dietary treatments during the experimentation, animals were fed to fixed predetermined ration, which was adjusted weekly relative to body weight, for 6 weeks. To determine the appropriate food ration, a preliminary short trial was implemented over a three-week period, where 15 rats of similar size were fed ad-libitum and total feed consumption was recorded. Then, using a regression equation comparing body weight (BW), the daily ration in grams, was estimated as:

$$\text{Ration}\,(\%\,\text{BW}) = -0.0283\text{BW} + 16.6 \quad (1)$$

Therefore, the experimental design for the rats in the Constant and Spike treatments was to consume exactly the same amount of fish oil (and therefore *n*-3 LC-PUFA) over a 7-day period, in order to establish if there was a difference in whole body bioavailability between these two feeding strategies (daily *vs.* weekly).

Throughout the 6-week trial period, the rats were weighed (twice per week), and faeces were collected every day during the last two weeks. After the 6 weeks, the rats were humanely sacrificed via CO_2 overdose. Six rats from each treatment (one per cage) were used for analysis of whole body lipids and the other six rats (one per cage) were used for the analysis of the individual tissue lipid contents. The collected faeces, whole body and tissues (liver, heart, white gastrocnemius muscle and perirenal adipose tissue) were analysed for fatty acid content.

Table 1. Experimental diet formulation, proximate composition and selected fatty acid concentrations.

Composition	No *n*-3 LC-PUFA Diet	Constant Diet	Spike Diet
(a) Diet Formulation and Proximate Composition *			
Diet formulation (%)			
Sucrose	10.00	10.00	10.00
Casein (acid)	20.00	20.00	20.00
Starch	37.44	37.44	37.44
Dextrinised starch	13.20	13.20	13.20
Safflower oil	0.05	0.13	0.64
Palm oil	9.88	9.11	4.45
Linseed oil	0.07	0.06	0.01
Fish oil **	0.00	0.70	4.90
Proximate Composition (mg/g of Diet)			
Protein	194.00	194.00	194.00
Fibre	84.00	84.00	84.00
Fat	100.00	100.00	100.00
(b) Fatty Acid Concentration of the Diet After Formulation(mg/g of Diet)			
16:0	43.00	38.50	26.40
18:0	4.00	3.81	3.10
18:1n-9	28.20	26.90	18.21
18:2n-6	7.71	7.82	7.20
20:4n-6	0.00	0.05	0.27
18:3n-3	0.50	0.50	0.30
18:4n-3	0.00	0.10	0.71
20:5n-3 (EPA)	0.00	0.90	4.50
22:5n-3 (DPA)	0.00	0.12	0.51
22:6n-3 (DHA)	0.00	0.60	2.92

EPA (eicosapentaenoic acid), DHA (docosahexaenoic acid), DPA (docosapentaenoic acid); * Diet formulation and proximate composition reported from data from the feed company; ** Fish oil was a mixture of fish oils used in diet manufacture. The mixture was made at the diet formulators premises before use; *n*-3 LC-PUFA, long chain omega-3 polyunsaturated fatty acids.

2.2. Lipid Analysis

The whole body, tissues and faeces samples were homogenized, and the lipids extracted by dichloromethane:methanol (2:1), a modification of the method described by Folch *et al.* [14]. Fatty acids derived from the lipids were methylated using an acid-catalysed trans-methylation [15]. In brief, an aliquot of fatty acids derived from the lipids plus a known amount of internal standard of tricosanoic acid (C23:0 >99%; Nu-Chek Prep Inc., Elysian, MN, USA) were reacted with acetyl chloride/methanol to form fatty acid methyl esters (FAME). The resulting FAME were separated, identified and quantified using an Agilent Technologies 7890A gas chromatography system (Agilent Technologies; Santa Clara,

CA, USA) equipped with a BPX70 capillary column (120 m, 0.25 mm internal diameter, 0.25 μm film thickness; SGE Analytical Science, Melbourne, Australia), an Agilent Technologies 7693 autosampler, a split injection system and a flame ionisation detector using established protocols [16].

2.3. *Lipid and Fatty Acid Apparent Digestibility*

Apparent digestibility of total lipid was measured according to Tou *et al.* [17] as ((lipid intake − faecal lipid)/(lipid intake)) × 100. Similarly, apparent digestibility of individual fatty acids was measured using the formula ((fatty acid intake − fatty acid excretion in faeces)/(fatty acid intake)) × 100. Lipid intake was determined as diet consumed per week × % lipid in the diet. Likewise, fatty acid intake was determined as diet consumed per week × % fatty acid in the diet. Faecal lipid and fatty acids were determined as total faeces excreted per week (pooled 7 days faecal samples) × % lipid and % fatty acids in the faeces respectively.

2.4. *Whole Body Fatty Acid Balance Method*

The fatty acid metabolism of rats was determined using the Whole Body Fatty Acid Balance Method, as conceived and described by Turchini *et al.* [18], with subsequent developments [19]. Briefly, the first step of the method required that the net appearance or disappearance of each individual fatty acid be determined by the difference between total fatty acid accumulation (=final fatty acid content-initial fatty acid content) and the net fatty acid intake (=total fatty acid intake-fatty acid excretion in faeces), as initially proposed by Cunnane's group [20–22]. Then, after the transformation of data from gram per animal per the duration of the trial to mol of fatty acid per gram of body weight per day, the subsequent second step involved a series of backwards computations along all the known fatty acid bioconversion pathways, therefore the fate of each individual fatty acid towards bioconversion, β-oxidation or deposition was determined and quantified. Eventually, data relative to apparent *in vivo* enzyme activity could be reported as nmol of enzyme's product per gram of body weight per day, and the *in vivo* metabolic fate (absorption, β-oxidation, bioconversion and deposition) of each dietary fatty acid could be reported as a % relative to the dietary intake.

2.5. *Statistical Analysis*

All data are reported as mean ± SD (standard deviation) of the six cages per treatment ($n = 6$, $N = 18$). The experimental unit was the cage (with two rats per cage). Significant differences between experimental treatments were tested using one-way analysis of variance (ANOVA), assessing the effects of diets, with an exception of using *t*-test for the *n*-3 LC-PUFA apparent digestibility (as only two treatments were considered). Paired tests were performed with Tukey's test. Statistical significance was considered for $p < 0.05$. Data analysis was performed with Minitab Statistical Software (Version 16; Minitab Inc., State College, PA, USA).

3. Results

3.1. *Feed and n-3 LC-PUFA Intake*

As described in the methods, rats were fed to fixed predetermined ration, which was adjusted weekly relative to body weight, for 6 weeks. Rats in the Control and Spike treatments consumed all the diet provided each week; however, rats in the Constant treatment left some food uneaten, especially in week three, and this was recorded and accounted for (Table 2).

Table 2. Actual feed intake over the six weeks of the experiment in the three treatments.

Total Diet Intake (g/rat/6 weeks)	Control	Constant	Spike
No *n*-3 LC-PUFA diet	938 ± 32	-	-
Constant diet	-	931 ± 44	804 ± 25
Spike diet	-	-	134 ± 11

Values are expressed as the mean ± SD of 6 cages per group; *n*-3 LC-PUFA, long chain omega-3 polyunsaturated fatty acids.

An important result that has to be noted and carefully considered was the fatty acid concentration of the experimental diets. Despite the prescribed formulation with 0.7% of fish oil in "Constant diet", and 4.9% fish oil in "Spike diet" (and fish oil being the only source of dietary *n*-3 LC-PUFA), the resulting manufactured diets had slightly different total amounts of *n*-3 LC-PUFA than expected (Table 1b). The "Constant diet" recorded EPA + DHA + DPA = 1.6 mg/g of diet, and the "Spike diet" recorded EPA + DHA + DPA = 8.0 mg/g of diet (a 5-fold difference, rather than the expected 7-fold difference).

3.2. *n-3 Fatty Acid Apparent Digestibility*

The effect of Constant and Spike treatments on apparent digestibility is shown in Table 3. There were small, but significant differences observed in EPA and DHA apparent digestibility between these two treatments, which was higher in the Constant, compared with the Spike treatment. However, DPA apparent digestibility was similar between Constant and Spike treatments.

Table 3. The effect of Constant and Spike treatments on the long chain omega-3 polyunsaturated fatty acids (*n*-3 LC-PUFA) apparent digestibility.

	Constant	Spike	*p*-Value
20:5n-3 (EPA)	99.4 ± 0.0	99.0 ± 0.9	0.021
22:5n-3 (DPA)	96.9 ± 1.0	96.5 ± 0.4	0.753
22:6n-3 (DHA)	98.8 ± 0.5	98.2 ± 0.2	0.042

Values are expressed as the mean ± SD of 6 cages per group; Control treatment not reported as no *n*-3 LC-PUFAwas provided by the diet; EPA, eicosapentaenoic acid; DPA, docosapentaenoic acid; DHA, docosahexaenoic acid.

3.3. *Growth and Biometrical Parameters*

There was no significant difference (p = 0.856) in the body weight of rats between the three experimental treatments during the six weeks of the experiment. The average body weights (±SD) of animals in the Control, Constant and Spike treatments were 412 ± 6 g, 413 ± 6 g, and 409 ± 11 g respectively, at the end of the experiment (Table 4).

In regard to the tissue weight, there was no significant difference in the tissue weight of rats between the three dietary treatments at the end of the experiment. In addition, the Hepatosomatic Index and Perirenal adipose-somatic index showed no significant difference in the Constant and Spike treatment compared with the Control (Table 4).

Table 4. The effect of Constant and Spike treatments on rat tissue weight and biometric parameters.

Weight (g)	Control	Constant	Spike	*p*-Value
Whole body	412.4 ± 6.2	412.6 ± 6.2	409.3 ± 10.8	0.714
Liver	17.9 ± 2.5	17.3 ± 2.1	17.0 ± 0.8	0.914
Heart	1.5 ± 0.2	1.5 ± 0.1	1.5 ± 0.1	0.547
Perirenal adipose	7.6 ± 2.9	6.8 ± 2.9	8.5 ± 1.9	0.225
Muscle	0.8 ± 0.1	0.7 ± 0.1	0.7 ± 0.1	0.856
HSI*	4.3 ± 0.6	4.2 ± 0.6	4.0 ± 0.3	0.432
PASI**	1.8 ± 0.7	1.7 ± 0.7	2.0 ± 0.4	0.543

Control, Constant and Spike treatments provided 0 mg, 9.2 mg and 8 mg per week of EPA + DPA + DHA, respectively; Values are expressed as the mean ± SD of 6 cages per group; * HSI (Hepatosomatic Index, liver weight/whole body weight × 100); ** PASI (Perirenal adipose-somatic index, Perirenal adipose weight/whole body weight × 100).

3.4. Lipid Content of Rat Whole Body and Tissues

Whole body and tissue lipid content (mg/g tissue wet weight) of all rats at the conclusion of the study were significantly higher compared with the baseline data ($p < 0.001$). There was no significant difference in the total lipid content of the whole body or tissues between the three dietary treatments (Table 5).

Table 5. Lipid content of tissues of rats fed the different experimental treatments.

Lipid Content	Control	Constant	Spike	*p*-Value
Whole Body (mg/g Whole Body)	133.7 ± 17.1	119.1 ± 12.6	111.4 ± 28.8	0.199
Tissues (mg/g Tissue)				
Liver	53.3 ± 16.9	51.6 ± 6.4	51.1 ± 8.1	0.942
Heart	29.8 ± 2.6	28.8 ± 0.8	30.7 ± 1.4	0.168
Perirenal adipose	831.2 ± 89.4	893.0 ± 27.4	931.2 ± 67.9	0.640
Muscle	19.5 ± 3.5	20.0 ± 2.8	24.7 ± 8.0	0.209

Values are expressed as the mean ± SD of 6 cages per group.

3.5. The Fatty Acid Concentration of the Rat Whole Body and Tissues

As shown in Table 6, the whole body fatty acid concentration for rats that received the Constant treatment was significantly higher for all *n*-3 LC-PUFA compared with rats on the Spike treatment at the end of experiment ($p < 0.05$). In addition, *n*-6 PUFA concentrations were significantly lower in the Spike compared with the Constant treatment at the end of the study period ($p = 0.003$). It should be recalled that rats in the Spike treatment received a relatively smaller amounts of *n*-3 LC-PUFA each week compared with the Constant treatment, because the manufactured diet slightly deviated from expected final fatty acid concentration.

Table 6. Selected fatty acid content of whole body (mg/g whole body) and tissues (mg/g tissue) from rats fed different dietary treatments.

	PUFA n-6	PUFA n-3	EPA	DPA	DHA	EPA + DPA + DHA
Whole Body(mg/g Whole Body)						
Control	11.23 ± 1.50^{b}	0.83 ± 0.12^{a}	n.d	0.06 ± 0.01^{a}	0.30 ± 0.08^{a}	0.37 ± 0.09^{a}
Constant	10.88 ± 1.12^{b}	1.76 ± 0.08^{c}	0.16 ± 0.02^{b}	0.22 ± 0.02^{c}	0.88 ± 0.06^{c}	1.26 ± 0.08^{c}
Spike	9.30 ± 1.38^{a}	1.49 ± 0.13^{b}	0.12 ± 0.02^{a}	0.19 ± 0.02^{b}	0.75 ± 0.05^{b}	1.07 ± 0.07^{b}
p-Value	0.003	0.001	0.001	0.001	0.001	0.001
Liver (mg/g Liver)						
Control	7.1 ± 1.7^{b}	1.1 ± 0.2^{a}	0.03 ± 0.01^{a}	0.05 ± 0.01^{a}	0.61 ± 0.19^{a}	0.68 ± 0.19^{a}
Constant	5.7 ± 1.1^{a}	2.2 ± 0.3^{b}	0.31 ± 0.03^{b}	0.14 ± 0.02^{b}	1.47 ± 0.32^{b}	1.92 ± 0.37^{b}
Spike	7.8 ± 1.0^{b}	2.6 ± 0.5^{b}	0.28 ± 0.08^{b}	0.19 ± 0.05^{c}	1.72 ± 0.50^{b}	2.20 ± 0.56^{b}
p-Value	0.049	0.001	0.001	0.001	0.001	0.001
Heart (mg/g Heart)						
Control	6.01 ± 0.34^{b}	0.96 ± 0.08^{a}	0.02 ± 0.01^{a}	0.08 ± 0.00^{a}	0.65 ± 0.07^{a}	0.74 ± 0.07^{a}
Constant	4.70 ± 0.32^{a}	2.34 ± 0.13^{b}	0.11 ± 0.01^{b}	0.25 ± 0.03^{b}	1.86 ± 0.11^{b}	2.21 ± 0.13^{b}
Spike	5.24 ± 0.39^{b}	2.27 ± 0.23^{b}	0.11 ± 0.00^{b}	0.29 ± 0.03^{b}	1.73 ± 0.21^{b}	2.12 ± 0.20^{b}
p-Value	0.001	0.001	0.001	0.001	0.001	0.001
Perirenal Adipose(mg/g Perirenal)						
Control	4.6 ± 0.7^{a}	0.3 ± 0.0^{a}	n.d	0.01 ± 0.01^{a}	0.01 ± 0.00^{a}	0.03 ± 0.01^{a}
Constant	7.7 ± 2.6^{a}	0.7 ± 0.2^{b}	0.06 ± 0.02^{a}	0.12 ± 0.06^{b}	0.09 ± 0.03^{b}	0.28 ± 0.09^{b}
Spike	7.1 ± 0.6^{a}	0.7 ± 0.1^{b}	0.07 ± 0.01^{a}	0.16 ± 0.03^{b}	0.11 ± 0.04^{b}	0.34 ± 0.06^{b}
p-Value	0.543	0.001	0.001	0.001	0.001	0.001
Muscle (mg/g Muscle)						
Control	3.37 ± 0.70^{b}	0.92 ± 0.38^{a}	0.08 ± 0.05^{a}	0.09 ± 0.01^{a}	0.34 ± 0.13^{a}	0.51 ± 0.19^{a}
Constant	2.37 ± 0.30^{a}	1.36 ± 0.14^{b}	0.14 ± 0.04^{b}	0.15 ± 0.02^{b}	0.92 ± 0.10^{b}	1.22 ± 0.15^{b}
Spike	2.91 ± 0.69^{b}	1.47 ± 0.06^{b}	0.13 ± 0.02^{b}	0.21 ± 0.02^{c}	0.95 ± 0.04^{b}	1.30 ± 0.05^{b}
p-Value	0.036	0.003	0.050	0.001	0.001	0.001

Values are expressed as the mean ± SD of 6 cages per group; a,b,c Values with different superscript letters in each column differ significantly ($p < 0.05$); n.d = not detected.

Supplementation with *n*-3 LC-PUFA diets (both Constant and Spike treatments) led to a significant increase ($p < 0.005$) in whole body EPA + DPA + DHAconcentrations compared with Control treatment and the baseline data, by a factor of 50% increase, over the six weeks of the experiment (data not shown).

In terms of tissue concentrations, no significant differences were observed in EPA and DHA concentration between these two feeding strategies in any of these four tissues. In contrast, rats on the Spike treatment had significantly higher concentrations of DPA than those on the Constant treatment in liver and muscle tissue, but not in heart or adipose tissue (Table 6).

Although EPA was the main *n*-3 LC-PUFA in the Constant and Spike diets, DHA was the predominant *n*-3 LC-PUFA in all tissues analysed except perirenal fat. DPA was the next most deposited *n*-3 LC-PUFA in tissues, except the in liver, where EPA levels were significantly higher than DPA levels.

3.6. EPA, DPA and DHA—Mass Balance

Intake and excretion: The Constant treatment provided significantly more EPA, DPA and DHA to rats compared with the Spike treatment over the duration of the experiment, as noted earlier. Rats under the Constant treatment excreted significantly more DPA ($p < 0.001$) and less EPA ($p < 0.001$) and DHA ($p < 0.001$) compared with those in the Spike treatment. In addition, *n*-6 PUFAintake and excretion were higher in rats in the Constant compared with the Spike treatment.

Accumulation: The total *n*-3 LC-PUFA content in whole body in both *n*-3 enriched treatments over the 6 weeks of the experiment was significantly higher compared with the Control treatment ($p < 0.05$), with no effect between the two feeding strategies being observed (Table 7).

Appearance/disappearance: There was a net disappearance of all *n*-3 LC-PUFA over the duration of the experiment (intake greater than accumulation) in both Spike and Constant treatments; with the exception of the Control treatment where a small net appearance was observed, due to formation from the dietary 18:3n-3 (Table 7). A statistically significant difference in the net disappearance of all *n*-3

LC-PUFA were observed as a result of dietary treatment, with values for the Constant treatment being higher than for the Spike treatment ($p < 0.05$).

Table 7. Selected fatty acids and fatty acid classes balance (mg/animal) in rats fed under the different dietary treatments.

	PUFA *n*-6	PUFA *n*-3	EPA	DPA	DHA	EPA + DPA +DHA
Total Intake (mg/Animal)						
Control	12812 ± 0 [a]	807 ± 0 [a]	n.d	n.d	n.d	n.d
Constant	14685 ± 84 [c]	4256 ± 24 [c]	1662 ± 10 [b]	237 ± 1 [b]	1104 ± 6 [b]	3003 ± 17 [b]
Spike	13115 ± 9 [b]	3161 ± 10 [b]	1208 ± 5 [a]	145 ± 1 [a]	779 ± 3 [a]	2132 ± 9 [a]
p-Value	0.001	0.001	0.001	0.001	0.001	0.001
Excretion (mg/Animal)						
Control	84 ± 0 [a]	4 ± 0 [a]	n.d	n.d	n.d	n.d
Constant	64 ± 0 [b]	46 ± 0 [c]	10 ± 0 [a]	8 ± 0 [b]	13 ± 0 [a]	31 ± 0 [a]
Spike	84 ± 0 [a]	45 ± 0 [b]	12 ± 0 [b]	5 ± 0 [a]	14 ± 0 [b]	31 ± 0 [b]
p-Value	0.001	0.001	0.001	0.001	0.001	0.001
Net Intake (mg/Animal)						
Control	12728 ± 0 [a]	807 ± 0 [a]	n.d	n.d	n.d	n.d
Constant	14621 ± 84 [c]	4210 ± 24 [c]	1652 ± 9 [b]	230 ± 1 [b]	1090 ± 6 [b]	2972 ± 17 [b]
Spike	13031 ± 9 [b]	3117 ± 10 [b]	1196 ± 5 [a]	140 ± 1 [a]	764 ± 3 [a]	2101 ± 9 [a]
p-Value	0.001	0.001	0.001	0.001	0.001	0.001
Initial Body Content (mg/Animal)						
Control	1331 ± 79 [a]	167 ± 10 [a]	4 ± 0 [a]	18 ± 1 [a]	44 ± 3 [a]	66 ± 4 [a]
Constant	1292 ± 107 [a]	162 ± 13 [a]	3 ± 0 [a]	18 ± 1 [a]	43 ± 4 [a]	64 ± 5 [a]
Spike	1274 ± 75 [a]	160 ± 9 [a]	3 ± 0 [a]	18 ± 1 [a]	42 ± 3 [a]	63 ± 4 [a]
p-Value	0.236	0.127	0.118	0.090	0.417	0.236
Final Body Content (mg/Animal)						
Control	5183 ± 1214 [a]	386 ± 108 [a]	3 ± 3 [a]	28 ± 9 [a]	144 ± 67 [a]	175 ± 76 [a]
Constant	4450 ± 384[a]	723 ± 28 [b]	66 ± 25 [b]	89 ± 30 [b]	360 ± 27 [b]	616 ± 36 [b]
Spike	4930 ± 1042 [a]	801 ± 204 [b]	67 ± 15 [b]	100 ± 21 [b]	416 ± 133 [b]	582 ± 168 [b]
p-Value	0.346	0.001	0.001	0.001	0.001	0.001
Accumulation (mg/Animal)						
Control	3852 ± 1285 [a]	219 ± 117 [a]	n.d	9.5 ± 10 [a]	100.2 ± 69 [a]	109 ± 80 [a]
Constant	3158 ± 227 [a]	561 ± 26 [b]	63 ± 9 [a]	71 ± 9 [b]	317 ± 28 [b]	452 ± 38 [b]
Spike	3656 ± 1045 [a]	641 ± 204 [b]	63 ± 15 [a]	82 ± 21 [b]	373 ± 133 [b]	519 ± 168 [b]
p-Value	0.476	0.001	0.001	0.001	0.001	0.001
Appearance/Disappearance (mg/Animal)						
Control	−8876 ± 1285 [a]	−584 ± 117 [a]	0.3 ± 3 [a]	10 ± 10 [a]	100 ± 69 [a]	109 ± 80 [a]
Constant	−11463 ± 441 [a]	−3649 ± 34 [c]	−1589 ± 13 [c]	−158 ± 9 [c]	−772 ± 23 [c]	−2520 ± 30 [c]
Spike	−9375 ± 1043 [a]	−2475 ± 198 [b]	−1133 ± 13 [b]	−58 ± 21 [b]	−391 ± 131 [b]	−1582 ± 162 [b]
p-Value	0.871	0.001	0.001	0.001	0.001	0.001

Values are expressed as the mean ± SD of 6 cages per group; [a,b,c] Values with different superscript letters differ significantly in each column ($p < 0.05$); n.d = not detected; PUFA (polyunsaturated fatty acid) n-6: 18:2n-6, 20:2n-6, 22:2n-6, 18:3n-6, 20:3n-6, 20:4n-6, 22:4n-6, 24:4n-6, 24:5n-6, 22:5n-6; PUFA *n*-3: 18:3n-3, 20:3n-3, 22, 3n-3, 18:4n-3, 20:4n-3, 20:5n-3, 22:5n-3, 24:5n-3, 24:6n-3, 22:6n-3.

3.7. EPA, DPA and DHA Apparentin Vivo Metabolism

The Whole Body Fatty Acid Balance Method allowed the calculation of apparent *in vivo* fatty acid metabolism (excretion, β-oxidation, bioconversion and deposition) as shown in Table 8. The two most important pathways identified for the *n*-3 LC-PUFA in this study were β-oxidation and deposition, which together accounted for more than 98% of the apparent *in vivo* metabolism (Table 8).

Based on calculation, the main fate of EPA, DPA and DHA in both *n*-3 LC-PUFA supplemented treatments was β-oxidation, except for DPA in rats fed the Spike treatment where deposition was observed as the main fate. β-oxidation was approximately 95% for EPA, while for DPA and DHA it ranged between 40% to 70%. There was a significant effect of the dietary treatment on the β-oxidation for EPA, DPA and DHA, which was higher for rats fed the Constant compared with Spike treatment.

Apart from β-oxidation, deposition was the next main fate of the EPA and DHA in both treatments and DPA in the Constant treatment. In the case of EPA, deposition amounted to less than 6% of the total metabolic activity, whereas in the case of DPA and DHA, deposition accounted for between 30% to 56% and 28% to 48%, respectively, depending on treatment (Table 8). The whole body deposition of all *n*-3 LC-PUFA was significantly higher ($p < 0.05$) in rats fed the Spike treatment compared with those fed the Constant treatment.

For EPA and DHA there were very similar trends between Spike and Constant treatments (for both treatments: β-oxidation > deposition > excretion); however, this was not the case for DPA since for the Constant treatment β-oxidation > deposition > excretion, while for the Spike treatment deposition > β-oxidation > excretion. DPA was likely not further bio-converted to other *n*-3 LC-PUFA (namely 24:5n-3, 24:6n-3 or DHA) in any treatment. In the control group, 18:3n-3 was bioconverted at a significantly higher rate compared with the other two treatments.

The *n*-6 fatty acid β-oxidation, bioconversion and deposition were similar between all three dietary treatments. However, the n-6 fatty acid excretion was significantly higher ($p < 0.001$) in the Spike compared with the Constant treatment. In the Constant and Spike treatments mostly 18:3n-6 and 20:4n-6 were bioconverted, 20:3n-6 was bioconverted only in the Spike treatment. In the Constant treatment, mostly 18:2n-6 and 20:4n-6 were deposited while in the Spike treatment, more n-6 fatty acids (18:2n-6, 20:4n-6, 22:4n-6, 22:5n-6) were deposited in the rat's whole body (data not shown).

Table 8. Metabolic fate of fatty acid (% of the intake) in rats under the three dietary treatments.

	PUFA *n*-6	PUFA *n*-3	EPA	DPA	DHA	EPA + DPA + DHA
Excreted (% of Intake)						
Control	0.65 ± 0.00^{c}	0.52 ± 0.00^{a}	n.d	n.d	n.d	n.d
Constant	0.43 ± 0.00^{a}	1.07 ± 0.00^{b}	0.57 ± 0.00^{a}	3.18 ± 1.01^{a}	1.23 ± 0.50^{a}	1.00 ± 0.00^{a}
Spike	0.62 ± 0.00^{b}	1.40 ± 0.00^{c}	1.02 ± 0.00^{b}	3.52 ± 0.00^{b}	1.84 ± 0.00^{b}	1.44 ± 0.00^{b}
p-Value	0.001	0.001	0.001	0.001	0.001	0.001
β-Oxidised (% of Intake)						
Control	69.78 ± 9.75^{a}	74.81 ± 12.84^{a}	n.d	n.d	n.d	n.d
Constant	78.23 ± 2.74^{a}	86.30 ± 0.74^{a}	95.66 ± 0.57^{b}	66.61 ± 3.62^{b}	69.98 ± 2.43^{b}	84.44 ± 1.20^{b}
Spike	71.80 ± 7.83^{a}	79.29 ± 6.11^{a}	93.78 ± 1.24^{a}	40.00 ± 14.60^{a}	50.21 ± 17.01^{a}	75.14 ± 7.49^{a}
p-Value	0.096	0.081	0.012	0.008	0.037	0.001
Bio-Converted (% of Intake)						
Control	4.90 ± 2.81^{b}	15.72 ± 10.10^{b}	n.d	n.d	n.d	n.d
Constant	1.56 ± 0.08^{a}	0.16 ± 0.02^{a}	n.d	n.d	n.d	n.d
Spike	$3.07 \pm 1.60^{a,b}$	0.05 ± 0.08^{a}	n.d	n.d	n.d	n.d
p-Value	0.026	0.001	-	-	-	-
Deposited (% of Intake)						
Control	24.67 ± 7.05^{a}	8.95 ± 3.28^{a}	n.d	n.d	n.d	n.d
Constant	19.78 ± 2.70^{a}	12.47 ± 0.75^{a}	3.76 ± 0.57^{a}	30.21 ± 3.87^{a}	28.79 ± 2.43^{a}	14.51 ± 1.21^{a}
Spike	24.51 ± 6.32^{a}	19.26 ± 6.04^{b}	5.24 ± 1.24^{b}	56.50 ± 14.60^{b}	47.9 ± 17.0^{b}	23.42 ± 7.49^{a}
p-Value	0.269	0.002	0.033	0.008	0.042	0.034

Values are expressed as the mean ± SD of 6 cages per group. [a,b,c] Values with different superscript letters differ significantly in each column ($p < 0.05$); n.d = not detected; PUFA (polyunsaturated fatty acid) n-6: 18:2n-6, 20:2n-6, 22:2n-6, 18:3n-6, 20:3n-6, 20:4n-6, 22:4n-6, 24:4n-6, 24:5n-6, 22:5n-6; PUFA n-3: 18:3n-3, 20:3n-3, 22:3n-3, 18:4n-3, 20:4n-3, 20:5n-3, 22:5n-3, 24:5n-3, 24:6n-3, 22:6n-3.

The apparent *in vivo* enzyme activities (expressed as mmol of product per g of body weight per day) are reported in Table 9. The apparent total elongase activity and desaturase activities (Δ-5 Desaturase and Δ-6 Desaturase) were similar in rats under the Constant and the Spike treatment. The apparent Δ-9 Desaturase enzyme activity was higher in rats under the Spike treatment compared with those on the Constant treatment.

Table 9. Apparent *in vivo* enzyme activities in rats fed the three dietary treatments.

	ξ Elongase	ξ Δ-9 Desaturase	ξ Δ-6 Desaturase	Δ-6 Desaturase for n-6	Δ-6 Desaturase for n-3	ξ Δ-5 Desaturase	Δ-5 Desaturase for n-6	Δ-5 Desaturase for n-3
Control	629 ± 335^{b}	1305 ± 245^{c}	298 ± 192^{b}	228 ± 142^{b}	69 ± 49	227 ± 147^{b}	195 ± 122^{b}	31 ± 24
Constant	97 ± 15^{a}	375 ± 134^{a}	48 ± 4^{a}	48 ± 4^{a}	n.d	56 ± 5^{a}	56 ± 5^{a}	n.d
Spike	219 ± 146^{a}	722 ± 240^{b}	$114 \pm 67^{a,b}$	$114 \pm 67^{a,b}$	n.d	$108 \pm 61^{a,b}$	$108 \pm 61^{a,b}$	n.d
p-Value	0.001	0.001	0.006	0.012	-	0.017	0.025	-

Values are expressed in mmol/g/day as the mean ± SD of 6 cages per group; [a,b,c] Values with different superscript superscript letters differ significantly in each column ($p < 0.05$); n.d = not detected. The Greek letter capital sigma (Σ) indicates summation.

4. Discussion

The present study sought to examine the whole body bioavailability and efficiency (as *n*-3 LC-PUFA metabolic fate) of the same overall dose of *n*-3 LC-PUFA, provided from the same source (fish oil), at the same overall weekly dose, but at different frequencies: daily*vs.* weekly. It was found that the growth of the animals was not different between treatments and no mortalities were recorded amongst the three experimental treatments (Constant, Spike and Control). There were significant but small differences in the excretion of the *n*-3 LC-PUFA between the Spike and Constant treatment groups, which are unlikely to be nutritionally relevant.

The results obtained by simply comparing tissue FA concentrations (mg/g tissue) were interesting, but they are admittedly of limited value towards achieving a better understanding of *n*-3 LC-PUFA "bioavailability". While the dietary intake of *n*-3 LC-PUFA provided by the two diets were similar, but not identical, there were some differences between treatments that might be independent of the difference in dietary intake. For example, the DPA concentration in liver and muscle was significantly greater in the Spike treatment than in the Constant treatment, despite the dietary DPA intake being significantly greater for the Constant treatment. This has no obvious explanation, but reveals that metabolic processing of dietary *n*-3 LC-PUFA is more complex than simply looking at dietary intake values or tissue levels.

A much greater and more accurate understanding of the actual metabolic fate of *n*-3 LC-PUFA provided by different oils can be achieved by observing the results of the Whole Body Fatty Acid Balance Method, which takes into account, and thus balances out, any differences in dietary intake.

This data showed that the major metabolic fate of the *n*-3 LC-PUFA (EPA + DPA + DHA) was towards catabolism (β-oxidation) accounting for over 70% of total dietary intake, whereas deposition accounted less than 25% of total dietary intake. It was found that significantly more *n*-3 LC-PUFA were β-oxidised when originating from the Constant treatment (84% of dose), compared with the Spike treatment (75% of dose). Conversely, it was found that significantly more *n*-3 LC-PUFA were deposited when originating from the Spike treatment (23% of dose), than from the Constant treatment (15% of dose). This result suggests that the *n*-3 LC-PUFA provided by the Spike treatment were more deposited (bioavailable), compared with those provided by the Constant treatment.

The differences in β-oxidation and deposition were not the same for each of EPA, DPA and DHA for either the Spike or Constant treatment. That is, EPA was more extensively β-oxidised than DPA and DHA on both treatments, but the differences between the 20 carbonand the 22 carbon PUFA were accentuated in the Spike treatment. In the case of β-oxidation, the Constant/Spike ratios were 1.7 for DPA and 1.4 for DHA, but only 1.0 for EPA. In terms of deposition, the Constant/Spike ratios were 0.5 for DPA, 0.6 for DHA, and 0.7 for EPA. This suggests that EPA is preferentially directed towards β-oxidation almost independent of whether the EPA is provided daily or once per week. This is consistent with data showing high affinity of EPA to catabolism (β-oxidation) in animal models [23]. It has been reported using Wistar rats that EPA-CoA was a good substrate for mitochondrial carnitine acyl-transferase-I and DHA was a poor substrate for both mitochondrial and peroxisomal β-oxidation, which could explain the high rate of β-oxidation for EPA [23].

In contrast to EPA, it would appear that DHA and DPA are somewhat spared from β-oxidation when consumed, as observed previously [24] but especially when a large dose of dietary *n*-3 LC-PUFA is provided weekly. This is consistent with the finding of Kaur *et al.* [24] in rodents who showed, using radiolabelled EPA, DPA and DHA in rats, that six hours after dosing 19% of the EPA was β-oxidized and expired as CO_2 compared with 5% in case of DPA and 7% of DHA. However, these data do not shed any light on why providing a bolus dose of *n*-3 LC-PUFA leads to a greater partitioning of DPA and DHA towards deposition. With the Spike treatment, it is therefore possible to speculate that this "flood" of *n*-3 LC-PUFA could have saturated the capacity of the mitochondria to β-oxidise any extra DPA and DHA, resulting in a greater retention and deposition of these fatty acids in tissues.

To our knowledge, this is the first study to compare the whole body bioavailability of *n*-3 LC-PUFA in rats fed a constant daily dose*vs.* a larger and less frequent dose of the same dietary source of *n*-3 LC-PUFA. From the two available human studies comparing a weekly dose of *n*-3 LC-PUFA with daily dose, only one study used the same source of *n*-3 LC-PUFA (capsules not fish meal) [12]. Both studies used blood levels (plasma, platelets or mononuclear cells) as a proxy for bioavailability. The limitations of these studies include a failure to provide the dose adjusted on a body weight basis, the failure to measure excretion and the failure to measure the EPA and DHA levels in the red blood cells (which are widely regarded as the best measure of EPA + DHA tissue status). Furthermore, because of the known high level of variability in the response of subjects to the same dose of fish oil (as noted by Kohler *et al.* [25]), these studies have limitations because the data was not adjusted for by gender, body weight or exercise level [26]. In the present rat study, rats were fed to fixed predetermined ration, which was adjusted weekly relative to body weight, for 6 weeks which helped to reduce the variability of the results achieved, increased the statistical power of the test (greater than 80% for the vast majority of data recorded), and ultimately contributed to obtaining more robust, substantiated and more easily interpretable findings.

The possible difference in bioavailability of *n*-3 LC-PUFA when provided in different edible sources has received some research attention. Specifically, the blood levels of *n*-3 LC-PUFA derived from daily fish oil capsules compared with either adaily fish meal or daily fish oil enriched food have been reported in a few studies [27–30].

In the current study, the Constant and the Spike treatment showed lower levels of apparent *in vivo* enzyme activity for elongase, Δ6 and Δ5 desaturase compared with the Control treatment. Lower Δ6 desaturase activity with fish oil feeding has been previously reported [31]; however, there is no data looking at a weekly*vs.* daily dose to compare with. These desaturases and elongases are required for the biosynthesis of LC-PUFA and their inter-conversion. High availability of these fatty acids in Constant and the Spike treatment can act via a negative feedback control mechanism and reduce the gene transcription rate and the actual activity of the desaturase and elongase enzymes in these treatments, possibly via sterol regulatory element binding protein (SREBP-1c) [32,33]. On the other hand, the lack of *n*-3 LC-PUFA intake in the diet of the Control rats has likely increased their elongase and desaturase enzyme activities in order to increase endogenous *n*-3 LC-PUFA synthesis. Dietary *n*-3 LC-PUFA deprivation has previously been shown to upregulate liver mRNA levels of Δ6 and Δ5 desaturases as well as activities of Δ6 and Δ5 desaturases [34,35].

Overall, there were no significant differences in the assessed enzyme activities between the Spike and Constant treatments, with the exception of Δ9 desaturase (required for the biosynthesis of monounsaturated fatty acids), which was significantly higher in the Spike treatment.

Admittedly, one of the limitations of the present study includes being an animal study in male rats. Nevertheless, these preliminary, novel and highly interesting findings warrant further investigations, and in particular the need to be substantiated by conducting appropriate trials in humans. It is worth noting that the dose of *n*-3 LC-PUFA used in the Constant treatment equates to 1012 mg/day for a 70 kg human [36], which is in the range of human recommendations for these fatty acids. Another limitation, as previously mentioned, was that the slightly different total amounts of *n*-3 LC-PUFA administered by the two *n*-3 LC-PUFA enriched dietary treatments used in this study. However, these differences are relatively minimal, and unlikely to be responsible of any major modification in the overall *n*-3 LC-PUFA metabolism, and have been accounted for in the Whole Body Fatty Acid Balance Method. A third limitation is that these results do not apply to comparative effects of consumption of daily fish oil capsules *vs.* a sporadic meal with fish or seafood, since the study investigated the bioavailability of the same food source of *n*-3 LC-PUFA; but this was intentional to exclude the possible effect of the matrix (food source) of the dietary *n*-3 LC-PUFA.

In conclusion, our data show that there was a significantly greater deposition of the *n*-3 LC-PUFA associated with a single large dose of dietary *n*-3 LC-PUFA compared with the smaller daily doses in rats, due to less β-oxidation and greater deposition, and not due to differences in excretion (digestibility). The results from this animal study provide a suitable platform for future human studies aimed at developing substantiated evidence for advising consumers on the most efficient way to increase their *n*-3 LC-PUFA status.These findings suggests that a large dose of *n*-3 LC-PUFA once per week is more effective in increasing whole body *n*-3 LC-PUFA content compared to a smaller dose delivered daily. This observation, if validated in humans, could have remarkable effects on the possible development of more effective and sustainable utilisation strategies of these limited and metabolically important nutrients, currently derived primarily from the dwindling oceanic fish stocks.

Acknowledgments: Authors wish to thank James Emery for his technical support. This study was supported by the Australian Research Council's Discovery Projects funding scheme (Project DP1093570). The views expressed herein are those of the authors and are not necessarily those of the Australian Research Council. The Molecular Medicine Strategic Research Centre, Deakin University is also acknowledged for their financial support.

Author Contributions: All authors contributed to this research. Samaneh Ghasemifard: contributed to the study design, conducted of the animal study, analysis of tissues and whole body of rats, conducted the statistical analysis, and preparation of the manuscript. Andrew J. Sinclair: contributed substantially to the conception and the experimental design, interpretation of findings and provided critical revision of the article. Paul Lewandowski: provided critical revision of the article. Gunveen Kaur: contributed to preparation of the manuscript and provided critical revision of the article. Giovanni M. Turchini: contributed substantially to the conception and the experimental design, diet analysis, data analysis, interpretation of findings and provided critical revision of the article.

Conflicts of Interest: The authors declare no conflict of interest.

References

1. Sherry, C.L.; Oliver, J.S.; Marriage, B.J. Docosahexaenoic acid supplementation in lactating women increases breast milk and plasma docosahexaenoic acid concentrations and alters infant omega 6:3 fatty acid ratio. *Prostaglandins Leukot. Essent. Fat. Acids* **2015**, *95*, 63–69. [CrossRef] [PubMed]
2. Guichardant, M.; Calzada, C.; Bernoud-Hubac, N.; Lagarde, M.; Véricel, E. Omega-3 polyunsaturated fatty acids and oxygenated metabolism in atherothrombosis. *Biochim. Biophys. Acta* **2015**, *1851*, 485–495. [CrossRef] [PubMed]
3. Turunen, A.W.; Suominen, A.L.; Kiviranta, H.; Verkasalo, P.K.; Pukkala, E. Cancer incidence in a cohort with high fish consumption. *Cancer Causes Control* **2014**, *25*, 1595–1602. [CrossRef] [PubMed]
4. Denis, I.; Potier, B.; Heberden, C.; Vancassel, S. Omega-3 polyunsaturated fatty acids and brain aging. *Curr. Opin. Clin. Nutr. Metab. Care* **2015**, *18*, 139–146. [CrossRef] [PubMed]
5. Salem, N., Jr.; Vandal, M.; Calon, F. The benefit of docosahexaenoic acid for the adult brain in aging and dementia. *Prostaglandins Leukot. Essent. Fat. Acids* **2015**, *92*, 15–22. [CrossRef] [PubMed]
6. Lorente-Cebrian, S.; Costa, A.G.; Navas-Carretero, S.; Zabala, M.; Laiglesia, L.M.; Martinez, J.A.; Moreno-Aliaga, M.J. An update on the role of omega-3 fatty acids on inflammatory and degenerative diseases. *J. Physiol. Biochem.* **2015**, *71*, 341–349. [CrossRef] [PubMed]
7. Skulas-Ray, A.C. Omega-3 fatty acids and inflammation: A perspective on the challenges of evaluating efficacy in clinical research. *Prostaglandins Other Lipid Mediat.* **2015**, *116–117*, 104–111. [CrossRef] [PubMed]
8. Mozaffarian, D.; Wu, J.H. (n-3) fatty acids and cardiovascular health: Are effects of EPA and DHA shared or complementary? *J. Nutr.* **2012**, *142*, 614S–625S. [CrossRef] [PubMed]

9. National Health and Medical Research Council (NHMRC). *Nutrient Reference Values for Australia and New Zealand. Including Recommended Dietary Intakes*; Commonwealth Department of Health and Ageing A, Ministry of Health NZ, Eds.; Canberra, Commonwealth of Australia and New Zealand Government: Canberra, Australia, 2006.
10. National heart foundation of australia. A review of the relationship between dietary fat and cardiovascular disease. *Aust. J. Nutr. Diet.* **1999**, *56*, 5–22.
11. William, S.H.; James, V.P.; Scott, A.S.; Philip, G.J. Comparison of the effects of fish and fish-oil capsules on the *n*-3 fatty acid content of blood cells and plasma phospholipids. *Am. J. Clin. Nutr.* **2007**, *86*, 1621–1625.
12. Browning, L.M.; Walker, C.G.; Mander, A.P.; West, A.L.; Gambell, J.; Madden, J.; Calder, P.C.; Jebb, S.A. Compared with daily, weekly *n*-3 PUFA intake affects the incorporation of eicosapentaenoic acid and docosahexaenoic acid into platelets and mononuclear cells in humans. *J. Nutr.* **2014**, *144*, 667–672. [CrossRef] [PubMed]
13. Ghasemifard, S.; Turchini, G.M.; Sinclair, A.J. Review: Omega-3 long chain fatty acid "bioavailability": A review of evidence and methodological considerations. *Prog. Lipid Res.* **2014**, *56*, 92–108. [CrossRef] [PubMed]
14. Folch, J.; Lees, M.; Stanley, G.H.S. A simple method for the isolation and purification of total lipids from animal tissues. *J. Biol. Chem.* **1957**, *226*, 497–509. [PubMed]
15. Christie, W.W. *Lipid Analysis. Isolation, Separation, Identification and structural Analysis of Lipids*, 3rd ed.; The Oily Press, PJ Barnes and Associates: Bridgwater, Somerset, UK, 2003; p. 416.
16. Norambuena, F.; Lewis, M.; Hamid, N.K.A.; Hermon, K.; Donald, J.A.; Turchini, G.M. Fish oil replacement in current aquaculture feed: Is cholesterol a hidden treasure for fish nutrition? *PLoS ONE* **2013**, *8*, e81705. [CrossRef] [PubMed]
17. Tou, J.C.; Altman, S.N.; Gigliotti, J.C.; Benedito, V.A.; Cordonier, E.L. Different sources of omega-3 polyunsaturated fatty acids affects apparent digestibility, tissue deposition, and tissue oxidative stability in growing female rats. *Lipids Health Dis.* **2011**, *10*, 179. [CrossRef] [PubMed]
18. Turchini, G.M.; Francis, D.S.; de Silva, S.S. A whole body, *in vivo*, fatty acid balance method to quantify pufa metabolism (desaturation, elongation and beta-oxidation). *Lipids* **2007**, *42*, 1065–1071. [CrossRef] [PubMed]
19. Turchini, G.M.; Francis, D.S. Fatty acid metabolism (desaturation, elongation and beta-oxidation) in rainbow trout fed fish oil- or linseed oil-based diets. *Br. J. Nutr.* **2009**, *102*, 69–81. [CrossRef] [PubMed]
20. Cunnane, S.C.; Ryan, M.A.; Craig, K.S.; Brookes, S.; Koletzko, B.; Demmelmair, H.; Singer, J.; Kyle, D.J. Synthesis of linoleate and alpha-linolenate by chain elongation in the rat. *Lipids* **1995**, *30*, 781–783. [CrossRef] [PubMed]
21. Cunnane, S.C.; Yang, J. Zinc deficiency impairs whole-body accumulation of polyunsaturates and increases the utilization of [1–14C]linoleate for *de novo* lipid synthesis in pregnant rats. *Can. J. Physiol. Pharmacol.* **1995**, *73*, 1246–1252. [CrossRef] [PubMed]
22. Cunnane, S.C.; Anderson, M.J. The majority of dietary linoleate in growing rats is beta-oxidized or stored in visceral fat. *J. Nutr.* **1997**, *127*, 146–152. [PubMed]
23. Madsen, L.; Rustan, A.C.; Vaagenes, H.; Berge, K.; Dyrøy, E.; Berge, R.K. Eicosapentaenoic and docosahexaenoic acid affect mitochondrial and peroxisomal fatty acid oxidation in relation to substrate preference. *Lipids* **1999**, *34*, 951–963. [CrossRef] [PubMed]
24. Kaur, G.; Molero, J.C.; Weisinger, H.S.; Sinclair, A.J. Orally administered [^{14}C] DPA and [^{14}C] DHA are metabolised differently to [^{14}C] EPA in rats. *Br. J. N.* **2013**, *109*, 441–448. [CrossRef] [PubMed]
25. Kohler, A.; Bittner, D.; Low, A.; von Schacky, C. Effects of a convenience drink fortified with *n*-3 fatty acids on the n-3 index. *Br. J. Nutr.* **2010**, *104*, 729–736. [CrossRef] [PubMed]
26. Flock, M.R.; Skulas-Ray, A.C.; Harris, W.S.; Etherton, T.D.; Fleming, J.A.; Kris-Etherton, P.M. Determinants of erythrocyte omega-3 fatty acid content in response to fish oil supplementation: A dose-response randomized controlled trial. *J. Am. Heart Assoc.* **2013**, *2*, e000513. [CrossRef] [PubMed]
27. Schram, L.B.; Nielsen, C.J.; Porsgaard, T.; Nielsen, N.S.; Holm, R.; Mu, H. Food matrices affect the bioavailability of (*n*-3) polyunsaturated fatty acids in a single meal study in humans. *Food Res. Int.* **2007**, *40*, 1062–1068. [CrossRef]
28. Visioli, F.; Risé, P.; Barassi, M.; Marangoni, F.; Galli, C. Dietary intake of fish *vs.* Formulations leads to higher plasma concentrations of *n*-3 fatty acids. *Lipids* **2003**, *38*, 415–418. [CrossRef] [PubMed]

29. Wallace, J.M.; McCabe, A.J.; Robson, P.J.; Keogh, M.K.; Murray, C.A.; Kelly, P.M.; Márquez-Ruiz, G.; McGlynn, H.; Gilmore, W.S.; Strain, J.J. Bioavailability of *n*-3 polyunsaturated fatty acids (PUFA) in foods enriched with microencapsulated fish oil. *Ann. Nutr. Metab.* **2000**, *44*, 157–162. [CrossRef] [PubMed]
30. Higgins, S.; Carroll, Y.L.; O'Brien, N.M.; Morrissey, P.A. Use of microencapsulated fish oil as a means of increasing *n*-3 polyunsaturated fatty acid intake. *J. Hum. Nutr. Diet.* **1999**, *12*, 265–271. [CrossRef]
31. Garg, M.L.; Sebokova, E.; Thomson, A.B.; Clandinin, M.T. Delta 6-desaturase activity in liver microsomes of rats fed diets enriched with cholesterol and/or omega 3 fatty acids. *Biochem. J.* **1988**, *249*, 351–356. [PubMed]
32. Kaur, G.; Sinclair, A.J.; Cameron-Smith, D.; Barr, D.P.; Molero-Navajas, J.C.; Konstantopoulos, N. Docosapentaenoic acid (22:5n-3) down-regulates the expression of genes involved in fat synthesis in liver cells. *Prostaglandins Leukot. Essent. Fat. Acids* **2011**, *85*, 155–161. [CrossRef] [PubMed]
33. Matsuzaka, T.; Shimano, H.; Yahagi, N.; Amemiya-Kudo, M.; Yoshikawa, T.; Hasty, A.H.; Tamura, Y.; Osuga, J.-I.; Okazaki, H.; Iizuka, Y. Dual regulation of mouse δ5-and δ6-desaturase gene expression by SREBP-1 and PPARα. *J. Lipid Res.* **2002**, *43*, 107–114. [PubMed]
34. Igarashi, M.; Ma, K.; Chang, L.; Bell, J.M.; Rapoport, S.I. Dietary n-3 PUFA deprivation for 15 weeks upregulates elongase and desaturase expression in rat liver but not brain. *J. Lipid Res.* **2007**, *48*, 2463–2470. [CrossRef] [PubMed]
35. Hofacer, R.; Jandacek, R.; Rider, T.; Tso, P.; Magrisso, I.J.; Benoit, S.C.; McNamara, R.K. Omega-3 fatty acid deficiency selectively up-regulates delta6-desaturase expression and activity indices in rat liver: Prevention by normalization of omega-3 fatty acid status. *Nutr. Res.* **2011**, *31*, 715–722. [CrossRef] [PubMed]
36. Reagan-Shaw, S.; Nihal, M.; Ahmad, N. Dose translation from animal to human studies revisited. *FASEB J.* **2008**, *22*, 659–661. [CrossRef] [PubMed]

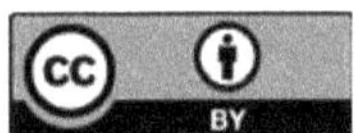

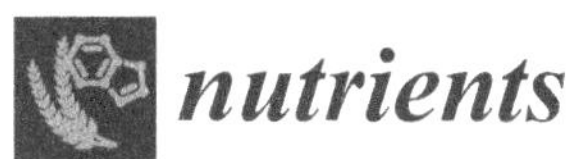

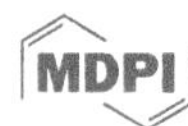

Article

The Pattern of Fatty Acids Displaced by EPA and DHA Following 12 Months Supplementation Varies between Blood Cell and Plasma Fractions

Celia G. Walker [1], Annette L. West [2], Lucy M. Browning [1], Jackie Madden [2], Joanna M. Gambell [1], Susan A. Jebb [1,3] and Philip C. Calder [2,4,5,*]

[1] MRC Human Nutrition Research, Elsie Widdowson Laboratory, Fulbourn Road, Cambridge CB1 9NL, UK; E-Mails: celia.walker@mrc-hnr.cam.ac.uk (C.G.W.); lmbrowning@btinternet.com (L.M.B.); j.m.gambell@gmail.com (J.M.G.); susan.jebb@phc.ox.ac.uk (S.A.J.)

[2] Human Development and Health Academic Unit, Faculty of Medicine, University of Southampton, Tremona Road, Southampton SO16 6YD, UK; E-Mails: A.West@soton.ac.uk (A.L.W.); jm24@soton.ac.uk (J.M.)

[3] Nuffield Department of Primary Care Health Sciences, University of Oxford, Woodstock Road, Oxford OX2 6GG, UK

[4] NIHR Southampton Biomedical Research Centre, University of Southampton and University Hospital Southampton NHS Foundation Trust, Tremona Road, Southampton SO16 6YD, UK

[5] Department of Biological Sciences, Faculty of Science, King Abdulaziz University, Jeddah 21589, Kingdom of Saudi Arabia

* Author to whom correspondence should be addressed; E-Mail: pcc@soton.ac.uk; Tel.: +44-23-8120-5250; Fax: +44-23-8120-4221.

Received: 26 May 2015 / Accepted: 27 July 2015 / Published: 3 August 2015

Abstract: Eicosapentaenoic acid (EPA) and docosahexaenoic acid (DHA) are increased in plasma lipids and blood cell membranes in response to supplementation. Whilst arachidonic acid (AA) is correspondingly decreased, the effect on other fatty acids (FA) is less well described and there may be site-specific differences. In response to 12 months EPA + DHA supplementation in doses equivalent to 0–4 portions of oily fish/week (1 portion: 3.27 g EPA+DHA) multinomial regression analysis was used to identify important FA changes for plasma phosphatidylcholine (PC), cholesteryl ester (CE) and triglyceride (TAG) and for blood mononuclear cells (MNC), red blood cells (RBC) and platelets (PLAT). Dose-dependent increases in EPA + DHA were matched by decreases in several n-6 polyunsaturated fatty acids (PUFA) in PC, CE, RBC and PLAT, but were predominantly compensated for by oleic acid in TAG. Changes were observed for all FA classes in MNC. Consequently the n-6:n-3 PUFA ratio was reduced in a dose-dependent manner in all pools after 12 months (37%–64% of placebo in the four portions group). We conclude that the profile of the FA decreased in exchange for the increase in EPA + DHA following supplementation differs by FA pool with implications for understanding the impact of n-3 PUFA on blood lipid and blood cell biology.

Keywords: EPA and DHA supplementation; n-3 fatty acid; n-6 fatty acid; fatty acid displacement; plasma fatty acid fractions; blood cell fatty acids

---

1. Introduction

A diet rich in oily fish containing high concentrations of the long-chain omega-3 (n-3) polyunsaturated fatty acids (PUFA) eicosapentaenoic acid (EPA; 20:5n-3) and docosahexaenoic acid (DHA; 22:6n-3) has been associated with health benefits, particularly a reduced risk of cardiovascular disease [1,2]. Studies with EPA and DHA in supplemental form report a wide range of effects on cardiovascular risk factors amongst other outcomes [2,3] that may explain the benefits of oily fish. EPA and DHA have been used clinically as an adjuvant therapy to prevent secondary myocardial infarction [4], to lower plasma triglycerides [5] and to prevent or alleviate inflammatory conditions including asthma, eczema and rheumatoid arthritis [6] with varying degrees of success [1–3]. Whilst not fully elucidated, the mechanisms underlying the health benefits of EPA and DHA, and of oily fish, have been partially attributed to EPA and DHA displacing other fatty acids (FA), notably the omega-6 (n-6) PUFA arachidonic acid (AA; 20:4n-6), in phospholipids of cell membranes [7]. Indeed, it has been well established that in response to supplementation with EPA and DHA, these fatty acids are incorporated in increased amounts into plasma phospholipids [8] and cell membranes including those of platelets [9], mononuclear cells [7], red blood cells [8,10] and other cells such as those of the myocardium [11]. This increased content of EPA and DHA in cell membranes alters the physical properties of the membrane such as its fluidity, which can impact on receptor migration and lipid raft formation, and alter cell signalling pathways which in turn influence cell and tissue responses linked to metabolism, hormone sensitivity, immune function and so on [12]. Furthermore, a decrease in cell membrane AA content and an increase in EPA and DHA alters the balance of eicosanoid and cytokine production from a generally pro-inflammatory profile to a less inflammatory and even inflammation resolving profile [7]. Because of the opposing actions of AA and of EPA and DHA in inflammation, immunity and blood clotting, there has been considerable focus on the ability of EPA and DHA to decrease the AA content of blood and cellular lipids. This has drawn attention away from effects that EPA and DHA might have on the content of other FA in blood lipids, cells and tissues. Consequently, the effect of increased EPA and DHA intake (and incorporation) on the proportions of FA other than AA in different plasma lipids and blood cells is not well described. It is possible that there are cell-specific differences in the FA that EPA and DHA replace which has implications for the metabolic and functional effects of EPA + DHA supplementation.

We previously reported the patterns of increased EPA and DHA incorporation seen in different plasma lipids and blood cells when individuals increased their intake of those fatty acids over the course of 12 months [13]. We now report the patterns of change in other FA observed in this study; we report findings for plasma phosphatidylcholine (PC), cholesteryl esters (CE) and triglycerides (TAG) and for blood mononuclear cells (MNC), red blood cells (RBC) and platelets (PLAT).

2. Experimental Section

2.1. Original Trial

Data used for this analysis were from a two-centre study examining changes in FA profiles of various blood and tissue fractions in response to 12 months supplementation equivalent to the amounts of marine n-3 PUFA provided by 0, 1, 2 and 4 portions of oily fish per week (one portion = 1.5 g EPA + 1.77 g DHA) [13]. Placebo capsules of high oleic sunflower oil balanced the intake of active capsules. The study was registered at www.controlled-trials.com as ISRCTN48398526 and is described in detail elsewhere [13]. All procedures were approved by the Suffolk Local Research Ethics Committee (approval 05/Q0102/181), and written informed consent was obtained from all participants. The study participants were all non-oily fish consumers and were stratified by age and sex [14], had a BMI range of 18.5–34.9 (median = 25.2) kg/m^2 and were all described as healthy.

Background diet was monitored by participants completing unweighed 4-day diet diaries recording intakes as estimated portions over three weekdays and one weekend day at 0, 6 and 12 months of the intervention period. At the nine study visits over the 12 month study period, participants were also asked specific questions relating to cooking oils and spreads and white fish consumption. Data were analysed using an in-house database [15] and, as reported previously, there were no significant differences between groups or between time points for total reported energy or macronutrient intake [13]. Compliance to the intervention was assessed by return of capsule blister packs and was high (mean: 98.1%; IQR: 2.2) as previously reported [13].

For this analysis, data for blood samples taken at baseline and after 12 months of supplementation were used. The preparation and analysis of samples has been described previously [13]. Briefly, plasma was prepared from fasting blood collected into heparin and the plasma lipid was further separated into the major fractions phosphatidylcholine (PC), cholesteryl esters (CE) and triglycerides (TAG) by solid-phase extraction on aminopropylsilica cartridges. Mononuclear cells (MNC) and red blood cells (RBC) were isolated from heparinised blood and platelets (PLAT) from citrated blood. FA were analysed as FA methyl esters by gas chromatography, performed on a Hewlett Packard 6890 gas chromatograph fitted with a BPX-70 column (30 m × 0.22 mm × 0.25 μm). The instrument was controlled by, and data were collected using, HPChemStation (Hewlett-Packard Co., Amsterdam, The Netherlands). Full details of lipid extraction methodology, FA methyl ester formation, and gas chromatography running conditions may be found elsewhere [13]. FA methyl esters were identified by comparison of retention times with those of authentic standards run previously [13]. FA are expressed as weight percentage of total fatty acids present in the lipid pool.

2.2. Data Analysis

Multinomial linear regression analysis was used to identify the important FA associated with the change in EPA and DHA. Median values for change in the proportion of the 37 FA within each pool were ranked. A threshold median change of 0.1% was set for each pool for inclusion in the model as an indication of potential change in proportion of FA in response to the intervention. A higher threshold of 0.2% median change was used for MNC and PLAT as the model was saturated by the inclusion of a large number of FA using a median change cut-off of 0.1%. A correlation matrix was used for each pool to identify highly correlated ($r > 0.7$) FA. In these situations only a single FA was added into the model at a time, in order to prevent colinearity destabilising the model, but both of the FA were considered important in further analyses. A multinomial regression model was built with change in EPA and DHA as the dependent variables and the FA which exceeded the threshold for each lipid pool as predictors. Other variables including age, sex and dietary change were tested as covariates. From this initial model a backward elimination procedure was used to find a more parsimonious model in order to identify the FA most influential in the change in EPA and DHA in each lipid pool.

In order to visualise patterns in FA classes which are important in each FA pool and the relative magnitude of FA changes, linear combinations were calculated of the coefficients of associations of each FA with EPA and with DHA for all the FA identified in each pool. The combined coefficient represents the change in EPA + DHA for a one unit increase in FA; therefore a FA which has a small magnitude of change has a large coefficient. In order to visualise the relative magnitude of FA changes the reciprocal of the combined coefficient was calculated and compared for each pool.

To determine whether the identified FA were reduced in a dose-dependent manner according to the EPA + DHA supplementation, the effect of dose on the change in each FA was assessed by linear regression analysis. Age and sex, and change in dietary fats (total SFA, MUFA, n-6 PUFA or n-3 PUFA) were tested as covariates in each model and retained if they had an effect.

The effect of the dose on the change in total n-6:n-3 PUFA ratio from baseline to 12 months in each of the pools was determined by mixed effect models adjusted for age and sex. The overall effect of dose over the 12 month visit was tested by a chi test (3 df) contrast of marginal linear predictions from mixed models for each pool.

All data were analysed with Stata version 13 (StataCorp, TX, USA). In all cases a value of $p < 0.05$ was taken to indicate statistical significance.

3. Results

3.1. Prevalence of FA in the Different Pools at Baseline

The relative proportions of FA in the different pools at baseline are shown in Table 1. The five most prevalent FA in each pool (palmitic acid (PA; 16:0), stearic acid (SA; 18:0), oleic acid (OA; 18:1n-9), linoleic acid (LA; 18:2n-6), and AA) are consistent between blood cells (MNC, PLAT, RBC). These five most abundant fatty acids make up 74%–91% of the total FA in each pool but differ in proportions between pools. PA, OA and LA, which are the most abundant FA in the average Western diet, are strongly represented in every lipid pool examined. AA is one of the most abundant FA in the blood cells and in plasma PC and CE. The n-6:n-3 PUFA ratio was high in plasma CE (median 37.3), low in RBC (5.44) but comparable in all other pools (MNC: 12.1; PLAT: 13.8; plasma PC: 15.0; plasma TAG 12.0). The AA:EPA + DHA ratio was higher in MNC (median 5.93) than in other pools (PLAT: 3.23; RBC: 2.22; plasma PC: 2.05; plasma CE: 4.09; plasma TAG: 1.65).

Table 1. Relative abundance of fatty acid (FA) in each lipid pool at baseline.

Fatty Acid	MNC	PLAT	RBC	CE	PC	TAG
10:0	0.14 (0.25)	0.03 (0.05)	0.00 (0.07)	0.06 (0.04)	0.00 (0.00)	0.00 (0.00)
12:0	0.05 (0.16)	0.08 (0.08)	0.00 (0.00)	0.06 (0.04)	0.00 (0.00)	0.06 (0.15)
13:0	0.03 (0.11)	0.00 (0.00)	0.00 (0.00)	0.13 (0.14)	0.00 (0.00)	0.00 (0.13)
14:0	0.41 (0.35)	0.74 (0.40)	0.25 (0.12)	0.49 (0.38)	0.27 (0.14)	1.49 (1.09)
14:1n-9	0.16 (0.21)	0.06 (0.09)	0.00 (0.00)	0.04 (0.02)	0.00 (0.00)	0.08 (0.10)
15:0	0.19 (0.14)	0.18 (0.07)	0.09 (0.14)	0.15 (0.07)	0.15 (0.21)	0.27 (0.08)
15:1	0.14 (0.36)	0.07 (0.21)	2.21 (1.99)	0.05 (0.03)	0.05 (0.03)	0.05 (0.04)
16:0	**18.2 (2.94)**	**20.7 (2.54)**	**19.3 (1.83)**	**11.3 (1.14)**	**28.9 (1.80)**	**25.6 (3.89)**
16:1n-7	1.13 (1.44)	1.97 (1.14)	0.38 (0.19)	**2.80 (1.74)**	0.70 (0.35)	**3.49 (1.50)**
17:0	0.32 (0.20)	0.26 (0.06)	0.27 (0.08)	0.07 (0.08)	0.35 (0.10)	0.30 (0.13)
17:1n-8	0.30 (0.37)	0.91 (0.90)	4.05 (0.63)	0.05 (0.05)	0.19 (0.11)	0.19 (0.10)
18:0	**17.4 (4.95)**	**8.67 (3.07)**	**16.2 (1.27)**	0.76 (0.25)	**12.8 (1.39)**	**3.07 (1.02)**
18:1n-9t	1.94 (1.33)	0.17 (0.07)	0.16 (0.22)	1.31 (0.43)	1.55 (0.32)	2.44 (0.62)
18:1n-9c	**16.2 (2.75)**	**19.9 (3.55)**	**13.1 (1.45)**	**19.1 (2.66)**	**11.2 (1.69)**	**39.8 (3.96)**
18:2n-6t	0.00 (0.19)	0.14 (0.12)	0.21 (0.26)	0.00 (0.00)	0.00 (0.00)	0.00 (0.00)
18:2n-6c	**11.4 (9.04)**	**25.1 (7.42)**	**9.93 (1.94)**	**51.7 (6.42)**	**22.4 (3.76)**	**16.6 (5.63)**
18:3n-6	0.20 (0.33)	0.43 (0.25)	0.09 (0.16)	0.95 (0.58)	0.11 (0.08)	0.34 (0.23)
18:3n-3	0.22 (0.30)	0.62 (0.31)	0.32 (0.33)	0.56 (0.25)	0.22 (0.15)	1.00 (0.49)
20:0	0.53 (0.62)	0.26 (0.19)	0.10 (0.16)	0.13 (0.05)	0.15 (0.07)	0.28 (0.16)
20:1n-9	0.60 (1.00)	0.35 (0.33)	0.36 (0.22)	0.06 (0.09)	0.20 (0.10)	0.29 (0.14)
20:2n-6	0.46 (0.60)	0.20 (0.07)	0.22 (0.18)	0.07 (0.05)	0.34 (0.11)	0.15 (0.09)
20:3n-3	0.04 (0.19)	0.10 (0.06)	0.15 (0.27)	0.00 (0.00)	0.00 (0.22)	0.00 (0.00)
20:3n-6	1.88 (1.42)	1.63 (0.50)	1.75 (0.56)	0.76 (0.26)	3.30 (1.11)	0.29 (0.14)
20:4n-6	**16.0 (9.19)**	**9.54 (4.18)**	**15.5 (2.14)**	**6.59 (2.10)**	**9.55 (2.39)**	1.55 (0.82)
20:4n-4	0.22 (0.50)	0.00 (0.00)	0.00 (0.00)	0.08 (0.04)	0.18 (0.11)	0.07 (0.11)
20:5n-3	0.57 (0.46)	1.00 (0.52)	1.42 (1.12)	0.91 (0.64)	1.05 (0.57)	0.22 (0.41)
21:0	0.30 (0.50)	0.13 (0.17)	0.37 (0.46)	0.03 (0.04)	0.06 (0.09)	0.00 (0.00)
22:0	0.18 (0.32)	0.23 (0.10)	0.20 (0.24)	0.00 (0.03)	0.03 (0.14)	0.00 (0.00)
22:2n-6	0.07 (0.21)	0.00 (0.00)	0.00 (0.00)	0.00 (0.00)	0.00 (0.00)	0.00 (0.08)
22:4n-6	0.76 (1.00)	0.46 (0.40)	2.80 (0.89)	0.03 (0.04)	0.34 (0.19)	0.14 (0.07)
22:5n-3	1.48 (0.84)	0.88 (0.26)	3.11 (0.60)	0.07 (0.08)	0.95 (0.28)	0.30 (0.43)
22:5n-6	0.37 (0.74)	0.13 (0.05)	0.47 (0.23)	0.04 (0.04)	0.23 (0.18)	0.17 (0.22)
22:6n-3	1.86 (0.76)	1.97 (0.71)	5.34 (1.88)	0.63 (0.34)	3.47 (1.51)	0.72 (0.46)
23:0	0.04 (0.17)	0.05 (0.07)	0.00 (0.00)	0.00 (0.00)	0.00 (0.00)	0.00 (0.26)
24:0	0.60 (1.16)	0.10 (0.05)	0.38 (0.13)	0.00 (0.00)	0.00 (0.00)	0.00 (0.00)
24:1n-9	0.20 (0.28)	0.00 (0.00)	0.00 (0.00)	0.04 (0.04)	0.25 (0.14)	0.00 (0.13)

Data are median (IQR). The five most prevalent FA in each pool are indicated in bold. MNC (mononuclear cells); PLAT (platelets); RBC (red blood cells); CE (plasma cholesteryl esters); PC (plasma phosphatidylcholine); TAG (plasma triglycerides).

3.2. Change in FA Profile in Each Lipid Pool

The FA identified by the multinomial models to be important for change in EPA and DHA are shown for plasma lipid pools in Figure 1a and for blood cells in Figure 1b. The FA displaced in PC were predominantly n-6 PUFA, whereas in TAG they were predominantly MUFA and SFA, and in CE SFA, MUFA and n-6 PUFA were all displaced following EPA and DHA supplementation. In RBC the FA predominantly decreased were n-6 PUFA, in PLAT predominantly SFA and n-6 PUFA, while in MNC there were a range of changes in FA from all classes. Docosapentaenoic acid (DPA; 22:5n-3) increased in most pools (plasma PC and TAG, RBC and MNC) with increased EPA and DHA intake.

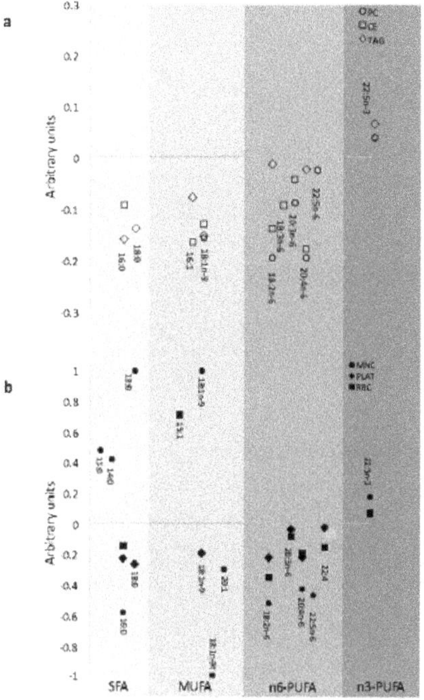

Figure 1. Patterns of modelled changes in fatty acids which occur with the increase in eicosapentaenoic acid (EPA) and docosahexaenoic acid (DHA) in (**a**) plasma and (**b**) blood cell fatty acid pools. Linear combinations of the co-efficients from the multinomial linear regression models were calculated for each fatty acid important for the change in EPA + DHA. As a small regression coefficient for the fatty acid of interest reflected a large change in the outcomes EPA + DHA and vice versa the data are the reciprocal of the co-efficients in order to portray the magnitude of effect, and this is presented in arbitrary units. Fatty acids are grouped according to class to depict the patterns of change in fatty acids for each pool.

3.3. *Effect of Dose of EPA and DHA on the Change in Identified FA in Each Pool*

The effect of the dose of EPA + DHA supplementation on the change in FA identified by the multinomial models is shown for each lipid pool in Figure 2. In plasma PC (Figure 2a) there was a clear dose response such that OA and three n-6 PUFAs (LA, di-homo-γ-linolenic acid (DGLA; 20:3n-6 and AA) were decreased in relation to an increasing dose (and increasing incorporation) of EPA + DHA. In plasma CE (Figure 2b) the n-6 PUFAs LA, γ-linolenic acid (GLA; 18:3n-6) and DGLA (when taking into account the change in dietary n-6 PUFA) decreased in a dose-dependent manner with increasing EPA + DHA. There was a dose-dependent decrease in OA, but this was not seen when changes in dietary MUFA intake were accounted for. PA was also increased in a dose-dependent manner in CE. In plasma TAG (Figure 2c) the only dose-dependent decreases were in MUFA (palmitoleic acid (POA; 16:1n-7) and OA). In RBC there was a significant dose-response decrease in the n-6 PUFAs DGLA, AA and docosatetraenoic acid (DTA; 22:4) (Figure 2d). In PLAT DGLA was decreased and there was also a trend (p = 0.09) for DTA to be decreased in a dose-dependent manner (Figure 2e). In both PLAT and MNC OA increased, but the magnitude of the increase was inversely proportional to dose. There was also a pattern for LA to be increased in MNC and PLAT in an inverse dose-responsive manner, although this was not significant (Figure 2d,e). DPA was increased in a dose-dependent manner in the four pools in which it was identified as an important contributor to change in EPA and DHA.

3.4. *Impact of EPA and DHA Supplementation on the FA Profile*

Although EPA and DHA increased in all pools, the most abundant FA remained the same as at baseline, even though the proportions of these FA were often changed. The only exception was in plasma CE, where EPA displaced POA at the highest intake of EPA + DHA as one of the five most abundant FA (at 12 months, EPA mean: 3.49, SD: 1.03; POA mean: 2.81, SD: 1.20).

The increase in EPA, DPA and DHA and the decrease in n-6 PUFAs resulted in a significant decrease in the n-6:n-3 PUFA ratio in each of the FA pools (Table 2). The ratio was decreased in the four portions group to 37%–64% compared to the placebo group across the FA pools (Table 2).

The AA:EPA + DHA ratio was also lower in all pools, such that after 12 months of the four portions dose the median values were MNC: 2.53; PLAT: 1.11; RBC: 1.13; plasma PC: 0.81; plasma CE: 1.21; plasma TAG: 0.40.

Table 2. The n-6:n-3 PUFA ratio in the 0 portions group and differences by dose in the change in the ratio after 12 months of EPA + DHA supplementation.

	n-6:n-3 PUFA Ratio	**Change in n-6:n 3 PUFA Ratio** ‡			**Overall Effect of Dose at 12 Months (p)**
	0 Portion Value †	**1 Portion**	**2 Portion**	**4 Portions**	
Plasma PC	14.4 ± 0.59	−3.32 (−4.90, −1.73)	−5.41 (−7.06, −3.77)	−7.48 (−9.09, −5.87)	<0.0001
Plasma CE	35.5 ± 1.50	−7.54 (−11.5, −3.51)	−14.5 (−18.7, −10.4)	−20.7 (−24.8, −16.6)	<0.0001
Plasma TAG	10.0 ± 0.49	−1.35 (−2.65, −0.05)	−2.88 (−4.23, −1.54)	−4.59 (−5.90, −3.27)	<0.0001
RBC	4.90 ± 0.27	−0.82 (−1.54, −1.04)	−1.31 (−2.06, −0.55)	−1.81 (−2.54, −1.07)	<0.0001
PLAT	15.3 ± 0.70	−4.17 (−5.69, −2.64)	−6.56 (−8.13, −4.99)	−9.76 (−11.3, −8.22)	<0.0001
MNC	16.2 ± 0.69	−3.20 (−5.04, −1.36)	−6.24 (−8.15, −4.33)	−8.71 (−10.6, −6.85)	<0.0001

Mixed-effects models for the change in n-6:n-3 PUFA ratio in each pool adjusted for age and sex. The overall effect of dose over the 12 month visit by 3df chi test contrast of marginal linear predictions from mixed model is presented for each pool. † 0 portion values are mean ± standard error; ‡ Adjusted mean differences (95% CI) between groups at 12 months calculated in the mixed effects models.

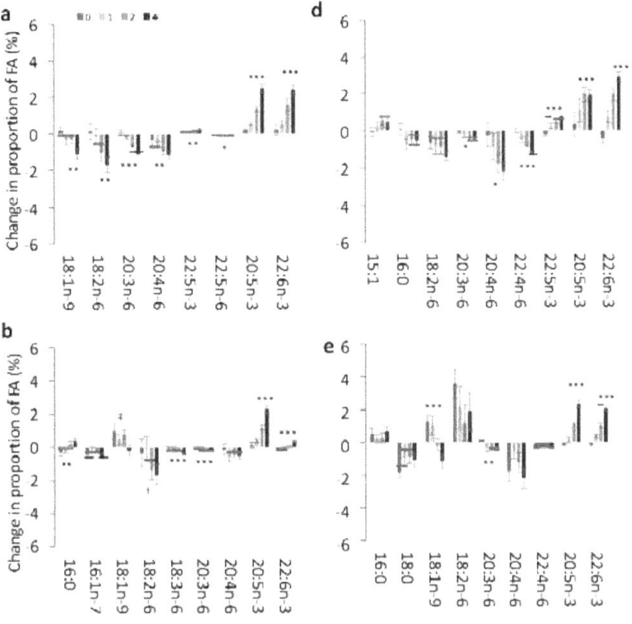

Figure 2. *Cont.*

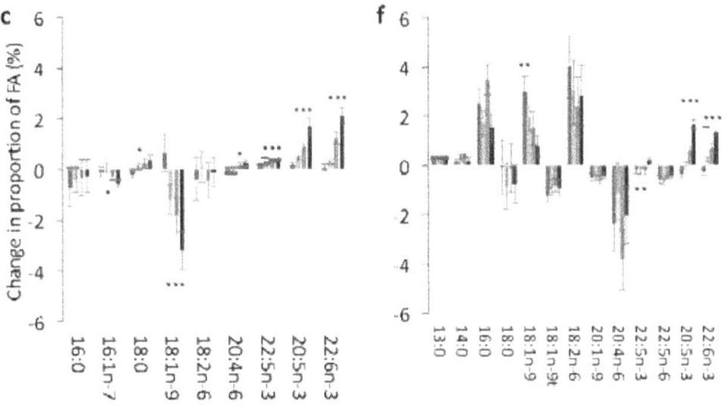

Figure 2. Mean change in key fatty acids in response to 12 months supplementation of EPA + DHA equivalent to 0, 1, 2 or 4 portions of fish per week in different plasma and blood cell pools. The observed mean ± SE change from baseline in the fatty acids identified as important in relation to change in EPA + DHA in the multinomial regression models in (**a**) Plasma PC; (**b**) Plasma CE; (**c**) Plasma TAG; (**d**) RBC; (**e**) PLAT; (**f**) MNC. The effect of dose was tested by linear regression models for each fatty acid. Each model was tested with and without age and sex which were included as covariates if significant. Change in dietary SFA, MUFA, n-3 PUFA or n-6 PUFA where relevant were also tested to determine if change in diet influenced the change in fatty acids with EPA + DHA dose. Significant effects of dose detected in these models are shown as: * $p < 0.05$; ** $p < 0.01$; *** $p < 0.0001$; † Effect of dose ($p = 0.05$) only when taking into account the change in dietary n-6 PUFA from baseline to 12 months; ‡ Effect of dose ($p < 0.05$) is no longer significant when taking into account the effect of change in dietary MUFA.

4. Discussion

In this study we show that the dose dependent incorporation of EPA and DHA following 12 months supplementation is matched by dose dependent decreases in other FA in all pools, but that the FA that change differ between pools. For the plasma fractions PC and CE, EPA and DHA predominantly displaced a range of n-6 PUFAs, whereas it was predominantly the MUFA OA which was displaced in TAG. In blood cells EPA and DHA displaced a range of n-6 PUFA, including but not limited to AA in RBC and PLAT, whereas in MNC a number of FA changes occurred across all classes of FA.

Decreases in n-6 PUFA were the most important compensatory FA changes in response to the increase in EPA and DHA in many pools and this was reflected in a change in total n-6:n-3 PUFA ratio in all pools. An increase in EPA and DHA intake equivalent to a dietary change of four portions of oily fish per week will reduce the n-6:n-3 PUFA ratio by around half in all of the FA pools. This effect on the n-6:n-3 PUFA ratio has been reported consistently from long-term (12 month) high dose (~10 g/day) n-3 PUFA supplementation [16] to comparatively low dose (0.8 g/day) n-3 PUFA for a comparatively short supplementation period of 10 weeks [17].

AA decreased in most pools, but significant dose-dependent decreases in AA were only observed in plasma PC and in RBC, although prominent non-dose dependent decreases were also observed in PLAT and MNC. There has been a longstanding interest in compensatory decreases in AA following EPA and DHA supplementation, due to the role of AA as a primary precursor of eicosanoids [7]. AA is one of the five most abundant FA in most of the pools, whereas significant dose-dependent changes of a comparable magnitude also were observed for DGLA in plasma PC and CE, RBC and PLAT where it was 3–10 fold less abundant, meaning these changes may have more biological impact. DGLA is itself important for eicosanoid synthesis and regulation of pathways involving other bioactive lipid compounds [7,18]. A significant decrease in DGLA but not AA was previously reported following supplementation with 3 g/day long chain n-3 PUFA for 10 weeks [17]. This was accompanied by a decrease in AA-derived pro-inflammatory mediators in plasma [17]. Likewise changes in other low abundance n-6 PUFA (Adrenic acid (AdA; 22:4n-6) in RBC and PLAT, and GLA in plasma CE) may be of biological importance. Changes to these other n-6 PUFA in response to EPA and DHA supplementation are not widely reported in the literature.

The AA:EPA + DHA ratio was higher in MNC than other blood cell types. This ratio may reflect the importance of AA as a precursor for eicosanoids involved as mediators and regulators of inflammation and the immune response [7]. Although AA:EPA + DHA was decreased in all lipid pools with increasing EPA + DHA intake, the decrease may have especially pronounced effects on the function of MNC and PLAT, where AA serves important roles as an eicosanoid precursor. The changes in the ratio of AA:EPA + DHA observed with increased consumption of EPA + DHA are strongly linked to the impact of the latter on inflammation [7] and thrombosis [2,3].

In addition to compensatory decreases in n-6 PUFA seen in most pools, prominent changes in MUFA and SFA were also observed in plasma TAG, plasma CE, MNC and PLAT. A FA profile change from MUFA or particularly SFA to n-3 PUFA is likely to have structural effects on membranes altering fluidity [19] and lipid raft formation with subsequent effects on membrane receptor function and cell signalling [12]. Thus these changes in FA class are also of interest, particularly in PLAT and MNC. Changes in FA class of membranes have not been consistently shown in response to EPA and DHA supplementation as summarised by Hodson *et al.* [20] although many previous studies tended to be of shorter duration (⩽12 weeks).

A pattern was evident in PLAT and MNC for OA and LA and in plasma CE for OA to be increased in an inverse dose-dependent manner (although this was not significant for LA), such that the increase was lowest for the highest dose of EPA and DHA. This is most likely explained by OA and LA provided by the placebo capsules, where the dose provided was inversely proportional to EPA and DHA (0 portions: 10.41 g OA + 1.92 g LA per week; four portions: 24.3 g OA + 4.48 g LA per week). A wide range of changes including increases in a number of SFA were noted in MNC. The incorporation of n-3 PUFA into the MNC membranes may have stimulated a number of FA changes in the membranes of these cells in order to maintain a constant membrane fluidity. It has previously been suggested that increased incorporation of n-3 PUFA into phospholipid membranes triggered changes in phospholipid class in cell membranes in order to maintain constant membrane fluidity [21]. There were clearly different patterns of FA displacement with the different pools studied here. In addition to a potential impact on membrane fluidity, altered FA composition of cell membranes can influence formation of lipid rafts and the activity of various types of membrane proteins and can alter signalling pathways that ultimately control cell and tissue responses linked to metabolism, hormone sensitivity, lipid mediator production, and function [12]. Thus, the FA changes described here are likely to be of functional relevance.

As this was a placebo-controlled trial, the potential impact of the high oleic sunflower oil placebo capsules (see Browning *et al.* [13] for full composition details) must be considered in the interpretation of the FA changes. Whilst this placebo was chosen to have minimal impact on FA composition of target lipid pools by closely mimicking the habitual diet, the inverse dose-response increase in OA (and trend in LA) noted in some pools indicate a potential impact. It is possible that changes in LA may also impact on changes in other n-6 PUFA. Dietary changes in FA would also contribute to changes in FA profiles and we attempted to account for this in our analyses. Although dietary data were collected at the start and the end of the 12 month study, these data only included total FA classes rather than individual FA contributions. Furthermore, this dietary information was captured by a four day food diary, which is not a robust indicator of habitual food intake. Whilst these measures, plus an additional assessment of diet conducted halfway through the trial, indicated no substantial changes in dietary habits at these three discrete time points [13], small changes in dietary fat intake in the intervening periods would none-the-less have an impact on the FA profile.

5. Conclusions

The profile of the FA decreased in compensation for the increase in EPA and DHA following supplementation differs by FA pool, and this may have important biological implications beyond the previously reported decreases in AA.

Acknowledgments: Acknowledgments

The UK Medical Research Council supported Celia G. Walker, Lucy M. Browning and Susan A. Jebb (grant code U1059.60.389) for this work. The original trial was funded by the UK Foods Standards Agency (N05065/66). The views expressed are those of the authors and do not necessarily reflect UK Government policy or advice. Equazen (Wallingford, Oxford, UK) supplied the capsules for the intervention.

The authors thank Adrian Mander and Jianhua Wu (statistical advice); Louise Timbers, Clionadh O'Reilly, Mariana Eberhard, Katey Bergstralh, and Sarah Gibbings (research assistants); Darren Cole (database manager); Laura Wang, Stephen Young, Sadiq Lula, Christine Clewes, Christiaan Gelauf, and Jade Pretorius (FA analysis); Alison Lennox, Birgit Teucher, Anna Gent, and Celia Greenberg (coding and analysis of dietary data); and Mario Siervo, Rosemary Hall, and Sue Fisher (clinical support).

Author Contributions: Philip C. Calder conceived the idea; Celia G. Walker designed and conducted the analysis; Celia G. Walker and Philip C. Calder drafted the manuscript. Lucy M. Browning, Susan A. Jebb and Philip C. Calder designed the original trial; Annette L. West, Lucy M. Browning, Jackie Madden and Joanna M. Gambell conducted the research on the original trial. All authors critically appraised the manuscript.

Conflicts of Interest: The authors declare no conflict of interest relevant to this paper.

References

1. Deckelbaum, R.; Torrejon, C. The omega-3 fatty acid nutritional landscape: Health benefits and sources. *J. Nutr.* **2012**, *142*, 587S–591S. [CrossRef] [PubMed]
2. Saravanan, P.; Davidson, N.C.; Schmidt, E.B.; Calder, P.C. Cardiovascular effects of marine omega-3 fatty acids. *Lancet* **2010**, *376*, 540–550. [CrossRef]

3. Calder, P.C. Very long chain omega-3 (n-3) fatty acids and human health. *Eur. J. Lipid Sci. Technol.* **2014**, *116*, 1280–1300. [CrossRef]
4. Hoy, S.; Keating, G. Omega-3 ethylester concentrate. *Drugs* **2009**, *69*, 1077–1105. [CrossRef] [PubMed]
5. Bradberry, J.C.; Hilleman, D.E. Overview of omega-3 fatty acid therapies. *P T.* **2013**, *38*, 681–691. [PubMed]
6. Yates, C.M.; Calder, P.C.; Ed Rainger, G. Pharmacology and therapeutics of omega-3 polyunsaturated fatty acids in chronic inflammatory disease. *P T.* **2014**, *141*, 272–282. [CrossRef] [PubMed]
7. Calder, P.C. Marine omega-3 fatty acids and inflammatory processes: Effects, mechanisms and clinical relevance. *Biochim. Biophys. Acta* **2015**, *1851*, 469–484. [CrossRef] [PubMed]
8. Arterburn, L.M.; Hall, E.B.; Oken, H. Distribution, interconversion, and dose response of n-3 fatty acids in humans. *Am. J. Clin. Nutr.* **2006**, *83*, S1467–1476S.
9. Lovegrove, J.A.; Lovegrove, S.S.; Lesauvage, S.V.; Brady, L.M.; Saini, N.; Minihane, A.M.; Williams, C.M. Moderate fish-oil supplementation reverses low-platelet, long-chain n-3 polyunsaturated fatty acid status and reduces plasma triacylglycerol concentrations in British Indo-Asians. *Am. J. Clin. Nutr.* **2004**, *79*, 974–982. [PubMed]
10. Krul, E.S.; Lemke, S.L.; Mukherjea, R.; Taylor, M.L.; Goldstein, D.A.; Su, H.; Liu, P.; Lawless, A.; Harris, W.S.; Maki, K.C. Effects of duration of treatment and dosage of eicosapentaenoic acid and stearidonic acid on red blood cell eicosapentaenoic acid content. *Prostaglandins Leukot. Essent. Fatty Acids* **2012**, *86*, 51–59. [CrossRef] [PubMed]
11. Harris, W.S.; Sands, S.A.; Windsor, S.L.; Ali, H.A.; Stevens, T.L.; Magalski, A.; Porter, C.B.; Borkon, A.M. Omega-3 fatty acids in cardiac biopsies from heart transplantation patients. *Circulation* **2004**, *110*, 1645–1649. [CrossRef] [PubMed]
12. Calder, P.C. Mechanisms of action of (n-3) fatty acids. *J. Nutr.* **2012**, *142*, 592S–599S. [CrossRef] [PubMed]
13. Browning, L.M.; Walker, C.G.; Mander, A.P.; West, A.L.; Madden, J.; Gambell, J.M.; Young, S.; Wang, L.; Jebb, S.A.; Calder, P.C. Incorporation of eicosapentaenoic and docosahexaenoic acids into lipid pools when given as supplements providing doses equivalent to typical intakes of oily fish. *Am. J. Clin. Nutr.* **2012**, *96*, 748–758. [CrossRef] [PubMed]
14. Walker, C.G.; Browning, L.M.; Mander, A.P.; Madden, J.; West, A.L.; Calder, P.C.; Jebb, S.A. Age and sex differences in the incorporation of EPA and DHA into plasma fractions, cells and adipose tissue in humans. *Br. J. Nutr.* **2014**, *111*, 679–689. [CrossRef] [PubMed]
15. Fitt, E.; Cole, D.; Ziauddeen, N.; Pell, D.; Stickley, E.; Harvey, A.; Stephen, A.M. DINO (Diet In Nutrients Out) – an integrated dietary assessment system. *Public Health Nutr.* **2014**, *18*, 234–241. [CrossRef] [PubMed]
16. Leaf, D.A.; Connor, W.E.; Barstad, L.; Sexton, G. Incorporation of dietary n-3 fatty acids into the fatty acids of human adipose tissue and plasma lipid classes. *Am. J. Clin. Nutr.* **1995**, *62*, 68–73. [PubMed]
17. Dawczynski, C.; Massey, K.A.; Ness, C.; Kiehntopf, M.; Stepanow, S.; Platzer, M.; Grün, M.; Nicolaou, A.; Jahreis, G. Randomized placebo-controlled intervention with n-3 LC-PUFA-supplemented yoghurt: Effects on circulating eicosanoids and cardiovascular risk factors. *Clin. Nutr.* **2013**, *32*, 686–696. [CrossRef] [PubMed]
18. Fan, Y.-Y.; Chapkin, R.S. Importance of dietary γ-linolenic acid in human health and nutrition. *J. Nutr.* **1998**, *128*, 1411–1414. [PubMed]
19. Lund, E.; Harvey, L.; Ladha, S.; Clark, D.; Johnson, I. Effects of dietary fish oil supplementation on the phospholipid composition and fluidity of cell membranes from human volunteers. *Ann. Nutr. Metab.* **1999**, *43*, 290–300. [CrossRef] [PubMed]
20. Hodson, L.; Skeaff, C.; Fielding, B. Fatty acid composition of adipose tissue and blood in humans and its use as a biomarker of dietary intake. *Prog. Lipid Res.* **2008**, *47*, 348–380. [CrossRef] [PubMed]
21. Popp-Snijders, C.; Schouten, J.A.; van Blitterswijk, W.J.; van der Veen, E.A. Changes in membrane lipid composition of human erythrocytes after dietary supplementation of (n-3) polyunsaturated fatty acids. Maintenance of membrane fluidity. *Biochim. Biophys. Acta* **1986**, *854*, 31–37. [CrossRef]

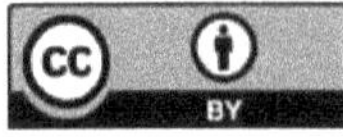

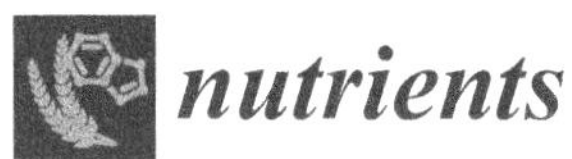

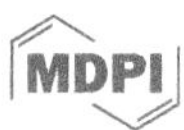

Article

Modification of Docosahexaenoic Acid Composition of Milk from Nursing Women Who Received Alpha Linolenic Acid from Chia Oil during Gestation and Nursing

Rodrigo Valenzuela [1,2,*], Karla A. Bascuñán [1], Rodrigo Chamorro [1], Cynthia Barrera [1], Jorge Sandoval [3], Claudia Puigrredon [3], Gloria Parraguez [1], Paula Orellana [1], Valeria Gonzalez [1] and Alfonso Valenzuela [2]

[1] Department of Nutrition, Faculty of Medicine, University of Chile, Av. Independencia 1027, Independencia, Santiago 8380453, Chile; E-Mails: kbascunan@med.uchile.cl (K.B.); rodrigochamorro@med.uchile.cl (R.C.); cynthia.barrera@gmail.com (C.B.); gparraguez@ug.uchile.cl (G.P.); p_orellana@ug.uchile.cl (P.O.); vale_elba@hotmail.com (V.G.)

[2] Lipid Center, Institute of Nutrition and Food Technology (INTA), University of Chile, Av. El Líbano 5524, Macul, Santiago 8380453, Chile; E-Mail: avalenzu@inta.uchile.cl

[3] Obstetrics and Gynecology Department, Clinical Hospital of the University of Chile, Av. Santos Dumont 999, Independencia, Santiago 8380453, Chile; E-Mails: jsandoval@hcuch.cl (J.S.); cpuigrredon@hcuch.cl (C.P.)

* Author to whom correspondence should be addressed; E-Mail: rvalenzuelab@med.uchile.cl; Tel.: +56-02-29786014; Fax: +56-02-29786182.

Received: 12 May 2015 / Accepted: 24 July 2015 / Published: 4 August 2015

Abstract: α-Linolenic acid (ALA) is the precursor of docosahexaenoic acid (DHA) in humans, which is fundamental for brain and visual function. Western diet provides low ALA and DHA, which is reflected in low DHA in maternal milk. Chia oil extracted from chia (*Salvia hispanica* L.), a plant native to some Latin American countries, is high in ALA (up to 60%) and thereby is an alternative to provide ALA with the aim to reduce DHA deficits. We evaluated the modification of the fatty acid profile of milk obtained from Chilean mothers who received chia oil during gestation and nursing. Forty healthy pregnant women (22–35 years old) tabulated for food consumption, were randomly separated into two groups: a control group with normal feeding (n = 21) and a chia group (n = 19), which received 16 mL chia oil daily from the third trimester of pregnancy until the first six months of nursing. The fatty acid profile of erythrocyte phospholipids, measured at six months of pregnancy, at time of delivery and at six months of nursing, and the fatty acid profile of the milk collected during the first six months of nursing were assessed by gas-chromatography. The chia group, compared to the control group, showed (*i*) a significant increase in ALA ingestion and a significant reduction of linoleic acid (LA) ingestion, no showing modification of arachidonic acid (AA), eicosapentaenoic acid (EPA) and DHA; (*ii*) a significant increase of erythrocyte ALA and EPA and a reduction of LA. AA and DHA were not modified; (*iii*) a increased milk content of ALA during the six months of nursing, whereas LA showed a decrease. AA and EPA were not modified, however DHA increased only during the first three months of nursing. Consumption of chia oil during the last trimester of pregnancy and the first three months of nursing transiently increases the milk content of DHA.

Keywords: pregnancy and nursing; chia oil; erythrocyte phospholipids; ALA and DHA in milk

---

1. Introduction

Several studies have established the important physiological role of n-3 fatty acids in infant growth and development, especially their importance for neuronal and visual development [1,2]. n-3 Fatty acids are a family of essential nutrients derived from alpha linolenic acid (C18:3 n-3, ALA), the precursor of the physiologically active n-3 long-chain polyunsaturated fatty acids (n-3 LCPUFA), eicosapentaenoic acid (C20:5, EPA) and docosahexaenoic acid (C22:6, DHA) [3]. ALA is an essential nutrient for humans, and its deficiency produces neurological alterations in infants [4] and dermatological disorders in adults [5]. Through a series of enzymatic reactions of elongation and desaturation, which occurs mainly in the liver, ALA is first transformed into EPA and then to DHA, which is the main metabolic end product. DHA is involved in multiple functions in the human body where it exerts a central role in the physiological and normal development of the individual from the embryonic stage on [6]. Accretion of DHA is critical during pregnancy and during the first year of life in humans, because the fatty acid is essential for the formation and function of the nervous and visual systems [7]. DHA comprises 10% of the dry weight of the human brain, the fatty acid making up 35%–40% of the total brain LCPUFA [8]. In the nervous tissue, and particularly in the brain, DHA is critical to all aspects of neurodevelopment and brain function, including neurogenesis, neurite proliferation and growth, nerve impulse transmission via the sodium-potassium pump, neuronal integrity and vitality, blood glucose transport and gene expression in the brain [9–11]. The pregnant and nursing woman has a physiological requirement of n-3 LCPUFA, and specifically of DHA, to assure the adequate and normal growth and development of the child [12]. Transformation of ALA into its metabolic products (EPA and DHA) mainly occurs in the hepatic tissue through enzymatic processes of elongation and desaturation [13]. EPA is primarily directed to the formation of eicosanoid derivatives, which have anti-inflammatory actions and regulatory effects on endothelial vascular activity [14]. Almost all the DHA is transported to the placenta during pregnancy and actively accreted at the fetal brain and visual tissues [15]. After birth, DHA is provided to the newborn through the maternal milk, which contains a small but significant amount of DHA (0.30%–0.32%) [16]. The Western diet provides very low amounts of DHA, because it only comprises small amounts of the main suppliers of this fatty acid (marine foods) [17]. Therefore DHA supplementation for women during pregnancy and nursing has been suggested [18]. However, this supplementation is not easily accepted during the perinatal period because some nutritional supplements of DHA are derived from fish oil of which mothers may show low tolerance [19]. Because ALA is the nutritional precursor of DHA, it has been proposed that the ingestion of foods containing ALA may compensate the chronically low ingestion of DHA by woman during the perinatal period, providing that ALA be ingested in high enough amounts because of its low metabolic transformation to DHA (less than 1%) [20]. A wide variety of vegetable oils having a high content of ALA (30%–65%) are available at present, such as camelina oil (*Camelina sativa* L., 36%), perilla oil (*Perilla frutescens* L., 53%), chia oil (*Salvia hispanica* L., 60%–65%), flaxseed oil (*Linum usitatissimun* L., 57%), sacha inchi oil (*Plukenetia volubilis* L., 49%) [3]. These oils, which are produced and commercially available in many countries, particularly in South America, are possibilities for dietary supplementation of ALA with the aim of increasing the DHA levels in breast milk. Previous research of our group has demonstrated that supplying ALA from chia oil to adult rats results in increased accretion of DHA in several tissues, particularly in the liver and brain [21], suggesting an efficient transformation of ALA into DHA. Chia seed and its oil have been very well characterized in their chemical composition and antioxidant value [22]. In the present report we evaluated the effect of chia oil as the main daily source of ALA by measuring the DHA content of erythrocyte phospholipids and breast milk obtained from women who received the oil during a period of gestation and nursing.

2. Subjects and Methods

2.1. Study Design and Subjects

The study was a randomized clinical trial that included 40 pregnant women currently attended at the Obstetrical and Gynecology Health Service of the University of Chile Hospital. It was conducted during the period from January 2012 to December 2013. Inclusion criteria were: an age of 22–35 years, a gestational age of at least 22 to 25 weeks according to the date of the last menstrual period and confirmed by ultrasound, 1–4 children and a history of successful nursing. Recruited women mainly belonged to the low and middle socioeconomic status according to the European Society for Opinion and Marketing Research (ESOMAR) [23]. All were of Hispanic origin. Women with a history of drugs or alcohol consumption, a diet including polyunsaturated fatty acids (PUFA, ALA supplements) or LCPUFA (EPA and or DHA supplements), with underweight as defined by the Chilean chart for pregnant women [24], with a history of twins or of suffering from chronic diseases such as diabetes, arterial hypertension, obesity, or other illness that could affect fetal growth, were excluded from the study. At the time of recruitment, all women fulfilling the inclusion criteria were given general information about the study, and a dietitian explained the objectives and main characteristics of the study design. The study protocol was reviewed and approved by the Institutional Review Board of the Faculty of Medicine, University of Chile (Protocol #073-2011) and by the Ethics Committee of the Clinical Hospital, University of Chile (Protocol #507/11). All information regarding the study was given to each participant who voluntarily agreed to participate and signed the informed consent.

During the first appointment for nutritional evaluations, the pregnant women were randomly assigned to either the control group (n = 21) or to the experimental group that received the dietary supplementation with chia oil (chia group, n = 19). The fatty acid profile and ALA content (65%–68%) of the oil has previously been assayed by our group [21]. All the pregnant women received a complete nutritional interview including nutritional diagnosis and counseling according to the dietary guidelines for pregnant women. Both groups were counseled to have a controlled intake of vegetable oil (sunflower/soybean oil, 80:20 v/v) at home. Each woman was given plastic teaspoons (4 mL) that allowed measuring her consumption of vegetable oil. A previous study had demonstrated a good tolerance of pregnant women of chia oil [25]. The specific indication for the control group was to consume four teaspoons of uncooked vegetable oil per day (16 mL/day) mainly in salads at lunch and dinner. The Chia group was instructed to replace their intake of usual oil with chia oil (16 mL/day; 10.1 g ALA/day). Women belonging to each group were given 4500 mL of each oil in 250 mL bottles. The control and chia groups consumed the respective oils from the 6th month of pregnancy until the 6th month of nursing (total intervention: 9 months). All women received a dietary record to register the daily consumption of vegetable oil and were visited weekly to assess oil consumption. Chia oil obtained by cold pressing of chia seeds was a gift of Benexia Co. (Santiago, Chile).

2.2. Assessment of Nutritional Status

Participants were subject to a clinical evaluation when incorporated into the study. A physician and a nurse assessed each participant regarding health following the standard clinical approach for pregnant women. Anthropometric data of weight (kg) and height (m) were assessed to determine body-mass index (BMI, kg/m^2). BMI was then used to establish maternal nutritional status according to gestational week following the Chilean reference [24]. Energy and nutrient requirements were established according to WHO criteria [26] and recommended dietary intakes according to the American Institute of Medicine, 2001 [27].

2.3. Dietary Intake of Mothers

All mothers were interviewed by a dietitian and asked to include all groups of consumed foods at the entry of the study, during the first week after delivery and six-months after delivery using a food frequency questionnaire. In addition to the food frequency questionnaire, dietitians used a photographic "Atlas of Commonly Consumed Foods in Chile" [28], a validated graphic instrument that helps to estimate the amount of each food consumed. Dietary data from the food-frequency questionnaire was grouped into nine food groups (cereals, fruits and vegetables, dairy, meats and eggs, legumes, fish and shellfish, high-lipid foods, oils and fats, sugars and processed foods). Cereals included all cereals and potatoes; fruits and vegetables included all kind of fruits, natural fruit juices and vegetables; dairy products included milk, cheese, fresh cheese and yogurts; meats and eggs included beef, chicken, pork and turkey meat, and all their derived products, and eggs; fish and shellfish included mackerel, tuna, salmon and shellfish (fresh and freeze); legumes included beans, chickpeas and lentils; high-lipid foods included olives, almonds, peanuts, walnuts, avocados, pistachios and hazelnuts; oils and fats included vegetable oils (mainly sunflower/soybean, canola, grape seed and olive oil) and fats (lard, butter, margarine, mayonnaise and cream); sugars and processes foods included sugar, honey, jam, delicacy, soft drinks, artificial juices, chocolates, cookies and sweet and savory snacks. Dietary data was analyzed using the software Food Processor SQL® (ESHA Research, Salem, OR, USA), to calculate energy and nutrient intake. Diet composition was obtained using a database from the USDA National Nutrient Database for Standard Reference, which also contained information from locally generated nutrient composition data.

2.4. Collection of Blood and Breast Milk Samples

Blood samples were obtained at the entry of the trial, immediately after delivery and six months after delivery. Butylated hydroxytoluene (BHT) was added to the blood samples as antioxidant and the samples were immediately centrifuged to obtain the erythrocyte fraction (3000$\times$ g for 10 min at 20 °C) and then frozen at −80 °C until further analysis. Breast milk (5 mL) was extracted by the mothers themselves after the infant had been fed for at least 2 minutes and was collected in plastic vials. Milk samples were immediately frozen at −80 °C until further analysis. Frozen erythrocytes and milk samples were transported to the Biochemical Nutritional Laboratory—Lipid Research Area at the Department of Nutrition, Faculty of Medicine, University of Chile, for analytical procedures.

2.5. Fatty Acid Analysis

2.5.1. Lipids Extraction from Erythrocytes and Breast Milk

Quantitative extraction of total lipids from erythrocytes and breast milk was carried out according to Bligh and Dyer [29] with the addition of BHT. Erythrocytes and breast milk samples were separately mixed with ice-cold chloroform/methanol (2:1 v/v, containing 0.01% BHT), magnesium chloride was added (0.5 N), and the mixture was homogenized in an Ultraturrax homogenizer (Janke & Kunkel, Stufen, Germany). The total lipids extracted from erythrocytes and milk were separated by think layer chromatography (TLC) (aluminum sheets 20 $\times$ 20 cm, silica gel 60 F-254; Merck), using the solvent system hexane/diethylether/acetic acid (80:20:1 v/v). After the development of the plates and solvent evaporation, lipid spots were visualized by exposing the plates to a Camag UV (250 nm) lamp designed for TLC. The solvent system allows the separation of phospholipids, triacylglycerols, cholesterol and cholesterol esters according to their relative mobility. Spots corresponding to phospholipids were scraped from TLC plates and extracted by elution with either diethylether or chloroform/methanol (2:1 v/v), according to Ruiz-Gutierrez *et al.* [30].

2.5.2. Preparation of Fatty Acid Methyl Esters (FAMEs)

Fatty acid methyl esters (FAMEs) from erythrocyte phospholipids and milk fatty acids were prepared according to Morrison and Smith [31]. Samples had previously been dissolved in chloroform/methanol (2:1 v/v) and were then evaporated under nitrogen stream until the volume was halved, then boron trifluoride (12% methanolic solution) and sodium hydroxide (0.5 N methanolic solution) were added and the mixture was cooled. FAMEs were extracted with 0.5 mL of hexane.

2.5.3. Gas Chromatographic Analysis of FAMEs

FAMEs were identified and quantified by gas-liquid chromatography in an Agilent equipment (model 7890B, Santa Clara, CA, USA) equipped with a capillary column (Agilent HP-88, 100 m × 0.250 mm; I.D. 0.25 μm) and flame ionization detector (FID). The injector temperature was set at 250 °C and the FID temperature at 300 °C. The oven temperature at sample injection was initially set at 120 °C and was programmed to increase to 220 °C at a rate of 5 °C per min. Hydrogen was utilized as the carrier gas at a flow rate of 35 cm per second in the column, and the inlet split ratio was set at 20:1. Identification and quantification of FAMEs were achieved by comparing the retention times and the peak area% values of unknown samples to those of commercial lipid standard (Nu-Chek Prep Inc., Elysian, MN, USA). C23:0 was used as internal standard (Nu-Chek Prep Inc., Elysian, MN, USA) and data was processed using the Hewlett-Packard Chemstation software system.

2.6. Statistical Analysis

Dietary data were checked by contrasting the energy/nutrient intake data composition with dietary questionnaires, identifying potential outliers. In the case if outliers, a careful review of each food frequency questionnaire was done. A descriptive analysis was conducted, and the analysis of the variable's distribution was done using a Shapiro–Wilk test. Results are expressed as the mean ± SD. Dietary nutrient intake and erythrocyte phospholipids and breast milk fatty acid composition at the three sampling points of the intervention were compared through one-way ANOVA and Newman-Keuls test. For all comparisons, statistical significance was set at α level $\leqslant 0.05$. The statistical software used was SPSS v.15.0 (Chicago, IL, USA) and GraphPad Prism v. 6.0 (GraphPad Software, San Diego, CA, USA) for figure processing.

3. Results

3.1. Background and Anthropometric Data of Groups

Table 1 shows the background and anthropometric data of the total sample and of each group. The total sample was composed of young women (28.6 ± 5.8 years), mainly of middle socioeconomic status (70.9%), and having very similar gestational periods, gender birth weight and height of their children. No significant differences were observed for the chia group when compared the control group for all background and anthropometric data.

Table 1. Background characteristics of both experimental groups.

Background characteristic	Group		
	Whole sample (n = 40)	Control (n = 21)	Chia (n = 19)
Age (mother), years [a]	28.6 ± 5.8	28.3 ± 6.7	29 ± 4.7
Pre-pregnancy weight, kg [a]	65.2 ± 11	65.9 ± 9.9	64.4 ± 12.4
Pre-pregnancy BMI, kg/m^2 [a]	24.9 ± 4.2	24.8 ± 3.7	24.9 ± 4.8
SES *			
High, %	13.9	19.0	5.3
Medium, %	70.9	66.7	73.7

Table 1. *Cont.*

Background characteristic	Group		
	Whole sample (*n* = 40)	**Control (*n* = 21)**	**Chia (*n* = 19)**
Low, %	15.2	14.3	21.1
Gestational age at birth, weeks	38.6 ± 1.1	38.6 ± 1.1	38.7 ± 1.2
Gender, masc %	53.3	53.8	52.6
Birth weight, g	4065.2 ± 481.9	4013.2 ± 587.9	4136.5 ± 279.8
Birth height, cm	48.6 ± 3.5	49.1 ± 3.4	48.0 ± 3.6

Data are expressed as mean ± S.D., or percentage (%) when indicated. * SES: socioeconomic status assessed by using the ESOMAR criteria [22]; BMI: body mass index = kg/m^2. [a] Anthropometric measures taken at the study enrollment.

3.2. Dietary Intake

The dietary intake of both groups is shown in Table 2. The energy and the macronutrient intake (carbohydrate, protein and fat), including fiber, of both groups was similar, with no significant differences. The exceptions were energy and carbohydrate consumption for the control group at the start (6th month of pregnancy) and at the end of the study (6th month of nursing). Total saturated fatty acid (SFA), monounsaturated fatty acid (MUFA) and polyunsaturated fatty acid (PUFA) ingestion were also similar in both experimental groups. However, as a result of the intervention, significant differences were observed for n-6, n-3 PUFA and some individual fatty acids (LA and ALA). At the point of delivery and at 6th month of nursing, compared to 6th month of pregnancy (start of intervention) a significant increase of ALA and a significant reduction of LA in the chia group was observed as expected from the chia oil intake. n-6/n-3 ratios were also significantly modified by chia oil ingestion. n-6 LCPUFA (AA) and n-3 LCPUFA (EPA and DHA) ingestion was not modified during the intervention.

3.3. Fatty Acid Profile of Erythrocyte Phospholipids

Table 3 shows the fatty acid composition of erythrocyte phospholipids obtained from woman during pregnancy and the nursing period. The first sampling (6th month of pregnancy) showed no differences in the fatty acid profiles when control and chia groups were compared. However, at the second sampling (at delivery) some significant differences were observed. Although total SFA, total MUFA and total PUFA showed no modifications, differences were observed when total n-6 and total n-3 PUFA and some individual fatty acids were compared. The chia group, compared to the control group, showed a significant reduction in total n-6 PUFA, with LA and AA not being modified. Total n-3 PUFA, ALA and EPA were increased in the chia group, but DHA was not modified. The n-6/n-3 PUFA ratio was significantly reduced in the chia group. The third sampling (6 months of nursing) showed similar levels for total and individual fatty acids and for the n-6/n-3 ratio, as was observed for the second sampling (at delivery).

Table 2. Energy and composition of diet ingested by mothers during pregnancy and nursing.

Energy/Nutrients	6th Month of Pregnancy		Delivery		6th Month of Nursing	
	Control group (a)	Chia group (b)	Control group (c)	Chia group (d)	Control group (e)	Chia group (f)
Energy (kcal)	2909 ± 426 (e)	2057 ± 642.8	2477 ± 764.4	2119 ± 444.1	2287 ± 593 (a)	1832 ± 510
Protein (g)	110.2 ± 30.1	94.6 ± 73	103.4 ± 30.1	81.7 ± 22.9	88.5 ± 37	74.2 ± 22.2
Carbohydrate (g)	400.7 ± 83.7 (e)	275.7 ± 108.2	330.9 ± 154.9	276.1 ± 78.4	283.5 ± 72.9 (a)	207.8 ± 54.2
Fat (g)	102.8 ± 30.5	85.0 ± 40.7	87.3 ± 24.9	66.8 ± 24.1	93.9 ± 31.4	66.1 ± 26.2
Cholesterol (mg)	312.2 ± 78.8	281.2 ± 190.2	328.4 ± 129.8	226.4 ± 79.9	277.4 ± 135.7	227.0 ± 61.6
Trans fatty acid (g)	2.2 ± 3.0	1.0 ± 0.7	1.3 ± 0.7	1.6 ± 1.1	1.5 ± 1.1	1.6 ± 0.9
Fiber (g)	35.4 ± 8.5	24.3 ± 10.4	25.9 ± 10.6	22.3 ± 7.6	24.8 ± 9.9	18.6 ± 8.2
SFA (g)	31.4 ± 11.0	24.7 ± 12.6	28.2 ± 11.2	24.9 ± 6.6	27.4 ± 11.5	20.6 ± 6.6
MUFA (g)	26.8 ± 11.0	22.9 ± 12.7	22.9 ± 8.2	24.6 ± 5.8	27.3 ± 14.5	23.8 ± 4.6
PUFA (g)	17.2 ± 5.2	19.3 ± 3.3	17.6 ± 3.9	21.5 ± 2.5	18.5 ± 2.7	17.9 ± 3.8
n-6 PUFA	15.4 ± 1.2 (d,f)	17.5 ± 2.3 (d,f)	16.3 ± 2.7 (d,f)	11.5 ± 2.1 (a,b,c,e)	16.9 ± 1.7 (d,f)	10.1 ± 1.3 (a,b,c,e)
n-3 PUFA	1.7 ± 0.05 (d,f)	1.6 ± 0.04 (d,f)	1.3 ± 0.2 (d,f)	10.0 ± 1.4 (a,b,c,f)	1.5 ± 0.04 (d,f)	7.8 ± 0.9 (a,b,c,e)
18:2, n-6 (LA) (g)	15.2 ± 3.0 (d,f)	17.3 ± 3.3 (d,f)	16.1 ± 2.6 (d,f)	10.9 ± 2.3 (a,b,c,e)	16.7 ± 3.3 (d,f)	9.8 ± 1.8 (a,b,c,e)
18:3, n-3 (ALA) (g)	1.1 ± 0.5 (d,f)	1.2 ± 0.6 (d,f)	1.1 ± 1.0 (d,f)	9.5 ± 4.9 (a,b,c,e)	0.9 ± 0.7 (d,e)	7.7 ± 4.3 (a,b,c,e)
20:4, n-6 (AA) (g)	0.08 ± 0.06	0.06 ± 0.06	0.09 ± 0.06	0.05 ± 0.02	0.08 ± 0.06	0.05 ± 0.02
20:5, n-3 (EPA) (g)	0.05 ± 0.07	0.03 ± 0.02	0.04 ± 0.05	0.03 ± 0.01	0.04 ± 0.02	0.005 ± 0.01
22:6, n-3 (DHA) (g)	0.1 ± 0.1	0.04 ± 0.05	0.07 ± 0.07	0.03 ± 0.03	0.04 ± 0.04	0.02 ± 0.03
n-6/n-3 PUFA ratio	9.1 ± 2.5 (d,f)	10.9 ± 2.3 (d,f)	12.5 ± 2.4 (d,f)	1.15 ± 4.0 (a,b,c,e)	11.3 ± 2.4 (d,f)	1.30 ± 0.3 (a,b,c,e)

Data are expressed as the mean ± SD for $n = 21$ women (Control group) and $n = 19$ (Chia group). Statistical significance ($p < 0.05$), [a]: significantly different from Control group at 6th month of pregnancy; [b]: significantly different from Chia group at 6th month of pregnancy; [c]: significantly different from Control group at delivery; [d]: significantly different from Chia group at delivery; [e]: significantly different from Control group at 6th month of nursing; [f]: significantly different from Chia group at 6th month. One-way ANOVA and Newman-Keuls test. Saturated fatty acids (SFA). Monounsaturated fatty acids (MUFA) Polyunsaturated fatty acids (PUFA).

Table 3. Fatty acid composition of erythrocyte phospholipids of mothers during pregnancy and nursing.

	6th Month Pregnancy		Delivery		6th Month Nursing	
Fatty acids (g/100 g of FAME)	**Control group (a)**	**Chia group (b)**	**Control group (c)**	**Chia group (d)**	**Control group (e)**	**Chia group (f)**
Total SFA	52.3 ± 4.5	53.6 ± 4.7	53.6 ± 3.3	50.2 ± 5.1	50.6 ± 4.1	49.7 ± 3.8
Total MUFA	12.3 ± 1.2	13.5 ± 0.9	11.7 ± 0.8	13.4 ± 1.1	15.9 ± 1.1	14.5 ± 0.9
Total PUFA	35.4 ± 3.0	32.9 ± 3.6	34.7 ± 2.9	36.4 ± 3.2	33.5 ± 3.3	35.8 ± 2.9
Total n-6 PUFA	28.7 ± 2.2	26.1 ± 3.3	27.1 ± 2.7	21.6 ± 1.8 (a,b,c,e)	27.2 ± 1.4	20.2 ± 1.4 (a,b,c,e)
Total n-3 PUFA	6.70 ± 0.8	6.80 ± 0.2	7.60 ± 0.9	14.8 ± 1.7 (a,b,c,e)	6.30 ± 1.1	15.6 ± 1.6 (a,b,c,e)
18:2, n-6 (LA)	13.4 ± 1.3	12.6 ± 1.5	12.1 ± 1.1	9.11 ± 1.4 (a,b,c,e)	12.8 ± 1.6	8.02 ± 1.3 (a,b,c,e)
18:3, n-3 (ALA)	1.03 ± 0.3	0.96 ± 0.2	1.02 ± 0.3	6.12 ± 2.3 (a,b,c,e)	0.94 ± 0.2	7.39 ± 1.3 (a,b,c,e)
20:4, n-6 (AA)	14.1 ± 1.6	13.2 ± 1.4	13.9 ± 1.2	12.2 ± 1.4	13.8 ± 1.4	11.9 ± 1.7
20:5, n-3 (EPA)	0.91 ± 0.1	0.89 ± 0.1	0.97 ± 0.3	2.58 ± 0.7 (a,b,c,e)	0.86 ± 0.2	2.13 ± 0.8 (a,b,c,e)
22:6, n-3 (DHA)	4.52 ± 0.8	4.68 ± 0.6	4.98 ± 1.0	5.33 ± 1.3	4.42 ± 1.1	5.10 ± 0.7
n-6/n-3 PUFA ratio	4.28 ± 0.9	3.83 ± 0.7	3.57 ± 0.7	1.46 ± 0.4 (a,b,c,e)	4.31 ± 1.0	1.30 ± 0.3 (a,b,c,e)

Data are expressed as g fatty acid per 100 g fatty acid methyl esters (FAME) and represent the mean ± SD for $n = 21$ women (Control group) and $n = 19$ (Chia group). Statistical significance ($p < 0.05$), [a]: significantly different from Control group at 6th month of pregnancy; [b]: significantly different from Chia group at 6th month of pregnancy; [c]: significantly different from Control group at delivery; [d]: significantly different from Chia group at delivery; [e]: significantly different from Control group at 6th month of nursing; [f]: significantly different from Chia group at 6th month. One-way ANOVA and Newman-Keuls test. Saturated fatty acids (SFA) correspond to 6:0, 8:0, 10:0, 12:0, 14:0, 16:0, 18:0, 20:0 and 22:0, 24:0. Monounsaturated fatty acids (MUFA) correspond to 14:1 n-5, 16:1 n-7 and 18:1, n-9. Polyunsaturated fatty acids (PUFA) correspond to 18:2 n-6, 18:3,n-3, 20:4 n-6, 20:5 n-3, 22:5 n-3 and 22:6 n-3; n-6/n-3 ratio is 20:4 n-6/ (20:5, n-3 + 22:5, n-3 + 22:6, n-3).

3.4. Fatty Acid Profile of Breast Milk

Total SFA, MUFA, PUFA, and total n-6 PUFA and n-3 PUFA of breast milk are shown in Figure 1A–E. Total SFA (Figure 1A), total MUFA (Figure 1B) and total PUFA (Figure 1C) were not modified during the dietary intervention with chia oil when compared to the control group. Total n-6 PUFA (Figure 1D) were significantly reduced and total n-3 PUFA (Figure 1E) were significantly increased after chia oil intake. Figure 2 shows the individual modification of the most relevant n-6 and n-3 fatty acids and the n-6/n-3 PUFA ratio after chia oil intake. LA was significantly reduced in the chia group (Figure 2A) whereas ALA was significantly increased (Figure 2B) during all the periods of chia oil intake. AA (Figure 2C) and EPA (Figure 2D) were not modified in these groups. However, DHA (Figure 2E) was significantly increased in the chia group only during the first, second and third month of nursing, returning to values similar to the control group after the initial three-month period. The n-6/n-3 PUFA ratio (Figure 2F) was significantly reduced in the chia group during the six months of nursing.

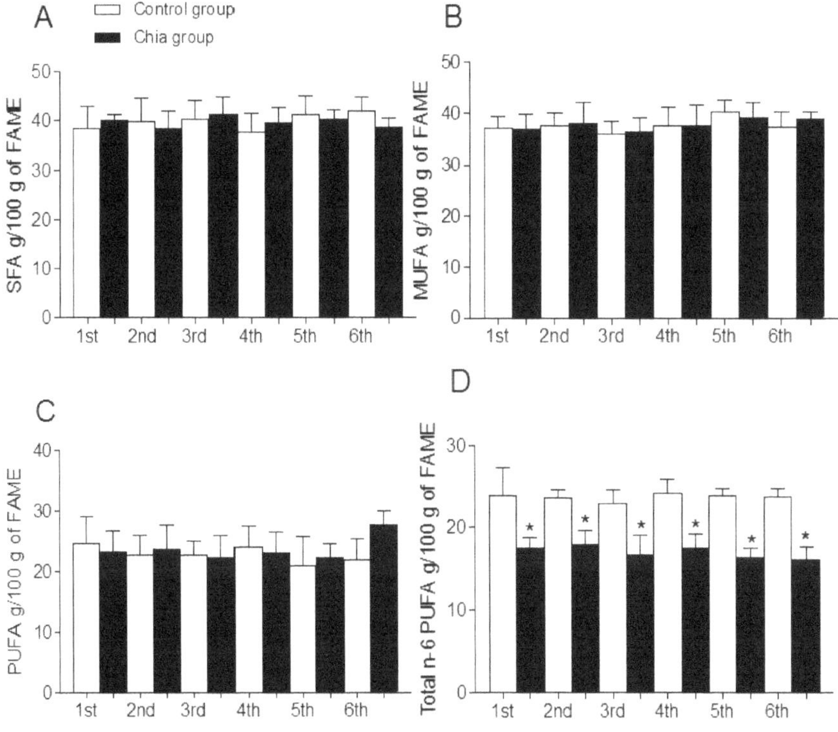

Figure 1. *Cont.*

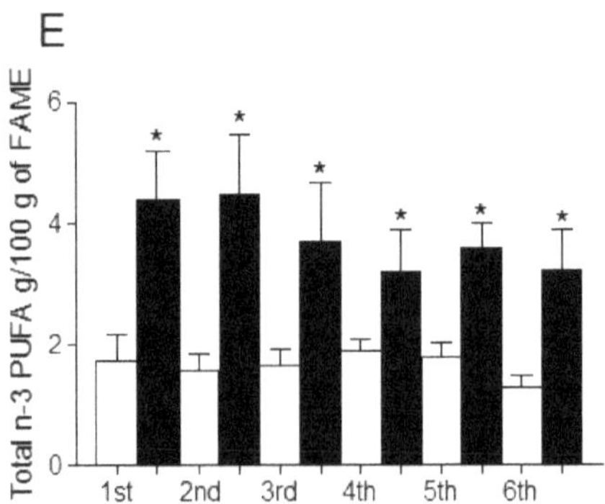

Figure 1. Total fatty acid composition of breast milk from mothers during nursing. Saturated fatty acids (SFA) (**A**); Monounsaturated fatty acids (MUFA) (**B**); Polyunsaturated fatty acids (PUFA) (**C**); Total n-6 PUFA (**D**); Total n-3 PUFA (E). Data are expressed as g fatty acid per 100 g FAME and represent the mean ± SD for $n = 21$ women (control group) and $n = 19$ (chia group). Statistical significance ($p < 0.05$); *: indicates significantly different when comparing the chia group with the control group for each month of nursing (*t*-test) and for all months of nursing (One-way ANOVA and Newman-Keuls test). SFA correspond to 6:0, 8:0, 10:0, 12:0, 14:0, 16:0, 18:0, 20:0 and 22:0, 24:0. MUFA correspond to 14:1 n-5, 16:1 n-7 and 18:1, n-9. PUFA correspond to 18:2 n-6, 18:3 n-3, 20:4 n-6, 20:5 n-3, 22:5 n-3 and 22:6 n-3.

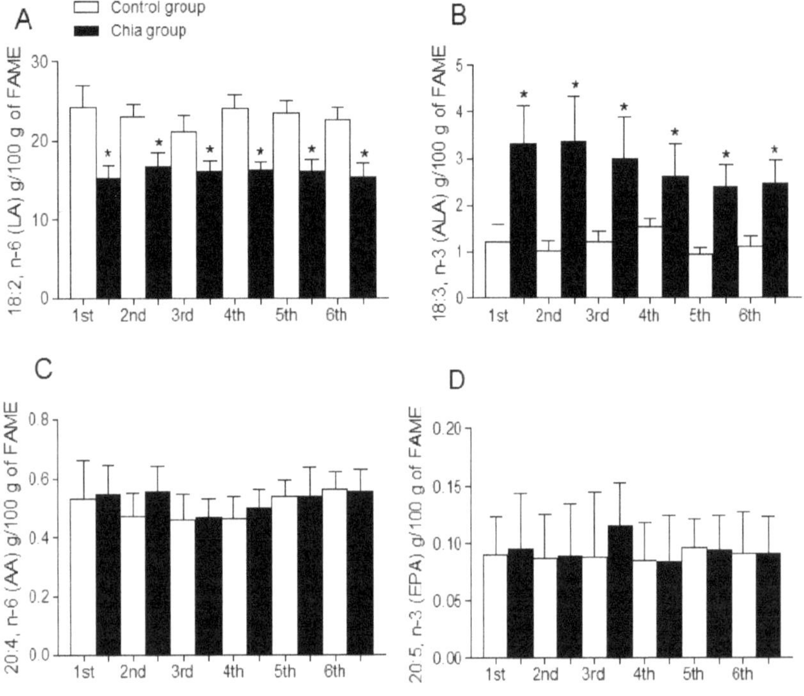

Figure 2. *Cont.*

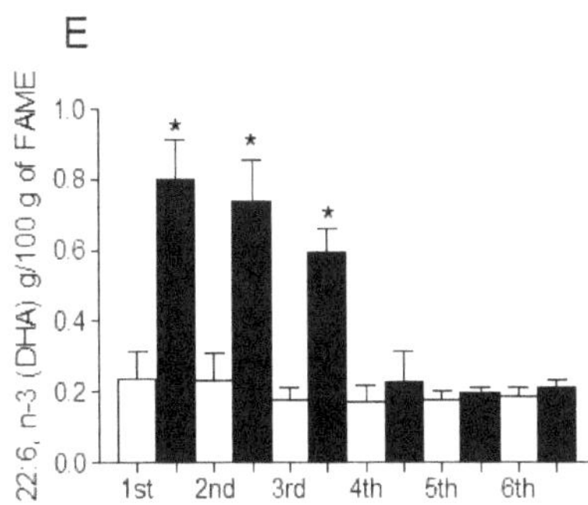

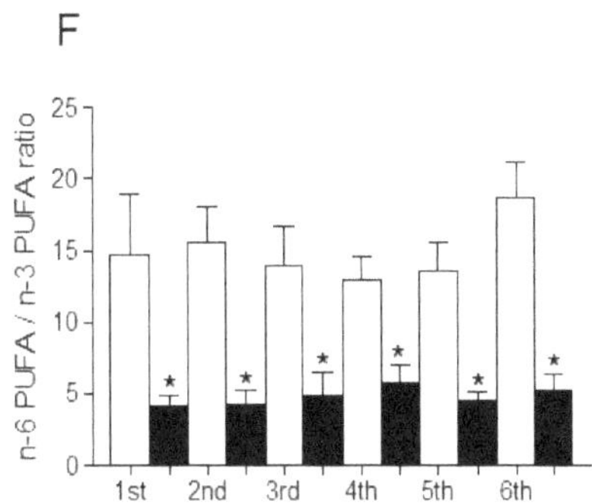

Figure 2. Individual fatty acid composition of breast milk from mothers during nursing. 18:2, n-6 (LA) (**A**); 18:3, n-3 (ALA) (**B**); 20:4, n-6 (AA) (**C**); 20:5, n-3 (EPA) (**D**); 22:6, n-3 (DHA) (E); (F). Data are expressed as g fatty acid per 100 g FAME and represent the mean ± SD for n = 21 women (control group) and n = 19 (chia group). Statistical significance ($p < 0.05$); *: indicates significant difference when comparing the chia group with the control group for each month of nursing (t-test) and for all months of nursing (One-way ANOVA and Newman-Keuls test). n-6 PUFA/n-3 PUFA ratio is (18:2, n-6 + 20:4, n-6)/(18:3, n-3 + 20:5, n-3 + 22:5, n-3 + 22:6, n-3).

4. Discussion

Dietary fatty acid intake by pregnant and nursing women in the supplementation periods studied is reflected in the fatty acid composition of erythrocyte phospholipids and also in the fatty acid composition of breast milk. Differences in the composition of fatty acids are particularly relevant for ALA, the precursor of n-3 LCPUFA, which in turn reflects the complex metabolism of polyunsaturated fatty acids and their conversion (through elongation and desaturation) to fatty acids of 20 and more carbon atoms [3,32]. In the same direction, our results demonstrate that ALA provided to pregnant and nursing women through chia oil increases (i) ALA and EPA content of erythrocyte phospholipids and (ii) ALA and DHA content of breast milk, but iii) does not modify DHA in erythrocyte phospholipids, which reflects that ALA conversion to n-3 LCPUFA and posterior accretion to cells or biological fluids, such as milk, is a highly regulated process [33]. Results for erythrocytes obtained from the chia group are in line with earlier observations by Arterburn *et al.*, (2006), who suggest that these cells are not metabolic reservoirs for DHA, as opposed to other tissues, such as brain cortex, sperm and retina [34]. However, erythrocytes are considered a good blood marker of the nutritional status of fatty acids [35]. Lauritzen and Carlson [36] have proposed that the maternal erythrocyte fatty acid profile during pregnancy and nursing is related to the fatty acid profile of the newborn's erythrocytes, which indicates an active role of the placenta during pregnancy and of breast milk during nursing [37]. It has been previously demonstrated that dietary ALA intake increases EPA accretion in erythrocytes [38]. However, it has been also demonstrated that ALA intake, supplied as sacha inchi oil (49% ALA), increases both fatty acids, EPA and DHA, in erythrocytes [39,40], thus introducing controversy regarding the metabolism of n-3 PUFA in humans.

During the six months of maternal milk analysis it was observed that daily intake of chia oil allowed a higher and more constant content of ALA. Similarly, an equal behavior for DHA was expected, as it is the product of the supposed continued transformation of ALA in the liver [41,42]. Both fatty acids are transported to the breast to be secreted in the milk [43]. Surprisingly, the increase of DHA in milk was only observed during the first, second and third months of nursing, reaching values similar to those of the control group after the third month of nursing in spite of the high and continuous ingestion of ALA. EPA did not increase either, as it has been shown to occur in populations were EPA ingestion via marine foods is high [34,44]. These observations lead to the hypothesis of a high control of the conversion of ALA to EPA and DHA, and of the presence of these fatty acids in breast milk. Breast milk does not contain EPA because this fatty acid competes with AA [45]. This is the reason why early formulas were enriched with DHA and AA from egg phospholipids excluding EPA [46]. We hypothesize that the physiological control of the conversion of ALA to DHA is produced: (i) through a high regulation in the activity of the enzymes involved in elongation and desaturation, which set DHA at physiological concentrations [47]; (ii) through the beta oxidation of exceeding ALA for energy production or carbon recycling [48]; (iii) due to the fact that excess of PUFA and LCPUFA may increase milk susceptibility to oxidative rancidity with the risk of tissue oxidative stress in the child, however this last proposal requires further demonstration.

Literature indicates that women's breast milk DHA values may vary from 0.2% to 1% of total fatty acids [34,49]. These values are highly dependent on the direct ingestion of DHA (*i.e.*, eating fish and/or taking n-3 LCPUFA supplements) as has been previously demonstrated [50]. In a recent study it was established that Chilean pregnant women who consistently show very low consumption of fish and other marine foods [51], as a result show a very low level of DHA in their breast milk as well as a low content of DHA in erythrocyte phospholipid fatty acids [51]. Populations that consume high amounts of fish, such as Philippine and Japanese women [52,53], show higher levels of DHA in milk compared to populations that consume less fish (e.g., Israel, Columbus, Ohio, USA) [54,55]. However the EPA content of the milk of women from these countries is very low and is not modified by fish consumption despite the presence of this fatty acid in marine food [34], indicating a physiological control in the transport and accretion of this fatty acid in the fat content of breast milk.

According to our results, ALA ingestion during the perinatal period only allows an increase of milk DHA during the first three months of nursing, suggesting either a limited further conversion and accretion of DHA in the liver and/or a regulated transport to the breast, as was postulated above. After the first three-month period of nursing, milk DHA reaches the estimated physiological levels for DHA (on average 0.3% to 0.32% of total fat) [56,57] despite the high nutritional availability of ALA. It is interesting that the content of AA and EPA of breast milk was not modified by ALA supplementation in our experimental model. This is highly relevant because of the close relationship of these two fatty acids with the control of vascular homeostasis and inflammatory responses in the infants [58]. In our study, AA was always present in erythrocytes of both experimental groups in the estimated physiological concentrations corroborating the important role of this fatty acid, such as for the brain development at early stages of life, as has been previously demonstrated [59].

Mothers that consumed chia oil were indicated to replace the habitual dietary vegetable oils (most commonly sunflower/soybean oil). This substitution which increases ALA consumption, allowed the replacement of a high proportion of LA for ALA, both in erythrocytes and in milk. It has been demonstrated that mothers that had a high dietary intake of LA and a low intake of ALA delivered children with subnormal scores of learning, where the high intake of LA was correlated with lower levels of DHA in breast milk [60]. A relevant result of the present study was the change in the total ratio of n-6/n-3 fatty acids in erythrocyte phospholipids and maternal milk. Ancestral modifications of this ratio in favor of n-3 fatty acids may have established a generic—evolutionary pattern, which at present characterizes the brain of humans [61].

Our results were obtained from non-obese mothers free of any chronic diseases, both aspects which are relevant because in obese women, mostly those suffering of nonalcoholic fatty liver disease, there is a reduction in the hepatic activity of desaturase enzymes (Δ-5 and Δ-6 desaturases) with a concomitant reduction in the formation of EPA and DHA from ALA [62]. Due the high prevalence of women obesity in western countries and comorbid nonalcoholic fatty liver disease [63], it is an interesting challenge for the future to evaluate the effect of ALA supplementation through chia oil and the presence of this fatty acid and of DHA in the milk secretion of these women. Our study did not evaluate the effect that the dietary intervention of pregnant and nursing women with chia oil had on their babies, such as length of gestational period, birth weight and cognitive and visual development. Other reports have studied the impact of DHA supplementation on these parameters [64,65], but not of ALA in concentrations as those used in our study. A previous study supplied canola oil (10% ALA) to pregnant women, showing an increase of the gestational period and birth weight [66].

5. Conclusions

Chia oil may constitute an available and inexpensive way to provide ALA in higher amounts to the population of many countries characterized by low fish consumption [51,67]. It is not of minor importance considering the actual low availability of fish and the increasing concerns about fish contamination with heavy metals and other toxic products that negatively influence fish consumption [68,69]. Our research has demonstrated that chia oil intake, a natural good source of ALA, allows an important modification in the EPA content of erythrocytes in pregnant mothers and an interesting increase of DHA in their milk. However, more research is necessary related to pre- and postnatal nutritional interventions with chia oil or other oils with a high content of ALA to scientifically support the recommendation of ALA consumption to increase the DHA content of breast milk. Chia oil supplementation may also contribute to improve the LA/ALA ratio in women during the perinatal period.

Acknowledgments: The authors are grateful to the Departments of Nutrition and of Obstetrics and Gynecology, Clinical Hospital, Faculty of Medicine, University of Chile, and to Benexia Company for the support of the research.

Author Contributions: Rodrigo Valenzuela, Karla A. Bascuñan, and Rodrigo Chamorro designed the study and analyzed and interpreted the data. Karla A. Bascuñan, Rodrigo Valenzuela, Cynthia Barrera, Gloria Parraguez, Paula Orellana, Valeria Gonzalez, Jorge Sandoval and Claudia Puigrredon performed clinical and nutritional evaluations. Karla A. Bascuñan and Rodrigo Chamorro conducted the dietary analysis. Rodrigo Valenzuela, Karla A. Bascuñan, Rodrigo Chamorro and Alfonso Valenzuela wrote the manuscript. All authors reviewed and approved the final version of the manuscript.

Conflicts of Interest: The authors declare no conflict of interest.

References

1. Innis, S.M. Dietary (n-3) fatty acids and brain development. *J. Nutr.* **2007**, *137*, 855–859. [PubMed]
2. Campoy, C.; Escolano-Margarit, M.V.; Anjos, T.; Szajewska, H.; Uauy, R. Omega 3 fatty acids on child growth, visual acuity and neurodevelopment. *Br. J. Nutr.* **2012**, *107*, S85–S106. [CrossRef] [PubMed]
3. Barceló-Coblijn, G.; Murphy, E.J. Alpha-linolenic acid and its conversion to longer chain n-3 fatty acids: Benefits for human health and a role in maintaining tissue n-3 fatty acid levels. *Prog. Lipid Res.* **2009**, *48*, 355–374. [CrossRef] [PubMed]
4. Holman, R.T.; Johnson, S.B.; Hatch, T.F. A case of human linolenic acid deficiency involving neurological abnormalities. *Am. J. Clin. Nutr.* **1982**, *35*, 617–623. [PubMed]
5. Bjerve, K.S.; Fischer, S.; Alme, K. Alpha-linolenic acid deficiency in man: Effect of ethyl linolenate on plasma and erythrocyte fatty acid composition and biosynthesis of prostanoids. *Am. J. Clin. Nutr.* **1987**, *46*, 570–576. [PubMed]
6. Janssen, C.I.; Kiliaan, A.J. Long-chain polyunsaturated fatty acids (LCPUFA) from genesis to senescence: The influence of LCPUFA on neural development, aging, and neurodegeneration. *Prog. Lipid Res.* **2013**, *53*, 1–17. [CrossRef] [PubMed]
7. Gustafson, K.M.; Colombo, J.; Carlson, S.E. Docosahexaenoic acid and cognitive function: Is the link mediated by the autonomic nervous system? *Prostaglandins Leukot. Essent. Fatty Acids* **2008**, *79*, 135–140. [CrossRef] [PubMed]
8. Makrides, M.; Neumann, M.A.; Byard, R.W.; Simmer, K.; Gibson, R.A. Fatty acid composition of brain, retina, and erythrocytes in breast- and formula-fed infants. *Am. J. Clin. Nutr.* **1994**, *60*, 189–194. [PubMed]
9. Harbeby, E.; Jouin, M.; Alessandri, J.M.; Lallemand, M.S.; Linard, A.; Lavialle, M.; Huertas, A.; Cunnane, S.C.; Guesnet, P. n-3 PUFA status affects expression of genes involved in neuroenergetics differently in the fronto-parietal cortex compared to the CA1 area of the hippocampus: Effect of rest and neuronal activation in the rat. *Prostaglandins Leukot. Essent. Fatty Acids* **2012**, *86*, 211–220. [CrossRef] [PubMed]

10. Ryan, A.S.; Astwood, J.D.; Gautier, S.; Kuratko, C.N.; Nelson, E.B.; Salem, N., Jr. Effects of long-chain polyunsaturated fatty acid supplementation on neurodevelopment in childhood: A review of human studies. *Prostaglandins Leukot. Essent. Fatty Acids* **2010**, *82*, 305–314. [CrossRef] [PubMed]
11. De Souza, A.S.; Fernandes, F.S.; do Carmo, M.D. Effects of maternal malnutrition and postnatal nutritional rehabilitation on brain fatty acids, learning, and memory. *Nutr. Rev.* **2011**, *69*, 132–144. [CrossRef] [PubMed]
12. Makrides, M.; Gould, J.F.; Gawlik, N.R.; Yelland, L.N.; Smithers, L.G.; Anderson, P.J.; Gibson, R.A. Four-year follow-up of children born to women in a randomized trial of prenatal DHA supplementation. *JAMA* **2014**, *311*, 1802–1804. [CrossRef] [PubMed]
13. Valenzuela, R.; Barrera, C.; Espinosa, A.; Llanos, P.; Orellana, P.; Videla, L.A. Reduction in the desaturation capacity of the liver in mice subjected to high fat diet: Relation to LCPUFA depletion in liver and extrahepatic tissues. *Prostaglandins Leukot. Essent. Fatty Acids* **2015**, *98*, 7–14. [CrossRef] [PubMed]
14. LeMieux, M.J.; Kalupahana, N.S.; Scoggin, S.; Moustaid-Moussa, N. Eicosapentaenoic acid reduces adipocyte hypertrophy and inflammation in diet-induced obese mice in an adiposity-independent manner. *J. Nutr.* **2015**, *145*, 411–417. [CrossRef] [PubMed]
15. Igarashi, M.; Santos, R.A.; Cohen-Cory, S. Impact of Maternal n-3 Polyunsaturated Fatty Acid Deficiency on Dendritic Arbor Morphology and Connectivity of Developing Xenopus laevis Central Neurons *in vivo*. *J. Neurosci.* **2015**, *15*, 6079–6092. [CrossRef] [PubMed]
16. Nishimura, R.Y.; Barbieiri, P.; Castro, G.S.; Jordão, A.A.; Perdoná, G.S.; Sartorelli, D.S. Dietary polyunsaturated fatty acid intake during late pregnancy affects fatty acid composition of mature breast milk. *Nutrition* **2014**, *30*, 685–689. [CrossRef] [PubMed]
17. Martin, M.A.; Lassek, W.D.; Gaulin, S.J.; Evans, R.W.; Woo, J.G.; Geraghty, S.R.; Davidson, B.S.; Morrow, A.L.; Kaplan, H.S.; Gurven, M.D. Fatty acid composition in the mature milk of Bolivian forager-horticulturalists: Controlled comparisons with a US sample. *Matern. Child. Nutr.* **2012**, *8*, 404–418. [CrossRef] [PubMed]
18. Sherry, C.L.; Oliver, J.S.; Marriage, B.J. Docosahexaenoic acid supplementation in lactating women increases breast milk and plasma docosahexaenoic acid concentrations and alters infant omega 6:3 fatty acid ratio. *Prostaglandins Leukot. Essent. Fatty Acids* **2015**, *95*, 63–69. [CrossRef] [PubMed]
19. Contreras, A.; Herrera, Y.; Rodriguez, L.; Pizarro, T.; Atalah, E. Acceptability and consumption of a dairy drink with omega-3 in pregnant and lactating women of the National Supplementary Food Program. *Rev. Chil. Nutr.* **2011**, *38*, 313–320.
20. Gillingham, L.G.; Harding, S.V.; Rideout, T.C.; Yurkova, N.; Cunnane, S.C.; Eck, P.K.; Jones, P.J. Dietary oils and FADS1-FADS2 genetic variants modulate [13C]α-linolenic acid metabolism and plasma fatty acid composition. *Am. J. Clin. Nutr.* **2013**, *97*, 195–207. [CrossRef] [PubMed]
21. Valenzuela, R.; Barrera, C.; González-Astorga, M.; Sanhueza, J.; Valenzuela, A. Alpha linolenic acid (ALA) from Rosa canina, sacha inchi and chia oils may increase ALA accretion and its conversion into n-3 LCPUFA in diverse tissues of the rat. *Food Funct.* **2014**, *5*, 1564–1572. [CrossRef] [PubMed]
22. Da Silva, R.; Aguiar, E.; Alves, S.; Teixeira, A.; Nogueira, M.; Maróstica, M. Chemical characterization and antioxidant potential of Chilean chia seeds and oil (Salvia hispanica L.). *LWT 416—Food Sci. Technol.* **2014**, *59*, 1304–1310.
23. European Society for Opinion and Marketing Research. *The ESOMAR Standard Demographic Classification*; ESOMAR: Amsterdam, The Netherlands, 1997.
24. Atalah, E.; Castillo, C.; Castro, R.; Aldea, A. Proposal of a new standard for the nutritional assessment of pregnant women. *Rev. Med. Chil.* **1997**, *125*, 1429–1436. [PubMed]
25. Valencia, A.; Valenzuela, R.; Bascuñán, K.; Chamorro, R.; Barrera, C.; Faune, M.; Jara, M.; Kuratomi, C.; Moraga, A.; Silva, D. Acceptability assessment of two vegetable oils with different level of alpha-linolenic acid in pregnant women from the Metropolitan Region of Chile. *Rev. Chil. Nutr.* **2014**, *41*, 85–89.
26. WHO/FAO/UNU. *Human Energy Requirements, Report of a Joint FAO/WHO/UNU Expert Consultation*; Food and Agriculture Organization: Rome, Italy, 2014.
27. Food and Nutrition Board, Institute of Medicine. *Dietary Reference Intakes: Guiding Principles for Nutrition Labeling and Fortification*; Institute of Medicine of the National Academies: Washington, DC, USA, 2001; pp. 1–224.
28. Cerda, R.; Barrera, C.; Arena, M.; Bascuñán, K.A.; Jimenez, G. *Atlas Fotográfico de Alimentos y Preparaciones Típicas Chilenas. Encuesta Nacional de Consumo Alimentario 2010*, 1st ed.; Gobierno de Chile, Ministerio de Salud: Santiago, Chile, 2010.

29. Bligh, E.G.; Dyer, W.J. A rapid method of total lipid extraction and purification. *Can. J. Biochem. Physiol.* **1959**, *37*, 911–917. [CrossRef] [PubMed]
30. Ruiz-Gutierrez, V.; Cert, A.; Rios, J.J. Determination of phospholipid fatty acid and triacylglycerol composition of rat caecal mucosa. *J. Chromatogr.* **1992**, *575*, 1–6. [CrossRef]
31. Morrison, W.R.; Smith, L.M. Preparation of fatty acid methyl esters and dimethylacetals from lipids with boron fluoride-Methanol. *J. Lipid Res.* **1964**, *5*, 600–608. [PubMed]
32. Domenichiello, A.F.; Chen, C.T.; Trepanier, M.O.; Stavro, P.M.; Bazinet, R.P. Whole body synthesis rates of DHA from α-linolenic acid are greater than brain DHA accretion and uptake rates in adult rats. *J. Lipid Res.* **2014**, *55*, 62–74. [CrossRef] [PubMed]
33. Das, U.N. Essential fatty acids: Biochemistry, physiology and pathology. *Biotechnol J.* **2006**, *1*, 420–439. [CrossRef] [PubMed]
34. Arterburn, L.M.; Hall, E.B.; Oken, H. Distribution, interconversion, and dose response of n-3 fatty acids in humans. *Am. J. Clin. Nutr.* **2006**, *83*, 1467S–1476S. [PubMed]
35. Gibson, R.A.; Muhlhausler, B.; Makrides, M. Conversion of linoleic acid and alpha-linolenic acid to long-chain polyunsaturated fatty acids (LCPUFAs), with a focus on pregnancy, lactation and the first 2 years of life. *Matern. Child. Nutr.* **2011**, *7*, 17–26. [CrossRef] [PubMed]
36. Lauritzen, L.; Carlson, S.E. Maternal fatty acid status during pregnancy and lactation and relation to newborn and infant status. *Matern. Child. Nutr.* **2011**, *7* (Suppl. 2), 41–58. [CrossRef] [PubMed]
37. Hanebutt, F.L.; Demmelmair, H.; Schiessl, B.; Larqué, E.; Koletzko, B. Long-chain polyunsaturated fatty acid (LC-PUFA) transfer across the placenta. *Clin. Nutr.* **2008**, *27*, 685–693. [CrossRef] [PubMed]
38. Finnegan, Y.E.; Minihane, A.M.; Leigh-Firbank, E.C.; Kew, S.; Meijer, G.W.; Muggli, R.; Calder, P.C.; Williams, C.M. Plant- and marine-derived n-3 polyunsaturated fatty acids have differential effects on fasting and postprandial blood lipid concentrations and on the susceptibility of LDL to oxidative modification in moderately hyperlipidemic subjects. *Am. J. Clin. Nutr.* **2003**, *77*, 783–795. [PubMed]
39. Gonzales, G.F.; Gonzales, C. A randomized, double-blind placebo-controlled study on acceptability, safety and efficacy of oral administration of sacha inchi oil (Plukenetia volubilis L.) in adult human subjects. *Food Chem. Toxicol.* **2014**, *65*, 168–176. [CrossRef] [PubMed]
40. Gonzales, G.F.; Gonzales, C.; Villegas, L. Exposure of fatty acids after a single oral administration of sacha inchi (Plukenetia volubilis L.) and sunflower oil in human adult subjects. *Toxicol. Mech. Methods* **2014**, *24*, 60–69. [CrossRef] [PubMed]
41. Sprecher, H.; Chen, Q.; Yin, F.Q. Regulation of the biosynthesis of 22:5n-6 and 22:6n-3: A complex intracellular process. *Lipids* **1999**, *34*, S153–S156. [CrossRef] [PubMed]
42. Sprecher, H.; Luthria, D.L.; Mohammed, B.S.; Baykousheva, S.P. Reevaluation of the pathways for the biosynthesis of polyunsaturated fatty acids. *J. Lipid Res.* **1995**, *36*, 2471–2477. [PubMed]
43. McManaman, J.L. Lipid transport in the lactating mammary gland. *J. Mammary Gland Biol. Neoplasia* **2014**, *19*, 35–42. [CrossRef] [PubMed]
44. Roy, S.; Dhar, P.; Ghosh, S. Comparative evaluation of essential fatty acid composition of mothers' milk of some urban and suburban regions of West Bengal, India. *Int. J. Food Sci. Nutr.* **2012**, *63*, 895–901. [CrossRef] [PubMed]
45. Much, D.; Brunner, S.; Vollhardt, C.; Schmid, D.; Sedlmeier, E.M.; Brüderl, M.; Heimberg, E.; Bartke, N.; Boehm, G.; Bader, B.L.; *et al.* Breast milk fatty acid profile in relation to infant growth and body composition: Results from the INFAT study. *Pediatr. Res.* **2013**, *74*, 230–237. [CrossRef] [PubMed]
46. Carlson, S.; Montalto, M.; Ponder, D.; Werkman, S.; Korones, S. Lower incidence of necrotizing enterocolitis in infant fed a preterm formula with egg phospholipids. *Ped. Res.* **1998**, *44*, 491–498. [CrossRef] [PubMed]
47. Kim, K.B.; Nam, Y.A.; Kim, H.S.; Hayes, A.W.; Lee, B.M. α-Linolenic acid: Nutraceutical, pharmacological and toxicological evaluation. *Food Chem. Toxicol.* **2014**, *70*, 163–178. [CrossRef] [PubMed]
48. Luxwolda, M.F.; Kuipers, R.S.; Koops, J.H.; Muller, S.; de Graaf, D.; Dijck-Brouwer, D.A.; Muskiet, F.A. Interrelationships between maternal DHA in erythrocytes, milk and adipose tissue. Is 1 wt% DHA the optimal human milk content? Data from four Tanzanian tribes differing in lifetime stable intakes of fish. *Br. J. Nutr.* **2014**, *111*, 854–866. [CrossRef] [PubMed]
49. Otto, S.J.; van Houwelingen, A.C.; Hornstra, G. The effect of supplementation with docosahexaenoic and arachidonic acid derived from single cell oils on plasma and erythrocyte fatty acids of pregnant women in the second trimester. *Prostaglandins Leukot. Essent. Fatty Acids* **2000**, *63*, 323–328. [CrossRef] [PubMed]

50. Dunstan, J.A.; Mori, T.A.; Barden, A.; Beilin, L.J.; Holt, P.G.; Calder, P.C.; Taylor, A.L.; Prescott, S.L. Effects of n-3 polyunsaturated fatty acid supplementation in pregnancy on maternal and fetal erythrocyte fatty acid composition. *Eur. J. Clin. Nutr.* **2004**, *58*, 429–437. [CrossRef] [PubMed]
51. Bascuñán, K.A.; Valenzuela, R.; Chamorro, R.; Valencia, A.; Barrera, C.; Puigrredon, C.; Sandoval, J.; Valenzuela, A. Polyunsaturated fatty acid composition of maternal diet and erythrocyte phospholipid status in Chilean pregnant women. *Nutrients* **2014**, *6*, 4918–4934. [CrossRef] [PubMed]
52. Tiangson, C.L.; Gavino, V.C.; Gavino, G.; Panlasigui, L.N. Docosahexaenoic acid level of the breast milk of some Filipino women. *Int. J. Food Sci. Nutr.* **2003**, *54*, 379–386. [CrossRef] [PubMed]
53. Wang, L.; Shimizu, Y.; Kaneko, S.; Hanaka, S.; Abe, T.; Shimasaki, H.; Hisaki, H.; Nakajima, H. Comparison of the fatty acid composition of total lipids and phospholipids in breast milk from Japanese women. *Pediatr. Int.* **2000**, *42*, 14–20. [CrossRef] [PubMed]
54. Smit, E.N.; Martini, I.A.; Mulder, H.; Boersma, E.R.; Muskiet, F.A. Estimated biological variation of the mature human milk fatty acid composition. *Prostaglandins Leukot. Essent. Fatty Acids* **2002**, *66*, 549–555. [CrossRef] [PubMed]
55. Auestad, N.; Halter, R.; Hall, R.T.; Blatter, M.; Bogle, M.L.; Burks, W.; Erickson, J.R.; Fitzgerald, K.M.; Dobson, V.; Innis, S.M.; *et al.* Growth and development in term infants fed long-chain polyunsaturated fatty acids: A double-masked, randomized, parallel, prospective, multivariate study. *Pediatrics* **2001**, *108*, 372–381. [CrossRef] [PubMed]
56. Kelishadi, R.; Hadi, B.; Iranpour, R.; Khosravi-Darani, K.; Mirmoghtadaee, P.; Farajian, S.; Poursafa, P. A study on lipid content and fatty acid of breast milk and its association with mother's diet composition. *J. Res. Med. Sci.* **2012**, *17*, 824–827. [PubMed]
57. Lassek, W.D.; Gaulin, S.J. Maternal milk DHA content predicts cognitive performance in a sample of 28 nations. *Matern. Child. Nutr.* **2013**. [CrossRef] [PubMed]
58. Calder, P.C. n-3 polyunsaturated fatty acids, inflammation, and inflammatory diseases. *Am. J. Clin. Nutr.* **2006**, *83*, 1505S–1519S. [PubMed]
59. Lauritzen, L.; Fewtrell, M.; Agostoni, C. Dietary arachidonic acid in perinatal nutrition: A commentary. *Pediatr. Res.* **2015**, *77*, 263–269. [CrossRef] [PubMed]
60. Lassek, W.D.; Gaulin, S.J. Linoleic and docosahexaenoic acids in human milk have opposite relationships with cognitive test performance in a sample of 28 countries. *Prostaglandins Leukot. Essent. Fatty Acids* **2014**, *91*, 195–201. [CrossRef] [PubMed]
61. Simopoulos, A.P. Evolutionary aspects of diet: The omega-6/omega-3 ratio and the brain. *Mol. Neurobiol.* **2011**, *44*, 203–215. [CrossRef] [PubMed]
62. Araya, J.; Rodrigo, R.; Pettinelli, P.; Araya, A.V.; Poniachik, J.; Videla, L.A. Decreased liver fatty acid delta-6 and delta-5 desaturase activity in obese patients. *Obesity (Silver Spring)* **2010**, *18*, 1460–1463. [CrossRef] [PubMed]
63. Brumbaugh, D.E.; Friedman, J.E. Developmental origins of nonalcoholic fatty liver disease. *Pediatr. Res.* **2014**, *75*, 140–147. [CrossRef] [PubMed]
64. Jiao, J.; Li, Q.; Chu, J.; Zeng, W.; Yang, M.; Zhu, S. Effect of n-3 PUFA supplementation on cognitive function throughout the life span from infancy to old age: A systematic review and meta-analysis of randomized controlled trials. *Am. J. Clin. Nutr.* **2014**, *100*, 1422–1436. [CrossRef] [PubMed]
65. Abu-Ouf, N.M.; Jan, M.M. The influence of fish oil on neurological development and function. *Can. J. Neurol. Sci.* **2014**, *41*, 13–18. [CrossRef] [PubMed]
66. Mardones, F.; Urrutia, M.T.; Villarroel, L.; Rioseco, A.; Castillo, O.; Rozowski, J.; Tapia, J.L.; Bastias, G.; Bacallao, J.; Rojas, I. Effects of a dairy product fortified with multiple micronutrients and omega-3 fatty acids on birth weight and gestation duration in pregnant chilean women. *Public Health Nutr.* **2008**, *11*, 30–40. [CrossRef] [PubMed]
67. Starling, P.; Charlton, K.; McMahon, A.T.; Lucas, C. Fish intake during pregnancy and fetal neurodevelopment—A systematic review of the evidence. *Nutrients* **2015**, *7*, 2001–2014. [CrossRef] [PubMed]

68. Miyashita, C.; Sasaki, S.; Saijo, Y.; Okada, E.; Kobayashi, S.; Baba, T.; Kajiwara, J.; Todaka, T.; Iwasaki, Y.; Nakazawa, H.; *et al*. Demographic, behavioral, dietary, and socioeconomic characteristics related to persistent organic pollutants and mercury levels in pregnant women in Japan. *Chemosphere* **2015**, *133*, 13–21. [CrossRef] [PubMed]
69. Nevárez, M.; Leal, L.O.; Moreno, M. Estimation of seasonal risk caused by the intake of lead, mercury and cadmium through freshwater fish consumption from urban water reservoirs in arid areas of northern Mexico. *Int. J. Environ. Res. Public Health* **2015**, *12*, 1803–1816. [CrossRef] [PubMed]

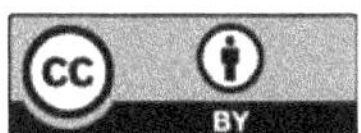

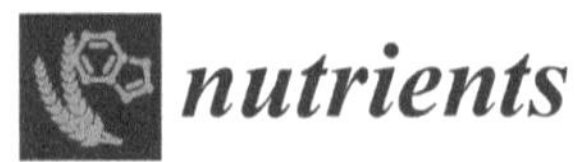

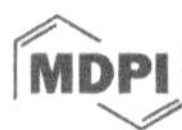

Article

Duality of *n*-3 Polyunsaturated Fatty Acids on *Mcp-1* Expression in Vascular Smooth Muscle: A Potential Role of 4-Hydroxy Hexenal

Kohji Nagayama [1], Katsutaro Morino [1,*], Osamu Sekine [1], Fumiyuki Nakagawa [1,2], Atsushi Ishikado [1,3,4], Hirotaka Iwasaki [1,5], Takashi Okada [1], Masashi Tawa [5], Daisuke Sato [1], Takeshi Imamura [5], Yoshihiko Nishio [6], Satoshi Ugi [1], Atsunori Kashiwagi [7], Tomio Okamura [5] and Hiroshi Maegawa [1]

[1] Department of Medicine, Shiga University of Medical Science, Shiga 520-2192, Japan; E-Mails: nagayama@belle.shiga-med.ac.jp (K.N.); sekine@belle.shiga-med.ac.jp (O.S.); f.nakagawa@jclbio.com (F.N.); atsushi.ishikado@jp.sunstar.com (A.I.); hiwasaki@belle.shiga-med.ac.jp (H.I.); tokada@belle.shiga-med.ac.jp (T.O.); dkst0310@belle.shiga-med.ac.jp (D.S.); sugi@belle.shiga-med.ac.jp (S.U.); maegawa@belle.shiga-med.ac.jp (H.M.)

[2] Osaka Laboratory, JCL Bioassay Corporation, 5-16-26, Minamisuita, Suita-shi, Osaka 564-0043, Japan

[3] Sunstar Inc., 3-1 Asahi-machi, Takatsuki, Osaka 569-1195, Japan

[4] Joslin Diabetes Centre, Harvard Medical School, MA 02115, USA

[5] Department of Pharmacology, Shiga University of Medical Science, Shiga 520-2192, Japan; E-Mails: tawa@belle.shiga-med.ac.jp (M.T.); timamura@belle.shiga-med.ac.jp (T.I.); okamura@belle.shiga-med.ac.jp (T.O.)

[6] Department of Diabetes and Endocrine Medicine, Kagoshima University, Kagoshima 890-8580, Japan; E-Mail: ynishio@m3.kufm.kagoshima-u.ac.jp

[7] Kusatsu General Hospital, 1660, Yabase-cho, Kusatsu, Shiga 525-8585, Japan; E-Mail: kashiwagi@kusatsu-gh.or.jp

* Author to whom correspondence should be addressed; E-Mail: morino@belle.shiga-med.ac.jp; Tel.: +81-77-548-2222; Fax: +81-77-543-3858.

Received: 22 May 2015 / Accepted: 31 August 2015 / Published: 21 September 2015

Abstract: *N*-3 polyunsaturated fatty acids such as docosahexaenoic acid (DHA) and eicosapentaenoic acid (EPA) have protective effects against atherosclerosis. Monocyte chemotactic protein (MCP)-1 is a major inflammatory mediator in the progression of atherosclerosis. However, little is known about the regulation of MCP-1 by DHA and EPA in vessels and vascular smooth muscle cells (VSMCs). In this study, we compared the effect of DHA and EPA on the expression of *Mcp-1* in rat arterial strips and rat VSMCs. DHA, but not EPA, suppressed *Mcp-1* expression in arterial strips. Furthermore, DHA generated 4-hydroxy hexenal (4-HHE), an end product of *n*-3 polyunsaturated fatty acids (PUFAs), in arterial strips as measured by liquid chromatography-tandem mass spectrometry. In addition, 4-HHE treatment suppressed *Mcp-1* expression in arterial strips, suggesting 4-HHE derived from DHA may be involved in the mechanism of this phenomenon. In contrast, *Mcp-1* expression was stimulated by DHA, EPA and 4-HHE through p38 kinase and the Keap1-Nuclear factor erythroid-derived 2-like 2 (Nrf2) pathway in VSMCs. In conclusion, there is a dual effect of *n*-3 PUFAs on the regulation of *Mcp-1* expression. Further study is necessary to elucidate the pathological role of this phenomenon.

Keywords: monocyte chemotactic protein 1; 4-hydroxy hexenal; docosahexaenoic acid; eicosapentaenoic acid

1. Introduction

Atherosclerosis is characterized by accumulation of oxidized fat, thickening of vessel walls by collagens secreted by proliferating vascular smooth muscle cells, and macrophage filtration [1]. There are several steps in the progression of atherosclerosis: (1) endothelial dysfunction, (2) migration of leukocytes and smooth muscle cells into the vessel wall, (3) foam cell formation, and (4) degradation of extracellular matrix. Epidemiologically, fish consumption negatively correlates with cardiovascular events, suggesting beneficial effects of *n*-3 polyunsaturated fatty acids (PUFA) [2,3]. Other clinical studies have indicated that *n*-3 PUFAs improved the carotid intima-media thickness and endothelial function [4,5], suggesting that *n*-3 PUFAs attenuate atherosclerosis by decreasing migration of leukocytes and proliferation of smooth muscle cells. This is supported by animal experiments that showed *n*-3 PUFAs attenuated VCAM-1 expression and macrophage filtration [6]. *N*-3 PUFAs mainly consist of eicosapentaenoic acid (EPA) and docosahexaenoic acid (DHA). However, the difference between EPA and DHA in terms of their anti-atherosclerotic effect is still unclear.

Monocyte chemotactic protein (MCP)-1/chemokine (C-C motif) ligand 2 (CCL2) is expressed in inflammatory cells and stromal cells such as endothelial and smooth muscle cells, and its expression is regulated by proinflammatory stimuli and tissue injury. MCP-1 is regulated both by the nuclear factor kappa-light-chain-enhancer of activated B cells (NF-κB) pathway and stress-activated kinases including p38, ERK and JNK [7]. There are several potential mechanisms that explain the anti-inflammatory effect of EPA and DHA. A recent report revealed that G-protein coupled receptor 120 (GPR120) is a receptor for DHA that mediates anti-inflammatory and insulin-sensitizing effects in rodents [8]. Other reports have suggested that resolvins and protectins—which are derived from EPA and DHA—are mediators of the anti-inflammatory effects [9]. We have recently reported that 4-hydroxy hexenal (4-HHE)—an end product of *n*-3 PUFA peroxidation—activates the nuclear factor erythroid 2-related factor 2 (Nrf2)-Kelch-like ECH-associated protein 1 (Keap1) pathway in human umbilical vein endothelial cells (HUVECs), contributing to endothelial function and antioxidative activity [10,11].

Nrf2 is a redox-sensitive master regulatory transcription factor regulated by Keap1. Electrophiles, shear stress, and reactive oxygen species (ROS) stimulate modification of the cysteine residues of Keap1, which allows its translocation to the nucleus. Nrf2 induces antioxidant enzymes such as heme oxygenase-1 (Hmox1) through the antioxidant response element (ARE) consensus sequence [12,13]. The 4-HHE induces Nrf2-mediated Hmox1 expression in multiple organs [14,15]. In addition, it has also been reported that DHA induces Nrf2-mediated Hmox1 expression in human vascular smooth muscle cells (VSMCs) isolated from small pulmonary artery or endothelial cells [16,17].

Therefore, we examined the regulation of MCP-1 by DHA and EPA in arterial strips and VSMCs. Furthermore, we measured the 4-HHE content by a liquid chromatography-tandem mass spectrometry (LC-MS/MS) and tested its role in these tissues.

2. Methods

2.1. Reagents

Dulbecco's Modified Eagle's Medium (DMEM) and fetal bovine serum (FBS) were obtained from Life Technologies (Grand Island, NY, USA). EPA, DHA, and 4-HHE were purchased from Cayman (Ann Arbor, MI, USA). The MTT assay kit, anti-β-actin (A5316) antibody and *N*-acetyl-L-cysteine were purchased from Sigma-Aldrich (St. Louis, MO, USA). Fatty acid-free bovine serum albumin (BSA) was purchased from Nacalai Tesque (Kyoto, Japan). Anti-p38 (#9112), anti-phospho-p38 (#9211), anti-ERK1/2 (#9102), anti-phospho-ERK1/2 (#9106), anti-JNK (#9252), anti-phospho-JNK (#9251), and anti-caspase-3 (#9661) antibodies were purchased from Cell Signaling (Danvers, MA, USA). Horseradish peroxidase-linked anti-mouse and anti-rabbit antibodies were purchased from Amersham Biosciences Corp. (Piscataway, NJ, USA). 2′7′-Dichlorodihydrofluorescein diacetate (H_2DCFDA) and small interfering RNA (SiRNA) reagents were purchased from Life Technologies (Tokyo, Japan). SB203580, PD98059 and SP600125 were purchased from Calbiochem (Cambridge, UK).

2.2. Animals and Experimental Procedures

All animal experimentation was approved by the committee for Animal Research of Shiga University of Medical Science (No. 2014-4-8, 7 May 2014). The experimental procedure for artery strips was performed as previously reported [18]. Briefly, eight-week-old male Sprague-Dawley rats (Japan SLC, Shizuoka, Japan) were housed in an environmentally controlled room with a 12 h light/dark cycle and free access to food and water. Rats were fed a regular diet (Dyets Inc., Bethlehem, PA, USA) for 12 weeks. After 12 h of fasting, rats were sacrificed by bleeding from the abdominal aorta under deep anesthesia. The thoracic aorta was dissected, excised, and cut into strips with special care being taken to preserve the endothelium. The strips were then fixed vertically between hooks in a muscle bath (10-mL capacity) containing modified Ringer-Locke solution bubbled with a gas mixture of 95% O_2 and 5% CO_2, pH 7.4 at 37 ± 0.3 °C. After treatment with DHA, EPA or 4-HHE for 6 h, the arterial strips were immediately freeze-clamped by liquid nitrogen, and stored at −80 °C. For lipid extraction, the frozen tissues were pulverized into a fine powder using a Cryo Press disruptor (Microtec Co., Ltd., Chiba, Japan). This fine powder was weighed on an ME235 electronic balance (Sartorius AG, Göttingen, Germany), homogenized in 490 μL of chloroform/methanol (1:1, v/v) and 10 μL of dibutylhydroxytoluene solution (10 mg/mL in ethanol), and incubated at 36 °C for 1 h [19]. The resulting solution was used for measuring the 4-HHE content.

2.3. Cell Culture

VSMCs were isolated from the aortas of male Sprague-Dawley rats (150–200 g) by enzymatic digestion as previously described [20]. Briefly, cells were maintained in DMEM supplemented with 10% FBS, and used between the 4th–12th passages except for primary cells, showing a dramatic growth rate because of transformation. Cells were grown to confluence in 12-well plates, and cell growth was arrested for 24 h in DMEM supplemented with 1% FBS before the real-time quantitative polymerase chain reaction (RT-qPCR) experiments.

2.4. Fatty Acid Treatment

DHA or EPA was administered as a complex with fatty acid-free BSA as previously described [15]. Briefly, 0.3 mM DHA or EPA was dissolved in ethanol (2.5 mL), and gradually solubilized in an 8.4% BSA solution (14.3 mL) at 37 °C. The 4-HHE was dissolved in dimethyl sulfoxide and then in serum-containing medium.

2.5. Messenger RNA (mRNA) Extraction and Real-Time RT-qPCR Analysis

Total RNA was extracted from cells and tissues using a Total RNA Mini Kit (Bio-Rad, Hercules, CA, USA). Single-stranded cDNA was synthesized from 1.5 μg of total RNA using the Prime Script RT Reagent Kit (Takara Bio, Shiga, Japan), and endogenous genomic DNA was degraded by DNase I (Life Technologies, CA, USA). RT-qPCR experiments were carried out with SYBR Green PCR master mix (Life Technologies, CA, USA) and the ABI 7500 Fast Real-Time PCR System (Applied Biosystems, Foster City, CA, USA). All the quantitative data were normalized against the expression levels of 18S rRNA (18S). RT-qPCR conditions were 95 °C for 10 min, followed by 40 cycles of 95 °C for 15 s and 60 °C for 1 min. The primers for the RT-qPCR are listed in Table 1.

Table 1. Candidate genes, primer sequences and accession numbers.

	Forward Primer	Reverse Primer	Accession Number
Mcp-1	GCTGCTACTCATTCACTGGCAA	TGCTGCTGGTGATTCTCTTGTA	NM_031530.1
Hmox-1	TCTATCGTGCTCGCATGAAC	AAGGCGGTCTTAGCCTCTTC	NM_012580.2
Nrf2	GGAGCAATTCAACGAAGCTC	ACAGTTCTGAGCGGCAACTT	NM_031789.2
18S	TTCCGATAACGAACGAGACTCT	TGGCTGAACGCCACTTGTC	NR_046237.1

2.6. Quantitative Analysis of 4-HHE in Biological Samples

The 4-HHE in aorta and VSMCs was quantitatively analyzed using LC-MS/MS procedure as described previously [15,21]. Briefly, a standard solution of 4-HHE (Cayman Chemical Co., Ann Arbor, MI, USA) was used for the calibration curve. Solid-phase extraction was done using a mixed-mode anion exchange solid-phase extraction (SPE) cartridge (Oasis MAX, Waters, Milford, MA, USA). An ACQUITY CSH C18 column (Waters) was used for separating 4-HHE. Electrospray ionization (ESI) was carried out with API4000 operating in the positive ionization and SRM mode. The SRM transitions for CHD-derivatized 4-HHE were m/z 284-216.

2.7. MTT Assay for Cell Viability

Rat VSMCs were seeded on 24-well plates. To determine the cell toxicity of DHA, EPA and 4-HHE, confluent cells were exposed to these reagents for 24 h, and then washed with phosphate-buffered saline (PBS). Cell viability was determined by the conventional MTT assay as previously described [11]. The absorbance of BSA-treated cells was used as the control.

2.8. Reactive Oxygen Species (ROS) Measurement Assay

Intracellular ROS production was determined using the fluorescent probe H_2DCFDA in VSMCs incubated with 20 μM H_2DCFDA for 20 min as previously described [11]. Following washing with PBS, cells were incubated with 50 μM DHA or 50 μM EPA. The fluorescence emitted from the cells was recorded immediately at 492 nm (excitation) and 525 nm (emission) using a fluorescent microplate reader (Tecan, Männedorf, Switzerland) over a 2-h period.

2.9. Western Blot Analysis

Total protein samples from VSMCs were prepared as previously descried [11], and were resolved by SDS-PAGE before being transferred to PVDF membranes. Membranes were incubated with antibodies against p38, ERK, JNK, their phosphorylated forms, caspase-3, or β-actin. Blots were then incubated with horseradish peroxidase-linked second antibody (Amersham, Buckinghamshire, UK), followed by chemiluminescence detection (PerkinElmer, Waltham, MA, USA).

2.10. Statistical Analysis

Data are presented as mean ± SE, unless otherwise stated. Differences between more than three groups were analyzed by Tukey–Kramer test. When two groups were compared, differences were analyzed by two-tailed Student's t-test. $P < 0.05$ was considered statistically significant.

3. Results

3.1. Docosahexaenoic Acid (DHA)—Though Not Eicosapentaenoic Acid (EPA)—Inhibits Mcp-1 mRNA Expression in Rat Aorta

To explore the direct effects of EPA and DHA on vessels, we examined the expression of *Mcp-1* mRNA in rat arterial strips. DHA (50–100 μM) but not EPA (50–100 μM) almost completely inhibited the expression of *Mcp-1* mRNA compared with BSA (Figure 1A). In contrast, DHA increased the expression of *heme oxygenase 1 (Hmox-1)* (Figure 1B), which is a known antioxidative gene in vessels. EPA also increased the expression of *Hmox-1*, but to a lesser extent than DHA did (Figure 1B). Because *Hmox-1* is a target gene of the Keap1-Nrf2 pathway, we measured the lipid peroxidation product levels in rat arterial strips by LC-MS/MS with or without *n*-3 PUFA incubation. We found that DHA but not EPA increased the tissue 4-HHE content, whereas it did not change the content of 4-hydroxy 2-noneral (4-HNE), a lipid peroxidation product derived from *n*-6 PUFA (Figure 1C). To test the role of 4-HHE, we exposed the arterial strips to 4-HHE and found that it inhibited the expression of *Mcp-1* (Figure 1D) and increased that of *Hmox-1* (Figure 1E) in rat aortic strips, suggesting that DHA regulates *Mcp-1* and *Hmox-1* expression through 4-HHE.

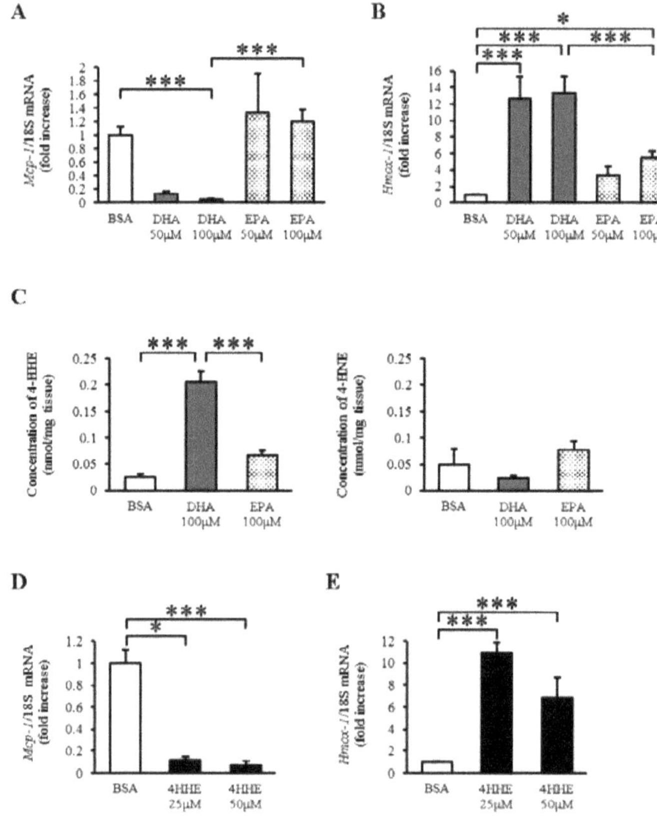

Figure 1. Docosahexaenoic acid (DHA)-derived DHA generated 4-hydroxy hexenal (4-HHE) inhibits the expression of *Mcp-1* Messenger RNA (mRNA), but induces *heme oxygenase 1* (*Hmox-1*) mRNA in rat aorta. Rat arterial strips were treated with bovine serum albumin (BSA), DHA (50–100 μM), EPA (50–100 μM) or 4-HHE (25–50 μM) for 6 h under *ex vivo* conditions. (**A**,**B**) Relative mRNA expression of *Mcp-1* (**A**) and *Hmox-1* (**B**) in arterial strips was quantitated using the real-time quantitative polymerase chain reaction (RT-qPCR). Results were normalized against 18S rRNA and expressed as fold increase over control. (**C**) 4-HHE and 4-HNE content were measured by a liquid chromatography-tandem mass spectrometry (LC-MS/MS). (**D**,**E**) Relative mRNA expression of *Mcp-1* (**D**) and *Hmox-1* (**E**) in arterial strips was quantitated using RT-qPCR. Results were normalized as above. Results are expressed as mean ± SE of 4–8 animals (n = 3–22; **A**,**B**,**D**,**E**), or a single experiment (n = 3; **C**). * $P < 0.05$, *** $P < 0.001$, compared with BSA control. NS, no significant difference.

3.2. Paradoxical Increase in Mcp-1 by DHA, EPA and 4-HHE in VSMCs

In contrast to the results observed for arterial strips, DHA, EPA and 4-HHE increased the expression of *Mcp-1* mRNA in a dose-dependent manner in rat VSMCs (Figure 2A). To clarify the differences in *Mcp-1* responses between rat arterial strips and VSMCs (Passage 4–12), we performed the same experiment using primary VSMCs (Passage 1). Similar to VSMCs (Passage 4–12), DHA, EPA, and 4-HHE increased the expression of *Mcp-1* in primary VSMCs (Figure 2B). Similar to rat arterial strips, DHA (50 μM), but not EPA (50 μM), increased the content of 4-HHE in VSMCs (Figure 2C), whereas it did not change the 4-HNE content.

Because *n*-3 PUFAs are known activators of the mitogen-activated protein kinase (MAPK) family, we assessed the phosphorylation levels of p38 kinase, ERK and JNK. DHA, EPA and 4-HHE increased the phosphorylation levels of p38, ERK and JNK (Figure 2D). To understand the effect of the MAPK family on the *Mcp-1* expression, we tested the effect of MAPK inhibitors on DHA-, EPA- or 4-HHE-induced *Mcp-1* expression. Pre-incubation with the p38 kinase inhibitor SB203580 completely suppressed the induction of *Mcp-1* expression (Figure 2E). The ERK inhibitor PD98059 had a partial inhibitory effect on *Mcp-1* expression, whereas the JNK inhibitor SP600125 did not (Figure 2E).

3.3. 4-HHE Derived from DHA Induces Mcp-1 Expression through the Nrf2 Pathway in Human Vascular Smooth Muscle Cells (VSMCs)

To evaluate the oxidative stress induced by DHA and 4-HHE, we used *N*-acetyl-L-cysteine (NAC), a known antioxidant that mimics glutathione. Pretreatment with NAC (10 mM) completely inhibited the DHA-, EPA- and 4-HHE-induced *Mcp-1* expression (Figure 3A). Furthermore, DHA and EPA increased ROS production measured by H_2DCFDA (Figure 3B). NAC pretreatment completely inhibited the DHA-induced ROS production in VSMCs (Figure 3B), supporting the role of oxidative stress in the DHA-induced *Mcp-1* expression.

To evaluate Nrf2 activation by DHA and 4-HHE, we examined the mRNA expression of *Hmox1*, a target of Nrf2, in VSMCs. We found that DHA and 4-HHE stimulated the expression of *Hmox1* mRNA in VSMCs, and that NAC inhibited the DHA- and 4-HHE-induced *Hmox-1* expression (Figure 3C). As expected, the 4-HHE-induced *Mcp-1* expression was decreased by siRNA against *Nrf2* (Figure 3D,E).

3.4. DHA Induces Apoptosis of VSMCs through 4-HHE

To test the toxicity of *n*-3 PUFA in VSMCs, VSMCs were incubated for 24 h with DHA, EPA or 4-HHE at a higher but physiological concentration, followed by measurement of cell viability by the MTT assay. DHA and 4-HHE only decreased cell viability at a high concentration (150 μM) compared with the BSA control (Figure 4A). In contrast, EPA did not decrease the cell viability of VSMCs (Figure 4A).

Apoptosis is a known downstream process of ROS production. Increased cleaved caspase-3 expression measured by Western blot analysis indicated that the cell toxicity of DHA and 4-HHE was caused by the induction of apoptosis (Figure 4B).

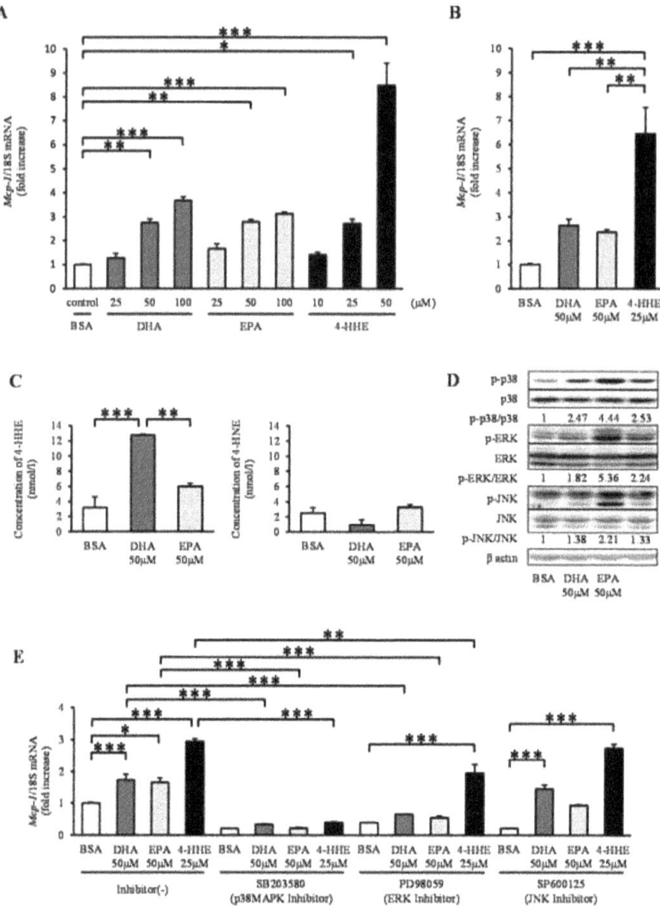

Figure 2. DHA, EPA, and 4-HHE induce *Mcp-1* expression through the p38 mitogen-activated protein kinase (MAPK) pathway in VSMCs. VSMCs (Passage 4–12) were treated with the indicated reagent for 6 h (**A**). (**B**) Primary vessels and vascular smooth muscle cells (VSMCs) (Passage 1) were treated with BSA, DHA (50 μM), EPA (50 μM) or 4-HHE (25 μM) for 6 h. Relative mRNA expression of *Mcp-1* was quantitated using RT-qPCR. The results were normalized against 18S rRNA and expressed as fold increase over control. (**C**) 4-HHE and 4-HNE content in VSMCs were measured using LC-MS/MS. (**D**) p38, ERK, JNK and their phosphorylated forms, and β-actin were determined by Western blotting. DHA (50 μM), EPA (50 μM) or 4-HHE (25 μM) were added for 10 min. (**E**) Pretreatment with p38 kinase inhibitor (SB203580; 10 μM), ERK inhibitor (PD98059; 25 μM) or JNK inhibitor (SP600125; 10 μM) was performed for 30 min before BSA, DHA, EPA or 4-HHE incubation. The results were normalized against 18S rRNA and expressed as fold increase over corresponding control. (**A**) Values represent the mean ± SE of four independent experiments (n = 9); (**B**) a single experiment (n = 3); (**C**) a single experiment (n = 3); or (**E**) three independent experiments (n = 3–9). * $P < 0.05$, ** $P < 0.01$, *** $P < 0.001$, compared with corresponding control.

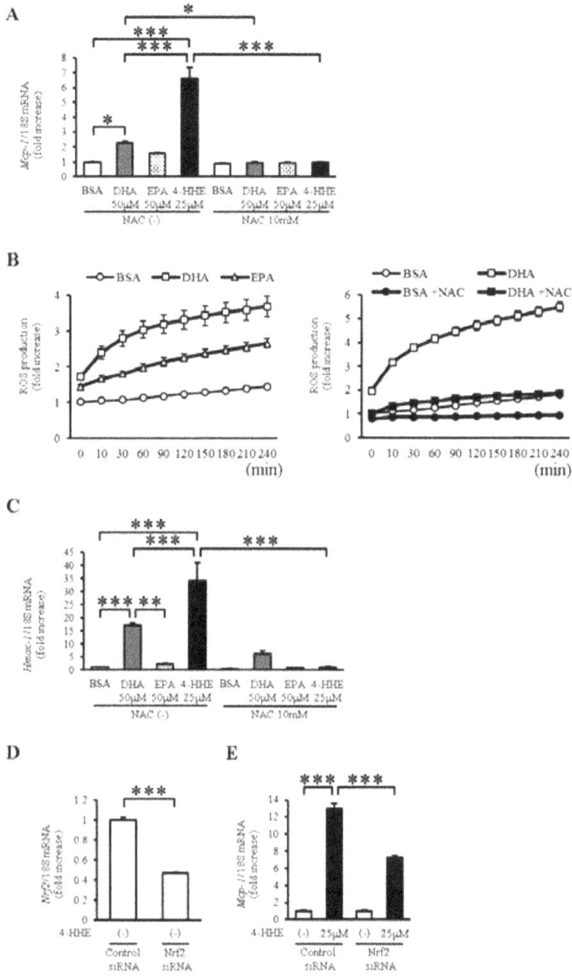

Figure 3. DHA-derived 4-HHE induces *Mcp-1* expression partially through the oxidative stress-induced Nrf2 pathway in VSMCs. (**A**,**C**) VSMCs were treated with *N*-acetyl-L-cysteine (NAC; 10 mM) for 1 h before incubation with BSA, DHA (50 μM), EPA (50 μM) or 4-HHE (25 μM) for 6 h. Relative mRNA expression of *Mcp-1* (**A**) and *Hmox-1* (**C**) in VSMCs was quantitated using RT-qPCR. Results were normalized against 18S rRNA and expressed as fold increase over control. (**B**) Reactive oxygen species (ROS) production was measured by 2′7′-Dichlorodihydrofluorescein diacetate (H_2DCFDA). BSA, DHA (50 μM) or EPA (50 μM) was added for 4 h (left panel). BSA or DHA (50 μM) was added with or without NAC (10 mM) for 4 h (right panel). (**D**,**E**) VSMCs were treated with *Nrf2* siRNA (40 nM) or control siRNA (40 nM). After 24 h, VSMCs were treated with vehicle or 4-HHE (25 μM) for 6 h. Relative mRNA of *Nrf2* (**D**) and *Mcp-1* (**E**) was quantitated using RT-qPCR. Values represent the mean ± SE of three independent experiments (n = 9; **A**,**C**); a single experiment (n = 3; **B**); and two independent experiments (n = 6; **D**,**E**). * $P < 0.05$, *** $P < 0.001$, compared with the corresponding control.

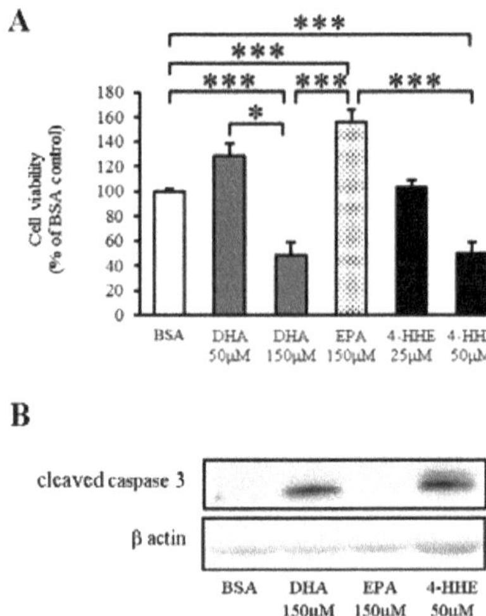

Figure 4. DHA-derived 4-HHE reduces cell viability through apoptosis in VSMCs. (**A**) VSMCs were treated with a high concentration of DHA (150 μM), EPA (150 μM) or 4-HHE (50 μM) for 24 h. Cell viability was determined by the MTT assay. Values are expressed as percentage of cell survival, and each value represents the mean ± SE of five experiments (n = 15). (**B**) Cleaved caspase-3 and β-actin were determined by Western blotting. DHA (150 μM), EPA (150 μM) or 4-HHE (50 μM) were added for 6 h. * P <0.05, *** P < 0.001, compared with BSA control.

4. Discussion

Our study has three important findings. First, DHA and 4-HHE, but not EPA, inhibited *Mcp-1* expression in rat arterial strips. Second, DHA and 4-HHE inhibited cell survival by promoting apoptosis in VSMCs. Third, DHA, EPA and 4-HHE stimulated *Mcp-1* expression via oxidative stress, p38 and the Keap1-Nrf2 pathway in VSMCs.

DHA and 4-HHE, but not EPA, inhibited *Mcp-1* expression in rat arterial strips. Previous studies have shown that *n*-3 PUFAs affect inflammation and plaque stability [22,23], which is consistent with the inhibitory effect of DHA on *Mcp-1* expression under *ex vivo* conditions in our study. In contrast, EPA had almost no effect on *Mcp-1* expression (Figure 1A). We assume this difference was the result of Nrf2 activation by 4-HHE, because we observed a similar difference between DHA and EPA in HUVECs, which was explained by the generation of 4-HHE [10,11,14–16]. As expected, DHA preferentially increased intracellular 4-HHE content in rat arterial strips compared with EPA (Figure 1C). In addition, 4-HHE directly inhibited *Mcp-1* expression in rat arterial strips (Figure 1D). Although the molecular mechanism underlying this phenomenon is not clear, 4-HHE may be a mediator of the anti-inflammatory effect of DHA.

We also found that DHA and 4-HHE at a higher concentration and longer incubation inhibited cell survival by promoting apoptosis in VSMCs. In agreement with our study, previous reports have shown that DHA induced apoptosis in VSMCs or cancer cells through p38 MAPK activation at 24 hours [24,25]. Another report demonstrated that 4-HHE induced cytotoxic and negative effects on YPEN-1 prostatic endothelial cells at 24 hours [26]. Because migration of transformed VSMCs is one of the main features of atherosclerosis [27], 4-HHE-induced apoptosis, followed by macrophage clearance via MCP-1 expression may be beneficial. Conversely, apoptosis in advanced plaque lesions may be detrimental. This discrepancy might explain the inconsistent effects of *n*-3 PUFAs on cardiovascular events in a secondary prevention study [28].

Both DHA and EPA stimulated *Mcp-1* expression in VSMCs. Our preliminary data suggest that other fatty acids including palmitic and arachidonic acid also stimulate *Mcp-1* expression. We speculate that this was due to oxidative stress induced by fatty acids—known as lipotoxicity [29,30]—rather than being an *n*-3 PUFA-specific effect. In addition to lipotoxicity, DHA preferentially degrades to 4-HHE via peroxidation. 4-HHE has an aldehyde residue that causes a Michael reaction with proteins, forming protein adducts [13]. *N*-acetyl-L-cysteine—a known antioxidant—protected VSMCs from 4-HHE-induced Nrf2 action through the formation of 4-HHE-NAC adducts. *Nrf2* siRNA inhibited the 4-HHE-induced *Mcp-1* expression, suggesting that DHA stimulated *Mcp-1*—at least in part—through the 4-HHE-Nrf2 pathway.

The opposite effects caused by DHA on *Mcp-1* mRNA expression between arterial strips and VSMCs were observed in this study. VSMCs were cultured in a different environment as compared to arterial strips: culture media, growth factors, and monolayer. These biological factors may explain the discrepancy between arterial strips and VSMCs. Other possibilities are that endothelial cells are a major source of *Mcp-1* mRNA and that endothelial cells induce smooth muscle cells to suppress *Mcp-1* mRNA in response to DHA. To test this possibility, DHA-induced *Mcp-1* expression were analyzed in VSMCs with the condition media from rat aortic endothelial cells, and aortic strips without endothelial cells. Our preliminary data suggest that DHA-induced *Mcp-1* is not affected by endothelial cells.

DHA but not EPA produces 4-HHE in rat arterial strips and VSMCs. Previous reports from our group and others have shown that the 4-HHE content or 4-HHE adducts increased after fish oil treatment in heart, liver and other tissues [15,31,32]. Furthermore, previous reports have shown that plasma 4-HHE levels increased following supplementation with DHA or fish-based diet intervention in humans [33,34]. The reason for the difference in 4-HHE generation between DHA and EPA is not clear; hence, further experiments are necessary to elucidate this phenomenon.

Concentrations of EPA and DHA (25–150 μM) used in this study are similar to previous studies [3,11,14,16]. These concentrations are relatively low compared to the reported concentrations in human plasma (200–400 μM) [3]. As shown in Figure 4, high concentrations of DHA had a cytotoxic effect compared to high concentrations of EPA. This phenomenon was consistent with a previous study that showed DHA but not EPA had a profound growth inhibitory effect on HPV16 immortalized cells but not on normal cells [35]. In addition, DHA has strong inhibitory effects on multiple cancer cell lines [26]. We speculated that 4-HHE preferentially generated by DHA might explain the difference between DHA and EPA.

There were some limitations in this study. First, we could not identify the molecular mechanism of the DHA-induced *Mcp-1* decrease in artery strips, although our data suggest that 4-HHE-induced Nrf2 activation may play a role. Second, the 4-HHE content measured was free 4-HHE. Because 4-HHE generates 4-HHE adducts—especially with glutathione—the total 4-HHE content in the tissues may be higher. We incubated VSMCs with 4-HHE at 25 μM based on its ability to stimulate Hmox1. Third, the clinical significance of the DHA-induced *Mcp-1* expression is still not clear.

5. Conclusions

DHA had contrasting effects on *Mcp-1* expression in vessels and VSMCs. We suggest a possible role for Nrf2 activation by DHA-derived 4-HHE. Furthermore, 4-HHE derived from DHA decreased cell viability by inducing apoptosis in VSMCs. These findings may explain the different effects of EPA and DHA on vessels.

Acknowledgments: Acknowledgments

We thank Chisato Kusunoki, Megumi Matsuo, Keiko Kosaka and Keiko Kondo for their technical help. Sources of founding: this study was funded by Shiga University of Medical Science. The Department of Medicine, Shiga University of Medical Science receives research promotion grants (Shogaku Kifukin) from Astellas Pharma, AstraZeneca, Boehringer-Mannheim, Daiichi-Sankyo, Dainippon-Sumitomo Pharma, MSD, Kowa, Sunstar, Takeda Pharmaceutical Company, Mitsubishi-Tanabe Pharma Corporation, Novartis, Novo Nordisk, Kyowa-Hakko-Kirin,

Taisho-Toyama, Teijin Pharma. However, the research topics of these grants are not restricted. This work was supported in part by a Grant-in-Aid from the Ministry of Education, Culture, Sports, Science and Technology of Japan to Y. Nishio (#23591336). This study was performed in collaboration between Shiga University of Medical Science and JCL Bioassay Corporation. F. Nakagawa is an employee of JCL Bioassay Corporation and a graduate student at Shiga University of Medical Science; however, this does not alter the authors' adherence to all of the policies of Nutrients regarding the sharing of data and materials.

Author Contributions: H.M. and Y.N. conceived and supervised the study; K.N, K.M. and O.S. designed experiments; K.N., F.N., A.I., H.I., T.O. and M.T. performed experiments; K.N., K.M. and D.S. wrote the manuscript; S.U., T.I., A.K., T.O. and H.M. made manuscript revisions.

Conflicts of Interest: The authors declare no conflict of interest.

Abbreviations

Monocyte chemotactic protein 1 (Mcp-1), nuclear factor erythroid 2-related factor 2 (Nrf2), 4-hydroxy hexenal (4-HHE), polyunsaturated fatty acids (PUFAs), docosahexaenoic acid (DHA), eicosapentaenoic acid (EPA), heme oxygenase-1 (Hmox1), vascular cell adhesion protein 1 (VCAM-1), extracellular signal-regulated kinase (ERK), c-JUN N-terminal kinase (JNK), p38 mitogen-activated protein kinase (p38).

References

1. Libby, P. Current concepts of the pathogenesis of the acute coronary syndromes. *Circulation* **2001**, *104*, 365–372. [CrossRef] [PubMed]
2. Kromhout, D.; Bosschieter, E.B.; de Lezenne Coulander, C. The inverse relation between fish consumption and 20-year mortality from coronary heart disease. *N. Engl. J. Med.* **1985**, *312*, 1205–1209. [PubMed]
3. Iso, H.; Kobayashi, M.; Ishihara, J.; Sasaki, S.; Okada, K.; Kita, Y.; Kokubo, Y.; Tsugane, S. Intake of fish and *n*-3 fatty acids and risk of coronary heart disease among Japanese: The Japan public health center-based (JPHC) study cohort I. *Circulation* **2006**, *113*, 195–202. [CrossRef]
4. Yagi, S.; Aihara, K.I.; Fukuda, D.; Takashima, A.; Hara, T.; Hotchi, J.; Ise, T.; Yamaguchi, K.; Tobiume, T.; Iwase, T.; *et al.* Effects of docosahexaenoic acid on the endothelial function in patients with coronary artery disease. *J. Atheroscler. Thromb.* **2015**, *22*, 447–454. [CrossRef] [PubMed]
5. Yamada, H.; Yoshida, M.; Nakano, Y.; Suganami, T.; Satoh, N.; Mita, T.; Azuma, K.; Itoh, M.; Yamamoto, Y.; Kamei, Y.; *et al.* *In vivo* and *in vitro* inhibition of monocyte adhesion to endothelial cells and endothelial adhesion molecules by eicosapentaenoic acid. *Arterioscler. Thromb. Vasc. Biol.* **2008**, *28*, 2173–2179. [CrossRef] [PubMed]
6. Matsumoto, M.; Sata, M.; Fukuda, D.; Tanaka, K.; Soma, M.; Hirata, Y.; Nagai, R. Orally administered eicosapentaenoic acid reduces and stabilizes atherosclerotic lesions in ApoE-deficient mice. *Atherosclerosis* **2008**, *197*, 524–533. [CrossRef] [PubMed]
7. Orr, A.W.; Hastings, N.E.; Blackman, B.R.; Wamhoff, B.R. Complex regulation and function of the inflammatory smooth muscle cell phenotype in atherosclerosis. *J. Vasc. Res.* **2010**, *47*, 168–180.
8. Oh, D.Y.; Talukdar, S.; Bae, E.J.; Imamura, T.; Morinaga, H.; Fan, W.; Li, P.; Lu, W.J.; Watkins, S.M.; Olefsky, J.M. Gpr120 is an omega-3 fatty acid receptor mediating potent anti-inflammatory and insulin-sensitizing effects. *Cell* **2010**, *142*, 687–698. [CrossRef] [PubMed]
9. Schwab, J.M.; Chiang, N.; Arita, M.; Serhan, C.N. Resolvin E1 and protectin D1 activate inflammation-resolution programmes. *Nature* **2007**, *447*, 869–874. [CrossRef] [PubMed]
10. Ishikado, A.; Nishio, Y.; Morino, K.; Ugi, S.; Kondo, H.; Makino, T.; Kashiwagi, A.; Maegawa, H. Low concentration of 4-hydroxy hexenal increases heme oxygenase-1 expression through activation of Nrf2 and antioxidative activity in vascular endothelial cells. *Biochem. Biophys. Res. Commun.* **2010**, *402*, 99–104. [CrossRef] [PubMed]
11. Ishikado, A.; Morino, K.; Nishio, Y.; Nakagawa, F.; Mukose, A.; Sono, Y.; Yoshioka, N.; Kondo, K.; Sekine, O.; Yoshizaki, T.; *et al.* 4-hydroxy hexenal derived from docosahexaenoic acid protects endothelial cells via Nrf2 activation. *PLoS ONE* **2013**, *8*, e69415. [CrossRef] [PubMed]

12. Itoh, K.; Tong, K.I.; Yamamoto, M. Molecular mechanism activating Nrf2-keap1 pathway in regulation of adaptive response to electrophiles. *Free Radic. Biol. Med.* **2004**, *36*, 1208–1213. [CrossRef] [PubMed]
13. Wakabayashi, N.; Dinkova-Kostova, A.T.; Holtzclaw, W.D.; Kang, M.I.; Kobayashi, A.; Yamamoto, M.; Kensler, T.W.; Talalay, P. Protection against electrophile and oxidant stress by induction of the phase 2 response: Fate of cysteines of the keap1 sensor modified by inducers. *Proc. Natl. Acad. Sci. USA* **2004**, *101*, 2040–2045. [CrossRef] [PubMed]
14. Kusunoki, C.; Yang, L.; Yoshizaki, T.; Nakagawa, F.; Ishikado, A.; Kondo, M.; Morino, K.; Sekine, O.; Ugi, S.; Nishio, Y.; *et al.* Omega-3 polyunsaturated fatty acid has an anti-oxidant effect via the Nrf-2/Ho-1 pathway in 3T3-L1 adipocytes. *Biochem. Biophys. Res. Commun.* **2013**, *430*, 225–230. [CrossRef] [PubMed]
15. Nakagawa, F.; Morino, K.; Ugi, S.; Ishikado, A.; Kondo, K.; Sato, D.; Konno, S.; Nemoto, K.; Kusunoki, C.; Sekine, O.; *et al.* 4-hydroxy hexenal derived from dietary *n*-3 polyunsaturated fatty acids induces anti-oxidative enzyme heme oxygenase-1 in multiple organs. *Biochem. Biophys. Res. Commun.* **2014**, *443*, 991–996. [CrossRef]
16. Stulnig, G.; Frisch, M.T.; Crnkovic, S.; Stiegler, P.; Sereinigg, M.; Stacher, E.; Olschewski, H.; Olschewski, A.; Frank, S. Docosahexaenoic acid (DHA)-induced heme oxygenase-1 attenuates cytotoxic effects of DHA in vascular smooth muscle cells. *Atherosclerosis* **2013**, *230*, 406–413. [CrossRef] [PubMed]
17. Yang, Y.C.; Lii, C.K.; Wei, Y.L.; Li, C.C.; Lu, C.Y.; Liu, K.L.; Chen, H.W. Docosahexaenoic acid inhibition of inflammation is partially via cross-talk between Nrf2/heme oxygenase 1 and IKK/NF-κB pathways. *J. Nutr. Biochem.* **2013**, *24*, 204–212. [CrossRef] [PubMed]
18. Okamura, T.; Tawa, M.; Geddawy, A.; Shimosato, T.; Iwasaki, H.; Shintaku, H.; Yoshida, Y.; Masada, M.; Shinozaki, K.; Imamura, T. Effects of atorvastatin, amlodipine, and their combination on vascular dysfunction in insulin-resistant rats. *J. Pharmacol. Sci.* **2014**, *124*, 76–85. [CrossRef] [PubMed]
19. Folch, J.; Lees, M.; Stanley, G.H.S. A simple method for the isolation and purification of total lipides from animal tissues. *J. Biol. Chem.* **1957**, *226*, 497–509. [PubMed]
20. Obata, T.; Kashiwagi, A.; Maegawa, H.; Nishio, Y.; Ugi, S.; Hidaka, H.; Kikkawa, R. Insulin signaling and its regulation of system A amino acid uptake in cultured rat vascular smooth muscle cells. *Circ. Res.* **1996**, *79*, 1167–1176. [CrossRef] [PubMed]
21. O'Brien-Coker, I.C.; Perkins, G.; Mallet, A.I. Aldehyde analysis by high performance liquid chromatography/tandem mass spectrometry. *Rapid. Commun. Mass Spectrom.* **2001**, *15*, 920–928. [CrossRef]
22. Calder, P.C. The role of marine omega-3 (*n*-3) fatty acids in inflammatory processes, atherosclerosis and plaque stability. *Mol. Nutr. Food Res.* **2012**, *56*, 1073–1080. [CrossRef] [PubMed]
23. Thies, F.; Garry, J.M.; Yaqoob, P.; Rerkasem, K.; Williams, J.; Shearman, C.P.; Gallagher, P.J.; Calder, P.C.; Grimble, R.F. Association of *n*-3 polyunsaturated fatty acids with stability of atherosclerotic plaques: A randomised controlled trial. *Lancet* **2003**, *361*, 477–485. [CrossRef]
24. Jeong, S.; Jing, K.; Kim, N.; Shin, S.; Kim, S.; Song, K.S.; Heo, J.Y.; Park, J.H.; Seo, K.S.; Han, J.; *et al.* Docosahexaenoic acid-induced apoptosis is mediated by activation of mitogen-activated protein kinases in human cancer cells. *BMC Cancer* **2014**, *14*, 481. [CrossRef] [PubMed]
25. Diep, Q.N.; Touyz, R.M.; Schiffrin, E.L. Docosahexaenoic acid, a peroxisome proliferator-activated receptor-alpha ligand, induces apoptosis in vascular smooth muscle cells by stimulation of p38 mitogen-activated protein kinase. *Hypertension* **2000**, *36*, 851–855. [CrossRef] [PubMed]
26. Lee, J.Y.; Je, J.H.; Kim, D.H.; Chung, S.W.; Zou, Y.; Kim, N.D.; Yoo, M. A.; Suck Baik, H.; Yu, B.P.; Chung, H.Y. Induction of endothelial apoptosis by 4-hydroxyhexenal. *Eur. J. Biochem.* **2004**, *271*, 1339–1347. [CrossRef] [PubMed]
27. Yoo, A.R.; Koh, S.H.; Cho, G.W.; Kim, S.H. Inhibitory effects of cilostazol on proliferation of vascular smooth muscle cells (VSMCs) through suppression of the ERK1/2 pathway. *J. Atheroscler. Thromb.* **2010**, *17*, 1009–1018. [CrossRef] [PubMed]
28. Kwak, S.M.; Myung, S.K.; Lee, Y.J.; Seo, H.G.; the Korean Meta-analysis Study Group. Efficacy of omega-3 fatty acid supplements (eicosapentaenoic acid and docosahexaenoic acid) in the secondary prevention of cardiovascular disease: A meta-analysis of randomized, double-blind, placebo-controlled trials. *Arch. Intern. Med.* **2012**, *172*, 686–694. [PubMed]
29. Dong, X.; Bi, L.; He, S.; Meng, G.; Wei, B.; Jia, S.; Liu, J. FFAs-ROS-ERK/P38 pathway plays a key role in adipocyte lipotoxicity on osteoblasts in co-culture. *Biochimie* **2014**, *101*, 123–131. [CrossRef] [PubMed]

30. Zhou, L.; Cai, X.; Han, X.; Ji, L. P38 plays an important role in glucolipotoxicity-induced apoptosis in INS-1 cells. *J. Diabetes Res.* **2014**, *2014*. [CrossRef] [PubMed]
31. Anderson, E.J.; Thayne, K.; Harris, M.; Carraway, K.; Shaikh, S.R. Aldehyde stress and up-regulation of Nrf2-mediated antioxidant systems accompany functional adaptations in cardiac mitochondria from mice fed *n*-3 polyunsaturated fatty acids. *Biochem. J.* **2012**, *441*, 359–366. [CrossRef] [PubMed]
32. Gladine, C.; Roy, N.C.; Rigaudière, J.P.; Laillet, B.; da Silva, G.; Joly, C.; Pujos-Guillot, E.; Morio, B.; Feillet-Coudray, C.; McNabb, W.C.; *et al.* Increasing intake of long-chain *n*-3 PUFA enhances lipoperoxidation and modulates hepatic gene expression in a dose-dependent manner. *Br. J. Nutr.* **2012**, *107*, 1254–1273. [CrossRef] [PubMed]
33. Calzada, C.; Colas, R.; Guillot, N.; Guichardant, M.; Laville, M.; Véricel, E.; Lagarde, M. Subgram daily supplementation with docosahexaenoic acid protects low-density lipoproteins from oxidation in healthy men. *Atherosclerosis* **2010**, *208*, 467–472. [CrossRef] [PubMed]
34. Kondo, K.; Morino, K.; Nishio, Y.; Kondo, M.; Nakao, K.; Nakagawa, F.; Ishikado, A.; Sekine, O.; Yoshizaki, T.; Kashiwagi, A.; *et al.* A fish-based diet intervention improves endothelial function in postmenopausal women with type 2 diabetes mellitus: A randomized crossover trial. *Metabolism* **2014**, *63*, 930–940. [CrossRef] [PubMed]
35. Chen, D.Z.; Auborn, K. Fish oil constituent docosahexa-enoic acid selectively inhibits growth of human papillomavirus immortalized keratinocytes. *Carcinogenesis* **1999**, *20*, 249–254. [CrossRef] [PubMed]

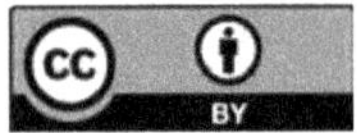

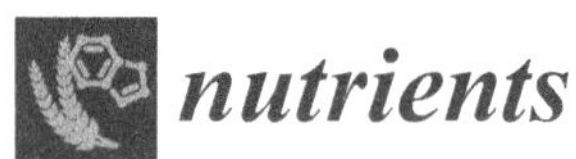

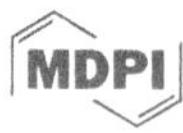

Article

Four Models Including Fish, Seafood, Red Meat and Enriched Foods to Achieve Australian Dietary Recommendations for *n*-3 LCPUFA for All Life-Stages

Flavia Fayet-Moore [1,*], Katrine Baghurst [2,†] and Barbara J. Meyer [3]

1 Nutrition Research Australia, Level 13/167 Macquarie St, Sydney, NSW 2000, Australia
2 CSIRO and consultant, Adelaide, SA 5000, Australia
3 School of Medicine, University of Wollongong, Northfields Ave, Wollongong, NSW 2522, Australia; bmeyer@uow.edu.au
* Correspondence: flavia@nraus.com; Tel.: +61-(2)-8667-3072; Fax: +61-(2)-8667-3200
† Deceased in December 2012.

Received: 31 August 2015 ; Accepted: 8 October 2015 ; Published: 16 October 2015

Abstract: Populations are not meeting recommended intakes of omega-3 long chain polyunsaturated fatty acids (*n*-3 LCPUFA). The aim was (i) to develop a database on *n*-3 LCPUFA enriched products; (ii) to undertake dietary modelling exercise using four dietary approaches to meet the recommendations and (iii) to determine the cost of the models. Six *n*-3 LCPUFA enriched foods were identified. Fish was categorised by *n*-3 LCPUFA content (mg/100 g categories as "excellent" "good" and "moderate"). The four models to meet recommended *n*-3 LCPUFA intakes were (i) fish only; (ii) moderate fish (with red meat and enriched foods); (iii) fish avoiders (red meat and enriched foods only); and (iv) lacto-ovo vegetarian diet (enriched foods only). Diets were modelled using the NUTTAB2010 database and *n*-3 LCPUFA were calculated and compared to the Suggested Dietary Targets (SDT). The cost of meeting these recommendations was calculated per 100 mg *n*-3 LCPUFA. The SDT were achieved for all life-stages with all four models. The weekly food intake in number of serves to meet the *n*-3 LCPUFA SDT for all life-stages for each dietary model were: (i) 2 "excellent" fish; (ii) 1 "excellent" and 1 "good" fish, and depending on life-stage, 3–4 lean red meat, 0–2 eggs and 3–26 enriched foods; (iii) 4 lean red meat, and 20–59 enriched foods; (iv) 37–66 enriched foods. Recommended intakes of *n*-3 LCPUFA were easily met by the consumption of fish, which was the cheapest source of *n*-3 LCPUFA. Other strategies may be required to achieve the recommendations including modifying the current food supply through feeding practices, novel plant sources and more enriched foods.

Keywords: omega-3 long chain polyunsaturated fatty acids (*n*-3 LCPUFA); recommended intakes; suggested dietary target intakes; omega-3 (*n*-3) enriched foods; dietary modelling

---

1. Introduction

There is a growing body of evidence worldwide that the consumption of omega-3 long-chain polyunsaturated fatty acids (*n*-3 LCPUFA), namely eicosapentaenoic acid (EPA), docosapentaenoic acid (DPA) and docosahexaenoic acid (DHA), is associated with numerous health outcomes, specifically in cardiovascular disease prevention [1,2]. The National Health and Medical Research Council (NHMRC) has set Nutrient Reference Values (NRV) for *n*-3 LCPUFA [3], which differ by life-stage and gender. The NHMRC Suggested Dietary Targets (SDT) is defined as "A daily average intake from food and beverages for certain nutrients that that may help in prevention of chronic disease". The SDT apply to adults and adolescents 14 years and over and the SDT for *n*-3 LCPUFA are set at 610 mg/day for men and 430 mg/day for women. The International Society for the Study of Fatty Acids and Lipids (ISSFAL) and the National Heart Foundation of Australia (NHFA) recommends that all Australians consume 500 mg of *n*-3 LCPUFA per day to lower the risk of heart disease [4,5]. Other countries recommend the consumption of two fish meals per week which is equivalent to 500 mg *n*-3 LCPUFA per day [6–11].

In recognition of the importance of DHA during pregnancy and lactation, the European Consensus statement [12], the World Health Organization guidelines [13] and a European consensus statement [14] all recommend 200 mg DHA/day for pregnant women, whilst the International Society for the Study of Fatty Acids and Lipids (ISSFAL) recommend 300 mg DHA during pregnancy and lactation [4]. Despite the international recommendation for DHA during pregnancy, many pregnant women lack the understanding and knowledge of the importance of DHA [15] and also do not meet the recommendation of 200 mg DHA per day [16]. A useful pamphlet has been developed specifically designed to increase awareness of DHA for pregnant women and consequently increase *n*-3 LCPUFA intake [17].

A small study in the Illawarra region of New South Wales, Australia showed that the median intake of *n*-6 and *n*-3 PUFA was 9.9 g and 1.2 g per day respectively [18]. Similar results were found from the National Nutrition Survey (NNS, *n* = 13,858) where the intakes of *n*-6 and *n*-3 PUFA were 10.9 and 1.36 g per day respectively [19], showing that Australians consume 8 times more *n*-6 PUFA than *n*-3 PUFA. Furthermore, the linoleic acid intakes were 10.64 g per day and the DHA intakes were only 0.1 g per day [20]. A study by Lassek *et al.* showed that DHA from breast milk was positively associated with cognitive performance, whilst LA from breastmilk was negatively associated with cognitive performance [21], suggesting that increased consumption of *n*-3 PUFA including DHA is warranted. The main dietary source of *n*-3 LCPUFA is fish/seafood (66%), followed by meat/poultry/game (29%) and eggs (5%) [18], with similar results from the NNS, with fish/seafood (71%), meat/poultry/game (20%) and eggs (6%) the major contributors to *n*-3 LCPUFA intakes [19]. Given that meat/poultry/game contributed at least 20% to *n*-3 LCPUFA intakes, this NNS was re-analysed after analytical fatty acid data became available on meat [22]. The re-analysed NNS showed that the previous reports under-estimated the contribution of meat to the *n*-3 LCPUFA intakes, as meat contributed close to 50% of *n*-3 LCPUFA intakes [20,23]. This is not because meat itself is a rich source of *n*-3 LCPUFA but because Australians consume at least 7 times more meat than fish/seafood [18–20]. Concurrently, recent reports on consumption show that Australians are not meeting *n*-3 LCPUFA recommendations [19,24–26]. Hence, there is a need to explore more practical options of achieving the recommended *n*-3 LCPUFA intake that provide consumers with a range of food-based choices to meet their dietary needs.

Although some groups have suggested the use of *n*-3 LCPUFA enriched foods [4,27–29] to meet recommendations, none have specified amounts of *n*-3 LCPUFA-enriched foods and beverages that need to be consumed to meet recommendations and that are commercially available. Food-based guidelines for meeting the recommended target of 500 mg per day of combined docosahexaenoic acid (DHA) and eicosapentaenoic acid (EPA) typically focus on: "*2–3 serves (150 g) of oily fish per week*" [5]. Whilst enriched foods and drinks are mentioned in recommendations, there is little dietary information available for consumers on alternative ways to meet daily or weekly *n*-3 LCPUFA intake. Despite many food products being enriched with *n*-3 LCPUFA in Australia, there is no comprehensive, up-to-date database on these foods.

Therefore, the aim of this study was (i) to develop a database on *n*-3 LCPUFA enriched foods and beverages; (ii) to undertake dietary modelling exercises using four dietary approaches to meet the nationally-set recommended *n*-3 LCPUFA intake for different life-stages; and (iii) to determine the cost of obtaining 100 mg of *n*-3 LCPUFA from the different food sources.

2. Experimental Section

2.1. Database

A supermarket trawl was undertaken to identify all *n*-3 LCPUFA enriched products available from four supermarkets in the metropolitan areas of Wollongong and Sydney in New South Wales, Australia. All *n*-3 LCPUFA enriched products were identified and the full name of the food, serving size, energy, macronutrient and total polyunsaturated fat, total *n*-6, total *n*-3, alpha-linoleic acid (ALA), EPA, DHA and total *n*-3 LCPUFA were recorded where available. In addition, the *n*-3 source was noted and cost per serve, as well as per 100 g, was calculated. A total of six products were identified and used in the modelling (see Appendix Table A1). These products included *n*-3 LCPUFA enriched bread, eggs, yoghurt, milk, flavoured beverage powder, and almond meal.

2.2. Models

Foods were included in the model if they met the Food Standards Australia New Zealand (FSANZ) Food Standards Code for voluntary *n*-3 fatty acid nutrition claims [30]. A claim that a food is a "source" of *n*-3 PUFA must contain no less than 200 g of ALA or 30 mg total EPA and DHA per serve, while a "good source" must contain no less than 60 mg total EPA and DHA per serve. Docosapentaenoic acid (DPA) is not included in the content claim recommendations, even though it contributes to *n*-3 LCPUFA intakes [2,19,23]. Serving sizes were consistent with National Dietary Guidelines for Australians [31] and set at 100 g of cooked fish or meat.

Diets were modelled using the NUTTAB2010 foods database [32]. Three subgroups of fish were developed based on *n*-3 LCPUFA content. Fish was categorized by *n*-3 LCPUFA content as "excellent" (⩾1200 mg/100 g), "good" (200–1200 mg/100 g) and "moderate" (<200 mg/100 g) (Table 1).

The average *n*-3 LCPUFA content of all meats were calculated using NUTTAB2010 by averaging *n*-3 LCPUFA content of all cooked lean cuts of meat. Red meat (beef, lamb, veal) and pork, met the FSANZ source claim of at least 30 mg of DHA and EPA per serve (100 g). Pork and chicken were not used in the dietary modelling due to their lower *n*-3 LCPUFA content compared to red meat. The average *n*-3 LCPUFA (DHA, EPA, DPA) for red meat, including beef, lamb and veal, was set at 119 mg/100 g, and a cut with approximately 119 mg/100 g serve was used in the model (e.g., beef mince, lamb shanks, scotch fillet).

Table 1. Types of fish and red meat used in the model categorized by content of *n*-3 LCPUFA.

Excellent Source of *n*-3 LCPUFA Fish	Good Source of *n*-3 LCPUFA Fish	Moderate Source of *n*-3 LCPUFA Fish and Red Meat
⩾1200 mg/100 g	*200–1200 mg/100 g*	*<200 mg/100 g*
Salmon, trout, silver perch, canned salmon (pink or red)	Smoked salmon, bream, anchovy, mullet, tinned tuna, snapper, flathead, calamari/squid, oysters, mussels	Barramundi, whiting, tilapia, prawn, fish fingers, shark (flake), fish cake, fish battered Beef, lamb, veal

Four dietary models were developed and calculated based on weekly intake. Model 1 included fish/seafood only (high fish consumers) equivalent of 2–3 "excellent/moderate" LC *n*-3 fish serves/week. Model 2 included some fish (moderate fish consumers) and equivalent to a maximum of 1 "excellent" LC *n*-3 fish serve/week in addition to lean red meat, eggs and *n*-3 LCPUFA enriched foods. Model 3 did not include fish, but did include lean red meat, eggs and *n*-3 LCPUFA enriched foods (non-fish consumers). Model 4 included only *n*-3 LCPUFA enriched foods (suitable for lacto-ovo vegetarian diets). Within each model, serves of red meat and fish as well as dairy and eggs were modelled based on the National Dietary Guidelines for Australians. Red meat was maximized at 3–4 weekly serves, fish at 2–3 weekly serves, dairy at three serves per day, eggs at six per week and bread at up to six slices or three serves per day.

2.3. Recommended Intake

The total n-3 LCPUFA in each model was calculated and compared to the NHMRC NRV SDT [3]. The SDT was multiplied by seven to calculate weekly target intakes. The NHMRC have SDT for n-3 LCPUFA for 14 year olds and older males at 610 mg/day and for females at 430 mg/day [3]. For the purposes of this modelling exercise, the SDT were adjusted for other age groups based on the age and sex-specific energy intakes for each age group [25]. For example, mean energy intake for 2–3 year old boys was 53% of that of 14–16 year olds [20], and hence the adjusted SDT (aSDT) for n-3 LCPUFA for 2–3 year old boys (323 mg/day) was set at 53% of the SDT for 14–16 year olds (610 mg/day). The other age groups were calculated according to their proportion of energy intake. Similar calculations were carried out for the various age groups for girls, using 430 mg per day for the 14–16 year old girls [26].

2.4. Cost Analysis

Average costs per pack in Australian dollars, per 100 g and per serve were recorded during the supermarket trawl and obtained online. The price for each popular lean cut of meat was obtained for supermarket-branded meats and averaged for beef, lamb and veal; lean red meat was calculated using the ratio of (beef + veal): lamb, or 4.3:1. Cost per 100 g (cooked weight) of lean red meat was then calculated. For fish and seafood, the average price of fresh, frozen and tinned/processed forms were obtained. The cost of obtaining 100 mg of n-3 LCPUFA for each diet modelled was calculated.

n-3 LCPUFA values for classification into "excellent", "good" and "moderate" were taken from NUTTAB 2010 (http://www.foodstandards.gov.au/consumerinformation/nuttab2010/).

3. Results

All four dietary models were able to meet the SDT for all life stages (Table 2). In model 1 the recommended SDT were easily met for all life-stages with two serves of "excellent" sources of n-3 LCPUFA (Table 1). At three serves of fish per week, SDT were met if one serve was an "excellent" source (Table 1) and the other two serves were "good" sources. Specifically for children, the SDT were met by a combination of "excellent" and "moderate" n-3 LCPUFA fish sources. For example, a 2–3 year old child could consume 100 g tinned salmon (an "excellent" source), and 100 g tinned tuna (a "good" source) to meet their weekly SDT.

In model 2 (Table 2), the type of fish was maximised at one serve of "excellent" fish per week and, therefore, a weekly intake of one "moderate" or "good" source of fish, four red meat serves (maximum serves per dietary guidelines) and the inclusion of three to 26 weekly serves of n-3 LCPUFA enriched foods (including enriched and non-enriched eggs) was necessary to meet the SDT recommendations. For children, where the SDT is lower than adults (see methods), a combination of "good" and "moderate" sources of fish was sufficient. The SDT for all children could be met with either: two fish serves per week (a "good" and a "moderate" source) and meat and enriched foods; or one serve of fish per week (an "excellent" source) and enriched foods. For 2–3 year old children as an example, 100 g of crumbed fish cake made with salmon (a "good" source), 100 g crumbed fish fingers (a "moderate" source), 300 g of mince, 3 n-3 LCPUFA enriched eggs and 7 × 90 g n-3 LCPUFA enriched yoghurts would be needed per week to meet their weekly SDT. For adult males using model 2, the SDT was reached with two serves of fish (an "excellent" and a "moderate" source), 400 g of lean beef, six enriched eggs, eight cups of milk and 10 slices of bread per week.

In model 3 (Table 2), where individuals do not consume fish, the maximum recommended four serves of red meat intake was necessary to meet the SDT for all life stages. All egg intake had to be n-3 LCPUFA enriched and up to 59 weekly serves, or about 8 serves per day of n-3 LCPUFA enriched products per day were also necessary. For a 2–3 year old child, this translates to 400 g mince, 6 n-3 LCPUFA enriched eggs and 3 cups of n-3 LCPUFA enriched milk a week, and approximately two slices of n-3 LCPUFA enriched bread and just over 100 g of n-3 LCPUFA enriched yoghurt per day. A sample diet to meet the SDT for adults of all life stages would be 400 g beef, six enriched eggs, two kilograms of yoghurt, 28 slices of bread and 11 cups of milk per week.

Table 2. Weekly food intake to meet the Suggested Dietary Target (SDT) *n*-3 LCPUFA intakes for all life-stages (2y+).

Food	**Model 1** *Fish Only*		**Model 2** *Moderate Fish*		**Model 3** *No fish*		**Model 4** *Vegetarian*	
	Serves	**Sample Diet**	**Serves**	**Sample Diet**	**Serves**	**Sample Diet**	**Serves**	**Sample Diet**
Fish	2 serves of "excellent" fish	100 g Atlantic salmon 200 g fish cake made with salmon	1 serve of "excellent" fish plus 1 serve of "good" or "moderate" fish	100 g Atlantic salmon 100 g King prawns	Nil	Nil	Nil	1
Lean red meat	Nil	Nil	3–4 serves	400 g beef	4 serves	400 g beef	Nil	Nil
Eggs [1]	Nil	Nil	0–2 serves	Nil	Nil	Nil	Nil	Nil
n-3 LCPUFA enriched foods [2]	Nil	Nil	3–26 serves	6 eggs 10 slices bread 8 cups milk	20–59 serves (3–8 serves per day)	6 eggs 21 × 90 g tubs of yoghurt 28 slices bread 10.5 cups milk 7 serves beverage powder	37–66 serves (5–9 serves)	6 *n*-3 eggs 21 × 90 g tubs of yoghurt 28 slices bread 2 Friands made with DHA almond meal 16 cups milk 7 serves of beverage powder

Model 1—2–3 serves of fish serves per week only (no red meat or *n*-3 LCPUFA enriched foods); Model 2—Maximum of 1 "excellent" source of *n*-3 LCPUFA fish per week with red meat and *n*-3 LCPUFA enriched foods; Model 3—Red meat and *n*-3 LCPUFA enriched foods only (no fish); Model 4—*n*-3 LCPUFA enriched foods only suitable for lacto-ovo vegetarians. [1] Whole non-enriched eggs; [2] Includes *n*-3 LCPUFA enriched eggs.

Model 4, the lacto-ovo vegetarian diet (Table 2) excludes two significant sources of n-3 LCPUFA, namely fish and red meat (beef/veal/lamb) and therefore the remaining source of n-3 LCPUFA in the diet included only n-3 LCPUFA enriched foods and eggs, which are maximised at six eggs per week by the National Heart Foundation recommendation. In order to meet the SDT for all life stages, a minimum of 37 and a maximum of 66 n-3 LCPUFA enriched food serves need to be consumed in one week. This translates to all milk, bread and egg consumption to be in the n-3 LCPUFA enriched form. An adult would need to consume enriched foods in model 3 plus 2 Friands (a type of muffin traditionally made with almond meal and popular in Australia) made with DHA almond meal and 5.5 cups of milk per week to meet their SDT.

The amount of n-3 LCPUFA (g per 100 g), the average cost per 100 g of food (fish or enriched food) and the cost per 100 mg of n-3 LCPUFA is shown in Figure 1. Excellent sources of fish (sardines and salmon) are amongst the most expensive foods but they provide the most n-3 LCPUFA and hence are the least expensive when expressed as cost per delivery of 100 mg n-3 LCPUFA. Lean meats are comparable in cost to excellent sources of fish but contain far less n-3 LCPUFA than fish and therefore are amongst the highest cost per delivery of 100 mg n-3 LCPUFA. The n-3 enriched foods have very low levels of n-3 LCPUFA per 100 g of food and hence the cost per delivery of 100 mg n-3 LCPUFA is much higher than fish. Excellent sources of fish provide the greatest amount of n-3 LCPUFA and the cost per 100 mg n-3 LCPUFA is the least (Figure 1). Fish oil supplements also provide high levels of n-3 LCPUFA and the cost per delivery of 100 mg n-3 LCPUFA is approximately 0.04 AUD. Unlike supplements that only provide vitamin E, the foods provide other nutrients in addition to n-3 LCPUFA: fish provides selenium, iodine, zinc; eggs provide iodine, selenium and biotin; meats provide iron, vitamin B_{12} and zinc; yoghurt and milk provide calcium; and bread provides fibre.

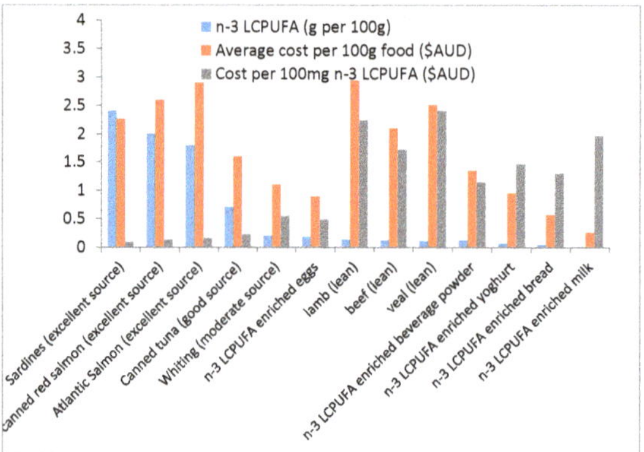

Figure 1. The amount of n-3 PUFA in fish and enriched foods, average cost * per 100 g of food and per 100 mg of n-3 LCPUFA. (* Cost estimated in December 2012.) Almond meal was excluded from the figure due to very low n-3 LCPUFA content.

4. Discussion

The nutritional intakes of n-3 LCPUFA (and DHA) of Australian men is 0.298 g per day (0.117 g per day); of Australian women is 0.195 g per day (0.083 g per day); of Australian elderly people is 0.219 g per day (0.096 g per day) [20] and of pregnant women 0.263 g per day (0.099 g per day) [16]. The SDT for n-3 LCPUFA were achieved for all life-stages with all four dietary models. The weekly food intake to meet the n-3 LCPUFA SDT for all life-stages for each dietary model was: 2 serves of an "excellent" source of n-3 LCPUFA fish (Model 1), 1 serve of an "excellent" and 1 serve of a "good" source of n-3 LCPUFA fish, 3–4 serves of lean red meat, 0–2 serves of eggs and 3–26 serves of n-3 LCPUFA enriched foods (Model 2), 4 serves of lean red meat, and 20–59 serves of n-3 LCPUFA enriched foods (Model 3), 37–66 serves of n-3 LCPUFA enriched foods (Model 4).

In the Australian diet, the median *n*-3 LCPUFA intake in adults (*n* = 10,851) was approximately 125 mg/day [22], which is well under the target of 500 mg/day [5]. A more recent Australian National Nutrition Survey conducted in 4487 children aged 2–16 years old showed that the median intakes ranged from 56 mg/day (2–3 years old) to 98 mg/day (14–16 years old) and only 6% of children met the SDT for *n*-3 LCPUFA per day [26]. Therefore, there is a need to increase *n*-3 LCPUFA in the diets of Australian adults and children in order to meet the SDT.

Fish/seafood, meat, eggs, *n*-3 LCPUFA enriched products and supplements are virtually the only sources of *n*-3 LCPUFA in Australia. Despite fish and seafood being the richest source of *n*-3 LCPUFA, they are not widely consumed by adults and children [33]. Based on the 1995 National Nutrition Survey and the 2007 Australian National Children's Nutrition and Physical Activity, the mean daily fish consumption in Australia was approximately 27 g for adults [33] and 13 g for children, whilst the median fish intake was zero [26]. Only 20% of children consumed fish or seafood and of the children that did consume fish and seafood, these children were originally born in countries where fish/seafood is traditionally eaten, like Japan, Korea and the Seychelles [26]. However the vast majority of Australians consume meat in quantities at least 7 times greater than fish/seafood [18–20,26], hence meat has been shown to be a major contributor of *n*-3 LCPUFA intake (47%) to the Australian diet [19,20,22,25,26]. In the model for fish avoiders (model 3), approximately half of the *n*-3 LCPUFA was derived from lean red meat and half from *n*-3 LCPUFA enriched products. Interestingly, increased meat consumption has been shown to be associated with lower odds of depression [34].

Diets that exclude fish, red meat and eggs are usually lower in *n*-3 LCPUFA [35]. The plant-based *n*-3 PUFA ALA can be converted into EPA and DHA, but the conversion rate is very inefficient [36,37]. Therefore, a lacto-ovo vegetarian diet would need to include *n*-3 LCPUFA enriched products or, alternatively, take encapsulated fish oil or micro-algal oil. However, long-term consumption of encapsulated fish oil may not be feasible for many individuals due to compliance, while enriched foods have been shown to be effective in increasing LC *n*-3 intake and status [27,38]. Therefore, the food industry is encouraged to develop a wider range of enriched staple food products with higher concentrations of *n*-3 LCPUFA that include both algal and fish sources of *n*-3 LCPUFA.

It is possible to meet *n*-3 LCPUFA intake with enriched foods, but it may not be feasible or practical long-term, due to the source of *n*-3 LCPUFA and the increased cost associated with enriched foods. Some enriched foods such as the almond meal, bread and the powdered beverage drink all use tuna oil as the source of *n*-3 LCPUFA. Therefore, these products would only be suitable for vegetarians that include fish in their diets. In addition, there is the burden of increased cost associated with a diet high in *n*-3 LCPUFA enriched products, as these products are more expensive than the un-enriched varieties. Lacto-ovo vegetarians may need to take algal supplements containing *n*-3 LCPUFA in order to meet SDT due to the unrealistic goal of consuming up to 66 serves of enriched foods per week. Furthermore, a recent Australian population based study by Rahmawaty *et al.* [39] showed that replacement of actual bread, milk, egg, and yoghurt consumption with *n*-3 LCPUFA enriched varieties, doubled the *n*-3 LCPUFA median intakes in non-fish consumers, without major dietary changes [39]. This doubling of intakes in non-fish consumers, still falls far short of the SDT, and hence there is a need for a wider range of enriched foods and supplements for lacto-ovo-vegetarians that include algal sources of *n*-3 LCPUFA.

The majority of Australians with low *n*-3 LCPUFA intake are people that do not consume fish/seafood since there are more non-fish consumers than consumers who do not meet the SDT for the prevention of chronic disease [40]. Furthermore, vegans have much lower *n*-3 status compared to omnivores [35], as they do not consume preformed *n*-3 LCPUFA in their diets and solely rely on the conversion of ALA to *n*-3 LCPUFA.

In terms of cost, on average the cost of quality lean red meat is similar to that of "excellent" and "good" sources of fish (Table 3). Fish is one of the cheapest sources when expressing the cost per 100 mg *n*-3 LCPUFA. Atlantic Salmon costs approximately 29 AUD per kilogram, but only costs

16 cents per 100 mg *n*-3 LCPUFA (equivalent to 80 cents per 500 mg *n*-3 LCPUFA). Meat is on average 25 AUD per kilogram, but costs 2 AUD per 100 mg *n*-3 LCPUFA (equivalent to $10 per 500 mg *n*-3 LCPUFA), which is more than 10-fold higher than Atlantic salmon. In terms of providing 100 mg *n*-3 LCPUFA, the *n*-3 LCPUFA enriched foods are comparable to, or slightly cheaper than, lean red meat, but are more expensive when compared to fish. Australians consume at least seven times more meat than fish [18] and on average consume 160 g per day [18], which demonstrates their willingness to pay for it. Given the similarities in cost per kilogram, fish is by far the better option when assessing the amount of *n*-3 LCPUFA per cost. However Australians do not consume fish for a variety of reasons including the smell, bones, pollutants, family members not liking it, taste, the preparation and price [41]. Amongst the fish consumers, price was the main negative effect for consuming fish [40,41], however, this study clearly shows that the average cost of fish is similar to that of lean red meat, yet fish supplies 10 times more *n*-3 LCPUFA than lean red meat.

Based on Australian food culture and eating patterns, non-fish sources of *n*-3 LCPUFA are increasingly important for meeting SDT for *n*-3 LCPUFA. The modelling research highlights the difficulties in currently meeting the SDT for *n*-3 LCPUFA if you are a non-fish or low-fish consumer, as very high and regular consumption of enriched food products are required. This may not be feasible for many consumers due to cost implications, compliance issues and availability of enriched products. Therefore, there is a need for a greater variety of staple foods enriched with *n*-3 LCPUFA, such as spreads, oils, breads and cereals, to make it easier for consumers to meet the SDT.

Better use of waste in existing fisheries [42,43] will contribute to sustainable sources of *n*-3 LCPUFA and a range of new research projects are underway to provide a range of sustainable long-term dietary solutions to meet *n*-3 LCPUFA needs. This includes research on land plant sources of *n*-3 LCPUFA [44] for use as feedstock in livestock production and aquaculture and novel plant sources of *n*-3 LCPUFA [45].

The easiest way of achieving the SDT for *n*-3 LCPUFA, is the consumption of two "excellent" or "good" fish meals per week. Furthermore, in addition to *n*-3 LCPUFA, fish also contains other vital nutrients like iodine, selenium, zinc, and is a good source of protein. Hence further research is required on how to encourage more frequent consumption of fish and seafood amongst Australian consumers.

5. Conclusions

The SDT can be achieved for adults and children with two serves of fish containing 2000 mg/100 g *n*-3 LCPUFA per week without red meat and enriched foods. Fish avoiders who consume red meat can meet SDT recommendations via four serves of red meat/week and at least 20 serves of enriched foods per week, while lacto-ovo vegetarians need at least 37 serves of enriched foods per week. These 4 modelled diets meet the SDT for all life stages. Therefore, Australians are encouraged to meet their *n*-3 LCPUFA intake by either: an increase in fish/seafood consumption from sustainable sources, or ensure that they meet *n*-3 LCPUFA recommendations by consuming a combination of red meat, *n*-3 LCPUFA enriched products and/or fish/algal supplements. Further research is required on how to encourage more frequent consumption of fish and seafood amongst Australian consumers.

Acknowledgments: This work received partial financial support from The Omega-3 Centre, Australia.

Author Contributions: All authors contributed to data analysis, interpretation and writing the manuscript. The authors' responsibilities were as follows—FFM developed the dietary models and calculated *n*-3 LC PUFA; KB provided guidance on model development and estimated age-specific SDT where necessary; BM provided guidance on dietary models and conducted the supermarket trawl and cost analysis; FFM drafted the manuscript with support from BM and KB; and FFM and KB critically reviewed and finalised the manuscript.

Conflicts of Interest: The authors declare no conflict of interest.

Appendix

Table A1. *n*-3 LCPUFA enriched products and the non-enriched varieties.

Food Type	Full Name of Food (Including Brand Name)	Serve Size (g)	Units per Serve	Serve Unit Name	Total FAT/100 g	*n*-3 LC PUFA mg/100 g	*n*-3 Source	Pack Size	Units per Pack	Average Price $/Pack	Average Price AUD/100 g AUD/Serve
Bread	Tip Top 1 Sunblest Up Omega-3 DHA wholemeal/sandwich bread	74–78 g	2	slice	3.5	44	Tuna oil 0.3%	700 g	18	3.98	0.57/100 g 0.45/serve
Bread	Tip Top 1 Sunblest Up Wholemeal Bread/White Sandwich	74–78 g	2	slice	3.5	N/A	N/A	650 g	18	3.99	0.57/100 g
Egg	Pace Farm Omega-3 Free Range Body Egg	102	2	egg	9.9	200	N/S	700 g	12	6.30	0.90/100 g 0.52/egg
Egg	Pace Farm Cage Eggs	102	2	egg	9.9	N/S	N/S	700 g	12	4.62	0.66/100 g 0.39/egg
Egg	Pace Farm Cage-Free Liberty Eggs	102	2	egg	9.9	N/S	N/S	700 g	12	5.35	0.76/100 g 0.45/egg
Egg	Veggs for Families Organic Grain Fed Hens	104	2	egg	10.1	110	N/S	700 g	12	5.99	0.90/100 g 0.50/egg
Egg	Farm Pride free range Omega 3 700 g	104	2	egg	9.4	110	Algal (Life's DHA)	700 g	12	6.49	0.93/100 g 0.54/egg
Egg	Farm Pride free range Omega 3 600 g	90	2	egg	9.15	50	Algal (Life's DHA)	600 g	12	6.49	1.08/100 g 0.54/egg
Eggs	Home Brand Woolworths	104	2	egg	9.9	110	N/S	700 g	12	2.69	0.38/100 g 0.22/egg
Eggs	Coles Free Range Eggs	104	2	egg	10.0	N/S	N/S	700 g	12	5.33	0.76/100 g 0.44/egg
Eggs	Ecoeggs	100	2	egg	10.1	230	N/S	550 g	10	6.42	0.64/egg 1.17/100 g
Yoghurt	Vaalia "My first yoghurt" for infants >6 months—Vanilla	60	1	cup	2.7	67	DHA algal oil	60 g	6	3.79	1.05/100 g 0.63/tub
Yoghurt	Vaalia for toddlers >12 months—Vanilla	90	1	cup	2.7	67	DHA algal oil	90 g	6	4.49	0.83/100 g 0.75/tub
Yoghurt	Vaalia for toddlers >12 months—Peach	90	1	cup	2.8	67	DHA algal oil	90 g	6	4.49	0.83/100 g 0.75/tub
Yoghurt	Vaalia for toddlers >12 months—Strawberry	90	1	cup	2.8	67	DHA algal oil	90 g	6	4.49	0.83/100 g 0.75/tub

Table A1. *Cont.*

Food Type	Full Name of Food (Including Brand Name)	Serve Size (g)	Units per Serve	Serve Unit Name	Total FAT/100 g	*n*-3 LC PUFA mg/100 g	*n*-3 Source	Pack Size	Units per Pack	Average Price $/Pack	Average Price AUD/100 g AUD/Serve
Yoghurt	Vaalia for toddlers yoghurt vanilla & peach	90	1	tub	3.1	N/A	N/A	90 g	6	4.89	0.91/100 g 0.82/tub
Yoghurt	baby Yoplait (for ages >6 months)—Pear/Peach	100	1	tub	3.1	N/A	N/A	100 g	4	3.99	1.00/100 g 1.00/tub
Milk	Dairy Farmers "Kids" Milk	250 mL	1	cup	3.4	120	*n*-3 DHA oil	1000 mL	4	2.69	0.27/100 mL 0.67/cup
Milk	Pura Kids Milk	250 mL	1	cup	8.5	30	Tuna oil	2000 mL	8	4.27	0.21/100 mL 0.53/cup
Milk	Dairy Farmers New Regular milk (2% fat)	250 mL	1	cup	2	N/A	N/A	1000 mL	4	2.24	0.56/cup 0.22/100 mL
Milk	Farmers Best—source of Omega-3	250 mL	1	cup	1.4	13.2	N/S	1000 mL	4	2.56	0.64/cup 0.26/100 mL
Milk	Farmers Best—Original	250 mL	1	cup	1.4	N/A	N/A	1000 mL	4	2.63	0.66/cup 0.26/100 mL
Milk beverage powder	Boost foods Nutriboost Chocolate	27	N/A	N/A	2.1	117	refined tuna oil	430 g	16	5.80	1.35/100 g 0.36/serve
Milk beverage powder	Boost foods Nutriboost Strawberry	43	N/A	N/A	1	117	refined tuna oil	430 g	10	5.80	1.35/100 g 0.58/serve
Baking	Lucky Almond Meal Omega 3	14 g *	N/A	N/A	50.6	0.12	tuna oil	100 g	N/A	3.73	3.73/100 g 0.52/serve
Baking	Lucky Almond Meal	14 g *	N/A	N/A	50.6	N/A	N/S	200 g	N/A	6.71	3.36/100 g 0.47/serve
Juice	Berri Australian Fresh Juice Orange Extra Pulp Omega	250 mL	1	cup	<1	50	fish oil	1000 mL	4	4.63	1.16/100 mL 1.16/serve
Juice	Berri Australian Fresh Orange Extra Pulp	250 mL	1	cup	<1	N/A	N/A	1000 mL	4	4.02	1.00/serve 1.00/100 mL

* 14 g is the equivalent used to make one Friand based on a standard Women's Weekly Magazine recipe. N/A—not applicable; N/S—not specified.

References

1. GISSI-Prevenzione Investigators (Gruppo Italiano per lo Studio della Sopravvivenza nell'Infarto miocardico). Dietary supplementation with *n*-3 polyunsaturated fatty acids and vitamin E after myocardial infarction: Results of the gissi-prevenzione trial. Gruppo Italiano per lo studio della sopravvivenza nell' infarto miocardico. *Lancet* **1999**, *354*, 447–455.
2. Yokoyama, M.; Origasa, H.; Matsuzaki, M.; Matsuzawa, Y.; Saito, Y.; Ishikawa, Y.; Oikawa, S.; Sasaki, J.; Hishida, H.; Itakura, H.; *et al.* Effects of eicosapentaenoic acid on major coronary events in hypercholesterolaemic patients (JELIS): A randomised open-label, blinded endpoint analysis. *Lancet* **2007**, *369*, 1090–1098. [CrossRef]
3. National Health and Medical Research Council. *Nutrient Refernce Values for Australia and New Zealand*; Commonwealth of Australia: Canberra, Australia, 2006.
4. Cunnane, S.; Drevon, C.; Harris, W.; Sinclair, A.; Spector, A. *Recommendations for Intake of Polyunsaturated Fatty Acids in Healthy Adults*; International Society for the Study of Fatty Acids (ISSFAL). Available online: http://www.issfal.org/statements/pufa-recommendations/statement-3 (accessed on 21 May 2013).
5. National Heart Foundation of Australia. *Position Statement. Dietary Fats and Dietary Cholesterol for Cardiovascular Health*; National Heart Foundation of Australia: Canberra, Australia, 2009.
6. American Heart Association Nutrition Committee; Lichtenstein, A.H.; Appel, L.J.; Brands, M.; Carnethon, M.; Daniels, S.; Franch, H.A.; Franklin, B.; Kris-Etherton, P.; Harris, W.S.; *et al.* Diet and lifestyle recommendations revision 2006: A scientific statement from the American Heart Association nutrition committee. *Circulation* **2006**, *114*, 82–96.
7. Brasseur, D.; Delzenne, N.; Henderickx, H.; Huyghebaert, A.; Kornitzer, M.; Ulens, M. *Recommendations and Claims Made on Omega-3 Fatty Acids*; Superior Health Council of Belgium: Brussel, Belgium, 2004.
8. Colquhoun, D.; Ferreira-Jardim, A.; Udell, T.; Eden, B. Nutrition andMetabolism Committee of the National Heart Foundation of Australia. In *National Heart Foundation of Australia Position Statement: Fish, Fish Oils, n-3 Polyunsaturated Fatty Acids and Cardiovascular Health*; National Heart Foundation of Australia: Canberra, Australia, 2008.
9. Kris-Etherton, P.M.; Innis, S.; Ammerican Dietetic Association; Dietitians of Canada. Position of the American Dietetic Association and Dietitians of Canada: Dietary fatty acids. *J. Am. Diet. Assoc.* **2007**, *107*, 1599–1611. [PubMed]
10. Health Council of Netherlands. *Guidelines for a Healthy Diet*; Health Council of the Netherlands: The Hague, The Netherlands, 2006.
11. Srinath Reddy, K.; Katan, M.B. Diet, nutrition and the prevention of hypertension and cardiovascular diseases. *Public Health Nutr.* **2004**, *7*, 167–186. [PubMed]
12. European Food Safety Authority. Scientific Opinion on Dietary Reference Values for fats, including saturated fatty acids, polyunsaturated fatty acids, monounsaturated fatty acids, trans fatty acids and cholesterol. *EFSA J.* **2010**, *8*, 1461. [CrossRef]
13. FAO/WHO. Interim summary of conclusions and dietary recommendations on total fat & fatty acids. In Proceedings of the Joint FAO/WHO Expert Consultation on Fats and Fatty Acids in Humen Nutrition, WHO HQ, Geneva, Switzerland, 10–14 November 2008.
14. Koletzko, B.; Cetin, I.; Brenna, J.T.; Perinatal Lipid Intake Working Group; Child Health Foundation; Diabetic Pregnancy Study Group; European Association of Perinatal Medicine; European Society for Clinical Nutrition and Metabolism; European Society for Paediatric Gastroenterology; Hepatology and Nutrition; *et al.* Dietary fat intakes for pregnant and lactating women. *Br. J. Nutr.* **2007**, *98*, 873–877. [PubMed]
15. Sinikovic, D.S.; Yeatman, H.R.; Cameron, D.; Meyer, B.J. Women's awareness of the importance of long-chain omega-3 polyunsaturated fatty acid consumption during pregnancy: Knowledge of risks, benefits and information accessibility. *Public Health Nutr.* **2009**, *12*, 562–569. [CrossRef] [PubMed]
16. Cosatto, V.F.; Else, P.L.; Meyer, B.J. Do pregnant women and those at risk of developing post-natal depression consume lower amounts of long chain omega-3 polyunsaturated fatty acids? *Nutrients* **2010**, *2*, 198–213. [CrossRef] [PubMed]
17. Emmett, R.; Akkersdyk, S.; Yeatman, H.; Meyer, B.J. Expanding awareness of docosahexaenoic acid during pregnancy. *Nutrients* **2013**, *5*, 1098–1109. [CrossRef] [PubMed]

18. Ollis, T.E.; Meyer, B.J.; Howe, P.R. Australian food sources and intakes of omega-6 and omega-3 polyunsaturated fatty acids. *Ann. Nutr. Metab.* **1999**, *43*, 346–355. [CrossRef] [PubMed]
19. Meyer, B.J.; Mann, N.J.; Lewis, J.L.; Milligan, G.C.; Sinclair, A.J.; Howe, P.R. Dietary intakes and food sources of omega-6 and omega-3 polyunsaturated fatty acids. *Lipids* **2003**, *38*, 391–398. [CrossRef] [PubMed]
20. Howe, P.; Meyer, B.; Record, S.; Baghurst, K. Dietary intake of long-chain omega-3 polyunsaturated fatty acids: Contribution of meat sources. *Nutrition* **2006**, *22*, 47–53. [CrossRef] [PubMed]
21. Lassek, W.D.; Gaulin, S.J. Linoleic and docosahexaenoic acids in human milk have opposite relationships with cognitive test performance in a sample of 28 countries. *Prostaglandins Leukot Essent. Fat. Acids* **2014**, *91*, 195–201. [CrossRef] [PubMed]
22. Williams, P. Nutritional composition of red meat. *Nutr. Diet.* **2007**, *64*, S113–S119. [CrossRef]
23. Howe, P.; Buckley, J.; Meyer, B. Long-chain omega-3 fatty acids in red meat. *Nutr. Diet.* **2007**, *64*, S135–S139. [CrossRef]
24. Meyer, B. Australian children dietary intakes with a focus on dietary fats. *Lipid Technol.* **2014**, *26*, 253–255. [CrossRef]
25. Meyer, B.J. Are we consuming enough long chain omega-3 polyunsaturated fatty acids for optimal health? *Prostaglandins Leukot Essent. Fat. Acids* **2011**, *85*, 275–280. [CrossRef] [PubMed]
26. Meyer, B.J.; Kolanu, N. Australian children are not consuming enough long-chain omega-3 polyunsaturated fatty acids for optimal health. *Nutrition* **2011**, *27*, 1136–1140. [CrossRef] [PubMed]
27. Murphy, K.J.; Meyer, B.J.; Mori, T.A.; Burke, V.; Mansour, J.; Patch, C.S.; Tapsell, L.C.; Noakes, M.; Clifton, P.A.; Barden, A.; *et al.* Impact of foods enriched with *n*-3 long-chain polyunsaturated fatty acids on erythrocyte *n*-3 levels and cardiovascular risk factors. *Br. J. Nutr.* **2007**, *97*, 749–757. [CrossRef] [PubMed]
28. Patch, C.S.; Tapsell, L.C.; Mori, T.A.; Meyer, B.J.; Murphy, K.J.; Mansour, J.; Noakes, M.; Clifton, P.M.; Puddey, I.B.; Beilin, L.J.; *et al.* The use of novel foods enriched with long-chain *n*-3 fatty acids to increase dietary intake: A comparison of methodologies assessing nutrient intake. *J. Am. Diet. Assoc.* **2005**, *105*, 1918–1926. [CrossRef] [PubMed]
29. Sioen, I.; Devroe, J.; Inghels, D.; Terwecoren, R.; de Henauw, S. The influence of *n*-3 PUFA supplements and *n*-3 PUFA enriched foods on the *n*-3 LC PUFA intake of flemish women. *Lipids* **2010**, *45*, 313–320. [CrossRef] [PubMed]
30. Food Standards Australia New Zealand. *Claims in Relation to Omega Fatty Acid Content of Foods*; Commonwealth of Australia: Canberra, Australia, 2000; pp. 68–69.
31. National Health & Medcial Research Council. *Dietary Guidelines for Australians*; Australian Government Publishing Service: Canberra, Australian, 2003.
32. Food Standards Australia New Zealand. *NUTTAB2010*; Food Standards Australia New Zealand: Canberra, Australia, 2006. Available online: http://www.foodstandards.gov.au/science/ monitoringnutrients/ nutrientables/pages/default.aspx (accessed on 10 October 2013).
33. McLennan, W.; Podge, A. *National Nutrition Nurvey Selected Highlights, Australia 1995*; Australian Government Publishing Service: Canberra, Australian, 1997.
34. Meyer, B.J.; Kolanu, N.; Griffiths, D.A.; Grounds, B.; Howe, P.R.; Kreis, I.A. Food groups and fatty acids associated with self-reported depression: An analysis from the australian national nutrition and health surveys. *Nutrition* **2013**, *29*, 1042–1047. [CrossRef] [PubMed]
35. Mann, N.; Pirotta, Y.; O'Connell, S.; Li, D.; Kelly, F.; Sinclair, A. Fatty acid composition of habitual omnivore and vegetarian diets. *Lipids* **2006**, *41*, 637–646. [CrossRef] [PubMed]
36. Burdge, G.C.; Finnegan, Y.E.; Minihane, A.M.; Williams, C.M.; Wootton, S.A. Effect of altered dietary *n*-3 fatty acid intake upon plasma lipid fatty acid composition, conversion of [13c]alpha-linolenic acid to longer-chain fatty acids and partitioning towards beta-oxidation in older men. *Br. J. Nutr.* **2003**, *90*, 311–321. [CrossRef] [PubMed]
37. Burdge, G.C.; Wootton, S.A. Conversion of alpha-linolenic acid to eicosapentaenoic, docosapentaenoic and docosahexaenoic acids in young women. *Br. J. Nutr.* **2002**, *88*, 411–420. [CrossRef] [PubMed]
38. Metcalf, R.G.; James, M.J.; Mantzioris, E.; Cleland, L.G. A practical approach to increasing intakes of *n*-3 polyunsaturated fatty acids: Use of novel foods enriched with *n*-3 fats. *Eur. J. Clin. Nutr.* **2003**, *57*, 1605–1612. [CrossRef] [PubMed]

39. Rahmawaty, S.; Lyons-Wall, P.; Charlton, K.; Batterham, M.; Meyer, B.J. Effect of replacing bread, egg, milk, and yogurt with equivalent omega-3 enriched foods on omega-3 LCPUFA intake of Australian children. *Nutrition* **2014**, *30*, 1337–1343. [CrossRef] [PubMed]
40. Rahmawaty, S.; Lyons-Wall, P.; Batterham, M.; Charlton, K.; Meyer, B.J. Food patterns of Australian children ages 9 to 13 y in relation to omega-3 long chain polyunsaturated intake. *Nutrition* **2014**, *30*, 169–176. [CrossRef] [PubMed]
41. Rahmawaty, S.; Charlton, K.; Lyons-Wall, P.; Meyer, B.J. Factors that influence consumption of fish and omega–3-enriched foods: A survey of Australian families with young children. *Nutr. Diet.* **2013**, *70*, 286–293. [CrossRef]
42. Naylor, R.L.; Hardy, R.W.; Bureau, D.P.; Chiu, A.; Elliott, M.; Farrell, A.P.; Forster, I.; Gatlin, D.M.; Goldburg, R.J.; Hua, K.; *et al.* Feeding aquaculture in an era of finite resources. *Proc. Natl. Acad. Sci. USA* **2009**, *106*, 15103–15110. [CrossRef] [PubMed]
43. Turchini, G.; Gunasekera, R.; de Silve, S. Effect of crude oil extracts from trout offal as a replacement for fish oil in the diets of the australian native fish murray cod maccullochella peelii peelii. *Aquac. Res.* **2003**, *34*, 697–708. [CrossRef]
44. Wu, G.; Truksa, M.; Datla, N.; Vrinten, P.; Bauer, J.; Zank, T.; Cirpus, P.; Heinz, E.; Qiu, X. Stepwise engineering to produce high yields of very long-chain polyunsaturated fatty acids in plants. *Nat. Biotechnol.* **2005**, *23*, 1013–1017. [CrossRef] [PubMed]
45. Turchini, G.M.; Nichols, P.D.; Barrow, C.; Sinclair, A.J. Jumping on the omega-3 bandwagon: Distinguishing the role of long-chain and short-chain omega-3 fatty acids. *Crit. Rev. Food Sci. Nutr.* **2012**, *52*, 795–803. [CrossRef] [PubMed]

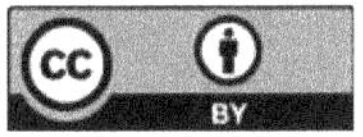

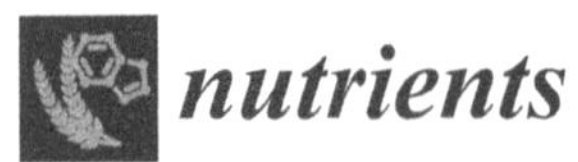

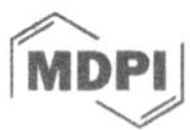

Article

DHA in Pregnant and Lactating Women from Coastland, Lakeland, and Inland Areas of China: Results of a DHA Evaluation in Women (DEW) Study

You Li [1,2,†], Hong-tian Li [1,2,†], Leonardo Trasande [3], Hua Ge [4], Li-xia Yu [5], Gao-sheng Xu [6], Man-xi Bai [7] and Jian-meng Liu [1,2,*]

1 Institute of Reproductive and Child Health/Ministry of Health Key Laboratory of Reproductive Health, Peking University Health Science Center, 38 Xueyuan Rd, Beijing 100191, China; liyou@pku.edu.cn (Y.L.); liht@bjmu.edu.cn (H.L.)
2 Department of Epidemiology and Biostatistics, School of Public Health, Peking University Health Science Center, 38 Xueyuan Rd, Beijing 100191, China
3 Department of Pediatrics, NYU School of Medicine, 227 East 30th Street, Room 735, New York, NY 10016, USA; Leonardo.Trasande@nyumc.org
4 Department of Obstetrics and Gynaecology, the First Affiliated Hospital of Baotou Medical School, 41 Linyin Rd, Baotou 014000, China; byyfygh2010@163.com
5 Department of Obstetrics and Gynaecology, Weihai Maternal and Child Health Hospital, 51 Guangming Rd, Weihai 264200, China; whyulixia@126.com
6 Department of Pediatrics, Yueyang Maternal and Child Health Hospital, 693 Baling Middle Rd, Yueyang 414000, China; xugaosheng0414@163.com
7 Wyeth Nutrition Science Center, 582 Wuzhong Rd, Shanghai 201103, China; Manxi.Bai@wyethnutrition.com
* Correspondence: liujm@pku.edu.cn; Tel.: +86-10-8280-1136; Fax: +86-10-8280-1141
† These authors contributed equally to this work.

Received: 13 August 2015 ; Accepted: 14 October 2015 ; Published: 21 October 2015

Abstract: Few studies have examined docosahexaenoic acid (DHA) in pregnant and lactating women in developing countries like China, where DHA-enriched supplements are increasingly popular. We aimed to assess the DHA status among Chinese pregnant and lactating women residing areas differing in the availability of aquatic products. In total, 1211 women in mid-pregnancy (17 $\pm$ 2 weeks), late pregnancy (39 $\pm$ 2 weeks), or lactation (42 $\pm$ 7 days) were enrolled from Weihai (coastland), Yueyang (lakeland), and Baotou (inland) city, with approximately 135 women in each participant group by region. DHA concentrations were measured using capillary gas chromatography, and are reported as weight percent of total fatty acids. Mean plasma DHA concentrations were higher in coastland (mid-pregnancy 3.19%, late pregnancy 2.54%, lactation 2.24%) and lakeland women (2.45%, 1.95%, 2.26%) than inland women (2.25%, 1.67%, 1.68%) (p values < 0.001). Similar differences were observed for erythrocyte DHA. We conclude that DHA concentrations of Chinese pregnant and lactating women are higher in coastland and lakeland regions than in inland areas. DHA status in the study population appears to be stronger than populations from other countries studied to date.

Keywords: docosahexaenoic acid; pregnant women; lactating women; plasma; erythrocyte; correlation

---

1. Introduction

Docosahexaenoic acid (DHA, 22:6n-3), as a fundamental constituent in cell membranes, is indispensable to the structure and function of the retina and central nervous system [1,2]. DHA is mainly contained in aquatic products, especially in seafood. Dietary DHA intake is a major source to meet human body requirements, since humans only synthesize a limited amount of DHA from α-linolenic acid [3]. It is widely acknowledged that pregnant and lactating women are more susceptible to DHA deficiency because they need to meet their own needs as well as those of the fetuses. Increased intake of DHA during pregnancy and lactation has been documented to benefit fetal and infant development [4–7].

The availability and consumption of aquatic products plays an important role in DHA status. In a study [8] conducted among women from four Tanzanian tribes differing in lifetime intakes of fish, Luxwolda *et al.* observed an obvious positive correlation between fish consumption and DHA levels. DHA status may also vary across ethnicities. In a study [9] comparing plasma DHA phospholipids between Dutch and ethnic minority pregnant women in Netherlands, van Eijsden *et al.* reported significant ethnic differences in maternal DHA status despite controlling for fish intake. Besides, in an earlier study [10] involving women from Ecuador and four European countries with different baseline phospholipid DHA status, Otto *et al.* observed consistent decreases in the DHA weight percentage of total fatty acids as women progress from early pregnancy to delivery.

In China, fish availability varies considerably in populations, and is greatest in coastland and lakeland regions in contrast to inland areas. In this study, we aimed to examine DHA status in a diverse population of Chinese pregnant and lactating women from coastland, lakeland, and inland areas.

2. Subjects and Methods

2.1. Settings and Subjects

The DHA Evaluation in Women (DEW) study was a cross-sectional survey conducted from May to July 2014 in three cities of China: Weihai (selected to represent the coastland population), Yueyang (selected to represent the lakeland population) and Baotou (selected to represent the inland population). Weihai is surrounded on three sides by the Huang Sea. Yueyang is near Dongting Lake, the second largest freshwater lake in China. Baotou is a typical inland city in the Mongolian Plateau. A total of 1211 apparently healthy women who were at mid-pregnancy (17 $\pm$ 2 gestational weeks), late pregnancy (39 $\pm$ 2 gestational weeks), or lactation (42 $\pm$ 7 days postpartum) were recruited approximately equally from the three regions, with on average 135 (127–138) women in each group per region. Eligible women were 18–35 years old, were local permanent residents, and had singleton pregnancies. An additional inclusion criterion for the lactating group was current breastfeeding. Women were excluded if they had been diagnosed with any cardiovascular, metabolic, and renal diseases, mental disorder, or aquatic food allergy; or had participated in other research projects in the past 30 days. Women with severe vomiting after 16 weeks of gestation were also excluded for the mid-pregnancy group. The research protocol was approved by the Institutional Review Boards/Human Subjects Committees at Peking University Health Science Center (IRB00001052-14012; date of approval: 22-04-2014), and all participating women signed informed consents.

2.2. Data and Sample Collection

Participants were enrolled from four local hospitals: one located in Weihai, one in Yueyang, and two in Baotou. Trained obstetricians or nurses from the hospitals completed enrolment and data collection. A structured questionnaire was used to collect maternal characteristics, including birthdate, ethnicity, height, pre-pregnancy weight, and educational attainment. For pregnant women, gestational age at enrolment was calculated according to the date of the last menstrual period. For lactating women, self-reported gestational age at delivery and parity were also collected.

Fasting venous blood (~5 mL) was collected from the antecubital vein into ethylenediaminetetraacetic acid (EDTA)-containing tubes. Samples were kept in the refrigerator at 5 °C for at least 30 min and then centrifuged at 3000$\times$ g for 10 min to separate plasma and erythrocytes. The erythrocytes were washed out with normal saline. Both plasma and erythrocyte samples were stored at −20 °C in the hospital for approximately 10 days, and then were transported on dry ice frozen at −80 °C to the central laboratory where samples were stored at a −80 °C freezer. Notably, the temporal storage of blood samples at −20 °C might have somewhat compromised DHA in erythrocyte [11,12].

To ensure data quality and to standardize data collection methodologies across sites, study staff attended training workshops and each site had a designated investigator who oversaw the standardized data collection procedures. In addition, senior investigators met weekly and provided additional oversight.

2.3. Sample Analysis

The extraction and derivatization of total lipids in plasma and erythrocyte samples were carried out using a modified method of Folch *et al.* [13]. The internal standard solution containing methyl undecanoate (C11:0) was added to the samples, and mixed with boron trifluoride and methanol. This mixture was heated at 115 °C for 20 min. After cooling to room temperature, the mixture was extracted with n-hexane. The n-hexane containing methyl esters of total lipids were analyzed by an Agilent 6890N gas chromatography (Agilent Technologies, Palo Alto, CA, USA) equipped with a flame ionization detector at 280 °C and a capillary column (CP-Sil 88, 50 m, 0.25 mm ID, 0.20 μm film thickness). The injector was set as a split mode at 250 °C, with the split ratio of 1:5. The oven temperature was programmed as follows: ramping from 120 °C to 166 °C at 2 °C/min, and holding at 166 °C for 10 min; then ramping to 200 °C at 2 °C/min and holding at 200 °C for 10 min. Individual fatty acids were identified against the reference standards. The data were collected and processed using Agilent OpenLAB software (Agilent Technologies, Santa Clara, CA, USA). Both absolute concentration (μg/mL) and the relative concentration (weight percent of total fatty acids, wt. %) of DHA were calculated.

2.4. Statistical Analysis

DHA concentrations are presented as means ± SDs. One-way analyses of variance were performed to compare overall differences in DHA concentrations among participant groups and regions. *T*-tests were used to examine the differences between women in inland and lakeland/coastland as well as between women in mid-pregnancy and late-pregnancy/lactation. Additionally, we explored whether DHA concentrations varied across subgroups based on maternal age (18.0–24.9, 25.0–29.9, and 30.0–34.9 years), pre-pregnancy BMI (<18.5, 18.5–23.9, and ⩾24.0 kg/m^2), and education attainment (middle school or less, high school, and college or above) by using multiple linear regression with adjustments for covariates including region and participant group.

To illustrate the relationship between plasma and erythrocyte DHA, we performed several sets of Pearson correlation analyses. We first estimated the overall correlation coefficient between plasma and erythrocyte relative DHA concentrations. Because the scatterplot indicated an obviously different correlation pattern between individuals with erythrocyte DHA concentrations ⩾3% and those <3%, separate correlation analyses for the two subgroups were then performed. We also repeated the above-mentioned correlation analyses within the 9 subgroups defined by region and participant group.

Significance was set at $p < 0.05$. All statistical analyses were performed by using SPSS version 20.0 (Chicago, IL, USA).

3. Results

3.1. Maternal Characteristics

Table 1 shows maternal characteristics by region and participant group. Overall, 87.8% women had high school or above education. In coastland and lakeland populations, 98.0% were of Han ethnicity, whereas the percentage was somewhat lower (89.8%) in inland, where 7.1% were Mongolian. The mean age, height, and pre-pregnancy BMI were comparable for the three participant groups residing coastland and inland, whereas women from the lakeland were younger, shorter in stature, and had lower pre-pregnancy BMI (p values < 0.001). In the lactating group, primiparous women accounted for 87.5%, 81.5%, and 86.0% in coastland, lakeland, and inland, respectively, and corresponding mean gestational age at delivery in the three regions was 39.3, 39.3, and 39.1 weeks, respectively.

Table 1. Maternal characteristics by region and participant group.

	Coastland			Lakeland			Inland		
Characteristic	**MP**	**LP**	**LA**	**MP**	**LP**	**LA**	**MP**	**LP**	**LA**
Number of participants	136	127	136	133	134	135	138	136	136
GA (week)/PP (day) at enrolment									
Mean	16.9	37.5	42.7	17.0	38.0	41.7	16.7	38.6	42.1
SD	0.9	0.7	2.3	1.1	0.9	4.1	1.1	1.2	3.9
Age (year)									
Mean	27.9	28.4	28.3	26.5	27.1	27.1	27.9	28.5	28.1
SD	2.4	2.7	2.7	3.1	3.1	3.0	2.9	3.3	3.0
Ethnics (%)									
Han	97.8	99.2	97.1	98.5	97.8	97.8	83.3	94.1	91.9
Mongolian	0	0	0	0	0	0	12.3	4.4	4.4
Hui	0	0	0.7	0	0	0	0.7	0.7	2.2
Others	2.2	0.8	2.2	1.5	2.2	2.2	3.6	0.7	1.5
Education (%)									
College or above	67.7	66.2	65.4	47.4	61.3	62.2	79.0	78.4	73.5
High school	15.4	24.4	25.0	36.8	24.6	23.7	13.8	16.2	19.1
Middle school or less	16.9	9.4	9.6	15.8	14.1	14.1	7.2	15.4	7.4
Height (cm)									
Mean	163.6	163.7	163.2	159.3	159.8	159.8	164.1	162.8	163.1
SD	4.9	4.6	5.0	4.5	3.9	4.3	4.9	4.7	4.6
Pre-pregnancy BMI (kg/m^2)									
Mean	21.1	21.3	21.9	20.2	19.8	20.1	21.3	21.6	21.2
SD	2.8	2.5	3.5	2.5	1.9	2.9	3.3	2.8	3.2

GA, gestational age; PP, postpartum; MP, mid-pregnancy; LP, late pregnancy; LA, lactation.

3.2. DHA Concentrations

Mean plasma and erythrocyte relative DHA concentrations of 9 region- and group-specific subgroups ranged 1.67%–3.19% and 5.06%–7.59%, respectively; corresponding absolute values ranged between 60.5 and 146.2 μg/mL and 89.3–127.7 μg/mL, respectively (Table 2).

Table 2. Docosahexaenoic acid (DHA) concentrations by region and participant group.

	Inland		Lakeland		Coastland		P ANOVA
	Mean	SD	Mean	SD	Mean	SD	
wt. %							
Plasma							
Mid-pregnancy	2.25	0.46	2.45 [a]	0.44	3.19 [a]	0.65	<0.001
Late pregnancy	1.67 [b]	0.35	1.95 [a,b]	0.45	2.54 [a,b]	0.60	<0.001
Lactation	1.68 [b]	0.48	2.26 [a,b]	0.53	2.24 [a,b]	0.70	<0.001
P ANOVA	<0.001		<0.001		<0.001		
Erythrocyte							
Mid-pregnancy	5.85	1.06	6.34 [a]	0.80	7.59 [a]	1.46	<0.001
Late pregnancy	5.06 [b]	1.25	6.23 [a]	1.09	7.09 [a,b]	1.93	<0.001
Lactation	5.20 [b]	1.15	6.20 [a]	0.92	6.07 [a,b]	1.59	<0.001
P ANOVA	<0.001		0.45		<0.001		
μg/mL							
Plasma							
Mid-pregnancy	93.4	25.2	86.2 [a]	20.5	118.4 [a]	30.8	<0.001
Late pregnancy	101.9 [b]	33.1	110.1 [a,b]	28.3	146.2 [a,b]	45.1	<0.001
Lactation	60.5 [b]	17.5	65.1 [b]	20.9	75.7 [a,b]	29.9	<0.001
P ANOVA	<0.001		<0.001		<0.001		
Erythrocyte							
Mid-pregnancy	108.0	22.1	103.2 [a]	13.6	127.7 [a]	27.2	<0.001
Late pregnancy	89.3 [b]	25.2	106.6 [a]	20.7	123.2 [a]	37.5	<0.001
Lactation	91.4 [b]	22.1	97.0 [a,b]	19.7	99.3 [a,b]	29.6	<0.05
P ANOVA	<0.001		<0.001		<0.001		

ANOVA, analyses of variance. [a]: Mean values were significant different compared with women from inland within the same participant group (by *t*-test, $p < 0.05$); [b]: mean values were significant different compared with women in mid-pregnancy within the same region (by *t*-test).

Plasma and erythrocyte DHA relative concentrations differed by region across participant groups (p values < 0.001). The concentrations were higher in coastland and lakeland women than in inland women. Similar regional differences in DHA absolute concentrations were observed (Table 2).

Plasma DHA relative concentrations differed significantly by participant groups across the regions (p values < 0.001); the concentrations were higher in mid-pregnancy than in late pregnancy and lactating women across regions (p values < 0.001). Similar patterns were also observed for erythrocyte DHA relative concentrations, although the difference was not significant among the three groups of lakeland women. In contrast, the plasma DHA absolute concentrations were highest in late-pregnancy women, followed by in mid-pregnancy, and lowest in lactating women. The erythrocyte DHA absolute concentrations were relatively higher in mid-pregnancy in inland, in mid- and late-pregnancy in lakeland and coastland women (Table 2).

In multiple linear regression analyses, maternal age and education were significantly associated with DHA concentrations; patterns for regional and inter-group DHA were similar to the aforementioned unadjusted analyses (Table 3).

3.3. Correlation between DHA in Plasma and Erythrocyte

The overall Pearson correlation coefficient between plasma and erythrocyte relative DHA concentrations was 0.625 ($p < 0.001$). The correlation profile was visually examined via a scatterplot and an obviously different correlation pattern was detected between women with erythrocyte DHA concentration ⩾3% and those <3% (Figure 1). The significant positive correlation persisted only in women with erythrocyte DHA concentrations ⩾3% ($n = 1175$; $r = 0.73$, $p < 0.001$), but not in those <3% ($n = 36$; $r = -0.13$, $p = 0.46$). After excluding women with erythrocyte DHA concentrations <3%, most of region- and group-specific correlation coefficients were substantially augmented by 18%–64% (Supplementary Table S1).

Table 3. Multiple linear regression of DHA concentrations on region, participant group and selected maternal characteristics.

Variables	Plasma DHA (wt. %)			Erythrocyte DHA (wt. %)			Plasma DHA (μg/mL)			Erythrocyte DHA (μg/mL)		
	Mean	β	*P*	**Mean**	β	*P*	**Mean**	β	*P*	**Mean**	β	*P*
Region												
Inland	1.87	0	Ref.	5.37	0	Ref.	85.3	0	Ref.	96.3	0	Ref.
Lakeland	2.22	0.36	<0.001	6.25	0.92	<0.001	87.0	3.6	0.091	102.2	6.7	<0.001
Coastland	2.66	0.80	<0.001	6.91	1.55	<0.001	112.7	28.4	<0.001	116.6	20.4	<0.001
Participant group												
Mid-pregnancy	2.63	0	Ref.	6.59	0	Ref.	99.4	0	Ref.	113.0	0	Ref.
Late pregnancy	2.04	−0.59	<0.001	6.10	−0.49	<0.001	118.8	19.4	<0.001	106.0	−7.0	<0.001
Lactation	2.06	−0.58	<0.001	5.82	−0.79	<0.001	67.1	−32.9	<0.001	95.9	−17.5	<0.001
Age(year)												
<25.0	2.15	0	Ref.	5.93	0	Ref.	88.2	0	Ref.	100.2	0	Ref.
25.0–29.9	2.27	0.02	0.623	6.24	0.17	0.129	94.7	1.7	0.499	106.1	2.8	0.191
⩾30.0	2.25	0.12	0.029	6.15	0.25	0.050	100.6	7.9	0.006	105.3	4.0	0.108
Education												
Middle school or less	2.18	0	Ref.	5.93	0	Ref.	90.1	0	Ref.	100.2	0	Ref.
High school	2.24	0.07	0.187	6.20	0.29	0.033	94.2	7.2	0.016	105.0	5.6	0.034
College or above	2.26	0.12	0.014	6.21	0.36	0.003	96.0	8.5	0.002	105.8	6.4	0.006
Pre-pregnancy BMI												
<18.5	2.26	0	Ref.	6.15	0	Ref.	90.7	0	Ref.	103.0	0	Ref.
18.5–23.9	2.27	−0.07	0.073	6.22	−0.06	0.546	96.0	−0.3	0.901	105.9	0.1	0.970
⩾24.0	2.12	−0.21	<0.001	5.97	−0.20	0.143	95.3	1.6	0.612	103.2	−1.7	0.523

β, regression coefficient; Ref, reference category.

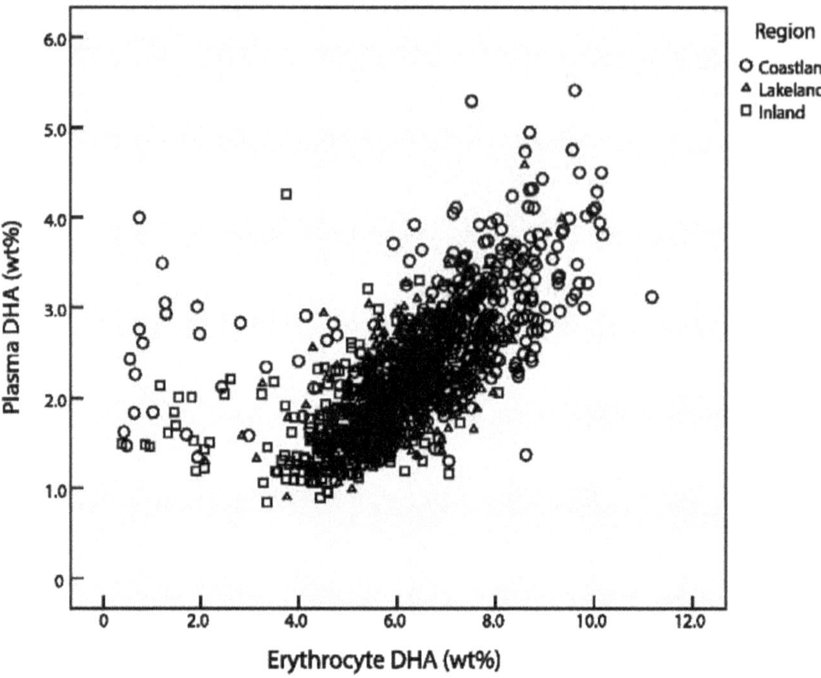

Figure 1. Correlation between plasma and erythrocyte DHA relative concentrations in 1211 participants.

4. Discussion

In this large cross-sectional study conducted in three typical urban areas of China, DHA concentrations measured by relative weight percent to total fatty acids in pregnant and lactating women were higher in coastland/lakeland women than in inland women as well as higher in mid-pregnancy than in late-pregnancy/lactation. Moreover, we observed a moderate to high degree of correlation between plasma and erythrocyte DHA.

Consistent with a previous study [8], we found DHA concentrations, whether in plasma or erythrocyte, for each participant group, were significantly higher in coastland/lakeland than in inland women, likely reflecting differences in consuming aquatic products. Relevant data of Chinese pregnant or lactating women are sparse. One small study [14] conducted in 138 late-pregnant Chinese women reported similar results for plasma choline phosphoglyceride DHA: highest in coastland, followed by lakeland, and lowest in inland. In addition, consistent with longitudinal studies [10,15], we observed that both plasma and erythrocyte DHA relative concentrations, despite the region, were significantly higher in mid-pregnancy than in late-pregnancy, probably in response to an increasing fetal needs for DHA and an increasing blood volume during pregnancy [16,17]. Meanwhile, we noticed that DHA absolute concentrations were higher in late-pregnancy than mid-pregnancy, which was probably due to an increasing synthesis during pregnancy [17]. Additionally, consistent with the findings from Stark *et al.* [18], DHA concentrations in plasma and erythrocytes increased with maternal age and education, possibly reflecting the difference in consuming aquatic products. We further compared DHA concentrations in total lipids (reported as wt. % of total fatty acids) with other populations worldwide, and found that the DHA concentrations of Chinese pregnant and lactating women were at relatively high level. Specifically, the concentrations of our inland women were higher than those of women residing in inland areas of India [19] or Germany [20], and close to or even higher than those of women residing in coastal areas of some nations like USA, United Kingdom, Denmark, Norway,

Japan, or Canada [17,21–25]; however, the concentrations of our coastland women were slightly lower than those of Spanish (mid-pregnancy: 3.19% *versus* 3.70% in plasma) [26] and Cubans (lactation: 2.24% *versus* 2.56% in plasma and 6.07% *versus* 6.80% in erythrocyte) [27]. Besides differences in consuming aquatic products or DHA enriched supplements, the potential explanations for ethnic differences also involve DHA synthesis and metabolism, for *FADS* genotypes influence maternal DHA concentrations [28,29].

As expected, we observed a moderate to high level of positive correlation between plasma and erythrocyte DHA (Pearson's $r = 0.63$). The correlation was even stronger ($r = 0.73$) in women with erythrocyte DHA ⩾3%, but not at all in those with erythrocyte DHA <3% ($n = 36$; $r = -0.13$, $p = 0.46$); interestingly, the plasma concentrations in the two subgroups of women (2.25% *versus* 2.04%) did not differ materially. One explanation regarding the inflection point in the correlation between plasma and erythrocyte DHA was that erythrocyte could serve as a reservoir and its DHA could be transported into plasma for body need in case of a lower DHA status [30]. Another explanation was that the storage of the blood samples at −20 °C might have compromised erythrocyte DHA, especially in those with lower DHA concentrations, whereas the storage probably had no impact on plasma DHA, which in turn resulted in a flawed deviation from the linear correlation [11,12]. Therefore, the correlation identified in our study should be interpreted with caution, which remains to be confirmed in further studies.

Our study has multiple strengths. We selected three typical regions with plausible differences in DHA intake due to differences in the availability of aquatic products, and recruited three groups of women to simultaneously assess DHA status in mid-pregnant, late-pregnant and lactating women by region. Procedures in data collection and sample analyses were intensively monitored. The region- and participant group-specified sample size (~135) was the largest compared to previous similar studies (~50). However, our study also has several limitations. Firstly, the study was not longitudinal, and was conducted only in urban areas of China, possibly confining the generalization of findings. Secondly, the mean erythrocyte DHA concentrations might be slightly lower than the true values due to the temporary storage of blood samples under −20 °C [11,12]. Thirdly, the regional differences in DHA concentrations for pregnant and lactating women could not be simply generalized to the non-pregnant because the increased DHA synthesis during pregnancy was likely more pronounced in individuals with lower DHA intakes [17]. Additionally, we only focused on DHA in this study as a preliminary step to understand maternal status of polyunsaturated fatty acids (PUFAs) in our population. Further studies regarding other PUFAs are encouraged, which are critical to the understanding of the entire profile of PUFAs as well as its relationship with dietary fatty acids.

In summary, DHA concentrations of Chinese pregnant and lactating women are higher in coastland and lakeland regions than in inland areas. DHA status in our population appears to be stronger than populations from other countries as reported in the literature. DHA concentrations varied by region and participant groups, which is likely due to differences in consumption of aquatic products or changes in physiological needs for DHA.

Supplementary Materials: Supplementary materials can be accessed at: http://www.mdpi.com/2072-6643/7/10/5428/s1.

Acknowledgments: The study was supported by a grant from Wyeth Nutrition Science Center (Project Number: 14.10.CN.INF). We thank all participants for their cooperation. We thank the dozens of physicians or nurses from Weihai Maternal and Child Health Hospital, Yueyang Maternal and Child Health Hospital, The First Affiliated Hospital of Baotou Medical School, and The Third Hospital of Baogang Group for their field work. We thank Lin-lin Wang, Ya-li Zhang, Zhao-xia Xiong, Yu-bo Zhou, and Meng-jiao Liu at the Peking University Institute of Reproductive and Child Health for their works on the project.

Author Contributions: The authors' responsibilities were as follows—Jian-meng Liu, Hong-tian Li and Man-xi Bai conceived and designed the study; Jian-meng Liu, Hong-tian Li, You Li, Hua Ge, Li-xia Yu, and Gao-sheng Xu conducted the field work; You Li and Hong-tian Li analyzed data; You Li, Hong-tian Li and Jian-meng Liu drafted the manuscript; Hong-tian Li, Jian-meng Liu, Leonardo Trasande and Man-xi Bai made critical reviews and revisions; All authors have reviewed and approved the final manuscript. Jian-meng Liu had primary responsibility for final content.

Conflicts of Interest: Jian-meng Liu has received a grant from Wyeth Nutrition Science Center and presented the part of the results at a scientific workshop organized by Wyeth Nutrition Science Center. Man-xi Bai is working for Wyeth Nutrition Science Center. All other authors declared no conflict of interest.

References

1. Heird, W.C.; Lapillonne, A. The role of essential fatty acids in development. *Ann. Rev. Nutr.* **2005**, *25*, 549–571. [CrossRef] [PubMed]
2. Lauritzen, L.; Hansen, H.S.; Jorgensen, M.H.; Michaelsen, K.F. The essentiality of long chain *n*-3 fatty acids in relation to development and function of the brain and retina. *Prog. Lipid Res.* **2001**, *40*, 1–94. [CrossRef]
3. FAO. *Fats and Fatty Acids in Human Nutrition*; Report of an Expert Consultation; Karger: Basel, Switzerland, 2010; Volume 91, pp. 1–166.
4. Carlson, S.E.; Colombo, J.; Gajewski, B.J.; Gustafson, K.M.; Mundy, D.; Yeast, J.; Georgieff, M.K.; Markley, L.A.; Kerling, E.H.; Shaddy, D.J.; *et al.* DHA supplementation and pregnancy outcomes. *Am. J. Clin. Nutr.* **2013**, *97*, 808–815. [CrossRef] [PubMed]
5. Hibbeln, J.R.; Davis, J.M.; Steer, C.; Emmett, P.; Rogers, I.; Williams, C.; Golding, J. Maternal seafood consumption in pregnancy and neurodevelopmental outcomes in childhood (ALSPAC study): An observational cohort study. *Lancet* **2007**, *369*, 578–585. [CrossRef]
6. Makrides, M.; Gibson, R.A.; McPhee, A.J.; Yelland, L.; Quinlivan, J.; Ryan, P.; Team, D.O.I. Effect of DHA supplementation during pregnancy on maternal depression and neurodevelopment of young children: A randomized controlled trial. *JAMA* **2010**, *304*, 1675–1683. [CrossRef] [PubMed]
7. Muthayya, S.; Dwarkanath, P.; Thomas, T.; Ramprakash, S.; Mehra, R.; Mhaskar, A.; Mhaskar, R.; Thomas, A.; Bhat, S.; Vaz, M.; *et al.* The effect of fish and omega-3 LCPUFA intake on low birth weight in Indian pregnant women. *Eur. J. Clin. Nutr.* **2009**, *63*, 340–346. [CrossRef] [PubMed]
8. Luxwolda, M.F.; Kuipers, R.S.; Koops, J.H.; Muller, S.; de Graaf, D.; Dijck-Brouwer, D.A.; Muskiet, F.A. Interrelationships between maternal DHA in erythrocytes, milk and adipose tissue. Is 1 wt % DHA the optimal human milk content? Data from four tanzanian tribes differing in lifetime stable intakes of fish. *Br. J. Nutr.* **2014**, *111*, 854–866. [CrossRef] [PubMed]
9. Van Eijsden, M.; Hornstra, G.; van der Wal, M.F.; Bonsel, G.J. Ethnic differences in early pregnancy maternal *n*-3 and *n*-6 fatty acid concentrations: An explorative analysis. *Br. J. Nutr.* **2009**, *101*, 1761–1768. [CrossRef] [PubMed]
10. Otto, S.J.; Houwelingen, A.C.; Antal, M.; Manninen, A.; Godfrey, K.; Lopez-Jaramillo, P.; Hornstra, G. Maternal and neonatal essential fatty acid status in phospholipids: An international comparative study. *Eur. J. Clin. Nutr.* **1997**, *51*, 232–242. [CrossRef] [PubMed]
11. Metherel, A.H.; Aristizabal Henao, J.J.; Stark, K.D. EPA and DHA levels in whole blood decrease more rapidly when stored at −20 °C as compared with room temperature, 4 and −75 °C. *Lipids* **2013**, *48*, 1079–1091. [CrossRef] [PubMed]
12. Metherel, A.H.; Stark, K.D. Cryopreservation prevents iron-initiated highly unsaturated fatty acid loss during storage of human blood on chromatography paper at −20 °C. *J. Nutr.* **2015**, *145*, 654–660. [CrossRef] [PubMed]
13. Folch, J.; Lees, M.; Sloane Stanley, G.H. A simple method for the isolation and purification of total lipides from animal tissues. *J. Biol. Chem.* **1957**, *226*, 497–509. [PubMed]
14. Zhang, J.; Wang, Y.; Meng, L.; Wang, C.; Zhao, W.; Chen, J.; Ghebremeskel, K.; Crawford, M.A. Maternal and neonatal plasma *n*-3 and *n*-6 fatty acids of pregnant women and neonates from three regions of China with contrasting dietary patterns. *Asia Pac. J. Clin. Nutr.* **2009**, *18*, 377–388. [PubMed]
15. Al, M.D.M.; van Houwelingen, A.C.; Hornstra, G. Relation between birth order and the maternal and neonatal docosahexaenoic acid status. *Eur. J. Clin. Nutr.* **1997**, *51*, 548–553. [CrossRef] [PubMed]
16. Koletzko, B.; Larque, E.; Demmelmair, H. Placental transfer of long-chain polyunsaturated fatty acids (LC-PUFA). *J. Perinat. Med.* **2007**, *35* (Suppl. S1), S5–S11. [CrossRef] [PubMed]
17. Stark, K.D.; Beblo, S.; Murthy, M.; Buda-Abela, M.; Janisse, J.; Rockett, H.; Whitty, J.E.; Martier, S.S.; Sokol, R.J.; Hannigan, J.H.; *et al.* Comparison of bloodstream fatty acid composition from African-American women at gestation, delivery, and postpartum. *J. Lipid Res.* **2005**, *46*, 516–525. [CrossRef] [PubMed]

18. Stark, K.D.; Beblo, S.; Murthy, M.; Whitty, J.E.; Buda-Abela, M.; Janisse, J.; Rockett, H.; Martier, S.S.; Sokol, R.J.; Hannigan, J.H.; *et al.* Alcohol consumption in pregnant, black women is associated with decreased plasma and erythrocyte docosahexaenoic acid. *Alcohol. Clin. Exp. Res.* **2005**, *29*, 130–140. [CrossRef] [PubMed]
19. Wadhwani, N.; Patil, V.; Pisal, H.; Joshi, A.; Mehendale, S.; Gupte, S.; Wagh, G.; Joshi, S. Altered maternal proportions of long chain polyunsaturated fatty acids and their transport leads to disturbed fetal stores in preeclampsia. *Prostaglandins Leukot. Essent. Fatty Acids* **2014**, *91*, 21–30. [CrossRef] [PubMed]
20. Enke, U.; Jaudszus, A.; Schleussner, E.; Seyfarth, L.; Jahreis, G.; Kuhnt, K. Fatty acid distribution of cord and maternal blood in human pregnancy: Special focus on individual trans fatty acids and conjugated linoleic acids. *Lipids Health Dis.* **2011**, *10*, 247. [CrossRef] [PubMed]
21. Markhus, M.W.; Skotheim, S.; Graff, I.E.; Froyland, L.; Braarud, H.C.; Stormark, K.M.; Malde, M.K. Low omega-3 index in pregnancy is a possible biological risk factor for postpartum depression. *PLoS ONE* **2013**, *8*. [CrossRef]
22. Olsen, S.F.; Hansen, H.S.; Sommer, S.; Jensen, B.; Sorensen, T.I.; Secher, N.J.; Zachariassen, P. Gestational age in relation to marine n-3 fatty acids in maternal erythrocytes: A study of women in the Faroe Islands and Denmark. *Am. J. Obstet. Gynecol.* **1991**, *164*, 1203–1209. [CrossRef]
23. Rioux, F.M.; Belanger-Plourde, J.; Leblanc, C.P.; Vigneau, F. Relationship between maternal DHA and iron status and infants' cognitive performance. *Can. J. Diet. Pract. Res.* **2011**, *72*, 76. [PubMed]
24. Stewart, F.; Rodie, V.A.; Ramsay, J.E.; Greer, I.A.; Freeman, D.J.; Meyer, B.J. Longitudinal assessment of erythrocyte fatty acid composition throughout pregnancy and post partum. *Lipids* **2007**, *42*, 335–344. [CrossRef] [PubMed]
25. Young, C.; Hikita, T.; Kaneko, S.; Shimizu, Y.; Hanaka, S.; Abe, T.; Shimasaki, H.; Ikeda, R.; Miyazawa, Y.; Nakajima, A. Fatty acid compositions of colostrum, cord blood, maternal blood and major infant formulas in Japan. *Acta Paediatr. Jpn.* **1997**, *39*, 299–304. [CrossRef] [PubMed]
26. Sanjurjo, P.; Matorras, R.; Ingunza, N.; Alonso, M.; Rodriguez-Alarcon, J.; Perteagudo, L. Cross-sectional study of percentual changes in total plasmatic fatty acids during pregnancy. *Horm. Metab. Res.* **1993**, *25*, 590–592. [CrossRef] [PubMed]
27. Krasevec, J.M.; Jones, P.J.; Cabrera-Hernandez, A.; Mayer, D.L.; Connor, W.E. Maternal and infant essential fatty acid status in Havana, Cuba. *Am. J. Clin. Nutr.* **2002**, *76*, 834–844. [PubMed]
28. Xie, L.; Innis, S.M. Genetic variants of the fads1 fads2 gene cluster are associated with altered (*n*-6) and (*n*-3) essential fatty acids in plasma and erythrocyte phospholipids in women during pregnancy and in breast milk during lactation. *J. Nutr.* **2008**, *138*, 2222–2228. [CrossRef] [PubMed]
29. Koletzko, B.; Lattka, E.; Zeilinger, S.; Illig, T.; Steer, C. Genetic variants of the fatty acid desaturase gene cluster predict amounts of red blood cell docosahexaenoic and other polyunsaturated fatty acids in pregnant women: Findings from the avon longitudinal study of parents and children. *Am. J. Clin. Nutr.* **2011**, *93*, 211–219. [CrossRef] [PubMed]
30. Ghebremeskel, K.; Min, Y.; Crawford, M.A.; Nam, J.H.; Kim, A.; Koo, J.N.; Suzuki, H. Blood fatty acid composition of pregnant and nonpregnant Korean women: Red cells may act as a reservoir of arachidonic acid and docosahexaenoic acid for utilization by the developing fetus. *Lipids* **2000**, *35*, 567–574. [CrossRef] [PubMed]

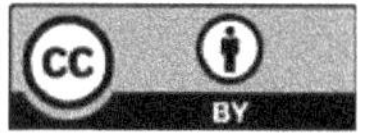

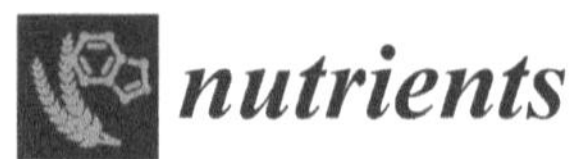

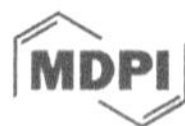

Article

Long-Term Effect of Docosahexaenoic Acid Feeding on Lipid Composition and Brain Fatty Acid-Binding Protein Expression in Rats

Marwa E. Elsherbiny [1], Susan Goruk [2], Elizabeth A. Monckton [1], Caroline Richard [2], Miranda Brun [1], Marwan Emara [3], Catherine J. Field [2] and Roseline Godbout [1,*]

1 Department of Oncology, Cross Cancer Institute, University of Alberta, 11560 University Avenue, Edmonton, AB T6G 1Z2, Canada; marwae@ualberta.ca (M.E.E.); eamonckton@shaw.ca (E.A.M.); mbrun@ualberta.ca (M.B.)

2 Department of Agricultural, Food and Nutritional Science, University of Alberta, Edmonton, AB T6G 2E1, Canada; sgoruk@ualberta.ca (S.G.); cr5@ualberta.ca (C.R.); cjfield@ualberta.ca (C.J.F.)

3 Centre for Aging and Associated Diseases, Zewail City for Science and Technology, Cairo 12588, Egypt; memara@zewailcity.edu.eg

* Correspondence: rgodbout@ualberta.ca; Tel.: +780-432-8901; Fax: +780-432-8892

Received: 15 August 2015 ; Accepted: 14 October 2015 ; Published: 22 October 2015

Abstract: Arachidonic (AA) and docosahexaenoic acid (DHA) brain accretion is essential for brain development. The impact of DHA-rich maternal diets on offspring brain fatty acid composition has previously been studied up to the weanling stage; however, there has been no follow-up at later stages. Here, we examine the impact of DHA-rich maternal and weaning diets on brain fatty acid composition at weaning and three weeks post-weaning. We report that DHA supplementation during lactation maintains high DHA levels in the brains of pups even when they are fed a DHA-deficient diet for three weeks after weaning. We show that boosting dietary DHA levels for three weeks after weaning compensates for a maternal DHA-deficient diet during lactation. Finally, our data indicate that brain fatty acid binding protein (FABP7), a marker of neural stem cells, is down-regulated in the brains of six-week pups with a high DHA:AA ratio. We propose that elevated levels of DHA in developing brain accelerate brain maturation relative to DHA-deficient brains.

Keywords: arachidonic acid; brain development; brain lipids; diet and dietary lipids; fatty acid/binding protein

---

1. Introduction

Human brain development starts at the fifth postmenstrual week and continues after birth with most of the brain's neurobiological processes fully developed by adolescence [1,2]. There is a spurt in brain growth during the last trimester of pregnancy, with the mass of the brain approaching that of adult brain by the time the child is about three years old [3]. The rapid growth of the brain during the last trimester requires a significant supply of long chain polyunsaturated fatty acids (PUFA), especially docosahexaenoic acid (DHA, C22:6, ω-3) and arachidonic acid (AA, C20:4, ω-6) which are the major PUFA components of brain lipids [4].

DHA accumulates in brain gradually over the course of its development specifically from the third trimester onwards [5]. Analysis of the phosphatidylethanolamine component of brain phospholipids revealed increases in ω-3 PUFA, contributed mainly by DHA, and in the ω-3:ω-6 PUFA ratio, in brains of children from six months to 8 years old compared to brains of zero to six month old infants. In turn, the latter had a higher ω-3 PUFA content and ω-3:ω-6 PUFA ratio than fetuses at 26 to 42 weeks of gestation [6]. Similarly, when rat brains were examined at postnatal day (P) 8 (comparable to 36–40 weeks of gestation in humans in terms of brain maturation [7]) and at embryonic days (E) 17 and E20, an increase in ω-3 PUFA was observed, with most of the increase being accounted for by DHA [8]. A similar scenario was reported for developing piglets, with increased DHA content at term and 14 weeks postnatally compared to mid-gestation [9].

Long chain ω-3 and ω-6 PUFAs can be endogenously synthesized from their precursors, alpha-linolenic acid (ALA) and linoleic acid (LA), respectively. However, these conversions are believed to be insufficient for the growing infant and must be supplemented by diet. Human breast milk contains about 13–22 wt% of its total fatty acid content as PUFA, with the DHA content varying widely depending on the mother's diet [10–13]. For example, in Japan, the average DHA content in breast milk is about 1% of total fatty acids while in Pakistan it is about 0.06% [14]. Studies in primate models have shown that maternal and neonatal diets deficient in ω-3 PUFAs result in altered brain and retinal fatty acid composition and are associated with impaired neural and visual function [15].

Fatty acid binding proteins (FABPs) are a family of 10 intracellular proteins that bind hydrophobic ligands including fatty acids [16,17]. Different members of the FABP family are expressed in the brain where they participate in the intracellular trafficking of different fatty acids [16]. Of these FABPs, brain fatty acid binding protein (B-FABP or FABP7) binds DHA with the highest affinity, although it can also bind other PUFAs such as AA [18]. FABP7 has well-established roles in brain development and has also been shown to be a key determinant of malignant glioma growth properties and prognosis [16,19–22]. It has been postulated that the relative levels of AA and DHA in brain may affect FABP7 expression [23]. A recent study suggests a link between FABP7, DHA and gene expression [24].

In this study, we explore the impact of DHA-rich maternal and weaning diets on brain fatty acid composition as well as FABP7 expression during the first six weeks of life. Although some reports have assessed the effect of feeding ω-3-rich diets to dams during pregnancy and lactation on brain fatty acid composition at embryonic and weanling stages [25,26], to our knowledge, there has been no follow-up at later developmental stages. The brains of three-week and six-week old rats correspond to that of 2–3 year old and 12–18 year old humans, respectively [7]. At these two developmental stages, the brains of rats and humans are thought to undergo fairly similar developmental processes [7]. Our model should therefore provide relevant information on brain fatty acid needs in humans at these two stages.

2. Experimental Section

2.1. Animals

Protocols involving animal use were approved by the University of Alberta Health Sciences Animal Care and Use Committee and were carried out following the Canadian Council on Animal Care guidelines and in compliance with the ARRIVE guidelines. Primiparous Sprague-Dawley rats (n = 20) were obtained from Charles River Laboratories (Montreal, Quebec, Canada) on day 14 of gestation. Dams were fed standard rat chow (Lab diet 5001; PMI Nutrition International, Brentwood, MO, USA) throughout gestation. Approximately 24 h before giving birth, dams were randomly allocated to one of two nutritionally adequate experimental diets. The composition of the diets, different only in fat composition, has been previously published [27]. The fatty acid composition of the control diet (Cnt, n = 12 dams) and the DHA-rich diet (ω-3, n = 8 dams) is described in Table 1. The fat content (20% w/w) and the polyunsaturated to saturated fatty acid (PUFA:SFA) ratio (0.5) did not differ between diets. All diets met the essential fatty acid requirements of the rodent. At birth, the litters were culled, leaving 10 pups per dam. Diets were fed *ad libitum* throughout the suckling period. Offspring were kept with their mothers until termination.

Three weeks postnatally, the dams and six pups/dam were weighed and sacrificed by CO_2 exposure and subsequent cervical dislocation. Their brains were carefully excised, snap frozen in liquid nitrogen and kept at −80 °C until assayed for fatty acid composition and FABP7 expression. Pup stomach content was also collected and assayed for fatty acid composition as an indicator of dietary effect on maternal milk composition [28]. The remaining pups from each dam (n = 4) were randomly assigned either the same diet as the dam (n = 2/dam) or crossed over to the other diet (n = 2/dam). The pups were fed this diet for an additional three weeks. This design resulted in four groups of six-week old pups: Cnt/Cnt, ω-3/Cnt, Cnt/ω-3, and ω-3/ω-3, based on the respective dam diet and final pup diet (dam diet/pup diet). At six weeks, rats were sacrificed and brain samples were collected as described previously. An outline of the experimental design is presented in (Figure 1).

Table 1. Fatty acid composition of control (Cnt) and docosahexaenoic acid (DHA)-rich (ω-3) diets. Data are presented as % of total fatty acids [a].

Fatty Acid	Control Diet (Cnt)	DHA Diet (ω-3)
	g/100 g of total fatty acids	
C14:0	0.1 ± 0.0	0.4 ± 0.0
C16:0	6.7 ± 0.3	6.2 ± 0.1
C16:1ω-7	0.2 ± 0.0	0.2 ± 0.1
C18:0	38.8 ± 1.2	40.6 ± 0.2
C18:1ω-9	29.0 ± 1.7	24.8 ± 0.3
C18:2ω-6 (LA)	21.2 ± 0.5	21.6 ± 0.0
C20:0	0.9 ± 0.0	0.9 ± 0.0
C18:3ω-3 (ALA)	1.7 ± 0.1	3.3 ± 0.1
C20:3ω-6	0.4 ± 0.1	0.4 ± 0.1
C20:4ω-6 (AA)	0.4 ± 0.0	0.4 ± 0.0
C22:6ω-3 (DHA)	0	0.9 ± 0.1

[a] Analysis by GLC of n = 2 batches, mean ± standard error of the mean (SEM); AA, arachidonic acid; ALA, α-linolenic acid; DHA, docosahexaenoic acid; ω, omega.

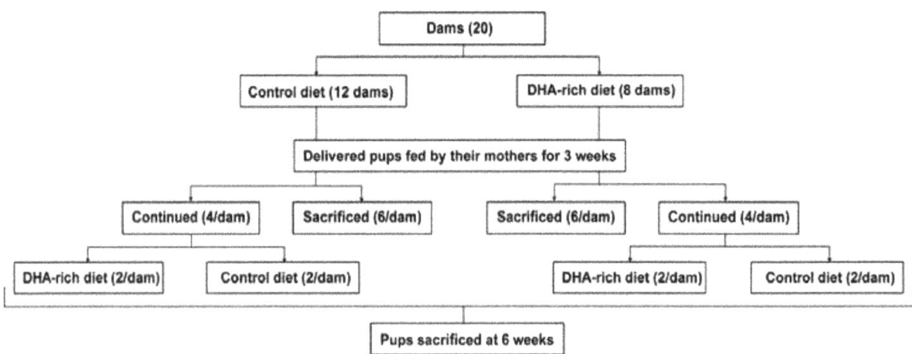

Figure 1. Outline of the study design. Dams were fed control (Cnt) or DHA-rich (ω-3) diets during lactation. Three weeks postnatally, dams and a portion of the pups were sacrificed and their brains were collected. Aliquots of dam breast milk and pup stomach content were collected to assess dietary effect on DHA content. The remaining pups were maintained on either control (Cnt) or DHA-rich (ω-3) diet for three more weeks until sacrificed and their brain samples were collected.

2.2. Brain Phospholipids Fatty Acid Composition

Brain lipids were extracted by a modified Folch method and total phospholipids were separated on silica G plates as previously described [29]. The bands were visualized with 8-anilino-1-naphthalenesulfonic acid under UV light. Appropriate standards were used for comparison. Fatty acid methyl esters were then prepared from the scraped silica bands and separated by automated gas liquid chromatography (Agilent Model 7890A, Agilent Technologies, Mississauga, ON, Canada) using a 100 m CP-Sil 88 fused capillary column (Agilent Technologies) with peaks identified by comparison with standards (NuChek Prep, Elysian, MN, USA). A total of 20 fatty acids were assessed and their values were expressed as g/100 g of total fatty acids.

2.3. Western Blot Analysis

Brain tissue was homogenized in modified RIPA buffer [50 mM Tris-HCl pH 7.0, 150 mM NaCl, 0.5% sodium deoxycholate, 1% NP40, 0.1% SDS, 1 mM sodium fluoride, 1× Complete Protease Inhibitor (Roche Diagnostics, Laval, Canada)]. Brain lysates (50 μg protein per lane) were electrophoresed in 12.5% SDS-polyacrylamide gels then transferred to nitrocellulose membranes and immunostained with rabbit anti-FABP7 antibody (1:500 dilution) [30] or goat anti-actin antibody (1:100,000) (Sigma-Aldrich, Oakville, Canada). Primary antibodies were detected with horseradish peroxidase-conjugated secondary antibodies (Jackson ImmunoResearch Laboratories Inc., Burlington, Canada) using the ECL detection system (GE Healthcare, Mississauga, Canada).

2.4. Statistical Analysis

Data are reported as mean ± standard error of the mean (SEM). In analyzing pup data, every dam was represented by one pup and pups were treated as individual experimental units. One-way analysis of variance, Duncan's multiple range *post hoc* test (4 groups) and Student's unpaired *t*-test (2 groups) were used to assess the significance of differences between groups. Where data did not conform to normality, Kruskal-Wallis one way analysis of variance on ranks and Dunn's test were used. Microsoft Excel (Microsoft, Redmond, WA, USA) and SigmaPlot 12.0 (Systat software, Inc. Chicago, IL, USA) were used in the statistical analysis of data. The level of significance was set at $p < 0.05$.

3. Results

3.1. Effect of a DHA-Rich Diet on Dam and Pup Brain Fatty Acid Composition

3.1.1. Dam Brain Fatty Acid Composition: DHA-Rich Diet Does Not Alter AA and DHA Levels

Dams were divided into two groups: those fed a control diet (Cnt) consisting of 1.7% total ω-3 PUFA (no added DHA), and those fed a DHA-rich diet (ω-3) consisting of 0.9% DHA with a total ω-3 PUFA content of 4.2% (Figure 1; Table 1). The ω-6:ω-3 ratios of the control and DHA-rich diets were 13.3:1 and 5.3:1, respectively. Dams were fed the diets until they were sacrificed 21 days after delivery. Litter size and body weights of Cnt and ω-3 dams did not differ significantly with average values being 323 ± 12.0 g and 299 ± 4.23 g at termination, respectively.

There were no significant differences in total saturated fatty acids (SFA), total monounsaturated fatty acids (MUFA), and total PUFA between the Cnt and ω-3 dam brains (Table 2) although a borderline ($p = 0.053$) reduction (by 8.2%) in ω-6 PUFA was observed in ω-3 dam brains compared to controls. Of note, LA (C18:2ω-6) was significantly increased (by 9.4%) whereas adrenic acid (C22:4ω-6) was significantly decreased (by 55.6%) in ω-3 dam brains. C22:4ω-6, a major PUFA in myelin, is formed from C20:4ω-6 by a 2-carbon chain elongation.

The ratio of C18:2ω-6:C20:4ω-6 was significantly increased (by 17.2%) in ω-3 dam brains compared to controls, indicating reduced conversion of LA to AA in dams fed a DHA-rich diet. A DHA diet also reduced the ω-6:ω-3 PUFA ratio by 12.5% ($p = 0.046$), and there was a trend towards a reduced AA:DHA ratio (by 12.3%, $p = 0.065$). Thus, the most dramatic effect of a DHA-rich diet on dam brain fatty acid composition is about a two-fold reduction in C22:4ω-6 levels, with no change in ω-3 PUFA levels and a borderline decrease in overall ω-6 PUFA levels.

3.1.2. Three-Week Old Pup Brain Fatty Acid Composition: DHA-Rich Diet Increases DHA and Decreases AA Content

At three weeks, pups weaned from Cnt or ω-3 dams showed no significant difference in body weight, with weights being 50.5 ± 0.74 g and 50.7 ± 1.3 g, respectively. DHA content was higher in milk samples collected from ω-3 dams compared to controls (1.43% ± 0.12% *vs.* 0.19% ± 0.02%, $p < 0.05$) with no change in AA content (2.9% ± 0.6% *vs.* 2.5% ± 0.3%, full composition not shown). The stomach contents of three-week pups were also collected as these should reflect the fatty acid composition of dams' milk. The increase in DHA observed in the breast milk of dams fed a DHA-rich diet was mirrored by pup stomach content with a DHA content of 1.1% ± 0.03% in ω-3 samples compared to 0.24% ± 0.18% in Cnt samples.

Table 2. Fatty acid composition of total phospholipids isolated from brains of dams fed either control (Cnt) or DHA-rich (ω-3) diet.

Fatty Acids	Cnt (n = 9)	ω-3 (n = 4)	p-Value *
		% of total fatty acids	
14:0	0.22 ± 0.07	0.29 ± 0.16	0.63
15:0	0.45 ± 0.15	0.52 ± 0.29	0.82
16:0	22.2 ± 0.15	22.9 ± 0.17 *	0.03
16:1ω-9	0.49 ± 0.03	0.51 ± 0.03	0.63
18:0	25.0 ± 0.22	25.1 ± 0.68	0.94
18:1ω-9	17.7 ± 0.25	17.5 ± 0.65	0.81
18:1c11	4.5 ± 0.38	4.4 ± 0.59	0.88
18:2ω-6	0.70 ± 0.01	0.77 ± 0.02 *	0.004
20:0	0.37 ± 0.02	0.37 ± 0.04	0.94
18:3ω-3	1.1 ± 0.05	1.1 ± 0.07	0.74
20:2ω-6	0.09 ± 0.008	0.09 ± 0.003	0.64
20:3ω-6	0.81 ± 0.05	0.77 ± 0.06	0.62
20:4ω-6	8.9 ± 0.25	8.3 ± 0.11	0.12
24:0	1.2 ± 0.07	1.2 ± 0.15	0.86
24:1ω-9	2.7 ± 0.12	2.5 ± 0.06	0.14
22:4ω-6	0.53 ± 0.04	0.24 ± 0.09 *	0.004
22:5ω-6	0.05 ± 0.008	0.06 ± 0.01	0.32
20:5ω-3	0.73 ± 0.05	0.73 ± 0.1	0.99
22:5ω-3	0.12 ± 0.01	0.16 ± 0.01	0.07
22:6ω-3	12.0 ± 0.28	12.6 ± 0.30	0.19
Total MUFA	25.3 ± 0.32	24.8 ± 0.07	0.16
Total SFA	49.5 ± 0.33	50.3 ± 0.44	0.18
ω-3 PUFA	13.9 ± 0.27	14.6 ± 0.36	0.19
ω-6 PUFA	11.1 ± 0.27	10.2 ± 0.13	0.05
Total PUFA	25.1 ± 0.34	24.8 ± 0.35	0.65
18:2ω-6:20:4ω-6	0.08 ± 0.003	0.09 ± 0.003 *	0.02
ω-6:ω-3 PUFA	0.8 ± 0.03	0.7 ± 0.02 *	0.046

Data are presented as mean ± standard error of the mean (SEM). * indicates significant difference between the two groups. MUFA: monounsaturated fatty acid; SFA: saturated fatty acid; PUFA: polyunsaturated fatty acids. * $p < 0.05$ indicates significant difference between the fatty acid levels in brain phospholipids of dams fed control diet *versus* ω-3 diet. Two-tailed unpaired t-test.

The brain composition of three-week old pups showed no change in terms of total SFA, total MUFA, and total PUFA content with DHA-rich diet. However, significant differences were observed within the PUFA category, with ω-6 PUFAs decreasing by 9.9%, and ω-3 PUFAs increasing by 15.3% in three-week old pups whose dams were fed a DHA-rich diet (Table 3). For ω-6 PUFA, C22:4 and C20:4 were significantly decreased by 64.4% and 9.0%, respectively, in keeping with the results observed for dams. As well, the C18:2ω-6:C20:4ω-6 ratio was significantly increased (by 22.1%). Thus, 3-week pup brains mimics dam brains in that conversion of LA to AA is decreased under DHA-rich conditions.

The increase in ω-3 PUFA observed in the brains of pups from dams fed a DHA-rich diet was mainly due to a 13.6% increase in C22:6 (Table 3). These changes in ω-6 and ω-3 PUFAs resulted in a 21.9% decrease in the ω-6:ω-3 PUFA ratio and a 20.1% decrease in the AA:DHA ratio (Table 3). We also observed a 13.4% decrease in the MUFA, C24:1ω-9 (nervonic acid), in pup brains as a consequence of high levels of DHA in the maternal diet (Table 3). The effect of a DHA-rich diet on C24:1ω-9 in pup brains is of potential significance as nervonic acid is a major component of myelin. These results demonstrate that pup brain fatty acid composition prior to weaning is highly dependent on dam diet, with significant increases observed in DHA content, as well as decreases in 22:4ω-6, C20:4ω-6 and 24:1ω-9 content.

Table 3. Fatty acid composition of total phospholipids isolated from brains of three-week old pups weaned from dams fed either control (Cnt) or DHA-rich (ω-3) diet.

Fatty Acids	Cnt (n = 15)	ω-3 (n = 9)	* p-Value
		% of total fatty acids	
14:0	0.42 ± 0.01	0.37 ± 0.02	0.05
15:0	0.77 ± 0.09	0.61 ± 0.12	0.29
16:0	27.5 ± 0.23	26.1 ± 0.69	0.08
16:1ω-9	1.1 ± 0.03	1.0 ± 0.04	0.20
18:0	23.7 ± 0.16	23.7 ± 0.3	0.99
18:1ω-9	13.3 ± 0.17	14.4 ± 0.79	0.22
18:1c11	2.7 ± 0.09	2.9 ± 0.20	0.16
18:2ω-6	1.1 ± 0.03	1.2 ± 0.04	0.07
20:0	0.25 ± 0.02	0.36 ± 0.08	0.23
18:3ω-3	0.38 ± 0.03	0.58 ± 0.15	0.21
20:2ω-6	0.18 ± 0.008	0.20 ± 0.02	0.19
20:3ω-6	0.70 ± 0.03	0.99 ± 0.14	0.07
20:4ω-6	11.6 ± 0.16	10.6 ± 0.43 *	0.04
24:0	0.31 ± 0.04	0.53 ± 0.16	0.19
24:1ω-9	3.2 ± 0.04	2.8 ± 0.04 *	<0.0001
22:4ω-6	1.4 ± 0.03	0.49 ± 0.02 *	<0.0001
22:5ω-6	0.03 ± 0.003	0.05 ± 0.01	0.14
20:5ω-3	0.39 ± 0.04	0.52 ± 0.14	0.42
22:5ω-3	0.14 ± 0.006	0.14 ± 0.01	0.88
22:6ω-3	10.8 ± 0.23	12.3 ± 0.43 *	0.003
Total MUFA	20.3 ± 0.23	21.2 ± 0.98	0.40
Total SFA	52.9 ± 0.31	51.6 ± 0.78	0.14
ω-3 PUFA	11.7 ± 0.21	13.5 ± 0.27 *	<0.0001
ω-6 PUFA	14.9 ± 0.13	13.5 ± 0.28 *	<0.0001
Total PUFA	26.7 ± 0.31	27.0 ± 0.44	0.56
ω-6 PUFA:ω-3 PUFA	1.3 ± 0.02	0.99 ± 0.02 *	<0.0001
20:4ω-6:22:6ω-3	1.1 ± 0.02	0.86 ± 0.02 *	<0.0001

Data are presented as mean ± standard error of the mean (SEM). MUFA: monounsaturated fatty acid; SFA: saturated fatty acid; PUFA: polyunsaturated fatty acids. One to two pups per dam were used for the fatty acid analyses. * $p < 0.05$ indicates significant difference between the fatty acid levels in brain phospholipids of three-week old pups from dams fed control diet *versus* ω-3 diet. Two-tailed unpaired t-test.

3.1.3. Six-Week Old Pup Brain Fatty Acid Composition: DHA-Rich Diet Maintains Elevated DHA Content after Pups Are Transferred to a Cnt Diet

In six week pups, there were no significant changes in the body weights among the four dietary groups, with values being 159.5 ± 4.1, 163.3 ± 4.5, 158.2 ± 4.8, 156.5 ± 4.7 g, for Cnt/Cnt, ω-3/Cnt, Cnt/ω-3, and ω-3/ω-3 groups, respectively. Similarly, total SFA, total MUFA and total PUFA were not significantly different among the four groups (Table 4). Although total PUFA content was not significantly different, statistically significant increases in ω-3 PUFA were observed when comparing Cnt/ω-3 and ω-3/ω-3 treatment groups to the Cnt/Cnt group, with increases of 15.5% and 18.9%, respectively. The 9% increase observed upon comparing the ω-3 PUFA content in the ω-3/Cnt group to that of the Cnt/Cnt group was not statistically significant (Figure 2A and Table 4). A trend towards reduced ω-6 PUFA content was apparent in ω-3/Cnt (5.7%) compared to Cnt/Cnt group, with significant reductions observed in the Cnt/ω-3 (7.6%) and ω-3/ω-3 (10.1%) groups (Figure 2A and Table 4)

Table 4. Fatty acid composition of total phospholipids isolated from brains of six-week old pups fed control diet (Cnt) or DHA-rich (ω-3) diet for three weeks after being weaned from dams that were fed either Cnt or ω-3 diets.

Fatty Acids	Treatment Groups (Dam diet/Pup Diet)			
	Cnt/Cnt (n = 10)	ω-3/Cnt (n = 7)	Cnt/ω-3 (n = 8)	ω-3/ω-3 (n = 8)
	% of Total Fatty Acids			
14:0	0.17 ± 0.006	0.17 ± 0.004	0.17 ± 0.004	0.16 ± 0.005
15:0	0.61 ± 0.21	0.77 ± 0.27	0.74 ± 0.22	1.1 ± 0.17
16:0	22.9 ± 0.28	24.5 ± 1.1	23.6 ± 0.34	21.8 ± 0.72
16:1ω-9	0.48 ± 0.01	0.55 ± 0.03	0.50 ± 0.02	0.48 ± 0.02
18:0	25.2 ± 0.46	24.5 ± 0.89	25.4 ± 0.49	23.7 ± 0.62
18:1ω-9	16.5 ± 0.39	16.4 ± 0.74	16.0 ± 0.21	18.3 ± 0.86
18:1c11	4.0 ± 0.31	3.2 ± 0.32	3.3 ± 0.34	3.1 ± 0.21
18:2ω-6	0.78 ± 0.04 a	0.80 ± 0.03 a	0.82 ± 0.03 a,b	0.94 ± 0.06 b
20:0	0.48 ± 0.05 a,b	0.45 ± 0.06 a,b	0.38 ± 0.01 a	0.58 ± 0.09 b
18:3ω-3	0.99 ± 0.12	0.78 ± 0.11	0.78 ± 0.05	1.4 ± 0.28
20:2ω-6	0.16 ± 0.02	0.13 ± 0.008	0.15 ± 0.009	0.19 ± 0.03
20:3ω-6	0.87 ± 0.07 a,b	0.83 ± 0.11 a,b	0.77 ± 0.02 a	1.1 ± 0.09 b
20:4ω-6	9.4 ± 0.23	9.3 ± 0.15	9.2 ± 0.25	8.7 ± 0.35
24:0	1.1 ± 0.11	0.95 ± 0.19	0.79 ± 0.03	1.3 ± 0.27
24:1ω-9	3.1 ± 0.06 a	2.7 ± 0.04 b	2.7 ± 0.1 b	2.7 ± 0.08 b
22:4ω-6	1.3 ± 0.08 a	0.81 ± 0.32 a,b	0.68 ± 0.08 a,b	0.28 ± 0.03 b
22:5ω-6	0.03 ± 0.003	0.04 ± 0.005	0.03 ± 0.001	0.05 ± 0.01
22:5ω-3	0.11 ± 0.007 a	0.13 ± 0.009 a,b	0.15 ± 0.02 a,b	0.16 ± 0.009 b
22:6ω-3	10.7 ± 0.15 a	12.1 ± 0.25 b	13.0 ± 0.35 b	12.4 ± 0.45 b
Total MUFA	24.1 ± 0.37 a,c	22.9 ± 0.56 a,b	22.4 ± 0.44 b	24.7 ± 0.75 c
Total SFA	50.4 ± 0.36	51.4 ± 0.42	51.1 ± 0.58	48.7 ± 0.90
ω-3 PUFA	12.6 ± 0.13 a	13.7 ± 0.14 a,b	14.6 ± 0.29 b	15.0 ± 0.40 b
ω-6 PUFA	12.6 ± 0.21 a	11.9 ± 0.31 a,b	11.6 ± 0.32 b	11.3 ± 0.23 b
Total PUFA	25.2 ± 0.19	25.6 ± 0.34	26.2 ± 0.58	26.3 ± 0.34
18:2ω-6:20:4ω-6	0.08 ± 0.006 a	0.09 ± 0.005 a,b	0.09 ± 0.004 a,b	0.11 ± 0.01 b
ω-6 PUFA:ω-3 PUFA	0.99 ± 0.02 a	0.87 ± 0.02 b	0.79 ± 0.01 b,c	0.76 ± 0.03 c
20:4ω-6:22:6ω-3	0.88 ± 0.02 a	0.77 ± 0.01 a,b	0.71 ± 0.01 b	0.71 ± 0.03 b

Data are presented as mean ± standard error of the mean (SEM). Differences were assessed for significance using one-way analysis of variance followed by Duncan's multiple range post hoc test for normally distributed data. Where the ranked data did not conform to normality, Kruskal-Wallis one way analysis of variance on ranks and Dunn's test were used. Significant difference ($p < 0.05$) between the different treatment groups is indicated by different letters across a row. One pup per dam was included in the analyses of the fatty acid composition for each group.

A significant reduction in the ω-6:ω-3 PUFA ratio was observed in ω-3/Cnt (13.5%), Cnt/ω-3 (20.1%), and ω-3/ω-3 (24.0%) compared to Cnt/Cnt pups (Figure 2B and Table 4). The ratio of AA:DHA was reflective of the overall change in ω-6:ω-3 PUFA ratio and was also decreased in ω-3/Cnt (12.6%), Cnt/ω-3 (19.5%), and ω-3/ω-3 (19.7%) compared to Cnt/Cnt pups; however, statistical significance was not attained when ω-3/Cnt pups were compared to Cnt/Cnt pups (Figure 2B and Table 4).

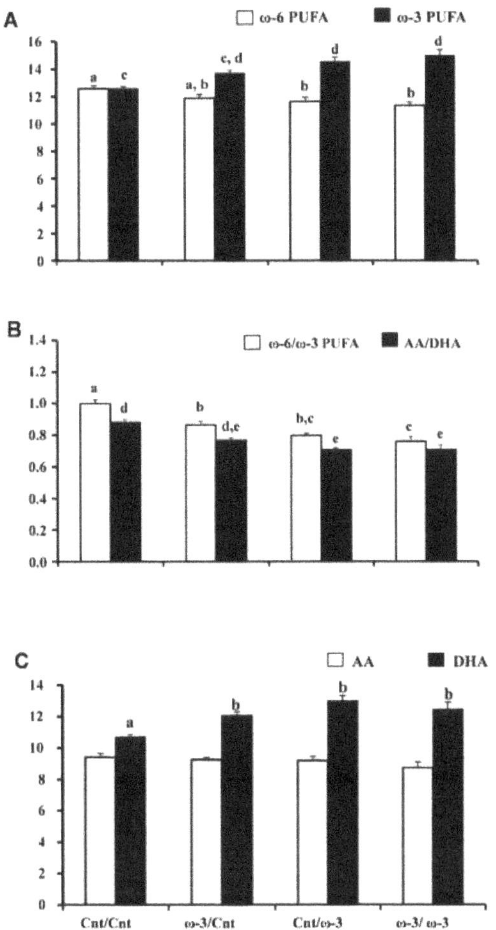

Figure 2. Effect of docosahexaenoic acid (DHA)-rich (ω-3) diet on brain long chain polyunsaturated fatty acids (PUFA) content in 6-week pups. The four sets of columns represent the Cnt/Cnt, ω-3/Cnt, Cnt/ω-3, and ω-3/ω-3 groups. Panel **A** shows ω-6 PUFA content and ω-3 PUFA content. Panel **B** shows ω-6:ω-3 PUFA and arachidonic acid (AA):DHA ratios. Panel **C** shows AA content and DHA content. Different letters indicate that groups are significantly different. Differences were assessed for significance using one-way analysis of variance followed by Duncan's multiple range *post hoc* test for normally distributed data. Where the ranked data did not conform to normality, Kruskal-Wallis one way analysis of variance on ranks and Dunn's test were used; $p < 0.05$. Numbers of pups included in the fatty acid assay at six weeks were 10, 7, 8 and 8 for the Cnt/Cnt, ω-3/Cnt, Cnt/ω-3, and ω-3/ω-3 groups, respectively. In all dietary groups, one pup per dam was used for the fatty acid analyses.

The increase in ω-3 PUFA content observed in six week pups was primarily due to increased DHA content (Figure 2C and Table 4). DHA was significantly increased in ω-3/Cnt, Cnt/ω-3, and ω-3/ω-3, by 12.5%, 21.2%, and 16.2%, respectively, when compared to Cnt/Cnt pups (Figure 2C and Table 4). C22:5ω-3 (EPA), a precursor of DHA that is normally found at very low levels in brain, was significantly increased by 51.2% in ω-3/ω-3 compared to Cnt/Cnt pups, with a trend towards increased EPA levels observed for ω-3/Cnt (21.9% increase) and Cnt/ω-3 pups (37.2% increase) (Table 4).

As previously noted for dam and three-week pup brains, the ω-6 PUFA, C22:4 was significantly decreased (by 79%) in ω-3/ω-3 brains, with a non-significant trend towards decreased levels observed in ω-3/Cnt (by 38.6%) and Cnt/ω-3 (by 48.6%) pups, compared to Cnt/Cnt pups (Table 4). LA (C18:2ω-6) was increased by 21.2% and 17.3% in the brains of ω-3/ω-3 pups compared to Cnt/Cnt and ω-3/Cnt pups, respectively, with the C18:2ω-6:C20:4ω-6 ratio being significantly increased in ω-3/ω-3 pups (by 32.2%) compared the Cnt/Cnt pups (Table 4). A trend towards an increased C18:2ω-6:C20:4ω-6 ratio was also observed in ω-3/Cnt (by 4.4%) and Cnt/ω-3 (by 12.9%) pups compared to Cnt/Cnt pups (Table 4).

The MUFA, C24:1ω-9, was significantly decreased in the brains of pups exposed to a DHA-rich diet, with percentage reductions of 11.7%, 13.1%, and 10.5% in ω-3/Cnt, Cnt/ω-3, and ω-3/ω-3 pups, respectively, compared to Cnt/Cnt pups (Table 4). Thus, our diet crossover experiment indicates that DHA feeding during lactation maintains a brain environment that favors ω-3 PUFA enrichment even after the pups are transferred to a low-DHA diet post weaning. Our data also show that continued feeding of a DHA-rich diet is needed for inhibition of the ω-6 metabolic conversion of LA to AA.

3.2. FABP7 Expression in Three-Week and Six-Week Pups

We next assessed the relationship between DHA intake and FABP7 protein levels as it has previously been postulated that the increase in the AA:DHA ratio observed in malignant glioma tumor tissue might be associated with changes in FABP7 expression [23]. Dam diet had no significant effect on FABP7 protein levels in three-week pups (Figure 3A, B). As expected, a significant reduction (69%) in FABP7 expression was observed in six-week pups compared to three-week pups fed a Cnt diet (Figure 3C, D). However, at six weeks, when FABP7 levels are generally low, a DHA-rich diet did have an effect on FABP7 levels, with significant reductions observed whether DHA was provided through the dam or as a three-week long dietary supplement starting when the pups were weaned. Percent reductions were 65%, 50%, and 70% in ω-3/Cnt, Cnt/ω-3 and ω-3/ω-3 pups compared to Cnt/Cnt pups, respectively (Figure 4A–E).

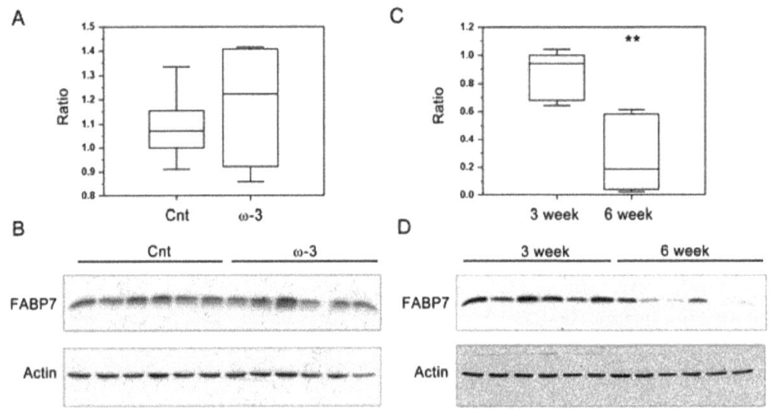

Figure 3. Effect of docosahexaenoic acid (DHA)-rich (ω-3) diet and age on brain fatty acid binding protein expression (FABP7). Box-plots represent band intensities of FABP7/actin (Y-axis) in the brains of three-week old pups fed a control diet (Cnt, $n = 6$; one pup per dam) or DHA-rich (ω-3, $n = 6$; one pup per dam) diet (**A**), and in the brains of three-week old pups ($n = 6$; one pup per dam) and six-week ($n = 6$; one pup per dam) fed a Cnt diet (**C**). Panels B and D are Western blots showing FABP7 and actin levels in the brains of three-week old pups fed control and DHA-rich diets (**B**), and three and six-week old pups fed a Cnt diet (**D**). ** indicates $p < 0.01$. Differences were assessed for significance using two-tailed unpaired t-test.

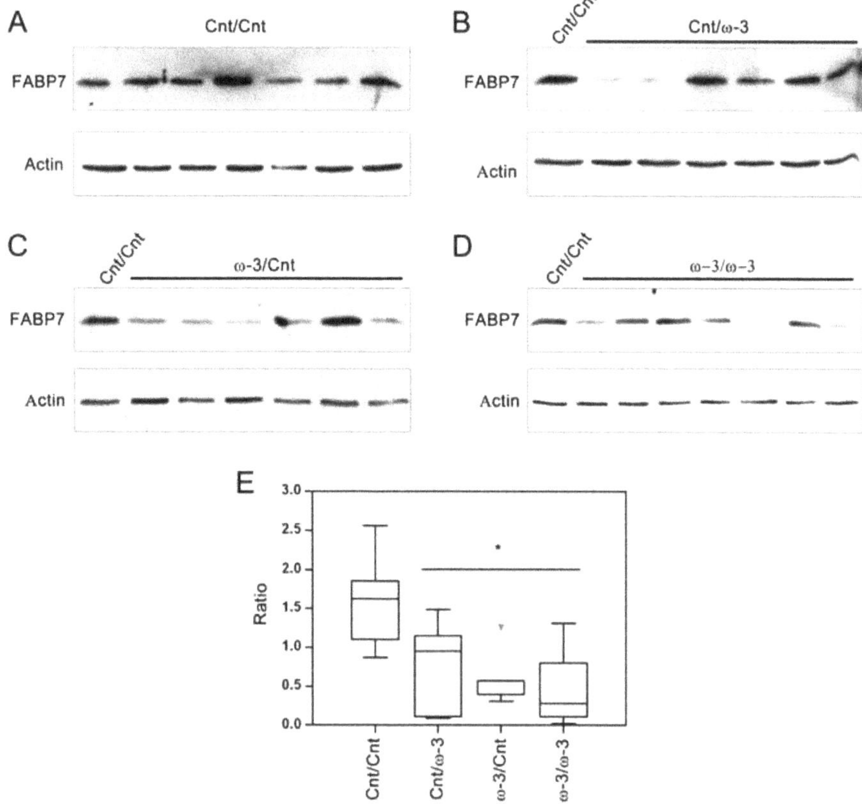

Figure 4. Effect of a docosahexaenoic acid (DHA)-rich (ω-3) diet on brain fatty acid binding protein expression (FABP7) at six weeks. Panels **A**, **B**, **C** and **D** are western blots showing FABP7 and actin levels in the brains of six-week old Cnt/Cnt ($n = 7$; one pup per dam), Cnt/ω-3 ($n = 6$; one pup per dam), ω-3/Cnt ($n = 6$; one pup per dam), and ω-3/ω-3 ($n = 6$; one pup per dam) pups, respectively. Panel **E** represents a Box-Plot of band intensities of FABP7 (Y-axis, normalized to actin and a Cnt/Cnt sample that was loaded in lane 1 of all gels to normalize for any differences in gel handling and electro-blotting) in different dietary groups. * indicates significant difference ($p < 0.05$) from the Cnt/Cnt with groups under the line being statistically equivalent.

4. Discussion

DHA-induced improvement in brain function is believed to be due to its modulation of synaptic proteins and overall activity [31]. Our results indicate that the developing brain readily incorporates DHA supplied during toddler/juvenile stages since the brains of six-week old rats are developmentally equivalent to 12–18 year-old human brains [32]. Furthermore, early introduction of DHA (during lactation) maintains high DHA levels in the brain even after the pups are switched to low-DHA weaning diet. Importantly, boosting brain DHA levels is still achievable through direct dietary supply at weaning in cases where DHA was not provided during suckling. Finally, we report that DHA down-regulates the expression of FABP7, a key factor associated with neural proliferation and differentiation [33,34]; however, this effect is only apparent later in brain development.

Diets were designed to provide an adequate supply of ω-6 (including AA) and ω-3 PUFA in the absence (Cnt) or presence of DHA (ω-3). Our dietary ratios of total ω-6 to total ω-3 PUFA are within the previously reported range in human breast milk samples, as well as milk fatty acid profiles of rats [10,12,35]. We observed the following effects of DHA feeding on brain lipid composition at the toddler and juvenile stages: (i) increased brain total ω-3 PUFA content (especially DHA), (ii) reduced brain total ω-6 PUFAs, (iii) reduced ω-6:ω-3 ratio and AA:DHA ratio, and (iv) reduced brain adrenic (C22:4ω-6) and nervonic acid (C24:1ω-9) content.

It is well known that adult brains are more resistant than juvenile brains to diet-induced changes in fatty acid composition [36]. Minor increases in brain DHA and total ω-3 PUFA content (~5%) with concomitant decreases in AA and total ω-6 PUFA (5–6%) have previously been reported in adult rats fed DHA-rich diet for eight weeks [37]. These observations are consistent with our results in lactating dams that were fed a DHA-rich diet for three weeks. We did observe increases in LA (C18:2ω-6) and in the LA:AA ratio (C18:2ω-6:C20:4ω-6), along with a decrease in C22:4ω-6 (adrenic acid), in the brains of dams fed a DHA-rich diet. These changes likely indicate DHA-mediated inhibition of LA metabolism through Δ-6 and Δ-5 desaturases or inhibition of AA elongation, as previously reported [38–40]. The lack of effect on AA levels is likely due to the adequate supply of AA in the DHA-rich (ω-3) diet.

In keeping with previous work, we observed more pronounced DHA-rich diet-induced changes in brain fatty acid composition at three weeks [26,41]. Human infant brains have been reported to be similarly susceptible to changes in dietary fatty acids, with higher (39%) brain DHA accumulation in six-month old breast-fed infants compared to infants fed formula that did not contain AA or DHA [42]. Our results indicate that the DHA-rich diet increases total ω-3 PUFA (mainly DHA) by 14.7% and decreases total ω-6 PUFA (mainly AA and C22:4ω-6) and ω-6:ω-3 ratio by 12.8% and 24%, respectively. Since the brain of a three-week old rat is at a comparable stage as that of a human toddler (2-3 years), our results suggest that DHA accretion in human brain may well extend beyond 6 months. As with the dams, decreases in LA metabolic products (C22:4ω-6 and AA), together with an increase in the LA:AA ratio, were observed at three weeks, indicating inhibition of Δ-6 and Δ-5 desaturases by DHA [43–46].

At six weeks, changes in brain fatty acid composition were most marked in pups born to Cnt dams and fed a DHA-rich diet (Cnt/ω-3) or born to ω-3 dams and maintained on a DHA-rich diet (ω-3/ω-3). There is clear indication of inhibition of the ω-6 PUFA desaturation and elongation pathway in these pups. Unlike changes in ω-6 PUFA which were readily reversible, increases in the levels of DHA in six-week old pup brains were not reversed when DHA was discontinued. In fact, brain DHA levels in ω-3/Cnt pups showed increases that were equivalent to pups fed a DHA-rich diet for three weeks post-weaning (Cnt/ω-3) or those exposed to DHA from birth up to six postnatal weeks (ω-3/ω-3 group). In comparison, DHA-induced decreases in ω-6 PUFA were readily reversible and disappeared when DHA was discontinued (ω-3/Cnt group). It will be important to determine whether the effect of a maternal DHA-rich diet on pup brain DHA levels can be extended past six weeks.

Levels of nervonic acid (C24:1ω-9) in three-week and six-week pup brains were significantly reduced by increased levels of DHA in the diet. Nervonic acid is the major very long chain fatty acid found in sphingomyelin, one of the main components of myelin [47,48]. Although studies show that there is postnatal accretion of nervonic acid in sphingomyelin, there are no systematic reports assessing the effect of a DHA-rich diet on myelination [6,49]. Interestingly, a diet high in DHA results in longer latencies of the auditory startle response (a functional indicator of myelination) [50]. In contrast to MUFA such as nervonic acid, PUFA content in myelin phospholipids is low, consisting of 1/6 to 1/3 of the PUFA content of gray matter phospholipid [48]. Adrenic acid (C22:4ω-6) is a major PUFA of myelin [6]. As our DHA-rich diet also significantly decreased adrenic acid levels in the brains of three-week and six-week pups, it will be important to carry out follow-up studies on the effect of a DHA-rich diet on the myelination of juvenile brain.

The mammalian brain has elevated levels of DHA and AA compared to other tissues, with the DHA:AA ratio increasing as a function of brain maturation [6,9]. Analysis of human brain at different stages has revealed different ratios of DHA:AA in the different phospholipid classes, with phosphotidylserine having the highest DHA:AA ratio and phosphotidylcholine having the lowest DHA:AA ratio [6]. The DHA:AA ratio in phosphotidylethanolamines changes over the course of brain maturation, from <1:1 to >1:1. It has been estimated that phosphotidylserine and phosphotidylethanolamine contain ~92% of the esterified DHA in total brain phospholipids of one-week old rat pups [8].

Different regions of the brain as well as the different phospholipid classes show different susceptibilities to diet-induced changes in fatty acid composition. For example, the DHA-rich frontal cortex appears to be particularly sensitive to ω-3 PUFA deficiency [51,52]. Phosphatidylethanolamines prepared from neuronal cells isolated from frontal cortex, cerebellum and hippocampus of pups whose dams were fed various diets during lactation showed differential accretion of DHA and AA over time depending on diet [53]. For example, one-week to three-week old pups born from dams fed either a diet with an LA to ALA ratio of 4:1 or a DHA-supplemented (0.8 g/100 g fat) diet showed steady increases in DHA levels, especially in the cerebellum. Extending the dam diet to weaned pups for an additional three weeks resulted in further accretion of DHA in the cerebellum, but not in the frontal lobe or hippocampus [53]. In comparison, DHA supplementation (0.8 g/100 g fat) had no effect on DHA levels in phosphotidylcholine in all three regions tested, although six-week old pups did show increased accretion of DHA in this phospholipid subclass in the frontal lobe and to a lesser extent in cerebellum [53]. Thus, results from the phosphotidylethanolamine analysis are in general agreement with our results, with the exception that we did not observe a further increase in DHA levels in whole brain phospholipids at six weeks compared to three weeks in pups fed a continuous DHA-rich diet for six weeks.

We have previously noted associations between the AA:DHA ratio and FABP7 in normal brain and brain tumors [23]. For example, FABP7 levels are high during normal brain development when the AA:DHA ratio is relatively high [8,9,19]. FABP7 expression decreases from birth onwards, a period that coincides with high brain DHA accumulation and a lower AA:DHA ratio [9,19]. Furthermore, the AA:DHA ratio in human malignant glioma tumors is increased compared to that of normal brain [54], with FABP7 expression also up-regulated in these tumors [21,55]. During brain development, FABP7 is expressed in radial glial cells, neural stem/progenitor cells that have self-renewal capacity and can differentiate into both neuronal and glial cells [19,56,57]. Radial glial cells form the fiber network along which neurons migrate in developing brain. Although radial glial cells are primarily found in developing brain, these cells are also retained in the centers of the brain that undergo neurogenesis in the adult [57]. *In vitro* binding studies indicate that FABP7 has a special affinity for PUFAs, including DHA and AA [18,58].

In this study, we tested the hypothesis that increased FABP7 levels are associated with a high AA:DHA ratio in a normally developing brain. Interestingly, we found that boosting brain DHA levels (thus decreasing the AA:DHA ratio) was associated with significant reductions in FABP7 levels at six weeks. The correlation between high levels of FABP7 and AA suggests a role for FABP7/AA in processes related to radial glial cell function such as formation of the fiber network that guide neuronal migration. Thus, there may be a reduced need for FABP7/AA-mediated events in the brains of six-week old pups exposed to a DHA-rich diet. In general agreement with our observation that changes in FABP7 levels were noted at six weeks but not at three weeks, Pelerin *et al.* reported little if any change in *FABP7* RNA levels in the cortex and microvessels of P14 pups whose dams were fed a DHA-supplemented diet [59]. Brains from older pups were not analyzed by these investigators.

Studies involving humans and pigs have shown that brain DHA content increases postnatally (up to eight years and 14 weeks, respectively) while brain AA plateaus or decreases postnatally [6,9]. Similar patterns have been observed in rats at ED17, ED20, and P8, with AA:DHA ratios of ~2 and ~1 observed in total brain lipids at E17 and P8, respectively [8]. While we didn't observe an increase in DHA content from three weeks to six weeks, there was a decrease in AA content during this period (by 19%) (Supplemental Figure S1), resulting in an overall decrease in the AA:DHA ratio as the brain assumes higher levels of structural and functional maturation. Along with this change in the AA:DHA ratio, we observed a significant reduction (69%) in brain FABP7 levels from three weeks to six weeks. Thus, we propose that a DHA-rich diet during lactation and/or weaning may enhance or accelerate brain maturation, as suggested by the observed: (i) increase in ω-3 PUFA; (ii) decrease in ω-6 PUFA; (iii) decrease in ω-6:ω-3 PUFA (and AA:DHA) ratio; and (iv) decrease in FABP7 protein levels.

5. Conclusions

We have examined the impact of DHA-rich maternal and weaning diets on brain fatty acid composition and FABP7 expression in developing rat brains. The study was carried out at two developmental stages: three weeks postnatal, which is developmentally equivalent to that of a 2–3-year old human, and six weeks postnatal, which is developmentally equivalent to that of a 12–18-year old human. Our data suggest that high levels of DHA in the maternal diet during lactation increases its levels in the infant brain and seems to have a protective effect since levels of DHA in brain can potentially be maintained up to adolescence even when the offspring is weaned to and maintained on a diet that is deficient in DHA. Furthermore, our data suggest that in cases where DHA is not supplied during lactation, it may still be possible to increase its levels in the brain by direct feeding perhaps until adolescence. Finally, there may be an association between brain DHA levels and FABP7 expression, with levels of FABP7 potentially reflecting brain maturation. The relevance of this observation to human health remains to be explored.

Supplementary Materials: Supplementary materials can be accessed at: http://www.mdpi.com/2072-6643/7/10/5433/s1.

Acknowledgments: We thank Nicole Coursen for her assistance with the animal studies. This work was supported by a discovery grant to Catherine J. Field from National Sciences and Engineering Research Council of Canada (NSERC) and a grant to Roseline Godbout from the Canadian Institutes of Health Research (CIHR) grant-Funding Reference Number 130314.

Author Contributions: Marwa E. Elsherbiny, Catherine J. Field and Roseline Godbout conceived and designed the experiments; Marwa E. Elsherbiny, Susan Goruk, Elizabeth A. Monckton and Miranda Brun performed the experiments; Marwa E. Elsherbiny, Caroline Richard and Marwan Emara analysed the data and performed statistical analysis; Marwa E. Elsherbiny and Roseline Godbout wrote the paper. All authors read and approved the paper.

Conflicts of Interest: The authors declare that they have no conflicts of interest.

References

1. De Graaf-Peters, V.B.; Hadders-Algra, M. Ontogeny of the human central nervous system: What is happening when? *Early Hum. Dev.* **2006**, *82*, 257–266. [CrossRef] [PubMed]
2. Tau, G.Z.; Peterson, B.S. Normal development of brain circuits. *Neuropsychopharmacology* **2010**, *35*, 147–168. [CrossRef] [PubMed]
3. Dekaban, A.S. Changes in brain weights during the span of human life: Relation of brain weights to body heights and body weights. *Ann. Neurol.* **1978**, *4*, 345–356. [CrossRef] [PubMed]
4. Clandinin, M.T. Brain development and assessing the supply of polyunsaturated fatty acid. *Lipids* **1999**, *34*, 131–137. [CrossRef] [PubMed]
5. Clandinin, M.T.; Chappell, J.E.; Leong, S.; Heim, T.; Swyer, P.R.; Chance, G.W. Intrauterine fatty acid accretion rates in human brain: Implications for fatty acid requirements. *Early Hum. Dev.* **1980**, *4*, 121–129. [CrossRef]
6. Martinez, M.; Mougan, I. Fatty acid composition of human brain phospholipids during normal development. *J. Neurochem.* **1998**, *71*, 2528–2533. [CrossRef] [PubMed]
7. Semple, B.D.; Blomgren, K.; Gimlin, K.; Ferriero, D.M.; Noble-Haeusslein, L.J. Brain development in rodents and humans: Identifying benchmarks of maturation and vulnerability to injury across species. *Prog. Neurobiol.* **2013**, *106–107*, 1–16. [CrossRef] [PubMed]
8. Green, P.; Yavin, E. Fatty acid composition of late embryonic and early postnatal rat brain. *Lipids* **1996**, *31*, 859–865. [CrossRef] [PubMed]
9. Purvis, J.M.; Clandinin, M.T.; Hacker, R.R. Fatty acid accretion during perinatal brain growth in the pig. A model for fatty acid accretion in human brain. *Comp. Biochem. Physiol. B* **1982**, *72*, 195–199. [CrossRef]
10. Xiang, M.; Alfven, G.; Blennow, M.; Trygg, M.; Zetterstrom, R. Long-chain polyunsaturated fatty acids in human milk and brain growth during early infancy. *Acta Paediatr.* **2000**, *89*, 142–147. [CrossRef] [PubMed]

11. Ruan, C.; Liu, X.; Man, H.; Ma, X.; Lu, G.; Duan, G.; DeFrancesco, C.A.; Connor, W.E. Milk composition in women from five different regions of China: The great diversity of milk fatty acids. *J. Nutr.* **1995**, *125*, 2993–2998. [PubMed]
12. Pedersen, L.; Lauritzen, L.; Brasholt, M.; Buhl, T.; Bisgaard, H. Polyunsaturated fatty acid content of mother's milk is associated with childhood body composition. *Pediatr. Res.* **2012**, *72*, 631–636. [CrossRef] [PubMed]
13. Sherry, C.L.; Oliver, J.S.; Marriage, B.J. Docosahexaenoic acid supplementation in lactating women increases breast milk and plasma docosahexaenoic acid concentrations and alters infant omega 6:3 fatty acid ratio. *Prostaglandins Leukot. Essent. Fatty Acids* **2015**, *95*, 63–69. [CrossRef] [PubMed]
14. Brenna, J.T.; Varamini, B.; Jensen, R.G.; Diersen-Schade, D.A.; Boettcher, J.A.; Arterburn, L.M. Docosahexaenoic and arachidonic acid concentrations in human breast milk worldwide. *Am. J. Clin. Nutr.* **2007**, *85*, 1457–1464. [PubMed]
15. Neuringer, M.; Connor, W.E.; Lin, D.S.; Barstad, L.; Luck, S. Biochemical and functional effects of prenatal and postnatal omega 3 fatty acid deficiency on retina and brain in rhesus monkeys. *Proc. Natl. Acad. Sci. USA* **1986**, *83*, 4021–4025. [CrossRef] [PubMed]
16. Liu, R.Z.; Mita, R.; Beaulieu, M.; Gao, Z.; Godbout, R. Fatty acid binding proteins in brain development and disease. *Int. J. Dev. Biol.* **2010**, *54*, 1229–1239. [CrossRef] [PubMed]
17. Liu, R.Z.; Li, X.; Godbout, R. A novel fatty acid-binding protein (FABP) gene resulting from tandem gene duplication in mammals: Transcription in rat retina and testis. *Genomics* **2008**, *92*, 436–445. [CrossRef] [PubMed]
18. Balendiran, G.K.; Schnutgen, F.; Scapin, G.; Borchers, T.; Xhong, N.; Lim, K.; Godbout, R.; Spener, F.; Sacchettini, J.C. Crystal structure and thermodynamic analysis of human brain fatty acid-binding protein. *J. Biol. Chem.* **2000**, *275*, 27045–27054. [CrossRef] [PubMed]
19. Feng, L.; Hatten, M.E.; Heintz, N. Brain lipid-binding protein (BLBP): A novel signaling system in the developing mammalian CNS. *Neuron* **1994**, *12*, 895–908. [CrossRef]
20. Mita, R.; Beaulieu, M.J.; Field, C.; Godbout, R. Brain fatty acid-binding protein and omega-3/omega-6 fatty acids: Mechanistic insight into malignant glioma cell migration. *J. Biol. Chem.* **2010**, *285*, 37005–37015. [CrossRef] [PubMed]
21. Liang, Y.; Bollen, A.W.; Aldape, K.D.; Gupta, N. Nuclear FABP7 immunoreactivity is preferentially expressed in infiltrative glioma and is associated with poor prognosis in EGFR-overexpressing glioblastoma. *BMC Cancer* **2006**. [CrossRef] [PubMed]
22. Mita, R.; Coles, J.E.; Glubrecht, D.D.; Sung, R.; Sun, X.; Godbout, R. B-FABP-expressing radial glial cells: The malignant glioma cell of origin? *Neoplasia* **2007**, *9*, 734–744. [CrossRef] [PubMed]
23. Elsherbiny, M.E.; Emara, M.; Godbout, R. Interaction of brain fatty acid-binding protein with the polyunsaturated fatty acid environment as a potential determinant of poor prognosis in malignant glioma. *Prog. Lipid Res.* **2013**, *52*, 562–570. [CrossRef] [PubMed]
24. Maximin, E.; Langelier, B.; Aioun, J.; Al-Gubory, K.H.; Bordat, C.; Lavialle, M.; Heberden, C. Fatty acid binding protein 7 and *n*-3 poly unsaturated fatty acid supply in early rat brain development. *Dev. Neurobiol.* **2015**. [CrossRef] [PubMed]
25. Ozias, M.K.; Carlson, S.E.; Levant, B. Maternal parity and diet (*n*-3) polyunsaturated fatty acid concentration influence accretion of brain phospholipid docosahexaenoic acid in developing rats. *J. Nutr.* **2007**, *137*, 125–129. [PubMed]
26. Anderson, G.J. Developmental sensitivity of the brain to dietary *n*-3 fatty acids. *J. Lipid Res.* **1994**, *35*, 105–111. [PubMed]
27. Robinson, L.E.; Field, C.J. Dietary long-chain (*n*-3) fatty acids facilitate immune cell activation in sedentary, but not exercise-trained rats. *J. Nutr.* **1998**, *128*, 498–504. [PubMed]
28. Lien, E.L.; Boyle, F.G.; Yuhas, R.J.; Kuhlman, C.F. Effect of maternal dietary arachidonic or linoleic acid on rat pup fatty acid profiles. *Lipids* **1994**, *29*, 53–59. [CrossRef] [PubMed]
29. Layne, K.S.; Goh, Y.K.; Jumpsen, J.A.; Ryan, E.A.; Chow, P.; Clandinin, M.T. Normal subjects consuming physiological levels of 18:3 (*n*-3) and 20:5 (*n*-3) from flaxseed or fish oils have characteristic differences in plasma lipid and lipoprotein fatty acid levels. *J. Nutr.* **1996**, *126*, 2130–2140. [PubMed]
30. Godbout, R.; Bisgrove, D.A.; Shkolny, D.; Day, R.S., 3rd. Correlation of B-FABP and GFAP expression in malignant glioma. *Oncogene* **1998**, *16*, 1955–1962. [CrossRef] [PubMed]

31. Sidhu, V.K.; Huang, B.X.; Kim, H.Y. Effects of docosahexaenoic acid on mouse brain synaptic plasma membrane proteome analyzed by mass spectrometry and (16)O/(18)O labeling. *J. Proteome Res.* **2011**, *10*, 5472–5480. [CrossRef] [PubMed]
32. Sengupta, P. The laboratory rat: Relating its age with human's. *Int. J. Prev. Med.* **2013**, *4*, 624–630. [PubMed]
33. Arai, Y.; Funatsu, N.; Numayama-Tsuruta, K.; Nomura, T.; Nakamura, S.; Osumi, N. Role of FABP7, a downstream gene of PAX6, in the maintenance of neuroepithelial cells during early embryonic development of the rat cortex. *J. Neurosci.* **2005**, *25*, 9752–9761. [CrossRef] [PubMed]
34. Matsumata, M.; Sakayori, N.; Maekawa, M.; Owada, Y.; Yoshikawa, T.; Osumi, N. The effects of FABP7 and FABP5 on postnatal hippocampal neurogenesis in the mouse. *Stem Cells* **2012**, *30*, 1532–1543. [CrossRef] [PubMed]
35. Priego, T.; Sanchez, J.; Garcia, A.P.; Palou, A.; Pico, C. Maternal dietary fat affects milk fatty acid profile and impacts on weight gain and thermogenic capacity of suckling rats. *Lipids* **2013**, *48*, 481–495. [CrossRef] [PubMed]
36. Bourre, J.M.; Dumont, O.S.; Piciotti, M.J.; Pascal, G.A.; Durand, G.A. Dietary alpha-linolenic acid deficiency in adult rats for 7 months does not alter brain docosahexaenoic acid content, in contrast to liver, heart and testes. *Biochim. Biophys. Acta* **1992**, *1124*, 119–122. [CrossRef]
37. Lin, Y.H.; Shah, S.; Salem, N., Jr. Altered essential fatty acid metabolism and composition in rat liver, plasma, heart and brain after microalgal DHA addition to the diet. *J. Nutr. Biochem.* **2010**, *22*, 758–765. [CrossRef] [PubMed]
38. Gibson, R.A.; Muhlhausler, B.; Makrides, M. Conversion of linoleic acid and alpha-linolenic acid to long-chain polyunsaturated fatty acids (LCPUFAs), with a focus on pregnancy, lactation and the first 2 years of life. *Matern. Child Nutr.* **2011**, *7*, 17–26. [CrossRef] [PubMed]
39. Wainwright, P.E.; Huang, Y.S.; Simmons, V.; Mills, D.E.; Ward, R.P.; Ward, G.R.; Winfield, D.; McCutcheon, D. Effects of prenatal ethanol and long-chain *n*-3 fatty acid supplementation on development in mice. 2. Fatty acid composition of brain membrane phospholipids. *Alcohol. Clin. Exp. Res.* **1990**, *14*, 413–420. [CrossRef] [PubMed]
40. Wijendran, V.; Lawrence, P.; Diau, G.Y.; Boehm, G.; Nathanielsz, P.W.; Brenna, J.T. Significant utilization of dietary arachidonic acid is for brain adrenic acid in baboon neonates. *J. Lipid Res.* **2002**, *43*, 762–767. [PubMed]
41. Anderson, G.J.; Connor, W.E.; Corliss, J.D. Docosahexaenoic acid is the preferred dietary *n*-3 fatty acid for the development of the brain and retina. *Pediatr. Res.* **1990**, *27*, 89–97. [CrossRef] [PubMed]
42. Cunnane, S.C.; Francescutti, V.; Brenna, J.T.; Crawford, M.A. Breast-fed infants achieve a higher rate of brain and whole body docosahexaenoate accumulation than formula-fed infants not consuming dietary docosahexaenoate. *Lipids* **2000**, *35*, 105–111. [CrossRef] [PubMed]
43. Garg, M.L.; Sebokova, E.; Thomson, A.B.; Clandinin, M.T. Delta 6-desaturase activity in liver microsomes of rats fed diets enriched with cholesterol and/or omega 3 fatty acids. *Biochem. J.* **1988**, *249*, 351–356. [CrossRef] [PubMed]
44. Garg, M.L.; Thomson, A.B.; Clandinin, M.T. Effect of dietary cholesterol and/or omega 3 fatty acids on lipid composition and delta 5-desaturase activity of rat liver microsomes. *J. Nutr.* **1988**, *118*, 661–668. [PubMed]
45. Njoroge, S.W.; Laposata, M.; Katrangi, W.; Seegmiller, A.C. DHA and EPA reverse cystic fibrosis-related FA abnormalities by suppressing FA desaturase expression and activity. *J. Lipid Res.* **2012**, *53*, 257–265. [CrossRef] [PubMed]
46. Wadhwani, N.S.; Manglekar, R.R.; Dangat, K.D.; Kulkarni, A.V.; Joshi, S.R. Effect of maternal micronutrients (folic acid, vitamin B12) and omega 3 fatty acids on liver fatty acid desaturases and transport proteins in wistar rats. *Prostaglandins Leukot. Essent. Fatty Acids* **2012**, *86*, 21–27. [CrossRef] [PubMed]
47. Yao, J.K.; Holman, R.T.; Lubozynski, M.F.; Dyck, P.J. Changes in fatty acid composition of peripheral nerve myelin in essential fatty acid deficiency. *Arch. Biochem. Biophys.* **1980**, *204*, 175–180. [CrossRef]
48. O'Brien, J.S.; Sampson, E.L. Fatty acid and fatty aldehyde composition of the major brain lipids in normal human gray matter, white matter, and myelin. *J. Lipid Res.* **1965**, *6*, 545–551. [PubMed]
49. Sargent, J.R.; Coupland, K.; Wilson, R. Nervonic acid and demyelinating disease. *Med. Hypotheses.* **1994**, *42*, 237–242. [CrossRef]

50. Haubner, L.; Sullivan, J.; Ashmeade, T.; Saste, M.; Wiener, D.; Carver, J. The effects of maternal dietary docosahexaenoic acid intake on rat pup myelin and the auditory startle response. *Dev. Neurosci.* **2007**, *29*, 460–467. [CrossRef] [PubMed]
51. Delion, S.; Chalon, S.; Herault, J.; Guilloteau, D.; Besnard, J.C.; Durand, G. Chronic dietary alpha-linolenic acid deficiency alters dopaminergic and serotoninergic neurotransmission in rats. *J. Nutr.* **1994**, *124*, 2466–2476. [PubMed]
52. Carrie, I.; Clement, M.; de Javel, D.; Frances, H.; Bourre, J.M. Specific phospholipid fatty acid composition of brain regions in mice. Effects of *n*-3 polyunsaturated fatty acid deficiency and phospholipid supplementation. *J. Lipid Res.* **2000**, *41*, 465–472. [PubMed]
53. Jumpsen, J.; Lien, E.L.; Goh, Y.K.; Clandinin, M.T. Small changes of dietary (*n*-6) and (*n*-3)/fatty acid content ration alter phosphatidylethanolamine and phosphatidylcholine fatty acid composition during development of neuronal and glial cells in rats. *J. Nutr.* **1997**, *127*, 724–731. [PubMed]
54. Martin, D.D.; Robbins, M.E.; Spector, A.A.; Wen, B.C.; Hussey, D.H. The fatty acid composition of human gliomas differs from that found in nonmalignant brain tissue. *Lipids* **1996**, *31*, 1283–1288. [CrossRef] [PubMed]
55. Kaloshi, G.; Mokhtari, K.; Carpentier, C.; Taillibert, S.; Lejeune, J.; Marie, Y.; Delattre, J.Y.; Godbout, R.; Sanson, M. FABP7 expression in glioblastomas: Relation to prognosis, invasion and EGFR status. *J. Neurooncol.* **2007**, *84*, 245–248. [CrossRef] [PubMed]
56. Anthony, T.E.; Klein, C.; Fishell, G.; Heintz, N. Radial glia serve as neuronal progenitors in all regions of the central nervous system. *Neuron* **2004**, *41*, 881–890. [PubMed]
57. Kurtz, A.; Zimmer, A.; Schnutgen, F.; Bruning, G.; Spener, F.; Muller, T. The expression pattern of a novel gene encoding brain-fatty acid binding protein correlates with neuronal and glial cell development. *Development* **1994**, *120*, 2637–2649. [PubMed]
58. Xu, L.Z.; Sanchez, R.; Sali, A.; Heintz, N. Ligand specificity of brain lipid-binding protein. *J. Biol. Chem.* **1996**, *271*, 24711–24719. [PubMed]
59. Pelerin, H.; Jouin, M.; Lallemand, M.S.; Alessandri, J.M.; Cunnane, S.C.; Langelier, B.; Guesnet, P. Gene expression of fatty acid transport and binding proteins in the blood-brain barrier and the cerebral cortex of the rat: Differences across development and with different DHA brain status. *Prostaglandins. Leukot. Essent. Fatty Acids* **2014**, *91*, 213–220. [CrossRef] [PubMed]

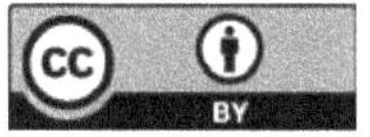

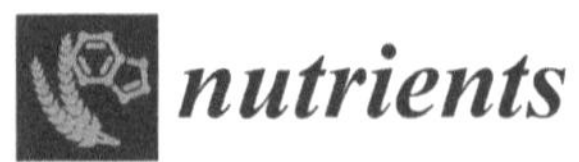

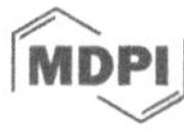

Article

Association between Blood Omega-3 Index and Cognition in Typically Developing Dutch Adolescents

Inge S. M. van der Wurff [1,*], Clemens von Schacky [2], Kjetil Berge [3], Maurice P. Zeegers [4,5], Paul A. Kirschner [1] and Renate H. M. de Groot [1,4]

1 Welten Institute, Research Centre for Learning, Teaching, and Technology, Open University of the Netherlands, Heerlen 6419 AT, The Netherlands; Paul.Kirschner@ou.nl (P.A.K.); renate.degroot@ou.nl (R.H.M.G.)

2 Omegametrix, Martinsried 82 152, Germany; Clemens.vonSchacky@med.uni-muenchen.de

3 Aker BioMarine Antarctic AS, Lysaker NO-1327, Norway; kjetil.berge@akerbiomarine.com

4 NUTRIM School of Nutrition and Translational Research in Metabolism, Maastricht University, Maastricht 6200 MD, The Netherlands; Zeegerm.zeegers@maastrichtuniversity.nl

5 CAPHRI School for Public Health and Primary Care, Maastricht University, Maastricht 6200 MD, The Netherlands

* Correspondence: inge.vanderwurff@ou.nl; Tel.: +31-45-576-2909

Received: 17 November 2015; Accepted: 15 December 2015; Published: 2 January 2016

Abstract: The impact of omega-3 long-chain polyunsaturated fatty acids (LCPUFAs) on cognition is heavily debated. In the current study, the possible association between omega-3 LCPUFAs in blood and cognitive performance of 266 typically developing adolescents aged 13–15 years is investigated. Baseline data from Food2Learn, a double-blind and randomized placebo controlled krill oil supplementation trial in typically developing adolescents, were used for the current study. The Omega-3 Index was determined with blood from a finger prick. At baseline, participants finished a neuropsychological test battery consisting of the Letter Digit Substitution Test (LDST), D2 test of attention, Digit Span Forward and Backward, Concept Shifting Test and Stroop test. Data were analyzed with multiple regression analyses with correction for covariates. The average Omega-3 Index was 3.83% (SD 0.60). Regression analyses between the Omega-3 Index and the outcome parameters revealed significant associations with scores on two of the nine parameters. The association between the Omega-3 Index and both scores on the LDST ($\beta = 0.136$ and $p = 0.039$), and the number of errors of omission on the D2 ($\beta = -0.053$ and $p = 0.007$). This is a possible indication for a higher information processing speed and less impulsivity in those with a higher Omega-3 Index.

Keywords: docosahexaneoic acid (DHA); eicosapentaenoic acid (EPA); adolescents; cognition; Omega-3 fatty acids; Omega-3 Index

1. Introduction

In recent decades, an increasing interest in the health benefits of long-chain polyunsaturated fatty acids (LCPUFAs) has been developed. Aside from its influence on cardiovascular health, it has also attracted attention because of its association with mental health (ADHD, autism, dyslexia) [1], cognitive functioning of healthy individuals [2–4] and cognitive decline in the elderly [5–7]. LCPUFAs and especially docosahexaneoic acid, 22:6*n*-3 (DHA), and eicosapentaenoic acid 20:5*n*-3 (EPA) are involved in many aspects of brain functioning such as neuronal membrane fluidity, neurotransmission, signal transduction, brain blood flow, and blood-brain barrier integrity [8,9]. The interest in the possible positive influence of LCPUFAs on brain functioning has led to a large number of both observational and experimental studies (for a review see [10,11]). These studies have, however, mainly focused on either diseased populations of infants, children, adults, and the elderly. Studies in typically developing adolescents are limited. The current study addresses this deficit.

Adolescence is a period in which LCPUFAs could be of special importance. During adolescence, the brain, especially the prefrontal cortex, undergoes development which continues until after age 20 [12,13]. The development of the prefrontal cortex is of utmost importance, since this development lays the basis for higher order cognitive functions that have been associated with academic achievements [14]. Moreover, the prefrontal cortex is a brain region especially enriched in DHA [15], and higher DHA intake has been associated with changes in the functional activity of the prefrontal cortex in boys aged 8–10 [16].

To our knowledge, three observational studies looking at the association between fish intake (the most important source of omega-3 LCPUFAs) and cognitive functioning in adolescents have been executed. Kim and colleagues showed that adolescents aged 15 years who regularly consumed fish had significantly better academic performance than peers who never or hardly ever consumed fish [17]. Aberg *et al.* demonstrated that high fish consumption in boys at age 15 was associated with better cognitive performance at age 18 [18]. Lastly, de Groot *et al.* studied 700 Dutch high school students aged 12–18 years. Fish consumption data, end term grades in Dutch, English and Math, scores on the Amsterdam Vocabulary Test, and scores on the Youth Self-Report (a self-reported measure for attention problems) were collected [19]. Results revealed that 13.6% of the Dutch adolescents never ate fish, 63.1% ate fish but too little to meet at least half of the recommended amount, 16.9% reached half of the recommended amount, and 6.4% met national guidelines (fish twice per week). Analysis of the variance showed significant differences between the four fish consumption groups (never, <1 per week (e.g., 1 time per month), 1 to 2 times per week, ⩾2 times per week) in vocabulary, and a trend for significance was found for the average end term grade. Significant quadratic associations (u-shape association) between fish consumption, vocabulary ($p = 0.01$), and average end term grades ($p = 0.001$) were shown. Higher fish intake was associated with a more advanced vocabulary and an almost significantly higher average end term grade. However, eating more fish than the recommended amount (>2 fish portions/week) seemed to no longer be beneficial. Overall, the observational studies in adolescents point to a beneficial association between fish intake (the main source of the omega-3 LCPUFAs DHA and EPA) and school grades.

Fish consumption is the most important dietary source of LCPUFAs but not the only source [20]. Moreover, there is a large interpersonal variability in the uptake of LCPUFAs [21]. Thus, to be sure about the association between LCPUFAs and cognition in adolescents, measurement of LCPUFAs in blood is needed. Therefore, the main objective of this study is to investigate the association between the Omega-3 Index (EPA + DHA in erythrocytes as percentage of total fatty acids measured [22]) measured in blood and cognitive performance in typically developing adolescents of lower general secondary education (LGSE). Cognition is a very broad term that includes both lower order simple responses and higher order processes. The higher order processes are also called the executive functions, and it is generally agreed that there are three core executive functions namely: (i) inhibition and interference; (ii) working memory; and (iii) cognitive flexibility [23]. These executive functions are used to build higher order skills such as reasoning and problem solving. Therefore, the executive functions are important for academic success and cognitive development [23]. These executive functions are located in the prefrontal cortex, the brain area most in development during adolescence [24]. The cognitive tasks used in the current study are standard tasks of cognitive/executive functioning for this age group and have previously been shown to increase activation of the frontal cortex, the area of the brain associated with the accumulation of DHA [16].

In addition to the main objective, two sub-objectives will be addressed. A number of earlier studies have shown differences in the LCPUFA status between typically developing participants and participants with disorders such as ADHD, autism, and dyslexia [25,26]. However, to our knowledge, whether LCPUFAs are associated with cognition in participants with learning disorders differently than in those without learning disorders has not yet been assessed. The second objective of the current study is, therefore, to explore whether the association between the Omega-3 Index and cognitive ability is different between adolescents with and without learning disorders.

Social economic status, often operationalized as educational level, has been shown to be associated with diet quality (*i.e.*, people with a higher SES have better diet quality) [27]. Moreover, in adults, higher social economic status has been found to be associated with higher fish consumption [28]. However, even though it is known that students from lower general secondary education (LSGE) levels have a less healthy diet and lifestyle than students from the higher levels [29], how much fish students from the LSGE consume has, to our knowledge, not yet been assessed. Therefore, the third objective of this study is to explore the fish consumption of second year students of the LSGE.

2. Materials and Methods

2.1. Design

This study was part of a larger randomized controlled clinical trial (Food2Learn) studying the influence of omega-3 LCPUFA supplementation on cognitive performance, mental wellbeing, and academic achievement scores in adolescents attending LGSE. Baseline data of Food2Learn were used to study the association between the Omega-3 Index measured in whole blood and cognition. Food2Learn has been approved by the Medical Ethical Committee of Atrium-Orbis-Zuyd Hospital (now Zuyderland), Heerlen, The Netherlands (NL45803.096.13). Food2Learn has been registered at the Netherlands Trial Register (NTR4082), which is connected to Clinicaltrials.gov (registered as NCT02240264.)

2.2. Procedure and Participants

Participants were recruited from 17 schools in the south of the Netherlands. For students who wanted to participate, an informed consent form had to be signed by themselves as well as by both parents and/or guardians. After informed consent was received, students underwent a finger prick to measure their Omega-3 Index. Inclusion criteria for Food2Learn were: 1 Omega-3 Index <5%, as it was expected that omega-3 fatty acid supplementation will be especially beneficial for participants with a very low baseline Omega-3 Index [22]; and 2 attending the second year of LSGE because Richardson *et al.* showed that omega-3 supplementation was especially beneficial in the 20% lowest performing students [30]. Therefore, the choice for students at one of the lowest educational levels in The Netherland's LGSE was made. In the Netherlands, secondary education is divided into three levels: pre-university, higher general secondary education, and LGSE. Approximately 38% of all adolescents follow LGSE [31]. LGSE is further divided up into four sublevels. For this study, students from the highest sublevel, the theoretical learning pathway (TLP), were recruited. Approximately 40% of students attending LGSE are in the TLP [31]. No other inclusion criteria were applied, thus, all second year students of the LSGE with an Omega-3 Index <5% could participate. After inclusion, participants underwent a neuropsychological test battery in a small group setting (10 students max) consisting of: Letter Digit Substitution Task (LDST), D2 test of Attention (D2), Digit Span Forward (DSF), and Backward (DSB). In addition, they filled out a number of questionnaires to collect important background information. The tests were led by one researcher via a standardized protocol, while one or two other researchers (depending on the group size) were monitoring to ensure that participants understood the tests and complied with the protocol. Before continuing with the real tests, students received a practice version of the tests, feedback was given, and the students confirmed they understood the tests. After this group test session, all participants filled out a questionnaire individually (data not used in the current study), during which participants were called one by one to perform the individual neuropsychological tests: Stroop Test and Concept Shifting Test (CST) under the supervision of one researcher.

2.3. Dependent Variable—Blood Analysis

Whole blood was obtained from a finger prick with an automated lancet and directly transferred to a filter paper (Whatman 903, General Electric, Frankfurt, Germany) pre-treated with a stabilizer. Filter papers were shipped immediately to Omegametrix, Martinsried, Germany for analysis. Whole blood fatty acid compositions were analyzed according to the HS-Omega-3 Index methodology [32]. Fatty acid methyl esters are generated by acid transesterification and analyzed by gas chromatography using a GC2010 Gas Chromatograph (Shimadzu, Duisburg, Germany) equipped with a SP2560, 100-m column (Supelco, Bellefonte, PA, USA) using hydrogen as a carrier gas. Fatty acids are identified by comparison with a standard mixture of fatty acids. Results are given as EPA plus DHA expressed as a percentage of total identified fatty acids after response factor correction. Since the Omega-3 Index is defined as EPA + DHA in erythrocytes, it was calculated using a sliding correction factor. The coefficient of variation for EPA plus DHA typically is 5%. Analyses are quality-controlled according to DIN ISO 15189.

2.3.1. Independent Variables—Cognitive Measures

The LDST is a paper-pencil task used to measure speed of information processing [33]. A nine letter/digit key is noted at the top of a page. Below this key, rows of letters are printed, and participants are asked to write the corresponding number in the box underneath the letter as quickly as possible. The number of correctly filled in numbers in 60 s is used as a measure of speed of information processing.

2.3.2. D2 Test of Attention

The D2 test is a paper-pencil task used to measure selective attention [34]. Participants are presented with 14 rows each consisting of 47 stimuli. Stimuli are the letters d and p with a varying number of dashes (between 1 and 4), below, above, or on both sides. Participants are instructed to only cross out the d with two dashes (2 above, 2 below or one on both sides) and ignore all other stimuli. Participants have to process as many stimuli as possible in 20 s per line after which they have to continue with the next row without pausing. The following measures per row and in total are noted after completion: total number of stimuli processed, number of correctly crossed out d2's, number of d2's not crossed out, and number of stimuli wrongly crossed out (thus, non d2). The total number of stimuli processed is used as a measure for information processing speed. The number of target stimuli not crossed out (*i.e.*, errors of omission) and non-target stimuli crossed out (*i.e.*, errors of commission) are used as a measure for impulsivity and inattention, respectively.

2.3.3. Digit Span Forward and Backward

The DSF is a measure for short-term memory that primarily activates the phonological loop. The DSB activates the executive component directly and shows the dynamic relationship between passive storage and active manipulation or transformation of information held in the memory [35] and is thus a measure for working memory (the ability to hold information in the mind and work with it). The DSF consists of 12 sequences of digits varying in length from three to eight digits (each length twice). Digits are announced by the researcher at a rate of approximately one digit per second. After completion of the digit sequence, participants are asked to write down the sequence. The DSB is similar to the DSF, except for the fact that it consists of 12 digit sequences varying in length from two to seven digits (each length twice) and after completion of the sequence by the researcher, students are asked to write down the sequence backwards, starting with the last number announced. The longest sequence of numbers of which participants had correctly written down at least one of the two rows was used as a measure for working memory.

2.3.4. Concept Shifting Task

The CST is a measure for cognitive shifting [36]. Cognitive shifting is the ability to adapt to changes in the environment by switching from one mental set to another [33]. The task consists of four parts. All parts consist of a sheet of paper with 16 small circles grouped in one large circle. In task A, the small circles are randomly filled with numbers, in task B the circles are filled with letters, and in task C the circles are filled with both. Participants are asked to cross out the items in the correct order (A: 1 to 12; B: A to P; C: 1–A–2–B to 8-H). Lastly, there is Task Zero, which consists of empty circles, where participants are asked to cross out the circles as quickly as possible. Task Zero is administered twice, and the average of these times is used to correct for basic motor speed in the other tasks. For all tasks, the time taken to complete and the number of errors are noted. The average of motor-speed corrected time needed for A and B was subtracted from the motor speed corrected time needed for C and used as a measure for shifting.

2.3.5. Stroop Test

The Stroop test provides a measure for cognitive inhibition. Cognitive inhibition is the ability to inhibit an overlearned response in favor of a more unusual one [37]. The Stroop task, as used in Food2Learn, consists of three cards containing 40 stimuli each: color names printed in black (Task 1), colored patches (Task 2), and color names printed in congruent or incongruent color (Task 3). For Task 1, participants are asked to read the name out loud. For Task 2, participants name the color of the patches, and for Task 3, participants name the ink color the word is printed in. Task 3 is a measure of mental flexibility and the ability to inhibit a dominant response (reading). The time needed for Task 2 was subtracted from the time needed for Task 1, the result of this sum was subtracted from the time needed for Task 3. The result of this sum was used as a measure for inhibition.

2.3.6. Additional Measures

Students filled out a questionnaire to assess covariates. The following covariates were assessed as they are known to correlate with cognition: BMI (weight/length^2, self-reported) [36], sex [37], age [38], alcohol consumption [39], smoking [40], and parental level of education [41]. Alcohol consumption was assessed with two questions: the number of days/week the participant generally drank alcohol and the number of units the participant drinks on a day that (s)he drinks alcohol. Alcohol consumption was defined as the number of alcohol units/time multiplied by the number of drinking days/week, and the measurement was used as a continuous measure. Smoking was assessed with the question: "How many cigarettes do you smoke per week?". If the participant indicated consuming cigarettes, (s)he was classified as smoker. Parental level of education was filled out by the parents on an ordinal eight-point scale [42]. Parental level of education was defined as the parent with the highest level of education, which is an indication for social economic status [43]. Additionally, fish consumption was assessed with a short, validated, and self-reported questionnaire [3]. Different kinds of fish were divided based on their DHA content: low (fish fingers, prawns, pickled herring, cod, mussels, plaice, tuna, tilapia); medium (trout, raw herring, smoked eel, smoked salmon, canned salmon); and high (smoked herring, herring and tomato sauce, mackerel, canned sardines, salmon). The consumption (never, once a month, two to three times a month, once a week or more than once a week) was used to calculate the fish consumption score. For the low DHA fish 0, 1, 2, 4, 8 points; for the medium DHA fish, 0, 2, 4, 8, 16 points; and for the high DHA fish, 0, 3, 6, 12, 24 points. The score for fish consumption could thus vary between 0 and 48 points. Lastly students were asked to indicate whether they had a disorder which could influence learning (examples were given) and who had made that diagnosis.

2.4. Quality Control

To ensure the quality of the data, all tests were scored by two independent researchers. Any discrepancies were solved by discussion. Furthermore, in order to prevent typing mistakes, all data were entered in the database twice, after which the two files were automatically compared. Any discrepancies between the two data files were checked and corrected by a third researcher.

2.5. Statistical Analyses

Data were checked for normality and if necessary, transformation was applied. Data were analyzed with linear regression or generalized linear regression (Poisson) for count data and data with a skewed distribution. For all analyses, first, a model with all covariates (*i.e.*, smoking, alcohol consumption units per week), BMI, age, level of parental education, sex, and diagnosis) was built; Model A. In Model B, the Omega-3 Index was added. In a separate analysis, potential moderation between the Omega-3 Index and diagnosis was tested. If results were significant, a sub-group analysis for typically developing adolescents and those who had indicated to have some sort of learning disorder (autism, dyslexia, ADHD, *etc.*) were executed in the same way (diagnosis was not entered as a covariate). For all analyses, a *p*-value below 0.05 was considered to be significant. All analyses were carried out using SPSS statistics version 22.

3. Results

3.1. Participants

A total of 286 students consented to participate in the study. Of these, four dropped out before blood sampling due to personal reasons and 16 had an Omega-3 Index > 5%. Thus, the associations between the Omega-3 Index and cognition of 266 participants (127 boys, 139 girls; M_{age} = 14.1 years) are discussed in this paper. Characteristics of the participants can be found in Table 1. Omega-3 Index and LCPUFAs as determined in blood can be found in Table 2. Scores on the cognitive tests can be found in Table 3. In this sample, 69 participants indicated having a disorder which can impact learning; 14 indicated having Attention Deficit Hyperactivity Disorder (ADHD) or Attention Deficit Disorder (ADD); 45 indicated having dyslexia or dyscalculia; eight reported an autism spectrum disorder; and two indicated a depression. In the total sample of 266 adolescents, 13.8% indicated never consuming fish, 77% indicated eating fish very irregularly (*i.e.*, less than half of the recommend amount of 450 mg DHA + EPA per day), 8.4% consumed at least half of the recommended amount (once a week), and 1% indicated consuming fish more than once a week. There was a significant difference in fish consumption between boys and girls ($p = 0.024$), with boys consuming more fish than girls. However, this did not result in significant differences in the Omega-3 Index ($p = 0.561$). The total score on the fish questionnaire correlated significantly with both the Omega-3 Index ($n = 216$, $r = 0.294$, $p < 0.001$) and DHA concentration ($n = 216$, $r = 0.287$, $p < 0.001$).

3.2. Cognitive Performance

Analyses revealed a significant association between the Omega-3 Index and score on the LDST ($\beta = 0.136$, $p = 0.039$). The addition of the Omega-3 Index to the model increased the r^2 with 0.017 (Table 4), *i.e.*, an additional 1.7% of the variance was explained. Furthermore, a significant association between the Omega-3 Index and errors of omission on the D2 was shown ($\beta = -0.053$, $p = 0.007$) (Table 5). The analysis for errors of omission also showed a significant moderator effect ($p = 0.005$). No other significant associations between the Omega-3 Index and any of the other cognitive measures were found.

Table 1. Participant characteristics.

Characteristic	All Participants		With Diagnosis [1]		Without Diagnosis [2]		p-Value [5]
	Mean ± SD or N (%)	N	Mean ± SD or N (%)	N	Mean ± SD or N (%)	N	
Age (years)	14.10 ± 0.49	266	14.26 ± 0.51	69	14.05 ± 0.47	196	**0.002**
Male/Female	127/139 (47.7/52.3%)	266	36/33 (52.2/47.8%)	69	93/103 (47.5/52.5%)	196	0.499
Smoking no/yes [3]	239/26 (90.2/9.8%)	265	59/10 (85.5/14.5%)	69	179/16 (91.8/8.2%)	195	0.132
Body Mass Index (BMI)	19.92 ± 3.00	248	20.34 ± 3.61	65	19.77 ± 2.74	183	0.187
Alcohol units per week [4]	0.46 ± 1.77	266	0.69 ± 2.85	69	0.39 ± 1.19	196	0.218
Level of Parental Education (LPE)	5.07 ± 1.52	248	5.21 ± 1.40	66	5.02 ± 1.56	182	0.371

[1] Diagnosis was defined as a diagnosis possible to influence learning; this was indicated by students themselves and included (but not limited to) dyslexia, dyscalculia, depression, autism, and Attention Deficit Hyperactivity Disorder (ADHD); [2] without diagnosis was defined as all students who did not indicate to have a diagnosis; [3] smoking was defined as anybody who indicated to smoke more than 0 cigarettes per week; [4] alcohol units per week was operationalized as number of day per week that alcohol is consumed times units per consumption moment; [5] comparison between those with and those without diagnoses. ANOVA was used for age, BMI, LPE and alcohol units per week, Chi Square for smoking, and sex. Significant differences ($p < 0.05$) are noted in bold.

Table 2. Fatty acid blood.

Fatty Acid (% wt/wt of Total FA)	All Participants	With Diagnosis [1]	Without Diagnosis [2]	p-Value [3]
	N = 261	N = 68	N = 193	
	Mean ± SD	Mean ± SD	Mean ± SD	
Omega-3 Index	3.83 ± 0.60	3.79 ± 0.61	3.84 ± 0.60	0.537
DHA 22:6n-3	2.58 ± 0.49	2.56 ± 0.50	2.59 ± 0.49	0.667
EPA 20:5n-3	0.39 ± 0.16	0.38 ± 0.13	0.39 ± 0.16	0.356
AA 20:4n-6	11.19 ± 1.25	11.49 ± 1.34	11.08 ± 1.20	**0.022**
ObA 22:5n-3	0.43 ± 0.10	0.43 ± 0.11	0.44 ± 0.10	0.725

[1] Diagnosis was defined as a diagnosis possible to influence learning; this was indicated by students themselves and included (but not limited to) dyslexia, dyscalculia, depression, autism and ADHD; [2] without diagnosis was defined as all students who did not indicate to have a diagnosis; [3] Comparison between those with and those without diagnoses. Significant differences ($p < 0.05$) are noted in bold. DHA: docosahexaneoic acid; EPA: eicosapentaenoic acid.

Table 3. Scores on the cognitive tests.

Measures	All Participants	With Diagnosis [1]	Without Diagnosis [2]	p-Value [3]
	N = 261	N = 68	N = 196	
	Mean ± SD	Mean ± SD	Mean ± SD	
LDST (number)	34.47 ± 5.46	33.52 ± 6.51	34.80 ± 5.02	0.094
D2-correct (number)	163.13 ± 22.95	160.04 ± 24.24	164.22 ± 22.45	0.194
D-error of omission (number)	11.83 ± 10.73	11.25 ± 8.07	12.04 ± 11.53	0.598
D2-error of commission (number)	1.31 ± 10.73	1.54 ± 1.96	1.22 ± 1.43	0.161
D2-Total (number)	417.33 ± 56.46	408.93 ± 55.11	420.29 ± 56.77	0.151
Shifting score (s)	11.70 ± 6.83	11.69 ± 6.50	11.71 ± 6.96	0.980
Inhibition score (s)	31.35 ± 8.50	34.85 ± 9.19	30.12 ± 7.91	**0.000**
Digit span Forward (digits)	5.58 ± 0.88	5.26 ± 0.87	5.70 ± 0.85	0.616
Digit Span Backward (digits)	4.56 ± 0.98	4.51 ± 0.93	4.58 ± 1.00	**0.000**

[1] Diagnosis was defined as a diagnosis possible to influence learning; this was indicated by students themselves and included (but not limited to) dyslexia, dyscalculia, depression, autism, and ADHD; [2] without diagnosis was defined as all students who did not indicate to have a diagnosis; [3] Comparison between those with and those without diagnoses. Significant differences ($p < 0.05$) are noted in bold.

Table 4. Results of multiple linear regression analyses between the Omega-3 Index and score on the Letter Digit Substitution Test (LDST) in the complete sample.

Predictor Variable	B (Standardized) [1]	Significance [2]
Model A (r^2 = 0.058, df = 7, p = 0.051)		
Smoking	0.028	0.679
Alcohol consumption	0.031	0.649
BMI	0.089	0.171
Age	0.047	0.477
Sex	0.177	**0.007**
Highest LPE	−0.056	0.387
Diagnosis	−0.104	0.113
Model B (r^2 = 0.075, df = 8, p = 0.019)		
Smoking	0.031	0.643
Alcohol consumption	0.045	0.500
BMI	0.080	0.218
Age	0.036	0.584
Sex	0.172	**0.008**
Highest LPE [3]	−0.084	0.203
Diagnosis	−0.094	0.147
Omega-3 Index	0.136	**0.039**

[1] Standardized beta refers to how many standard deviations the dependent variable will change per standard deviation change in the predictor variable. Smoking, sex, and diagnosis were not standardized as they are dichotomous variables; [2] Significant results ($p < 0.05$) are printed in bold; [3] LPE = level of parental education.

Table 5. Results of generalized linear model analyses between the Omega-3 Index and number of errors of omission on the D2 test in the complete sample.

Predictor Variable	B (Standardized) [1]	Significance [2]
Model A (χ^2 = 47.90, df = 7, p < 0.001)		
Smoking	0.066	0.310
Alcohol consumption	0.036	**0.030**
BMI	0.043	**0.026**
Age	0.036	0.068
Sex	−0.047	0.226
Highest LPE	−0.087	**0.000**
Diagnosis	−0.071	0.109
Model B (χ^2 = 51.852, df = 8, p < 0.001)		
Smoking	0.062	0.349
Alcohol consumption	0.030	0.078
BMI	0.043	**0.028**
Age	0.041	0.037
Sex	−0.052	0.181
Highest LPE [3]	−0.077	**0.000**
Diagnosis	−0.083	0.063
Omega-3 Index	−0.053	**0.007**

[1] Standardized beta refers to how many standard deviations the dependent variable will change per standard deviation change in the predictor variable. Smoking, sex, and diagnosis were not standardized as they are dichotomous variables; [2] Significant results ($p < 0.05$) are printed in bold; [3] LPE = level of parental education.

3.3. Sub-Group Analyses

When participants were divided into those without learning disorders and those who indicated having one or more learning disorders, differences between the two groups arose. Those with a diagnosis were significantly older (Table 1, p = 0.002, 14.26 ± 0.51, and 14.05 ± 0.47, respectively) than those without a diagnosis. Furthermore, they had a slightly higher AA status (Table 2, 11.08 ± 1.20, and 11.49 ± 1.34, respectively). With regard to the test scores, there was a significant difference in average score between those with and those without a diagnoses in inhibition as measured with the

Stroop test (p = 0.000, 34.85 ± 9.19, and 30.12 ± 7.91, respectively) and on the digit span backwards (p = 0.000, 5.26 ± 0.869, and 5.7 ± 0.851, respectively).

When a moderation term was added to the regression analysis, a moderation effect was seen for the number of errors of omission (p = 0.005), *i.e.*, the association between the Omega-3 Index and score on the D2—the errors of omission were different between those with and those without diagnosis. Therefore, a separate group regression analysis was executed. This analysis showed no significant associations in adolescents with one or more learning disorders between the Omega-3 Index and errors of omission (p = 0.073). For typically developing adolescents, a significant association between the Omega-3 Index and errors of omission was seen (Table 6), students with a higher Omega-3 Index had a lower number of errors.

Table 6. Results of generalized linear model analyses between the Omega-3 Index and number of errors of omission on the D2 test in the typically developing participant sample.

Predictor Variable	B (Standardized) [1]	Significance [2]
Model A (χ^2 = 42.11, df = 6, p < 0.001)		
Smoking	0.032	0.685
Alcohol consumption	0.036	0.277
BMI	0.091	**0.000**
Age	0.002	0.914
Sex	−0.136	**0.003**
Highest LPE	−0.085	**0.000**
Model B (χ^2 = 55.642, df = 7, p < 0.001)		
Smoking	0.029	0.714
Alcohol consumption	0.027	0.410
BMI	0.089	**0.000**
Age	0.015	0.515
Sex	−0.138	**0.002**
Highest LPE [3]	−0.067	**0.003**
Omega-3 Index	−0.083	**0.000**

[1] Standardized beta refers to how many standard deviations the dependent variable will change per standard deviation change in the predictor variable. Smoking and sex were not standardized as they are dichotomous variables; [2] Significant results (p < 0.05) are printed in bold; [3] LPE = level of parental education.

4. Discussion

The main aim of this study was to investigate the association between the Omega-3 Index measured in blood and cognitive performance of 14-year-old Dutch adolescents. The Omega-3 Index was significantly associated with information processing operationalized as LDST score. This indicates that a higher Omega-3 Index was associated with better information processing speeds. Every 1% increase in the Omega-3 Index was associated with an increase of 1.23 digits on the LDST. Also, students with a higher Omega-3 Index had fewer errors of omission on the D2 test of attention, an indicator of inattention/impulsivity (*i.e.*, they paid more attention than students with a lower Omega-3 Index). An increase of 1% in the Omega-3 Index was associated with a decrease of 0.94 stimuli forgotten to cross out. Associations with all other cognitive measures were not significant.

To our knowledge, this is the first study assessing the association between the Omega-3 Index measured in blood and cognition in typically developing adolescents from the general population. There are a number of observational studies of adolescents that found positive associations between fish consumption, the most important source of omega-3 LCPUFAs, and school grades [17–19]. However, even though cognition/executive functioning and school performance are correlated, they are not equal. School performance depends on additional factors such as time spent on homework [44] and personality [45]. Although we are not aware of studies looking at the association/relationship between LCPUFA status and cognition in adolescents, multiple studies of children are available. For example, Portillo-Reyes *et al.* found an improvement in processing speed in their supplementation study (180 mg DHA and 270 mg EPA per day for three months) of marginally malnourished children age 8–12 years [46]. Parletta *et al.* also found a positive effect of supplementation (750 mg EPA + DHA per school day for 40 weeks) on a non-verbal cognitive test [47]. However, there are also a number of studies that do not show an association or relationship between omega-3 LCPUFAs and cognition in children [48–50]. Overall, results remain mixed, and a number of possible explanations for these differences have been proposed [50,51]. For example, it has been suggested that an effect of LCPUFAs on cognition might be more likely to be demonstrated in underperforming children and adolescents, as shown in the study of Richardson *et al.* [30]. We tried to address this in the current study by recruiting students from one of the lowest educational levels in the Netherlands. Additionally, it has been suggested that LCPUFAs might only be beneficial in certain periods of life when the brain is developing, the so-called windows of opportunity. We tried to address this by including adolescents because the brain undergoes profound development in adolescence [12].

A number of earlier studies have shown a positive relationship between LCPUFAs and cognition in people with learning disorders [30,52–54]. Therefore, a moderator analysis was executed to check whether the association between the Omega-3 Index and score on the cognitive test was different between those with and those without a learning disorder. If a moderator effect was shown, separate analyses for adolescents who indicated to have a learning disorder *versus* typically developing adolescents were executed. There was a significant association between the covariate diagnosis and score on errors of commission and on the interference score. The moderator effect could, however, only be shown for errors of omission. Firstly, the number of students with a diagnosis was relatively low ($n = 69$), which could have led to a reduced statistical power. Secondly, the self-reporting of diagnosis and the fact that many adolescents did not know who made the diagnosis could have led to attenuation of the associations. Thus, the measure of diagnosis might not be accurate. However, when the test scores of those with and those without a diagnosis were compared, students with a diagnosis score lower on the test of interference (Stroop). This would suggest that the assessment of a learning disorder is accurate, since it has been shown before that patients with ADHD and other psychiatric problems have impaired performance on this test [55]. Moreover, the variation in the Omega-3 Index (inherent to our pre-selection of participants with an Omega-3 Index < 5%) was relatively low (SD = 0.61), which makes the appearance of associations less likely. In contrast, even though this spread was also low (SD = 0.60) in typically developing adolescents, a significant association between Omega-3 Index and cognitive measures could be shown. This could be explained by the fact that the number of students with a diagnosis was only 69; therefore, the power to detect an association was not sufficient [56].

The Omega-3 Index (3.83%) in this sample was relatively low (well below the recommended range of 8%–11% [22]). This could be due to the exclusion of participants with a high Omega-3 Index, although if these were included the mean was still only 3.89 (SD 0.67). The low Omega-3 Index in this sample is no surprise since 13.9% of the students did not consume any fish and 77% consumed fish rarely, as measured by the fish consumption questionnaire. This frequency of fish consumption is somewhat lower than the consumption of the adolescents in the sample of de Groot *et al.* [19]. However, the study of de Groot *et al.* was carried out with students in higher general secondary education or pre-university education with a somewhat higher social economic status (assessed by level of education of the parents) than the students in the current study. The number of students that never consume fish is also in line with the results from the National Dutch Consumption Survey, which indicates that 11% of boys and 18% of girls never consume fish [57]. Similarly in our sample, girls also consumed significantly less fish than boys. However, the number of adolescents who consumed fish twice or more a week was in only 1% in this sample, while in the survey 9% of the boys and 7% of the girls consumed the recommended amount of fish.

The main strength of the current study is that the Omega-3 Index was measured in blood. Furthermore, standardized and validated cognitive tests that assess several aspects of executive functioning were used. The main limitation of the study is that it is an observational study and can, therefore, not prove causality. Also, the variation in the Omega-3 Index was rather small. Furthermore, no Bonferroni correction for multiple statistical was applied, with correction significant results were not present anymore, which weakens the certainty of the associations found. However, the data presented here are part of a large intervention study, which will elucidate the effect of LCPUFA supplementation on cognition, mood, and academic achievement in adolescence. Furthermore, the supplementation study will achieve a higher Omega-3 Index and a larger spread in the Omega-3 Index, which could lead to more significant results (a number of associations were borderline significant).

In conclusion, this study has revealed a positive association between the Omega-3 Index measured in blood from typically developing adolescents and two of the nine cognitive measures. The results of the supplementation study will further elucidate the effect of LCPUFA supplementation on cognition. If a positive effect of LCPUFA supplementation on cognition is shown, this could help improve cognitive functioning and possibly the school performance of adolescents in a relatively inexpensive and easy way.

Acknowledgments: We like to thank all participants and schools who participated in Food2Learn. Furthermore, we like to thank the dedicated research assistants: Marije Broens-Paffen, Denise Hofman and Annemarijn Weber. The study is funded by the grant Food, Cognition and Behaviour from the Dutch Scientific Organisation (grant number 057-13-002), Aker Biomarine (Norway) who provided the krill and placebo capsules, and Omegametrix (Germany) who was responsible for the blood analyses.

Author Contributions: R.G., C.v.S., K.B. and P.A.K. were responsible for the study design and resource acquisition R.G. and I.W. were responsible for execution of the trial, data collection and logistics. I.W. was responsible for data analyses. All authors contributed to the writing of the paper.

Conflicts of Interest: C.v.S. is owner of Omegametrix, who is partly funding the study. K.B. is an employee of Aker Biomarine, who is partly funding the study. All other authors declare no conflict of interest. The sponsors had no role in in the collection, analyses, or interpretation of data.

References

1. Richardson, A. Clinical trials of fatty acid treatment in ADHD, dyslexia, dyspraxia and the autistic spectrum. *Prostaglandins Leukot. Essent. Fat. Acids* **2004**, *70*, 383–390. [CrossRef] [PubMed]
2. Gale, C.R.; Robinson, S.M.; Godfrey, K.M.; Law, C.M.; Schlotz, W.; O'Callaghan, F.J. Oily fish intake during pregnancy—Association with lower hyperactivity but not with higher full-scale IQ in offspring. *J. Child Psychol. Psychiatry* **2008**, *49*, 1061–1068. [CrossRef] [PubMed]
3. De Groot, R.; Hornstra, G.; Jolles, J. Exploratory study into the relation between plasma phospholipid fatty acid status and cognitive performance. *Prostaglandins Leukot. Essent. Fat. Acids* **2007**, *76*, 165–172. [CrossRef] [PubMed]
4. Stonehouse, W.; Conlon, C.A.; Podd, J.; Hill, S.R.; Minihane, A.M.; Haskell, C.; Kennedy, D. DHA supplementation improved both memory and reaction time in healthy young adults: A randomized controlled trial. *Am. J. Clin. Nutr.* **2013**, *97*, 1134–1143. [CrossRef] [PubMed]
5. Konagai, C.; Yanagimoto, K.; Hayamizu, K.; Han, L.; Tsuji, T.; Koga, Y. Effects of krill oil containing *n*-3 polyunsaturated fatty acids in phospholipid form on human brain function: A randomized controlled trial in healthy elderly volunteers. *Clin. Interv. Aging* **2013**, *8*, 1247–1257. [CrossRef] [PubMed]
6. Fotuhi, M.; Mohassel, P.; Yaffe, K. Fish consumption, long-chain omega-3 fatty acids and risk of cognitive decline or Alzheimer disease: A complex association. *Nat. Clin. Pract. Neurol.* **2009**, *5*, 140–152. [CrossRef] [PubMed]
7. Danthiir, V.; Burns, N.R.N.; Nettelbeck, T.; Wilson, C.; Wittert, G. The older people, omega-3, and cognitive health (EPOCH) trial design and methodology: A randomised, double-blind, controlled trial investigating the effect of long-chain omega-3 fatty acids on cognitive ageing and wellbeing in cognitively healthy older adults. *Nutr. J.* **2011**, *10*, 117. [PubMed]
8. Parletta, N.; Milte, C.; Meyer, B.J. Nutritional modulation of cognitive function and mental health. *J. Nutr. Biochem.* **2013**, *24*, 725–743. [CrossRef] [PubMed]
9. Assisi, A.; Banzi, R.; Buonocore, C.; Capasso, F.; di Muzio, V.; Michelacci, F.; Renzo, D.; Tafuri, G.; Trotta, F.; Vitocolonna, M.; *et al.* Fish oil and mental health: The role of *n*-3 long-chain polyunsaturated fatty acids in

cognitive development and neurological disorders. *Int. Clin. Psychopharmacol.* **2006**, *21*, 319–336. [CrossRef] [PubMed]

10. Cooper, R.E.; Tye, C.; Kuntsi, J.; Vassos, E.; Asherson, P. Omega-3 polyunsaturated fatty acid supplementation and cognition: A systematic review and meta-analysis. *J. Psychopharmacol.* **2015**, *29*, 753–763. [CrossRef] [PubMed]
11. Karr, J.E.; Alexander, J.E.; Winningham, R.G. Omega-3 polyunsaturated fatty acids and cognition throughout the lifespan: A review. *Nutr. Neurosci.* **2011**, *14*, 216–225. [CrossRef] [PubMed]
12. Gogtay, N.; Giedd, J.N.; Lusk, L.; Hayashi, K.M.; Greenstein, D.; Vaituzis, A.C.; Nugent, T.F.; Herman, D.H.; Clasen, L.S.; Toga, A.W.; *et al.* Dynamic mapping of human cortical development during childhood through early adulthood. *Proc. Natl. Acad. Sci. USA* **2004**, *101*, 8174–8179. [CrossRef] [PubMed]
13. Crone, E.A. Executive functions in adolescence: Inferences from brain and behavior. *Dev. Sci.* **2009**, *12*, 825–830. [CrossRef] [PubMed]
14. Bull, R.; Espy, K.; Wiebe, S. Short-term memory, working memory, and executive functioning in preschoolers: Longitudinal predictors of mathematical achievement at age 7 years. *Dev. Neuropsychol.* **2008**, *33*, 205–228. [CrossRef] [PubMed]
15. McNamara, R.K.; Carlson, S.E. Role of omega-3 fatty acids in brain development and function: Potential implications for the pathogenesis and prevention of psychopathology. *Prostaglandins. Leukot. Essent. Fat. Acids* **2006**, *75*, 329–349. [CrossRef] [PubMed]
16. McNamara, R.K.; Able, J.; Jandacek, R.; Rider, T.; Tso, P.; Eliassen, J.; Alfieri, D.; Weber, W.; Jarvis, K.; Delbello, M.; *et al.* Docosahexaenoic acid supplementation increases prefrontal cortex activation during sustained attention in healthy boys: A placebo-controlled, dose-ranging, functional magnetic resonance imaging study. *Am. J. Clin. Nutr.* **2010**, *91*, 1060–1067. [CrossRef] [PubMed]
17. Kim, J.; Winkvist, A.; Äberg, M.; Äberg, N.; Sundberg, R.; Torén, K.; Brisman, J. Fish consumption and school grades in Swedish adolescents: A study of the large general population. *Acta Paediatr. Int. J. Paediatr.* **2010**, *99*, 72–77. [CrossRef] [PubMed]
18. Äberg, M.; Äberg, N.; Brisman, J.; Sundberg, R.; Winkvist, A.; Torén, K. Fish intake of Swedish male adolescents is a predictor of cognitive performance. *Acta Paediatr.* **2009**, *98*, 555–560. [CrossRef] [PubMed]
19. De Groot, R.; Ouwehand, C.; Jolles, J. Eating the right amount of fish: Inverted U-shape association between fish consumption and cognitive performance and academic achievement in Dutch adolescents. *Prostaglandins Leukot. Essent. Fat. Acids* **2012**, *86*, 113–117. [CrossRef] [PubMed]
20. Meyer, B.J.; Mann, N.J.; Lewis, J.L.; Milligan, G.C.; Sinclair, A.J.; Howe, P.R.C. Dietary intakes and food sources of omega-6 and omega-3 polyunsaturated fatty acids. *Lipids* **2003**, *38*, 391–398. [CrossRef] [PubMed]
21. Köhler, A.; Bittner, D.; Löw, A.; von Schacky, C. Effects of a convenience drink fortified with *n*-3 fatty acids on the *n*-3 index. *Br. J. Nutr.* **2010**, *104*, 729–736. [CrossRef] [PubMed]
22. Von Schacky, C. Omega-3 fatty Acids in cardiovascular disease—An uphill battle. *Prostaglandins Leukot. Essent. Fat. Acids* **2014**, *92*, 41–47. [CrossRef] [PubMed]
23. Diamond, A. Executive functions. *Annu. Rev. Psychol.* **2013**, *64*, 135–168. [CrossRef] [PubMed]
24. Crone, E.A.; Dahl, R.E. Understanding adolescence as a period of social–affective engagement and goal flexibility. *Nat. Rev. Neurosci.* **2012**, *13*, 636–650. [CrossRef] [PubMed]
25. Bell, J.G.; Sargent, J.R.; Tocher, D.R.; Dick, J.R. Red blood cell fatty acid compositions in a patient with autistic spectrum disorder: A characteristic abnormality in neurodevelopmental disorders? *Prostaglandins. Leukot. Essent. Fat. Acids* **2000**, *63*, 21–25. [CrossRef] [PubMed]
26. Antalis, C.J.; Stevens, L.J.; Campbell, M.; Pazdro, R.; Ericson, K.; Burgess, J.R. Omega-3 fatty acid status in attention-deficit/hyperactivity disorder. *Prostaglandins Leukot. Essent. Fat. Acids* **2006**, *75*, 299–308. [CrossRef] [PubMed]
27. Giskes, K.; Kunst, A.; Benach, J.; Borrell, C.; Costa, G.; Dahl, E.; Dalstra, J.; Federico, B.; Helmert, U.; Judge, K.; *et al.* Trends in smoking behaviour between 1985 and 2000 in nine European countries by education. *J. Epidemiol. Community Health* **2005**, *59*, 395–401. [CrossRef] [PubMed]
28. Hulshof, K.; Brussaard, J.H.; Kruizinga, A.G.; Telman, J.; Löwik, M.R.H. Socio-economic status, dietary intake and 10 year trends: The Dutch National Food Consumption Survey. *Eur. J. Clin. Nutr.* **2003**, *57*, 128–137. [CrossRef] [PubMed]

29. Schrijvers, C.T.M.; Schoemaker, C.G. *Spelen Met Gezondheid Leefstijl en Psychische Gezondheid van de Nederlandse Jeugd (Playing with Your Health Lifestyle and Mental Health in the Dutch Youth Population)*; National Institute for Public Health and the Environment: Bilthoven, The Netherlands, 2008.
30. Richardson, A.; Burton, J.; Sewell, R.; Spreckelsen, T.; Montgomery, P. Docosahexaenoic acid for reading, cognition and behavior in children aged 7–9 years: A randomized, controlled trial (the DOLAB Study). *PLoS ONE* **2012**, *7*, e43909. [CrossRef] [PubMed]
31. Centraal Bureau Voor de Statistiek (Statistics Netherlands). VO; Leerlingen, Onderwijssoort in Detail, Leerjaar (Secondary Education, Students, Type of Education in Detail Per Teaching Year). Available online: http://statline.cbs.nl/StatWeb/publication/?VW=T&DM=SLnl&PA=80040NED&LA=nl (accessed on 22 July 2015).
32. Harris, W.S.; von Schacky, C. The omega-3 Index: A new risk factor for death from coronary heart disease? *Prev. Med.* **2004**, *39*, 212–220. [CrossRef] [PubMed]
33. Moriguchi, Y.; Hiraki, K. Neural origin of cognitive shifting in young children. *Proc. Natl. Acad. Sci. USA* **2009**, *106*, 6017–6021. [CrossRef] [PubMed]
34. Brickenkam, R.; Zillmerr, E. *The d2 Test of Attention*; Hogrefe & Huber Publishers: Seattle, WA, USA, 1998.
35. Hale, J.B. Analyzing digit span components for assessment of attention processes. *J. Psychoeduc. Assess.* **2002**, *20*, 128–143. [CrossRef]
36. Li, Y.; Dai, Q.; Jackson, J.C.; Zhang, J. Overweight is associated with decreased cognitive functioning among school-age children and adolescents. *Obesity* **2008**, *16*, 1809–1815. [CrossRef] [PubMed]
37. Satterthwaite, T.D.; Wolf, D.H.; Roalf, D.R.; Ruparel, K.; Erus, G.; Vandekar, S.; Gennatas, E.D.; Elliott, M.A.; Smith, A.; Hakonarson, H.; *et al.* Linked sex differences in cognition and functional connectivity in youth. *Cereb. Cortex* **2014**. [CrossRef] [PubMed]
38. Steinberg, L. Cognitive and affective development in adolescence. *Trends Cogn. Sci.* **2005**, *9*, 69–74. [CrossRef] [PubMed]
39. Zeigler, D.W.; Wang, C.C.; Yoast, R.A.; Dickinson, B.D.; McCaffree, M.A.; Robinowitz, C.B.; Sterling, M.L. The neurocognitive effects of alcohol on adolescents and college students. *Prev. Med. (Baltim)* **2005**, *40*, 23–32. [CrossRef] [PubMed]
40. Jacobsen, L.K.; Krystal, J.H.; Mencl, W.E.; Westerveld, M.; Frost, S.J.; Pugh, K.R. Effects of smoking and smoking abstinence on cognition in adolescent tobacco smokers. *Biol. Psychiatry* **2005**, *57*, 56–66. [CrossRef] [PubMed]
41. Ardila, A.; Rosselli, M.; Matute, E.; Guajardo, S. The influence of the parents' educational level on the development of executive functions. *Dev. Neuropsychol.* **2005**, *28*, 539–560. [CrossRef] [PubMed]
42. De Bie, S.E. *Standaardvragen 1987: Voorstellen van Uniformering van Vraagstelling naar Achtergrondkenmerken en Interviews (Standard questions 1987: Proposal for Uniformisation of Questions Regarding Background Variables and Interviews)*; Leiden University Press: Leiden, The Netherlands, 1987.
43. Kaplan, G.A.; Keil, J.E. Socioeconomic factors and cardiovascular disease: A review of the literature. *Circulation* **1993**, *88*, 1973–1998. [CrossRef] [PubMed]
44. Cooper, H.; Robinson, J.C.; Patall, E.A. Does homework improve academic achievement? A synthesis of research, 1987–2003. *Rev. Educ. Res.* **2006**, *76*, 1–62. [CrossRef]
45. Poropat, A.E. A meta-analysis of the five-factor model of personality and academic performance. *Psychol. Bull.* **2009**, *135*, 322–338. [CrossRef] [PubMed]
46. Portillo-Reyes, V.; Pérez-García, M.; Loya-Méndez, Y.; Puente, A.E. Clinical significance of neuropsychological improvement after supplementation with omega-3 in 8–12 years old malnourished Mexican children: A randomized, double-blind, placebo and treatment clinical trial. *Res. Dev. Disabil.* **2014**, *35*, 861–870. [CrossRef] [PubMed]
47. Parletta, N.; Cooper, P.; Gent, D.N.; Petkov, J.; O'Dea, K. Effects of fish oil supplementation on learning and behaviour of children from Australian Indigenous remote community schools: A randomised controlled trial. *Prostaglandins Leukot. Essent. Fat. Acids* **2013**, *89*, 71–79. [CrossRef] [PubMed]
48. Bakker, E.; Ghys, A.; Kester, A.; Vles, J.; Dubas, J.; Blanco, C.; Hornstra, G. Long-chain polyunsaturated fatty acids at birth and cognitive function at 7 year of age. *Eur. J. Clin. Nutr.* **2003**, *57*, 89–95. [CrossRef] [PubMed]
49. Kairaluoma, L.; Närhi, V.; Ahonen, T.; Westerholm, J.; Aro, M. Do fatty acids help in overcoming reading difficulties? A double-blind, placebo-controlled study of the effects of eicosapentaenoic acid and carnosine supplementation on children with dyslexia. *Child Care Health Dev.* **2009**, *35*, 112–119. [CrossRef] [PubMed]

50. Kennedy, D.O.; Jackson, P.A.; Elliott, J.M.; Scholey, A.B.; Robertson, B.C.; Greer, J.; Tiplady, B.; Buchanan, T.; Haskell, C.F. Cognitive and mood effects of 8 weeks' supplementation with 400 mg or 1000 mg of the omega-3 essential fatty acid docosahexaenoic acid (DHA) in healthy children aged 10–12 years. *Nutr. Neurosci.* **2009**, *12*, 48–56. [CrossRef] [PubMed]
51. Frensham, L.J.; Bryan, J.; Parletta, N. Influences of micronutrient and omega-3 fatty acid supplementation on cognition, learning, and behavior: Methodological considerations and implications for children and adolescents in developed societies. *Nutr. Rev.* **2012**, *70*, 594–610. [PubMed]
52. Richardson, A.J.; Puri, B.K. A randomized double-blind, placebo-controlled study of the effects of supplementation with highly unsaturated fatty acids on ADHD-related symptoms in children with specific learning difficulties. *Prog. Neuropsychopharmacol. Biol. Psychiatry* **2002**, *26*, 233–239. [CrossRef]
53. Stevens, L.; Zhang, W.; Peck, L.; Kuczek, T.; Grevstad, N.; Mahon, A.; Zentall, S.S.; Arnold, L.E.; Burgess, J.R. EFA supplementation in children with inattention, hyperactivity, and other disruptive behaviors. *Lipids* **2003**, *38*, 1007–1021. [CrossRef] [PubMed]
54. Milte, C.; Parletta, N.; Buckley, J.; Coates, A.; Young, R.; Howe, P. Eicosapentaenoic and docosahexaenoic acids, cognition, and behavior in children with attention-deficit/hyperactivity disorder: A randomized controlled trial. *Nutrition* **2012**, *28*, 670–677. [CrossRef] [PubMed]
55. Lansbergen, M.M.; Kenemans, J.L.; van Engeland, H. Stroop interference and attention-deficit/hyperactivity disorder: A review and meta-analysis. *Neuropsychology* **2007**, *21*, 251–262. [CrossRef] [PubMed]
56. Tabachnick, B.G.; Fidell, L.S. *Using Multivariate Statistics*, 5th ed.; Pearson Education: New York City, NY, USA, 2007.
57. Van Rossum, C.T.M.; Fransen, H.P.; Verkaik-Kloosterman, J.; Buurma-Rethans, E.J.M.; Ocké, M.C. *Dutch National Food Consumption Survey 2007–2010—Diet of Children and Adults Aged 7 to 69 Years*; National Institute for Public Health and the Environment: Bilthoven, The Netherlands, 2011.

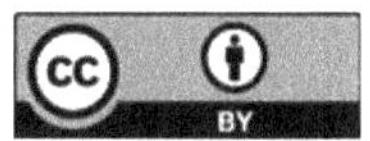

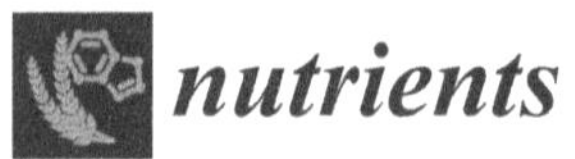 nutrients

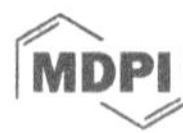

Review

DHA Effects in Brain Development and Function

Lotte Lauritzen [1,*], Paolo Brambilla [2,3], Alessandra Mazzocchi [4], Laurine B. S. Harsløf [1], Valentina Ciappolino [2] and Carlo Agostoni [4]

1 Department of Nutrition Exercise and Sports, University of Copenhagen, Rolighedsvej 26, 1958 Frederiksberg C, Denmark; laurinebs@gmail.com

2 Psychiatric Clinic, Department of Neurosciences and Mental Health, Fondazione IRCCS Ospedale Cà Granda-Ospedale Maggiore Policlinico, University of Milan, 20121 Milan, Italy; paolo.brambilla1@unimi.it (P.B.); valentina.ciappolino@libero.it (V.C.)

3 Department of Psychiatry and Behavioural Neurosciences, University of Texas at Houston, 2800 South Macgregor Way, Houston, TX 77021, USA

4 Pediatric Clinic, Fondazione IRCCS Ospedale Cà Granda-Ospedale Maggiore Policlinico, Department of Clinical Sciences and Community Health, University of Milan, 20121 Milan, Italy; alessandra.mazzocchi1@gmail.com (A.M.); carlo.agostoni@unimi.it (C.A.)

* Correspondence: ll@nexs.ku.dk; Tel.: +45-3533-2508; Fax: +45-3533-2483

Received: 3 November 2015; Accepted: 11 December 2015; Published: 4 January 2016

Abstract: Docosahexaenoic acid (DHA) is a structural constituent of membranes specifically in the central nervous system. Its accumulation in the fetal brain takes place mainly during the last trimester of pregnancy and continues at very high rates up to the end of the second year of life. Since the endogenous formation of DHA seems to be relatively low, DHA intake may contribute to optimal conditions for brain development. We performed a narrative review on research on the associations between DHA levels and brain development and function throughout the lifespan. Data from cell and animal studies justify the indication of DHA in relation to brain function for neuronal cell growth and differentiation as well as in relation to neuronal signaling. Most data from human studies concern the contribution of DHA to optimal visual acuity development. Accumulating data indicate that DHA may have effects on the brain in infancy, and recent studies indicate that the effect of DHA may depend on gender and genotype of genes involved in the endogenous synthesis of DHA. While DHA levels may affect early development, potential effects are also increasingly recognized during childhood and adult life, suggesting a role of DHA in cognitive decline and in relation to major psychiatric disorders.

Keywords: docosahexaenoic acid; brain development; desaturases; psychiatric disorders

---

1. Introduction

Long chain polyunsaturated fatty acid (LC-PUFA), including docosahexaenoic acid (DHA) and arachidonic acid (AA), are incorporated into membrane phospholipids and, apart from their structural role in these membranes, they also act as precursors of autocoid signaling molecules (e.g., docosanoids) and as potent activators of a number of gene transcription factors (e.g., peroxisome proliferator activated receptors). The essentiality of n-3 LC-PUFA is generally mainly contributed to the incorporation of DHA in uniquely high levels in the central nervous system—although DHA is incorporated in most other tissues where it may also have important functional effects.

Overall, membrane PUFA composition (the principal components of which are linoleic acid (LA), AA and DHA) seems to be more responsive to DHA in the diet than to intake of LA and AA [1]. Animal studies have demonstrated that an increase in dietary α-linolenic acid (ALA) is almost completely reflected in membrane n-3/n-6 PUFA-ratios at LA/ALA intakes of <10, whereas the dietary balance between ALA and LA has little influence at higher ALA intakes, and a similar biphasic response is also seen in diets that contain LC-PUFA [2]. These results show a high sensitivity of tissue membranes to dietary variations in the PUFA-supply within the normal range, strongly favoring incorporation of n-3 LC-PUFA over LA and AA. In the case of a dietary deficiency of n-3 PUFA, there is a trend for DHA to be replaced with the nearest n-6 PUFA equivalents, whereas few changes are seen for the reciprocal lack of dietary of n-6 PUFA [3,4]. Thus, n-3 PUFA seem to be the main determinant of membrane PUFA composition and unsaturation. Membrane DHA incorporation in different tissues, e.g., erythrocytes (RBC), has been shown to depend on diet, mainly fish intake and in infants also breastfeeding, but is also to some extent supported by DHA formed endogenously by desaturation and elongation of ALA. This conversion is limited by the delta-6 desaturase enzymatic step, which generally has a low efficiency, but the rate conversion has been shown to be affected by genetic setup in the fatty acid desaturase (*FADS*) gene cluster and to vary depending on age and circulating levels of sex hormones.

The present paper will give an update of the current literature and try to answer the following questions: (1) Does the high rate of DHA accumulation in the brain have any functional importance? (2) If yes, is the endogenous synthesis of DHA high enough to support optimal functional levels of DHA in the brain? Finally, we will also address whether DHA may contribute to normal brain functioning later in life.

2. Brain DHA Accumulation during Development Depending on Diet

The accumulation of DHA in the brain takes place during the brain growth spurt in the intrauterine and neonatal period up to two years of age and the high levels of DHA in the brain are maintained throughout life [5]. Due to the lack of *de novo* PUFA synthesis, the rate of membrane DHA incorporation in early life—in the brain as well as in other tissues—depends on maternal transfer, dietary supply (*i.e.*, breastfeeding) and endogenous LC-PUFA production. The DHA accumulation in the brain during the third trimester of pregnancy is substantially higher (in % of fatty acids (FA%)) than the overall body deposition rates, whereas brain incorporation of AA is more in line with that which occurs in other tissues [6]. Fetal LC-PUFAs accumulation occurs mainly during the last trimester, in which weight increase becomes more rapid and growth is accompanied by a deposition of fat tissue, which begins around the 30th week of gestation [7]. Fetal fat tissues contain relatively low levels of DHA and AA [8,9] compared to the large relative amounts of LC-PUFAs that are deposited in the brain [8,10]. However, the absolute amount of DHA in fetal adipose tissue exceeds that in the brain [7]. Based on *post-mortem* studies it has been calculated that whole-body DHA accretion during the third trimester amounts to around 50 mg/day while the accretion of AA is approximately twice as high (100 mg/day) [8]. It has been estimated that this fetal LC-PUFA accumulation is supported by a supply of approximately 50 mg/(kg × day) of n-3 LC-PUFA and 400 mg/(kg × day) of n-6 LC-PUFA [6].

The intrauterine PUFA supply occurs via transfer of non-esterified PUFA mainly derived from the maternal circulation across the placenta [10,11]. The overall fat concentration in maternal plasma increases throughout pregnancy [7], and placental fat transport is driven by a concentration gradient as the fetus has substantially lower fat concentrations [12], including the concentration of DHA and AA [7,13]. The relative proportion of DHA and AA is, however, consistently higher in circulating lipids of the neonate [14], whereas the concentrations of LA and ALA differ much less from that in the maternal blood [15,16], indicating a preferential transfer of LC-PUFA. The exact mechanisms involved in placental PUFA transfer remain unclear, but is generally considered to involve proteins with some specificity for LC-PUFA, especially DHA, over PUFAs with shorter chain length [17–19]. Additionally, DHA has been shown to be incorporated into triacylglycerol in human placental cells, whereas AA is primarily esterified in phospholipids [20,21], and this differential esterification may contribute to the preferential transport of DHA and accumulation of AA in the placenta itself. AA has been shown to be taken up from the maternal blood by the placenta at higher rates than DHA, while DHA accumulates in the fetal blood stream at a three-fold higher rate than AA [20]. Although other interpretations are plausible, the specificity for placental transfer of DHA over AA could be interpreted as a specific retention of AA on the maternal side possibly for prostaglandin production in relation to the initiation of delivery. Maternal dietary n-3 LC-PUFA has a slight gestation prolonging effect, which may be explained by a dampening of the AA-derived eicosanoid response [22], which results in an increase birth weight and intrauterine LC-PUFA accretion. In infants born preterm the progressive accumulation of LC-PUFA in fetal tissues is truncated at the end of pregnancy and accumulation is also strongly limited in growth-retarded fetuses [23].

Post-natal accumulation of LC-PUFA in infant tissues is supported by maternal transfer of PUFA through breastmilk, and blood levels of LC-PUFA in breast-fed infants remain higher than maternal levels for some time postnatally [24,25]. In neonate baboons, dietary DHA has been shown to consistently support greater brain DHA incorporation and maintenance of cortex DHA concentration, while brain AA is unaffected by dietary supply and decreases with age [26]. Moreover, brain autopsies from human infants have shown an around 25% higher mean FA% of DHA in cortical phospholipid of breast-fed (9.7%) compared to age-matched formula-fed infants (7.6%) [27]. The overall percentage of LC-PUFA was maintained in formula-fed infants by a compensatory increase in the incorporation of n-6 LC-PUFA, which however was incomplete in formula-fed preterm infants with the lowest concentration of cortical DHA, where an increase in the n-9 series PUFA was also detected [27]. A second autopsy study also showed an increase in cortex DHA with age in breast-fed but not in formula-fed infants, whereas the percentage of AA in the brain increased with age irrespective of diet [28] just as in the infant baboons. Similarly, the RBC DHA content of breast-fed infants has been found to be higher than that of formula-fed infants [28]. Breastmilk has been shown to be a main contributor to the DHA content in infant RBC [29], and infant RBC DHA has been shown to be associated with maternal n-3 LC-PUFA intake and RBC DHA status during lactation [30]. RBC DHA decrease after infancy as complementary feeding usually supplies less DHA [31]. The intake of n-3 LC-PUFA has been shown to be low in a number of studies in children [32] and European children have been shown to have whole blood n-3 LC-PUFA levels consistently below 2.5 FA% between 3 and 8 years of age [33].

The phenomenon of increasing LC-PUFA in fetal and infant blood and tissues relative to that of their mother has been described as "bio-magnification" [34], but could also be interpreted as a natural consequence of a dual liver system *i.e.*, the combined PUFA metabolism and conversion of LA and ALA to AA and DHA in both the mother and the fetus/infant. Both term and preterm infants have been shown to convert stable isotope labeled LA and ALA to AA and DHA, respectively [35–37], and the synthesis has been shown to decrease with post-conceptional age [38]. The desaturase capacity has been estimated to be in the order of 40 mg/(kg × day) of AA and 13 mg/(kg × day) of DHA in neonates born in the 32nd week of gestation, but to decrease to around 14 and 3 mg/(kg × day) at 1 month past expected term [39]. This synthetic rate may still provide a substantial contribution to fulfill infant needs, which, based on maintenance of plasma DHA homeostasis, have been estimated to be around 5 mg/(kg × day) of DHA [40]. However, this does not exclude that exogenous sources of DHA are needed in the diet to fulfill the requirements of the growing infant.

3. Effects of FADS Polymorphisms on LC-PUFA Levels

Overall, data suggest that n-6 PUFAs in breastmilk, plasma and RBC membranes across all ages are more affected by single nucleotide polymorphisms (SNPs) in the *FADS* gene cluster than n-3 PUFAs, typically with an increase in LA and a decrease in AA levels in minor allele carriers [29,41–45]. Minor allele homozygotes of various *FADS* SNPs have also been found to have lower blood (RBC and plasma) levels of AA and higher levels of LA and ALA during pregnancy [41,42]. *FADS* polymorphisms have been estimated to explain as much as 29% of the variation in serum AA contents in adults, in whom serum DHA concentrations are determined primarily by the dietary supply of preformed DHA [43]. Colostrum AA and DHA levels have been found to be decreased in minor allele carriers of a number of *FADS* SNPs [46], but studies in mature breastmilk have shown that the concentration of AA is influenced to a larger extent than that of DHA [41,47,48]. Findings in plasma from both mothers and neonates have shown strong inverse associations between the minor allele for two *FADS* SNPs and the concentrations of DHA and eicosapentaenoic acid (EPA) as well as AA in the newborn infants, thus confirming that synthesis of DHA provides a relevant contribution to status [49]. Curiously, a study of 2000 cord blood samples found that minor allele *FADS* SNPs in the mother gave rise to increased levels of n-6 PUFA before the delta-5 desaturation step (LA and di-homo-γ-linoleic acid), whereas minor allele SNPs in the child resulted in decreased levels of AA and other n-6 LC-PUFA beyond this point in the metabolic pathway [50]. More data on the biochemical effects of *FADS* polymorphisms are needed to derive a biologically plausible interpretation of their potential functional effects. Furthermore, both AA and DHA needs to be considered together since apart from the main determinants of their levels, either endogenous or exogenous, their balance may be critical for the functional outcomes in infancy and beyond.

We have recently found that some *FADS* polymorphisms may substantially contribute to RBC DHA levels in late infancy (to the same extent as breastfeeding) [29]. Some SNP minor alleles (rs1535 and rs3834458) were even found to dose-dependently up-regulate DHA status [29], whereas minor alleles of all the investigated SNPs lowered AA in a consistent way [51]. Interestingly, identical analyses did not reveal any effect of these SNPs on RBC DHA at 3 years of age [29], which could be explained by increased residual variation in the model due to a more diverse fish intake or could be interpreted as a decline in the endogenous DHA biosynthesis, consistent with other findings [39]. Furthermore, a longitudinal study of serum phospholipid fatty acid composition at 2 and 6 years of age in 331 children found higher tracking in n-3 LC-PUFA levels in children who were major allele carriers [52]. Instead tracking of n-6 LC-PUFA was lower in major allele homozygotes of various *FADS* SNPs compared to tracking in carriers of at least one minor allele [52]. More longitudinal outcome data may suggest plausible biological interpretations. However, although DHA may mainly be determined by variation in intake, mainly of preformed DHA, the genetic patterns also appear to be of relevance for tissue DHA levels in the perinatal phases, although probably less later in life as the rate of endogenous synthesis declines, thus increasing the importance of exogenous DHA.

4. Dietary DHA and Postnatal Development

The majority of the randomized controlled trials investigating the effect of dietary LC-PUFA supplementation in term infants have added both DHA and AA, and only few have investigated the effect of varying DHA intakes at a constant intake of AA. With respect to the functional effects of LC-PUFA supplementation in infancy, the most accepted developmental effect is an increased rate of visual acuity development [53]. This effect seems to be explained solely by DHA, as a meta-regression analysis found that variability in the effects on visual acuity between studies was explained by the dose of DHA [54]. However, little is known regarding the persistency of this effect on vision and the potential effects that this early visual deficit may have on cognitive development.

Overall, meta-analyses of the randomized controlled trials that have investigated the effect of LC-PUFA supplementation on neurodevelopmental outcomes throughout the first two years of life have not shown any clear benefit of LC-PUFA addition to infant formula on development of term or preterm infants [55–57]. However, a meta-analysis that combined all LC-PUFA formula supplementation trials in both term and preterm infants found a trend for an effect on the Bayley scale Mental Developmental Index at around 12 months of age, which were not affected by the maturity of the infant at birth [57]. This meta-analysis did not find any effect of LC-PUFA dose, although there was a trend towards an effect of the DHA dose, but no such trend for AA [57]. The studies that have supplemented the infants with DHA indirectly via n-3 LC-PUFA supplementation of their pregnant or lactating mothers, generally provide a more clean way to study effects of the early DHA supply as this has little effect on the AA supply to the infant. A meta-analysis of randomized trials that supplemented lactating mothers with n-3 LC-PUFA showed that infants of supplemented mothers had larger heads at 2 years of age [58]. Furthermore, the meta-analyses looking at the developmental effects of maternal n-3 LC-PUFA supplements in pregnancy and lactation have suggested some effects on neurodevelopment based on a few studies [58,59]. However, at the current stage, this does not provide any definite proof that an increase in the early DHA supply improves the mental development of infants.

So far, few studies have shown that the effect of perinatal n-3 LC-PUFA supplementation may be affected by the gender of the child. In two large investigations, the DINO and DOMInO trials [60,61], an increased early DHA supply was associated with different effects on cognitive outcomes in girls and boys. A gender-treatment interaction on cognitive outcomes was also observed in a small Danish trial of maternal fish oil supplementation during lactation [62], although no clear effects were observed when the children were followed up at 7 years of age [63]. The different effects of increased DHA supply on various outcomes in girls and boys all appear to counteract the normally observed gender differences in behavior. It is not clear if these effects should be interpreted as beneficial in one gender and adverse in the other or if it is due to some other effect of DHA that diminish the cultural gender differences which we have come to perceive as normal biological differences. Interestingly, in the Danish maternal fish oil supplementation trial treatment-gender interactions were found also on blood pressure at 7 years of age [64]. Blood pressure is not normally defined as cognitive outcome, but is nevertheless affected by the central nervous system in response to anxiety. As was the case with cognitive outcomes, boys and girls in the fish oil group were found to have comparable diastolic and mean arterial blood pressures, whereas girls had higher blood pressures than boys in the control group [64]. The intervention was also found to level out gender differences on energy intake and physical activity at 7 years of age [64]. Accordingly, these results indicate that early DHA intake could also have long-term health consequences, which might be mediated effects in the brain and lifestyle choices.

Many of the available studies on the effects of maternal or, more commonly, infant n-3 LC-PUFA supplementations on neurodevelopmental outcome during infancy have several limitations, which become more and more evident as our knowledge on the physiology of LC-PUFA, and DHA in particular, progresses. The vast majority of the studies, whether on cognition of other functional outcomes or if they provide the supplement during pregnancy, lactation or to the infant in various types of formula, show a great heterogeneity with respect to LC-PUFA sources, doses of DHA (and AA) and durations of interventions. It should be noted that the methodologies for primary outcome assessment as well as age of effect examination differed between trials, and the effects in the first few years of life and potential long-term effects may be quite different. For outcomes such as neurological and cognitive development, there may be a necessity to use different tests at different ages to accommodate changes in age and maturity level. However, many trials have investigated effects on numerous outcome measures, which are often internally inconsistent, or show no apparent pattern over time. In addition, studies often have low power in terms of the number of participants and sometimes also high rates of dropouts as well as lack of intention-to-treat analysis and a sufficient description of allocation concealment. Although baseline demographic characteristics are constantly reported, often baseline n-3 PUFA intake or status is not included in the characterization. This omission is critical for the interpretation, since baseline n-3 PUFA status will likely affects the response to changes in n-3 PUFA intake—both with respect to acute and persistent functional effect. Finally, as mentioned above, the effects of early n-3 LC-PUFA supply may vary in boys and girls, and this is not taken into account in the older studies. The emerging knowledge indicates that it is critical to take these aspects into account and that the variation in these aspects complicate attempts to combine data in meta-analyses to achieve conclusions with respect to the functional consequences of the addition of LC-PUFA, even beyond the single, specific effects of DHA.

5. Effects of FADS Polymorphisms on Cognition and Neurobehavioral Outcomes

Current knowledge about the functional effects of *FADS* polymorphism is limited and although the most clear effect on PUFA metabolism as mentioned is a decrease in AA production, functional associations with *FADS* genotype cannot be interpreted as a consequence of a reduction in AA. The influence of *FADS* polymorphisms on LC-PUFA status—and specifically the observed variations between specific SNPs and specific LC-PUFA over time—introduces new variables to be considered in the evaluation of the effects of *FADS* genotype on development and health of young children.

Several studies have showed that infant *FADS* genotype, examined by use of different individual SNPs, modifies the effect of breastfeeding on IQ-like neurodevelopmental outcomes in childhood [46,65,66], while other studies did not find any significant interaction [67,68] (Figure 1).

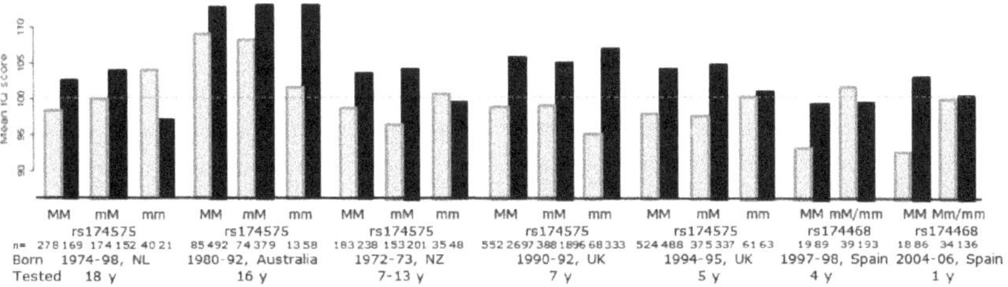

Figure 1. Results from studies examining the potential modifying effect of single nucleotide polymorphisms in the fatty acid desaturase gene cluster on the effect of breastfeeding on IQ-like neurodevelopmental outcomes in children. The figure is based on data from [46,65–68] and gives the average IQ in the SNP×feeding groups (breast-fed in black and formula-fed in light gray). The grey stippled line is the reference line for mean normal IQ.

As expected, based on the observed differences between breast-fed and formula-fed infants, all the studies have higher scores in breast-fed compared to formula-fed major allele carriers, but with no apparent differences between homozygotes and heterozygotes, which might be expected based on the additive effects of number of major alleles that is expected according to the observed effects on LC-PUFA. Thus, an interaction is dependent on a different pattern among the minor allele homozygotes (or the minor allele carriers in the Spanish study in which these were pooled with the heterozygotes). In the studies that found an interaction this is based on an equal "IQ" in breast-fed and formula-fed in the two cohorts in the Caspi study [66] and the two Spanish cohorts [46], whereas the largest of the studies found an even bigger difference between breast-fed and formula-fed among the minor allele homozygotes [65]. However, in all of the studies there were only few formula-fed minor allele carriers, and thus the largest variation in this group was likely skewed because of the scores of few children were at a high risk of chance effects. The studies differ with respect to breastfeeding frequency as well as the definition of breastfeeding, which in the large UK study was defined as >1 months [65] and ever having been breast-fed in the Dutch study [67], but was not clearly defined in other studies [46,66]. The Australian study tried to examine the effect of breastfeeding duration (not apparent in the figure in which we have pooled all the breast-fed groups), but they did not have the power to judge this due to a lack of a statistical (although visual indicated) dose-response between duration of breastfeeding and IQ [68]. The Dutch study found that the effect appeared to vary—although not significantly—between different cognitive functions and testing ages [67]. Furthermore, given the variation in the year of birth of the subjects in the studies, it is also reasonable to assume that there could have been differences in the PUFA composition of the formulas and presumably also in the maternal fish intake, and lifestyle in general, and thus in the DHA content of the breastmilk of the study populations. Little is known regarding interactions between the *FADS* polymorphisms and intake of AA and DHA from breastmilk and infant formula or the dietary ratio between the precursors, LA and ALA, but it is reasonable to suspect that this might have an influence on the functional response. Due to the increasing availability of micro-invasive methods for determination of blood fatty acid status, future Mendelian randomization studies should now be able to study effects of these potential sources of heterogeneity.

Additionally, the studies on interactions between breastfeeding and IQ used different *FADS* SNPs (mainly rs174575, rs1535 and rs174468), but, as indicated by the aforementioned study from Harsløf and coworkers, they may not all down-regulate the endogenous DHA synthesis in the infants [29]. This could contribute to the observed variable associations, and it is important to consider potential disequilibrium with other SNPs in the interpretation of the results from the *FADS* SNP studies. Interestingly, Steer *et al.* reported opposing effects of rs174574 and rs3834458 in the modulation of the association between breastfeeding and IQ [69]. Opposing effects of rs1535 and rs174448 have also been observed in problem solving and communication skills assessed by the Ages and Stages Questionnaire (ASQ) in a recent study among 3 year-olds [51]. None of the *FADS* SNP-breastfeeding interaction studies have considered whether the effect might differ between boys and girls. As in the DINO trials [60], the Mendelian randomization of *FADS* SNPs *versus* 3-year ASQ outcomes found that the effect of DHA increasing SNPs appeared to be negative in girls and positive in boys [51]. Due to the previously mentioned opposing effects of these SNPs on DHA in early life and the lack of opposing effects on AA plus the lack of association between *FADS* SNPs and DHA status at 3 years of age, these results might be interpreted as proof of a *programming effect* specifically of early DHA dietary intakes. However, the lack of effect of the *FADS* SNPs on DHA status later in life could be due to a blurring effect of a more diverse dietary intake of DHA from fish. Therefore, it is not possible to rule out that DHA supply contrary to the current hypothesis of an early window of vulnerability might have an effect on brain function at all stages of life.

6. Neurobehavioural Outcomes in Older Children

Brain DHA accretion continues into childhood, and although the accretion rate declines, the incorporation of DHA is still high at least during the preschool years. Once high levels of DHA are achieved in the brain these are maintained during later life, and this presumably also depends on an optimal dietary supply, as dietary intake of DHA from fish in adults has been shown to be the dominant determinant of DHA levels in various lipid pools [70]. However, to our knowledge no studies have examined the dietary requirements in order to achieve optimal brain DHA maintenance. Few studies have investigated the effect of *FADS* SNPs or n-3 LC-PUFA supplementation on cognitive development, emotions and behavior in toddlers and later in childhood or even in healthy adults.

A single study pooling data from three trials that randomized to LC-PUFA formulas immediately after birth or after breastfeeding for 6 weeks or 4–6 months, respectively and continued supplementation throughout the first year of life, found significant beneficial effects on problem solving at 9 months of age only in the two studies that started intervention early [71]. However, one study that examined the effects of DHA-enriched baby food also found an apparent improvement of cognitive outcomes [72]. Furthermore, a trial that provided a teaspoonful of cod liver oil (free of vitamin A and D) from 9 to 12 month of age found an increase in voluntary attention in a free play test after the intervention, especially in boys, compared with un-supplemented children [73].

Results from studies in schoolchildren in low-income countries have shown relatively convincing cognitive effects of fish oil supplementation. The effects have been shown to be stronger in children with low socioeconomic status or malnutrition-related health problems and a low consumption of fish and very little n-3 PUFA [74,75]. However, no overall cognitive effects were found after fish oil supplementation of 6–11 year-old South African children with poor iron and n-3 LC-PUFA status [75], but paradoxically an adverse effect of fish oil was observed on memory mainly in girls and specifically those with iron deficiency anemia. Little research has been performed on the effects of n-3 LC-PUFA on brain functions in school-aged children from high-income countries. One functional magnetic resonance imaging study showed that DHA supplementation was associated with increased activation of the prefrontal cortex and better reaction time during sustained attention in healthy 8–10 year-old boys [76]. In a cross-over intervention trial with more than 800 schoolchildren we have recently found that healthy school meals rich in fish improve school performance [77]. Some observational studies have also observed a positive association between n-3 LC-PUFA intake and cognitive performance. A study of 4000 American children found that the association between n-3 LC-PUFA intake and cognitive performance was stronger in girls than in boys [78]—again, an example of gender-related nutrition. Four randomized trials have supplied schoolchildren from high-income countries specifically with n-3 LC-PUFA [79–82]. Three of these studies found some beneficial effects on cognition or school performance of 0.4–1 g/day of n-3 LC-PUFA, while the study that did not find any effect supplied only around 0.2 g/day [79]. This dose-response effect is however not always consistent, as a three-armed study in 90 British 10–12 year-old children found a beneficial effect of 0.4 g/day of DHA on word recognition, but poorer performance in children who had 1 g/day [80].

In the last mentioned study, all the DHA supplemented children had a more relaxed mood compared to controls [80], which is consistent with another trial that found an apparent effect on mood, *i.e.*, a reduction in impulsivity and anti-social behavior, in 450 healthy 8–10 year-old children supplemented with fish oil *versus* olive oil [81]. Similar behavioral effects were also observed in one of the South African studies, which showed a decrease in physical activity during school hours, less oppositional behavior, inattention and lower scores on a rating scale of traits of attention-deficit hyperactivity disorder (ADHD) after fish oil supplementation [82]. Comparable behavioral effects have also been indicated, although not firmly proven, in children with ADHD [83] and in addition, one study has found an association between *FADS* SNPs and the development of ADHD, specifically in the context of prenatal alcohol exposure [84]. It is difficult to draw any firm conclusions based on the results of these trials and observational studies in schoolchildren due to differences in dose, duration and most of all the tested outcomes. Furthermore, the studies on behavioral conditions may be biased due to methodological flaws such as limited sample size and the large number of neurological tests that were performed in most of the studies (out of which only a few showed significant effects). More well-conducted studies, adjusted for multiple test administrations, are therefore needed in order to provide more convincing evidence for an effect of n-3 LC-PUFA intake on cognitive, behavioral and emotional effects in children.

So far, the effect of gender has not been given much attention in intervention trials with n-3 LC-PUFA in preschool and school-aged children. However, as was the case in the studies on the effects of DHA in the perinatal period, a gender-treatment effect has been observed on mean arterial blood pressure after fish oil supplementation from 9 to 18 month of age in healthy Danish infants, which just as in the previously mentioned maternal fish oil supplementation study was mostly affected in boys [85]. In this case, blood pressure was reduced in the boys, which however was still counteracting the observed gender difference in the control group, resulting in an almost similar mean arterial blood pressure in the girls and boys of the fish oil supplemented group [85]. A similar gender-equalizing effect was observed on the systolic blood pressure later in infancy in a study that compared fish oil *versus* no supplement during the complementary feeding period [86]. In that study, the observed changes in systolic blood pressure were found to correlate with the previously mentioned changes in free play attention [73], which could indicate a common emotional component. Furthermore, a recent randomized controlled cross-over trial in young adults also observed a gender-specific effect of fish oil supplementation on the sensation of appetite that abolished gender differences observed after a three week intervention in the soy oil control period [87].

7. Neurobehavioural Outcomes beyond Childhood

Only a few studies have examined if fish oil supplementation can affect brain functions in healthy young adults, but some studies indicate that DHA may be important for cognition and behavior during late adulthood. DHA supplementation improved memory in healthy, young adults whose habitual diets were low in DHA, and the response was still modulated by sex [88] suggesting consistence with the effects found in late infancy with the achievement of gross motor milestones [89]. An observational study conducted in 6158 individuals of >65 years found that high fish consumption, but not dietary n-3 LC-PUFA intake, had a protective effect on cognitive decline [90,91]. A systematic review and meta-analysis from 2006 gathered all available evidence from observational, preclinical and clinical studies to assess the effects of n-3 LC-PUFA on cognitive protection [92]. Four of the trials have shown a protective effect of n-3 LC-PUFA only among those with mild cognitive impairment conditions [93]. In another trial with 485 subjects with mild memory complaints, an improvement of memory was demonstrated after 0.9 g/day of DHA for 24 weeks [94]. A recent meta-analysis of all randomized trials that have investigated the effect of fish oil on cognitive decline also indicated a potential beneficial effect, but only in trials that had supplied >1 g/day of DHA in subjects who at the beginning of the trail exhibited some signs of cognitive decline [90]. There are nine separate observational studies that have suggest a possible link between increased fish consumption and reduced risk of Alzheimer's disease [95,96]. Furthermore, analysis of human cadaver brains has shown that people with Alzheimer disease have less DHA in their frontal lobe and hippocampus compared with unaffected individuals [97]. In addition, studies in mice provide support for the protective role of n-3 LC-PUFA, showing that a dietary intake of DHA induces an increase in DHA levels in the hippocampus with subsequent improvement of memory performances [98].

DHA has also been suggested to be effective in major psychiatric disorders. Most of the conducted studies have used n-3 LC-PUFA levels in RBC membranes as a measure of exposure, due to the objectivity of this measure and their high correlation with habitual dietary intake [99] in addition to their presumed reflection of brain LC-PUFA levels. Such studies have shown a significant correlation between DHA deficits and schizophrenia [100]. Life style in schizophrenia is characterized by heavy smoking, drinking, high-caloric diets, low physical activity and use of drugs that cause oxidative stress in the body. However, a recent study found no reduction of either DHA or AA in large groups of un-medicated Indian and Malaysian patients suffering from schizophrenia [101]. There is a tendency for RBC membrane levels of DHA and AA to diminish during storage, and this may happen abnormally rapidly in schizophrenia [102], possibly because of an increased oxidative stress [103]. Interestingly, several studies reported a better outcome in psychotic patients supplemented with n-3 LC-PUFA, either EPA or DHA [104].

Accumulating evidence also suggests that n-3 LC-PUFA supplementation may be efficacious for the treatment of positive and negative symptoms in patients with schizophrenia or at ultra-high risk for psychosis [105]. There is also some evidence that n-3 LC-PUFA may be relevant in relation to the pathophysiology of depression [106]. Cross-national studies indicate that higher intake of fish/seafood is correlated with lower lifetime prevalence rates of unipolar and bipolar depression [107]. In fact, depression may present with an increased production of pro-inflammatory cytokines and elevations in plasma homocysteine levels [108], and n-3 LC-PUFA have in randomized controlled trials been shown to be able to reduce both [109]. Thus, it can be speculated that n-3 PUFAs produce a positive effect on mood, partly because of the high brain content of DHA and its involvement in neurogenesis and neuroplasticity and partly due to their anti-inflammatory properties [110] as well as their effect on carbon metabolism, which is known to be of importance in relation to the metabolism of mono-aminergic neurotransmitters [111]. Some epidemiological studies have in the same way found that lower n-3 LC-PUFA intake is linked to an increased risk for emerging depressive symptoms [112]. Therefore, higher habitual dietary n-3 LC-PUFA intake may be protective against mood swings or even ultimately prevent mood dysregulation [113]. There is however a need for large well-performed randomized controlled trials in this area in order to confirm such effects.

8. Conclusions

The effects of DHA on brain and cognitive development have been extensively investigated in the last years. Its functional effects have been progressively, but not entirely, separated from those of AA. Clinical trials on maternal and infant dietary intakes are not entirely clear and consistent, but seem to indicate a complex interaction between the genotype pattern of *FADS*, gender, dietary intakes and lifestyle. For these reasons it is difficult to disentangle the effects of dietary DHA from the results of the randomized supplementation trials. In future studies an appropriate sample size should be calculated in order to adjust for the different variables. Mendelian trials provide a new tool to investigate the effects of LC-PUFA on cognitive development, but the interpretation of results from such trials requires an improved understanding of the biochemical effects of individual *FADS* SNPs and also needs to consider the potential differences between boys and girls.

Thus, our two questions, (1) Does the high rate of DHA accumulation in the brain have any functional importance? (2) If yes, is the endogenous synthesis of DHA high enough to support optimal functional levels of DHA in the brain? Regarding the first, there is clear evidence that DHA contributes to the visual development of infants, as also concluded by EFSA [53], but the associations with cognitive development are still not clearly interpreted [114,115], and one of the main problems could be that the effects differ between boys and girls, which needs to be considered in future trials. Due to the proposed early window of vulnerability, so far few studies have focused on the potential effects of n-3 LC-PUFA intake on cognitive and behavioral outcomes in children and young adults, but available studies indicate that the hypothesis might be worth challenging. Finally, there is preliminary evidence that DHA may ameliorate cognitive decline and affect behavioral symptoms in major neuropsychiatric disorders such as dementia, schizophrenia and depression. There is an extremely poor availability of trials on the effect of DHA supplementations that have investigated the changes in the fatty acid status as a function of the *FADS* polymorphisms. Most evidence indicates that the DHA accumulation is mainly affected by dietary intake, specifically of preformed DHA. However new studies indicate that the genetic make-up in the *FADS* gene cluster may contribute substantially to the current understanding, but that the effects may be SNP-specific and may even vary with age, or at least are most evident in the perinatal period, where the endogenous synthesis of LC-PUFA is upregulated and diet may be more easily controlled for, especially during lactation (or formula feeding).

Author Contributions: All the Authors contributed significantly to the paper. Lotte Lauritzen drafted the two sections about *FADS* and Neurobehavioural Outcomes in Older Children with assistance from Laurine BS Harsløf, the section on Dietary DHA and Postnatal Development and the background section on Brain DHA Accumulation during Development Depending on Diet was drafted by Lotte Lauritzen and Carlo Agostoni, and the section on Neurobehavioural Outcomes beyond Childhood was drafted by Paolo Brambilla and Valentina Ciappolino. Alessandra Mazzocchi and Valentina Ciappolino performed the literature search, commented on the manuscript, proof read and ordered the references.

Conflicts of Interest: The authors declare no conflict of interest. PB was partially supported by grants from the Italian Ministry of Health (GR-2010-2317873).

Abbreviations

AA: Arachidonic acid;
ADHD: Attention-Deficit Hyperactivity Disorder;
ALA: α-linolenic acid;
DHA: Docosahexaenoic acid;
EPA: Eicosapentaenoic acid;
FA%: % of the fatty acids;
FADS: Fatty acid desaturase gene;
LA: Linoleic acid;
LC-PUFA: Long chain PUFA;
PUFA: Polyunsaturated fatty acid;
RBC: Erythrocyte;
SNP: Single nucleotide polymorphism

References

1. Vlaardingerbroek, H.; Hornstra, G.; de Koning, T.J.; Smeitink, J.A.; Bakker, H.D.; de Klerk, H.B.; Rubio-Gozalbo, M.E. Essential polyunsaturated fatty acids in plasma and erythrocytes of children with inborn errors of amino acid metabolism. *Mol. Genet. Metab.* **2006**, *88*, 159–165. [CrossRef] [PubMed]

2. Abbott, S.K.; Else, P.L.; Atkins, T.A.; Hulbert, A.J. Fatty acid composition of membrane bilayers: Importance of diet polyunsaturated fat balance. *Biochim. Biophys. Acta* **2012**, *1818*, 1309–1317. [CrossRef] [PubMed]
3. Neuringer, M.; Connor, W.E.; Lin, D.S.; Barstad, L.; Luck, S. Biochemical and functional effects of prenatal and postnatal omega 3 fatty acid deficiency on retina and brain in rhesus monkeys. *Proc. Natl. Acad. Sci. USA* **1986**, *83*, 4021–4025. [CrossRef] [PubMed]
4. Carrie, I.; Clement, M.; de Javel, D.; Frances, H.; Bourre, J.M. Specific phospholipid fatty acid composition of brain regions in mice: Effects of n-3 polyunsaturated fatty acid deficiency and phospholipid supplementation. *J. Lipid Res.* **2000**, *41*, 465–472. [PubMed]
5. Carver, J.D.; Benford, V.J.; Han, B.; Cantor, A.B. The relationship between age and the fatty acid composition of cerebral cortex and erythrocytes in human subjects. *Brain Res. Bull.* **2001**, *56*, 79–85. [CrossRef]
6. Cetin, I.; Alvino, G.; Cardellicchio, M. Long chain fatty acids and dietary fats in fetal nutrition. *J. Physiol.* **2009**, *587*, 3441–3451. [CrossRef] [PubMed]
7. Haggarty, P. Effect of placental function on fatty acid requirements during pregnancy. *Eur. J. Clin. Nutr.* **2004**, *58*, 1559–1570. [CrossRef] [PubMed]
8. Kuipers, R.S.; Luxwolda, M.F.; Offringa, P.J.; Boersma, E.R.; Dijck-Brouwer, D.A.J.; Muskiet, F.A.J. Fetal intrauterine whole body linoleic, arachidonic and docosahexaenoic acid contents and accretion rates. *Prostaglandins Leukot. Essent. Fat. Acids* **2012**, *86*, 13–20. [CrossRef] [PubMed]
9. Kuipers, R.S.; Luxwolda, M.F.; Offringa, P.J.; Boersma, E.R.; Dijck-Brouwer, D.A.J.; Muskiet, F.A.J. Gestational age dependent changes of the fetal brain, liver and adipose tissue fatty acid compositions in a population with high fish intakes. *Prostaglandins Leukot. Essent. Fat. Acids* **2012**, *86*, 189–199. [CrossRef] [PubMed]
10. Clandinin, M.T.; Chappell, J.E.; Leong, S.; Heim, T.; Swyer, P.R.; Chance, G.W. Intrauterine fatty acid accretion rates in human brain: Implications for fatty acid requirements. *Early Hum. Dev.* **1980**, *4*, 121–129. [CrossRef]
11. Herrera, E. Implications of dietary fatty acids during pregnancy on placental, fetal and postnatal development—A review. *Placenta* **2002**, *23*, S9–S19. [CrossRef] [PubMed]
12. Campbell, F.M.; Gordon, M.J.; Dutta-Roy, A.K. Placental membrane fatty acid-binding protein preferentially binds arachidonic and docosahexaenoic acids. *Life Sci.* **1998**, *63*, 235–240. [CrossRef]
13. Haggarty, P. Fatty acid supply to the human fetus. *Annu. Rev. Nutr.* **2010**, *30*, 237–255. [CrossRef] [PubMed]
14. Montes, R.; Chisaguano, A.M.; Castellote, A.I.; Morales, E.; Sunyer, J.; Lopez-Sabater, M.C. Fatty acid composition of maternal and umbilical cord plasma and early childhood atopic eczema in a Spanish cohort. *Eur. J. Clin. Nutr.* **2013**, *67*, 658–663. [CrossRef] [PubMed]
15. Agostoni, C.; Galli, C.; Riva, E.; Rise, P.; Colombo, C.; Giovannini, M.; Marangoni, F. Whole blood fatty acid composition at birth: From the maternal compartment to the infant. *Clin. Nutr.* **2011**, *30*, 503–505. [CrossRef] [PubMed]
16. Oliveira, O.R.C.; Santana, M.G.; Santos, F.S.; Conceicao, F.D.; Sardinha, F.L.C.; Veiga, G.V.; do Carmo, M.G.T. Composition of fatty acids in the maternal and umbilical cord plasma of adolescent and adult mothers: Relationship with anthropometric parameters of newborn. *Lipids Health Dis.* **2012**, *11*, 157. [CrossRef] [PubMed]
17. Gil-Sanchez, A.; Larque, E.; Demmelmair, H.; Acien, M.I.; Faber, F.L.; Parrilla, J.J.; Koletzko, B. Maternal-fetal *in vivo* transfer of (^{13}C)docosahexaenoic and other fatty acids across the human placenta 12 h after maternal oral intake. *Am. J. Clin. Nutr.* **2010**, *92*, 115–122. [CrossRef] [PubMed]
18. Campbell, F.M.; Dutta-Roy, A.K. Plasma-membrane fatty acid binding protein ($FABP_{pm}$) is exclusively located in the maternal facing membranes of the human placenta. *FEBS Lett.* **1995**, *375*, 227–230. [CrossRef]
19. Dutta-Roy, A.K. Transfer of long-chain polyunsaturated fatty acids across the human placenta. *Prenat. Neonat. Med.* **1997**, *2*, 101–107.
20. Crabtree, J.T.; Gordon, M.J.; Campbell, F.M.; Dutta-Roy, A.K. Differential distribution and metabolism of arachidonic acid and docosahexaenoic acid by human placental choriocarcinoma (BeWo) cells. *Mol. Cell. Biochem.* **1998**, *185*, 191–198. [CrossRef] [PubMed]
21. Campbell, F.M.; Clohessy, A.M.; Gordon, M.J.; Page, K.R.; Dutta-Roy, A.K. Uptake of long chain fatty acids by human placental choriocarcinoma (BeWo) cells: Role of plasma membrane fatty acid binding protein. *J. Lipid Res.* **1997**, *38*, 2558–2568. [PubMed]
22. Allen, K.G.D.; Harris, M.A. The role of n-3 fatty acids in gestation and parturition. *Exp. Biol. Med.* **2001**, *226*, 498–506.

23. Cetin, I.; Giovannini, N.; Alvino, G.; Agostoni, C.; Riva, E.; Giovannini, M.; Pardi, G. Intrauterine growth restriction is associated with changes in polyunsaturated fatty acid fetal-maternal relationships. *Pediatr. Res.* **2002**, *52*, 750–755. [CrossRef] [PubMed]
24. Jørgensen, M.H.; Nielsen, P.K.; Michaelsen, K.F.; Lund, P.; Lauritzen, L. The composition of polyunsaturated fatty acids in erythrocytes of lactating mothers and their infants. *Mater. Child Nutr.* **2006**, *2*, 29–39. [CrossRef] [PubMed]
25. Koletzko, B.; Schmidt, E.; Bremer, H.J.; Haug, M.; Harzer, G. Effects of dietary long-chain polyunsaturated fatty acids on the essential fatty acid status of premature infants. *Eur. J. Pediatr.* **1989**, *148*, 669–675. [CrossRef] [PubMed]
26. Hsieh, A.T.; Brenna, J.T. Dietary docosahexaenoic acid but not arachidonic acid influences central nervous system fatty acid status in baboon neonates. *Prostaglandins Leukot. Essent. Fat. Acids* **2009**, *81*, 105–110. [CrossRef] [PubMed]
27. Farquharson, J.; Cockburn, F.; Patrick, W.A.; Jamieson, E.C.; Logan, R.W. Infant cerebral cortex phospholipid fatty-acid composition and diet. *Lancet* **1992**, *340*, 810–813. [CrossRef]
28. Makrides, M.; Neumann, M.A.; Byard, R.W.; Simmer, K.; Gibson, R.A. Fatty acid composition of brain, retina, and erythrocytes in breast- and formula-fed infants. *Am. J. Clin. Nutr.* **1994**, *60*, 189–194. [PubMed]
29. Harsløf, L.B.S.; Larsen, L.H.; Ritz, C.; Hellgren, L.I.; Michaelsen, K.F.; Vogel, U.; Lauritzen, L. *FADS* genotype and diet are important determinants of DHA status: A cross-sectional study in Danish infants. *Am. J. Clin. Nutr.* **2013**, *97*, 1403–1410. [CrossRef] [PubMed]
30. Lauritzen, L.; Carlson, S.E. Maternal fatty acid status during pregnancy and lactation and relation to newborn and infant status. *Mater. Child Nutr.* **2011**, *7*, 41–58. [CrossRef] [PubMed]
31. Rise, P.; Tragni, E.; Ghezzi, S.; Agostoni, C.; Marangoni, F.; Poli, A.; Catapano, A.L.; Siani, A.; Iacoviello, L.; Galli, C. Different patterns characterize omega-6 and omega-3 long chain polyunsaturated fatty acid levels in blood from Italian infants, children, adults and elderly. *Prostaglandins Leukot. Essent. Fat. Acids* **2013**, *89*, 215–220. [CrossRef] [PubMed]
32. Rahmawaty, S.; Charlton, K.; Lyons-Wall, P.; Meyer, B.J. Dietary intake and food sources of EPA, DPA and DHA in Australian children. *Lipids* **2013**, *48*, 869–877. [CrossRef] [PubMed]
33. Wolters, M.; Schlenz, H.; Foraita, R.; Galli, C.; Rise, P.; Moreno, L.A.; Molnar, D.; Russo, P.; Veidebaum, T.; Tornaritis, M.; *et al.* Reference values of whole-blood fatty acids by age and gender from European children aged 3–8 years. *Int. J. Obes.* **2014**, *38*, S86–S98. [CrossRef] [PubMed]
34. Crawford, M.A.; Hassam, G.A.; Williams, G.; Whitehouse, W.L. Essential fatty acids and fetal brain growth. *Lancet* **1976**, *1*, 452–453. [CrossRef]
35. Sauerwald, T.U.; Hachey, D.L.; Jensen, C.L.; Chen, H.; Anderson, R.E.; Heird, W.C. Intermediates in endogenous synthesis of C22:6 omega-3 and C20:4 omega-6 by term and preterm infants. *Pediatr. Res.* **1997**, *41*, 183–187. [CrossRef] [PubMed]
36. Salem, N., Jr.; Wegher, B.; Mena, P.; Uauy, R. Arachidonic and docosahexaenoic acids are biosynthesized from their 18-carbon precursors in human infants. *Proc. Natl. Acad. Sci. USA* **1996**, *93*, 49–54. [CrossRef] [PubMed]
37. Szitanyi, P.; Koletzko, B.; Mydlilova, A.; Demmelmair, H. Metabolism of C-13-labeled linoleic acid in newborn infants during the first week of life. *Pediatr. Res.* **1999**, *45*, 669–673. [CrossRef] [PubMed]
38. Uauy, R.D.; Mena, P.; Wegher, B.; Nieto, S.; Salem, N., Jr. Long chain polyunsaturated fatty acid formation in neonates: Effect of gestational age and intrauterine growth. *Pediatr. Res.* **2000**, *47*, 127–135. [CrossRef] [PubMed]
39. Carnielli, V.P.; Simonato, M.; Verlato, G.; Luijendijk, I.; de Curtis, M.; Sauer, P.J.; Cogo, P.E. Synthesis of long-chain polyunsaturated fatty acids in preterm newborns fed formula with long-chain polyunsaturated fatty acids. *Am. J. Clin. Nutr.* **2007**, *86*, 1323–1330. [PubMed]
40. Lin, Y.H.; Llanos, A.; Mena, P.; Uauy, R.; Salem, N., Jr.; Pawlosky, R.J. Compartmental analyses of H-2(5)-alpha-linolenic acid and C-13-U-eicosapentaenoic acid toward synthesis of plasma labeled 22:6 n-3 in newborn term infants. *Am. J. Clin. Nutr.* **2010**, *92*, 284–293. [CrossRef] [PubMed]
41. Xie, L.; Innis, S.M. Genetic Variants of the *FADS1 FADS2* gene cluster are associated with altered n-6 and n-3 essential fatty acids in plasma and erythrocyte phospholipids in women during pregnancy and in breast milk during lactation. *J. Nutr.* **2008**, *138*, 2222–2228. [CrossRef] [PubMed]

42. Koletzko, B.; Lattka, E.; Zeilinger, S.; Illig, T.; Steer, C. Genetic variants of the fatty acid desaturase gene cluster predict amounts of red blood cell docosahexaenoic and other polyunsaturated fatty acids in pregnant women: Findings from the Avon Longitudinal Study of Parents and Children. *Am. J. Clin. Nutr.* **2011**, *93*, 211–219. [CrossRef] [PubMed]
43. Schaeffer, L.; Gohlke, H.; Muller, M.; Heid, I.M.; Palmer, L.J.; Kompauer, I.; Demmelmair, H.; Illig, T.; Koletzko, B.; Heinrich, J. Common genetic variants of the *FADS1 FADS2* gene cluster and their reconstructed haplotypes are associated with the fatty acid composition in phospholipids. *Hum. Mol. Genet.* **2006**, *15*, 1745–1756. [CrossRef] [PubMed]
44. Mathias, R.A.; Vergara, C.; Gao, L.; Rafaels, N.; Hand, T.; Campbell, M.; Bickel, C.; Ivester, P.; Sergeant, S.; Barnes, K.C.; *et al.* *FADS* genetic variants and omega-6 polyunsaturated fatty acid metabolism in a homogeneous island population. *J. Lipid Res.* **2010**, *51*, 2766–2774. [CrossRef] [PubMed]
45. Bokor, S.; Dumont, J.; Spinneker, A.; Gonzalez-Gross, M.; Nova, E.; Widhalm, K.; Moschonis, G.; Stehle, P.; Amouyel, P.; de Henauw, S.; *et al.* Single nucleotide polymorphisms in the *FADS* gene cluster are associated with delta-5 and delta-6 desaturase activities estimated by serum fatty acid ratios. *J. Lipid Res.* **2010**, *51*, 2325–2333. [CrossRef] [PubMed]
46. Morales, E.; Bustamante, M.; Gonzalez, J.R.; Guxens, M.; Torrent, M.; Mendez, M.; Garcia-Esteban, R.; Julvez, J.; Forns, J.; Vrijheid, M.; *et al.* Genetic variants of the *FADS* gene cluster and *ELOVL* gene family, colostrum LCPUFA levels, breastfeeding, and child cognition. *PLoS ONE* **2011**, *6*, e17181. [CrossRef] [PubMed]
47. Moltó-Puigmartí, C.; Plat, J.; Mensink, R.P.; Müller, A.; Jansen, E.; Zeegers, M.P.; Thijs, C. *FADS1 FADS2* gene variants modify the association between fish intake and the docosahexaenoic acid proportions in human milk. *Am. J. Clin. Nutr.* **2010**, *91*, 1368–1376. [CrossRef] [PubMed]
48. Lattka, E.; Rzehak, P.; Szabo, E.; Jakobik, V.; Weck, M.; Weyermann, M.; Grallert, H.; Rothenbacher, D.; Heinrich, J.; Brenner, H.; *et al.* Genetic variants in the *FADS* gene cluster are associated with arachidonic acid concentrations of human breast milk at 1.5 and 6 mo postpartum and influence the course of milk dodecanoic, tetracosenoic, and trans-9-octadecenoic acid concentrations over the duration of lactation. *Am. J. Clin. Nutr.* **2011**, *93*, 382–391. [PubMed]
49. Steer, C.D.; Hibbeln, J.R.; Golding, J.; Smith, G.D. Polyunsaturated fatty acid levels in blood during pregnancy, at birth and at 7 years: Their associations with two common *FADS2* polymorphisms. *Hum. Mol. Genet.* **2012**, *21*, 1504–1512. [CrossRef] [PubMed]
50. Lattka, E.; Koletzko, B.; Zeilinger, S.; Hibbeln, J.R.; Klopp, N.; Ring, S.M.; Steer, C.D. Umbilical cord PUFA are determined by maternal and child fatty acid desaturase (*FADS*) genetic variants in the Avon Longitudinal Study of Parents and Children (ALSPAC). *Br. J. Nutr.* **2013**, *109*, 1196–1210. [CrossRef] [PubMed]
51. Jensen, H.A.R.; Harsløf, L.B.S.; Nielsen, M.S.; Christensen, L.B.; Ritz, C.; Michaelsen, K.F.; Vogel, U.; Lauritzen, L. *FADS* single-nucleotide polymorphisms are associated with behavioral outcomes in children, and the effect varies between genders and is dependent on PPAR genotype. *Am. J. Clin. Nutr.* **2014**, *100*, 826–832. [CrossRef] [PubMed]
52. Glaser, C.; Rzehak, P.; Demmelmair, H.; Klopp, N.; Heinrich, J.; Koletzko, B. LISA study group. Influence of *FADS* polymorphisms on tracking of serum glycerophospholipid fatty acid concentrations and percentage composition in children. *PLoS ONE* **2011**, *6*, e21933. [CrossRef] [PubMed]
53. European Food Safety Authority. The Panel on Dietetic Products, Nutrition and Allergies on a request from Mead Johnson Nutritionals. Scientific opinion on DHA and ARA and visual development. *EFSA J.* **2009**, *941*, 1–14. [CrossRef]
54. Uauy, R.; Hoffman, D.R.; Mena, P.; Llanos, A.; Birch, E.E. Term infant studies of DHA and ARA supplementation on neurodevelopment: Results of randomized controlled trials. *J. Pediatr.* **2003**, *143*, S17–S25. [CrossRef]
55. Simmer, K.; Patole, S.K.; Rao, S.C. Long-chain polyunsaturated fatty acid supplementation in infants born at term. *Cochrane Database Syst. Rev.* **2011**, *12*. [CrossRef]
56. Qawasmi, A.; Landeros-Weisenberger, A.; Leckman, J.F.; Bloch, M.H. Meta-analysis of long-chain polyunsaturated fatty acid supplementation of formula and infant cognition. *Pediatrics* **2012**, *129*, 1141–1149. [CrossRef] [PubMed]
57. Schulzke, S.M.; Patole, S.K.; Simmer, K. Long-chain polyunsaturated fatty acid supplementation in preterm infants. *Cochrane Database Syst. Rev.* **2011**, *2*. [CrossRef]

58. Delgado-Noguera, M.F.; Calvache, J.A.; Cosp, X.B. Supplementation with long chain polyunsaturated fatty acids (LCPUFA) to breastfeeding mothers for improving child growth and development. *Cochrane Database Syst. Rev.* **2010**, *12*. [CrossRef]
59. Gould, J.F.; Smithers, L.G.; Makrides, M. The effect of maternal omega-3 LCPUFA supplementation during pregnancy on early childhood cognitive and visual development: A systematic review and meta-analysis of randomized controlled trials. *Am. J. Clin. Nutr.* **2013**, *97*, 531–544. [CrossRef] [PubMed]
60. Makrides, M.; Gibson, R.A.; McPhee, A.J.; Collins, C.T.; Davis, P.G.; Doyle, L.W.; Simmer, K.; Colditz, P.B.; Morris, S.; Smithers, L.G.; *et al.* Neurodevelopmental outcomes of preterm infants fed high-dose docosahexaenoic acid: A randomized controlled trial. *JAMA* **2009**, *301*, 175–178. [CrossRef] [PubMed]
61. Makrides, M.; Gibson, R.A.; McPhee, A.J. Effect of DHA supplementation during pregnancy on maternal depression and neurodevelopment of young children: A randomized controlled trial. *JAMA* **2010**, *304*, 1675–1683. [CrossRef] [PubMed]
62. Lauritzen, L.; Jørgensen, M.H.; Olsen, S.F.; Straarup, E.M.; Michaelsen, K.F. Maternal fish oil supplementation in lactation: Effect on developmental outcome in breast-fed infants. *Reprod. Nutr. Dev.* **2005**, *45*, 535–547. [CrossRef] [PubMed]
63. Cheatham, C.L.; Nerhammer, A.S.; Asserhøj, M.; Michaelsen, K.F.; Lauritzen, L. Fish oil supplementation during lactation: Effects on cognition and behavior at 7 years of age. *Lipids* **2011**, *46*, 637–645. [CrossRef] [PubMed]
64. Asserhøj, M.; Nehammer, S.; Matthiessen, J.; Michaelsen, K.F.; Lauritzen, L. Maternal fish oil supplementation during lactation may adversely affect long-term blood pressure, energy intake, and physical activity of 7-year-old boys. *J. Nutr.* **2009**, *139*, 298–304. [CrossRef] [PubMed]
65. Steer, C.D.; Smith, G.D.; Emmett, P.M.; Hibbeln, J.R.; Golding, J. *FADS2* polymorphisms modify the effect of breastfeeding on child IQ. *PLoS ONE* **2010**, *5*. [CrossRef] [PubMed]
66. Caspi, A.; Williams, B.; Kim-Cohen, J.; Craig, I.W.; Milne, B.J.; Poulton, R.; Schalkwyk, L.C.; Taylor, A.; Werts, H.; Moffitt, T.E. Moderation of breastfeeding effects on the IQ by genetic variation in fatty acid metabolism. *Proc. Natl. Acad. Sci. USA* **2007**, *104*, 18860–18865. [CrossRef] [PubMed]
67. Groen-Blokhuis, M.M.; Franic, S.; van Beijsterveldt, C.E.M.; de Geus, E.; Bartels, M.; Davies, G.E.; Ehli, E.A.; Xiao, X.J.; Scheet, P.A.; Althoff, R.; *et al.* A prospective study of the effects of breastfeeding and *FADS2* polymorphisms on cognition and hyperactivity/attention problems. *Am. J. Med. Genet. B. Neuropsychiatr. Genet.* **2013**, *162*, 457–465. [CrossRef] [PubMed]
68. Martin, N.W.; Benyamin, B.; Hansell, N.K.; Montgomery, G.W.; Martin, N.G.; Wright, M.J.; Bates, T.C. Cognitive function in adolescence: Testing for interactions between breast-feeding and *FADS2* polymorphisms. *J. Am. Acad. Child Adolesc. Psychiatry* **2011**, *50*, 55–62. [CrossRef] [PubMed]
69. Steer, C.D.; Lattka, E.; Koletzko, B.; Golding, J.; Hibbeln, J.R. Maternal fatty acids in pregnancy, *FADS* polymorphisms, and child intelligence quotient at 8 y of age. *Am. J. Clin. Nutr.* **2013**, *98*, 1575–1582. [CrossRef] [PubMed]
70. Browning, L.M.; Walker, C.G.; Mander, A.P.; West, A.L.; Madden, J.; Gambell, J.M.; Young, S.; Wang, L.; Jebb, S.A.; Calder, P.C. Incorporation of eicosapentaenoic and docosahexaenoic acids into lipid pools when given as supplements providing doses equivalent to typical intakes of oily fish. *Am. J. Clin. Nutr.* **2012**, *96*, 748–758. [CrossRef] [PubMed]
71. Drover, J.; Hoffman, D.R.; Castaneda, Y.S.; Morale, S.E.; Birch, E.E. Three randomized controlled trials of early long-chain polyunsaturated fatty acid supplementation on means-end problem solving in 9-month-olds. *Child Dev.* **2009**, *80*, 1376–1384. [CrossRef] [PubMed]
72. Hoffman, D.R.; Theuer, R.C.; Castaneda, Y.S.; Wheaton, D.H.; Bosworth, R.G.; O'Connor, A.R.; Morale, S.E.; Wiedemann, L.E.; Birch, E.E. Maturation of visual acuity is accelerated in breast-fed term infants fed baby food containing DHA-enriched egg yolk. *J. Nutr.* **2004**, *134*, 2307–2313. [PubMed]
73. Harbild, H.L.; Harsløf, L.B.S.; Christensen, J.H.; Kannass, K.N.; Lauritzen, L. Fish oil-supplementation from 9 to 12 months of age affects infant attention in a free-play test and is related to change in blood pressure. *Prostaglandins Leukot. Essent. Fat. Acids* **2013**, *89*, 327–333. [CrossRef] [PubMed]
74. Parletta, N.; Cooper, P.; Gent, D.N.; Petkov, J.; O'Dea, K. Effects of fish oil supplementation on learning and behaviour of children from Australian Indigenous remote community schools: A randomised controlled trial. *Prostaglandins Leukot. Essent. Fat. Acids* **2013**, *89*, 71–79. [CrossRef] [PubMed]

75. Baumgartner, J.; Smuts, C.M.; Malan, L.; Kvalsvig, J.; van Stuijvenberg, M.E.; Hurrell, R.F.; Zimmermann, M.B. Effects of iron and n-3 fatty acid supplementation, alone and in combination, on cognition in school children: A randomized, double-blind, placebo-controlled intervention in South Africa. *Am. J. Clin. Nutr.* **2012**, *96*, 1327–1338. [CrossRef] [PubMed]
76. McNamara, R.K.; Able, J.; Jandacek, R.; Rider, T.; Tso, P.; Eliassen, J.C.; Alfieri, D.; Weber, W.; Jarvis, K.; DelBello, M.P.; *et al.* Docosahexaenoic acid supplementation increases prefrontal cortex activation during sustained attention in healthy boys: A placebo-controlled, dose-ranging, functional magnetic resonance imaging study. *Am. J. Clin. Nutr.* **2010**, *91*, 1060–1067. [CrossRef] [PubMed]
77. Sørensen, L.B.; Dyssegaard, C.B.; Damsgaard, C.T.; Petersen, R.A.; Dalskov, S.M.; Hjorth, M.F.; Andersen, R.; Tetens, I.; Ritz, C.; Astrup, A.; *et al.* The effect of Nordic school meals on concentration and school performance in 8 to 11 year-old children in the OPUS School Meal Study: A cluster-randomized controlled cross-over trial. *Br. J. Nutr.* **2015**, *113*, 1280–1291. [CrossRef] [PubMed]
78. Eilander, A.; Hundscheid, D.C.; Osendarp, S.J.; Transler, C.; Zock, P.L. Effects of n-3 long chain polyunsaturated fatty acid supplementation on visual and cognitive development throughout childhood: A review of human studies. *Prostaglandins Leukot. Essent. Fat. Acids* **2007**, *76*, 189–203. [CrossRef] [PubMed]
79. Osendarp, S.J.M.; Baghurst, K.I.; Bryan, J.; Calvaresi, E.; Hughes, D.; Hussaini, M.; Karyadi, S.J.M.; van Klinken, B.J.W.; van der Knaap, H.C.M.; Lukito, W.; *et al.* Effect of a 12-mo micronutrient intervention on learning and memory in well-nourished and marginally nourished school-aged children: 2 parallel, randomized, placebo-controlled studies in Australia and Indonesia. *Am. J. Clin. Nutr.* **2007**, *86*, 1082–1093. [PubMed]
80. Kennedy, D.O.; Jackson, P.A.; Elliott, J.M.; Scholey, A.B.; Robertson, B.C.; Greer, J.; Tiplady, B.; Buchanan, T.; Haskell, C.F. Cognitive and mood effects of 8 weeks' supplementation with 400 mg or 1000 mg of the omega-3 essential fatty acid docosahexaenoic acid (DHA) in healthy children aged 10–12 years. *Nutr. Neurosci.* **2009**, *12*, 48–56. [CrossRef] [PubMed]
81. Kirby, A.; Woodward, A.; Jackson, S.; Wang, Y.; Crawford, M.A. A double-blind, placebo-controlled study investigating the effects of omega-3 supplementation in children aged 8–10 years from a mainstream school population. *Res. Dev. Disabil.* **2010**, *31*, 718–730. [CrossRef] [PubMed]
82. Smuts, C.M.; Greeff, J.; Kvalsvig, J.; Zimmermann, M.; Baumgartner, J. Long-chain n-3 polyunsaturated fatty acid supplementation decrease physical activity during class in iron deficient South African school children. *Br. J. Nutr.* **2015**, *113*, 212–224. [CrossRef] [PubMed]
83. Rytter, M.J.H.; Andersen, L.B.B.; Houmann, T.; Bilenberg, N.; Hvolby, A.; Mølgaard, C.; Michaelsen, K.F.; Lauritzen, L. Diet in the treatment of ADHD in children-A systematic review of the literature. *Nord. J. Psychiatry* **2015**, *69*, 1–18. [CrossRef] [PubMed]
84. Brookes, K.J.; Chen, W.; Xu, X.; Taylor, E.; Asherson, P. Association of fatty acid desaturase genes with attention-deficit/hyperactivity disorder. *Biol. Psychiatry* **2006**, *60*, 1053–1061. [CrossRef] [PubMed]
85. Harsløf, L.B.; Damsgaard, C.; Hellgren, L.; Andersen, A.; Vogel, U.; Lauritzen, L. Effects on metabolic markers are modified by *PPARG2* and *COX2* polymorphisms in infants randomized to fish oil. *Genes Nutr.* **2014**, *9*, 1–11. [CrossRef] [PubMed]
86. Damsgaard, C.T.; Schack-Nielsen, L.; Michaelsen, K.F.; Fruekilde, M.B.; Hels, O.; Lauritzen, L. Fish oil affects blood pressure and the plasma lipid profile in healthy Danish infants. *J. Nutr.* **2006**, *136*, 94–99. [PubMed]
87. Damsbo-Svendsen, S.; Rønsholdt, M.D.; Lauritzen, L. Fish oil-supplementation increases appetite in healthy adults. A randomized controlled cross-over trial. *Appetite* **2013**, *66*, 62–66. [CrossRef] [PubMed]
88. Stonehouse, W.; Conlon, C.A.; Podd, J.; Hill, S.R.; Minihane, A.M.; Haskell, C.; Kennedy, D. DHA supplementation improved both memory and reaction time in healthy young adults: A randomized controlled trial. *Am. J. Clin. Nutr.* **2013**, *97*, 1134–1143. [CrossRef] [PubMed]
89. Agostoni, C.; Zuccotti, G.V.; Radaelli, G.; Besana, R.; Podesta, A.; Sterpa, A.; Rottoli, A.; Riva, E.; Giovannini, M. Docosahexaenoic acid supplementation and time at achievement of gross motor milestones in healthy infants: A randomized, prospective, double-blind, placebo-controlled trial. *Am. J. Clin. Nutr.* **2009**, *89*, 64–70. [CrossRef] [PubMed]
90. Yurko-Mauro, K.; Alexander, D.D.; van Elswyk, M.E. Docosahexaenoic acid and adult memory: A systematic review and meta-analysis. *PLoS ONE* **2015**, *10*. [CrossRef]
91. Morris, M.C.; Evans, D.A.; Tangney, C.C.; Bienias, J.L.; Wilson, R.S. Fish consumption and cognitive decline with age in a large community study. *Arch. Neurol.* **2005**, *62*, 1849–1853. [CrossRef] [PubMed]

92. Lim, W.S.; Gammack, J.K.; van Niekerk, J.; Dangour, A.D. Omega-3 fatty acid for the prevention of dementia. *Cochrane Database Syst. Rev.* **2006**, *1*. [CrossRef]
93. Chiu, C.C.; Su, K.P.; Cheng, T.C.; Liu, H.C.; Chang, C.J.; Dewey, M.E.; Stewart, R.; Huang, S.Y. The effects of omega-3 fatty acids monotherapy in Alzheimer's disease and mild cognitive impairment: A preliminary randomized double-blind placebo-controlled study. *Prog. Neuropsychopharmacol. Biol. Psychiatry* **2008**, *32*, 1538–1544. [CrossRef] [PubMed]
94. Yurko-Mauro, K.; McCarthy, D.; Rom, D.; Nelson, E.B.; Ryan, A.S.; Blackwell, A.; Salem, N., Jr.; Stedman, M. Beneficial effects of docosahexaenoic acid on cognition in age-related cognitive decline. *Alzheimers Dement.* **2010**, *6*, 456–464. [CrossRef] [PubMed]
95. Astarita, G.; Jung, K.M.; Berchtold, N.C.; Nguyen, V.Q.; Gillen, D.L.; Head, E.; Cotman, C.W.; Piomelli, D. Deficient liver biosynthesis of docosahexaenoic acid correlates with cognitive impairment in Alzheimer's disease. *PLoS ONE* **2010**, *5*, e12538. [CrossRef] [PubMed]
96. Bazan, N.G.; Molina, M.F.; Gordon, W.C. Docosahexaenoic acid Signal lipidomics in nutrition: Significance in aging, neuroinflammation, macular degeneration, Alzheimer's, and other neurodegenerative diseases. *Annu. Rev. Nutr.* **2011**, *31*, 321–351. [CrossRef] [PubMed]
97. De Mel, D.; Suphioglu, C. Fishy business: Effect of omega-3 fatty acids on zinc transporters and free zinc availability in human neuronal cells. *Nutrients* **2014**, *6*, 3245–3258. [CrossRef] [PubMed]
98. Labrousse, V.F.; Nadjar, A.; Joffre, C.; Costes, L.; Aubert, A.; Gregoire, S.; Bretillon, L.; Laye, S. Short-term long chain omega3 diet protects from neuroinflammatory processes and memory impairment in aged mice. *PLoS ONE* **2012**, *7*, e36861. [CrossRef] [PubMed]
99. Sands, S.A.; Windsor, S.L.; Reid, K.J.; Harris, W.S. The impact of age, body mass index, and fish intake on the EPA and DHA content of human erythrocytes. *Lipids* **2005**, *40*, 343–347. [CrossRef] [PubMed]
100. Hoen, W.P.; Lijmer, J.G.; Duran, M.; Wanders, R.J.; van Beveren, N.J.; de Haan, L. Red blood cell polyunsaturated fatty acids measured in red blood cells and schizophrenia: A meta-analysis. *Psychiatry Res.* **2013**, *207*, 1–12. [CrossRef] [PubMed]
101. Peet, M.; Shah, S.; Selvam, K.; Ramchand, C.N. Polyunsaturated fatty acid levels in red cell membranes of unmedicated schizophrenic patients. *World J. Biol. Psychiatry* **2004**, *5*, 92–99. [CrossRef] [PubMed]
102. Khan, M.M.; Evans, D.R.; Gunna, V.; Scheffer, R.E.; Parikh, V.V.; Mahadik, S.P. Reduced erythrocyte membrane essential fatty acids and increased lipid peroxides in schizophrenia at the never-medicated first-episode of psychosis and after years of treatment with antipsychotics. *Schizophr. Res.* **2002**, *58*, 1–10. [CrossRef]
103. Reyazuddin, M.; Azmi, S.A.; Islam, N.; Rizvi, A. Oxidative stress and level of antioxidant enzymes in drug-naive schizophrenics. *Indian J. Psychiatry* **2014**, *56*, 344–349. [PubMed]
104. Hashimoto, M.; Maekawa, M.; Katakura, M.; Hamazaki, K.; Matsuoka, Y. Possibility of polyunsaturated fatty acids for the prevention and treatment of neuropsychiatric illnesses. *J. Pharmacol. Sci.* **2014**, *124*, 294–300. [CrossRef] [PubMed]
105. Amminger, G.P.; Schafer, M.R.; Papageorgiou, K.; Klier, C.M.; Cotton, S.M.; Harrigan, S.M.; Mackinnon, A.; McGorry, P.D.; Berger, G.E. Long-chain omega-3 fatty acids for indicated prevention of psychotic disorders: A randomized, placebo-controlled trial. *Arch. Gen. Psychiatry* **2010**, *67*, 146–154. [CrossRef] [PubMed]
106. Machado-Vieira, R.; Mallinger, A.G. Abnormal function of monoamine oxidase-A in comorbid major depressive disorder and cardiovascular disease: Pathophysiological and therapeutic implications. *Mol. Med. Rep.* **2012**, *6*, 915–922. [CrossRef] [PubMed]
107. Weissman, M.M.; Bland, R.C.; Canino, G.J.; Faravelli, C.; Greenwald, S.; Hwu, H.G.; Joyce, P.R.; Karam, E.G.; Lee, C.K.; Lellouch, J.; *et al.* Cross-national epidemiology of major depression and bipolar disorder. *JAMA* **1996**, *276*, 293–299. [CrossRef] [PubMed]
108. Severus, W.E.; Littman, A.B.; Stoll, A.L. Omega-3 fatty acids, homocysteine, and the increased risk of cardiovascular mortality in major depressive disorder. *Harv. Rev. Psychiatry* **2001**, *9*, 280–293. [CrossRef] [PubMed]
109. Huang, T.; Zheng, J.; Chen, Y.; Yang, B.; Wahlqvist, M.L.; Li, D. High consumption of omega-3 polyunsaturated fatty acids decrease plasma homocysteine: A meta-analysis of randomized, placebo-controlled trials. *Nutrition* **2011**, *27*, 863–867. [CrossRef] [PubMed]
110. Bourre, J.M. Roles of unsaturated fatty acids (especially omega-3 fatty acids) in the brain at various ages and during ageing. *J. Nutr. Health Aging* **2004**, *8*, 163–174. [PubMed]

111. Assies, J.; Mocking, R.J.T.; Lok, A.; Ruhé, H.G.; Pouwer, F.; Schene, A.H. Effects of oxidative stress on fatty acid- and one-carbon- metabolism in psychiatric and cardiovascular disease comorbidity. *Acta Psychiatr. Scand.* **2014**, *130*, 163–180. [CrossRef] [PubMed]
112. Lin, P.Y.; Huang, S.Y.; Su, K.P. A meta-analytic review of polyunsaturated fatty acid compositions in patients with depression. *Biol. Psychiatry* **2010**, *68*, 140–147. [CrossRef] [PubMed]
113. McNamara, R.K.; Vannest, J.J.; Valentine, J.C. Role of perinatal long-chain omega-3 fatty acids in cortical circuit maturation: Mechanisms and implications for psychopathology. *World J. Psychiatry* **2015**, *5*, 15–34. [PubMed]
114. European Food Safety Authority. The Panel on Dietetic Products, Nutrition and Allergies on a request from Mead Johnson Nutritionals. Scientific Opinion on DHA and ARA and brain development. *EFSA J.* **2009**, *1000*, 1–13. [CrossRef]
115. European Food Safety Authority. The Panel on Dietetic Products, Nutrition and Allergies. Scientific Opinion on the substantiation of a health claim related to DHA and contribution to normal brain development pursuant to Article 14 of Regulation (EC) No 1924/2006. *EFSA J.* **1924**, *12*. [CrossRef]

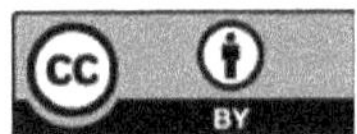

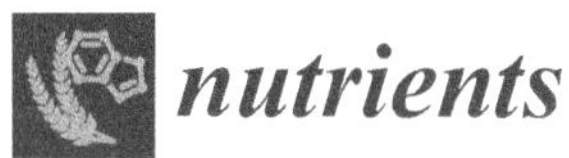

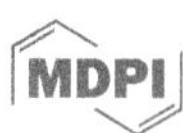

Article

Rise in DPA Following SDA-Rich Dietary Echium Oil Less Effective in Affording Anti-Arrhythmic Actions Compared to High DHA Levels Achieved with Fish Oil in Sprague-Dawley Rats

Mahinda Y. Abeywardena *, Michael Adams, Julie Dallimore and Soressa M. Kitessa

Commonwealth Scientific and Industrial Research Organisation (CSIRO) Food & Nutrition, Kintore Ave, Adelaide SA 5000, Australia; Michael.Adams@csiro.au (M.A.); Julie.Dallimore@csiro.au (J.D.); Soressa.Kitessa@csiro.au (S.M.K.)

* Correspondance: mahinda.abeywardena@csiro.au; Tel.: +61-08-8303-8889; Fax: +61-08-8303-8899

Received: 23 October 2015; Accepted: 18 December 2015; Published: 4 January 2016

Abstract: Stearidonic acid (SDA; C18:4*n*-3) has been suggested as an alternative to fish oil (FO) for delivering health benefits of C $\geqslant$ 20 long-chain *n*-3 polyunsaturated fatty acids (LC *n*-3 PUFA). Echium oil (EO) represents a non-genetically-modified source of SDA available commercially. This study compared EO and FO in relation to alterations in plasma and tissue fatty acids, and for their ability to afford protection against ischemia-induced cardiac arrhythmia and ventricular fibrillation (VF). Rats were fed (12 weeks) diets supplemented with either EO or FO at three dose levels (1, 3 and 5% *w*/*w*; $n = 18$ per group). EO failed to influence C22:6*n*-3 (DHA) but increased C22:5*n*-3 (DPA) in tissues dose-dependently, especially in heart tissue. Conversely, DHA in hearts of FO rats showed dose-related elevation; 14.8%–24.1% of total fatty acids. Kidney showed resistance for incorporation of LC *n*-3 PUFA. Overall, FO provided greater cardioprotection than EO. At the highest dose level, FO rats displayed lower ($p < 0.05$) episodes of VF% (29% *vs.* 73%) and duration (22.7 $\pm$ 12.0 *vs.* 75.8 $\pm$ 17.1 s) than the EO group but at 3% EO was comparable to FO. We conclude that there is no endogenous conversion of SDA to DHA, and that DPA may be associated with limited cardiac benefit.

Keywords: *n*-3 fatty acids; fish oil; Echium oil; stearidonic acid; docosapentaenoic acid; docosahexaenoic acid; eicosapentaenoic acid; cardiac arrhythmia; rat

---

1. Introduction

The influence of dietary fats on the pathogenesis of coronary heart disease, congestive heart failure as well as vulnerability to cardiac arrhythmias and sudden cardiac death has been well documented [1,2]. In this regard, both the "type" and the "amount" of dietary oils and fats have been identified as important determinants [3–5]. For example, a considerable body of supporting evidence shows that long chain (C $\geqslant$ 20) *n*-3 polyunsaturated fatty acids (LC *n*-3 PUFA) derived from marine sources (seafood, fish and microalgae) are particularly effective in affording cardiovascular protection [6,7] although more recent analyses have reported inconsistent outcomes [8]. In similar vein, a review of recent clinical trials (2007–2013 period) showed a lack of clear benefit of fish oil supplements although high dietary intake of fish was associated with lower incidence of sudden cardiac death, congestive heart failure, myocardial infarction and stroke [9]. Among the *n*-3 PUFA, the two major LC- *n*-3 PUFA are eicosapentaenoic acid (EPA, C20:5*n*-3) and docosahexaenoic acid (DHA, C22:6*n*-3).

A number of studies [10,11] have reported certain positive cardiovascular health outcomes from consumption of α-linolenic acid (ALA, C18:3*n*-3), an essential *n*-3 PUFA widely available from plant-based food sources including certain seed oils (e.g., flax, canola, perilla, chia, walnut, *etc.*). The primary mechanism by which ALA fosters cardiovascular health benefits is usually explained in terms of it being a precursor for endogenous LC n-3 PUFA biosynthesis of EPA and DHA, the two key fatty acid substrates for the synthesis of eicosanoid family of biological mediators. However, in humans, the conversion of ALA to EPA and DHA is inefficient, almost negligible in the case of conversion to DHA [12–14]. This is due to the lack of an efficient elongation and desaturation process to convert ALA to EPA by any more than 5%–7% [12]. The primary reason for this inefficiency is explained by the n-6 PUFA linoleic acid (LA) competing with ALA at the level of the Δ6-desaturase enzyme complex [12–14], which inserts additional double bonds to these precursor fatty acids. Accordingly, the conversion of ALA to stearidonic acid (SDA, C18:4n-3), facilitated by this enzyme, is considered the rate-limiting step in LC n-3 PUFA biosynthesis in vertebrates [15].

In order to address this limited bio-conversion of ALA to EPA and beyond, there has been interest in evaluating plant oils with better conversion to EPA and DHA than ALA-rich oils. In this regard, oils containing SDA have been the subject of much interest in feeding experiments involving farm animals [16,17], aquaculture fish [18], animal models [19] and humans [20–22]. SDA is relatively abundant in plants of the *Boraginaceae* family. One of the commercially available non-GM sources of SDA is extracted from *Echium plantagineum* [23]. SDA has been found to be further metabolised *in vivo* and lead to increased plasma and tissue levels of LC n-3 PUFA both in animal models [19] and in humans [24]. For example, increased EPA and DPA have been observed following supplementation of humans with Echium oil (EO) [24]. In parallel with such compositional alterations, modification of several biochemical and physiological markers for cardiovascular disease have also been observed [25]. For example, daily supplementation with 15 g EO for four weeks lowered serum triacylglycerols in hypertriglyceridemic subjects [24], whilst a longer feeding protocol (17 g/day EO for 8-weeks equating to 2 g/day SDA) in normal and overweight individuals was accompanied by reductions in serum cholesterol, LDL-cholesterol, oxidized-LDL, HDL-cholesterol and triacylglycerols [25]. In contrast, a more recent randomized controlled trial [26] of overweight and obese subjects found no change in serum triacylglycerols following EO (1.2 g/day SDA; 6-weeks). In subjects with metabolic syndrome, further to improving plasma lipid profiles, additional benefits of EO were noted by Khunt *et al.* [25] with reductions in blood pressure and plasma insulin. Interestingly, this latter study has concluded that the collective outcomes of EO on cardiovascular risk biomarkers are broader than that exerted by fish oil (1.9 g/day EPA) itself. These benefits of EO were observed in the absence of any increase in DHA in plasma and/or peripheral blood mononuclear cells.

Biochemical studies in animals, using apoB100-only LDLrKO mice, have shown that decreased lipogenic gene expression increased intravascular lipolysis and enhanced clearance of plasma very low density lipoprotein (VLDL) as potential mechanisms for the triglyceride lowering action of EO [27,28]. In addition to lipid lowering properties, anti-atherogenic actions of EO have also been reported [29]. For example, both EO and FO were equally effective in reducing plasma triglycerides, total plasma cholesterol, VLDL and LDL-cholesterols and apoB lipoproteins, as reflected in the form of reduced aortic deposition of cholesterol, and surface lesion formation leading to retardation in atherogenesis [29]. Such collective observations from both human and animal studies have led these investigators to suggest that EO may be useful as a botanical alternative to FO in reducing hypertriglyceridemia and affording athero-protection [29,30].

Most studies with EO have reported increased accumulation of EPA and DPA with no change in DHA in blood and cell lipids [25] suggesting incomplete metabolism (elongation/desaturation) of the precursor fatty acids in EO. However, compositional data following EO supplementation on major organs (heart, kidney, liver) is lacking and it is unknown whether or not further conversion/incorporation of SDA and its metabolites has taken place, for example, in tissue specific manner. Moreover, several recent studies have reported EO is able to mimic biochemical measures of cardiovascular risk reduction benefits of FO [24,25,27,28]. Nevertheless, except for an indirect or secondary observation [19] regarding blood pressure, no datum exists in relation to any direct measure(s) of a given endpoint of cardiovascular pathophysiology that may be influenced after ingesting EO. In this context, a unique characteristic of the two major LC n-3 PUFA in fish oils—EPA and DHA—is their ability to modify ischemia-induced ventricular fibrillation and sudden cardiac death [31]. The anti-arrhythmic actions of EPA and DHA first demonstrated in this laboratory over two decades ago in whole animal models have now been confirmed in large scale human clinical trials [32] which has also validated the experimental model employed. To this end, despite the presence of a sound body of evidence showing increased accumulation of LC *n*-3 PUFA following dietary EO (SDA), and claimed benefits on plasma lipids, its potential to facilitate any direct anti-arrhythmic benefit has not yet been evaluated. Therefore, this study was initiated with two main objectives: (A) to compare the impact of any dose-related outcomes of EO and FO on the LC *n*-3 PUFA contents of membrane phospholipids in major tissues, and (B) to provide comparative data on the anti-arrhythmic potential of these two sources of *n*-3 PUFA, using the well-established rat model of cardiac arrhythmia, ventricular fibrillation and sudden cardiac death [33].

2. Materials and Methods

2.1. Animals, Diet and Experimental Design

A total of 126 Sprague Dawley (SD) were obtained from the Animal Resource Centre, Western Australia, at 12 weeks of age. After arrival in the Animal House, they were fed with standard rat and mouse pellets (www.specialtyfeeds.com) containing 19.6% protein, 5% fat, 4.3% crude fibre and 14.3 megajoule/kg digestible energy for a period of two weeks (acclimatisation period). The test diets were prepared by supplementing the standard rat diet (Control,) with either Echium (EO) or fish oil (FO) at three different doses (1%, 3% and 5% *w*/*w*). Hence, the total dietary fat was 5%) for the Control, and 6%, 8% or 10% for the three supplement levels, respectively. The supplemented diets were iso-caloric at any given dose-level. At the age of 14 weeks, they were randomly assigned (n = 18 group) to their allotted treatment groups (Control, EO-1 or FO-1, EO-3 or FO-3 and EO-5 or FO-5). The initial weight (mean ± SEM) of rats for the groups were as follows: 403 ± 8.1, 425 ± 6.2, 401 ± 12.2, 420 ± 7.0, 403 ± 7.0, 473 ± 7.3, and 400 ± 8.7 g for Control, EO-1, FO-1, EO-3, FO-3, EO-5 and FO-5, respectively. The Echium oil (Crossential 5A14) was supplied by Croda Australia (Wetherill Park, New South Wales, NSW, Australia). The fish oil used was a tuna oil high in DHA supplied by Clover Corporation (Sydney, NSW, Australia). The major *n*-3 and *n*-6 PUFA composition of the oils used are shown in Table 1. Animals were caged in groups of 4 and were provided with food and water *ad libitum* with a 12-h light-dark cycle and maintained on their allocated treatment diets for a period of 12 weeks. Body weights were recorded weekly. At the completion of pre-feeding period, the rats were subjected to coronary artery ligation as detailed below. All experimental procedures, including housing and welfare were approved by the institutional Animal Ethics Committee (CSIRO Health Sciences and Nutrition) in accordance with the Australian (National Health & Medical Research Council) code for the care and use of animals for scientific purposes.

Table 1. Major *n*-3 and *n*-6 composition (% total fatty acids) of Echium oil, Fish oil and Control diet used in the study.

Fatty Acid	Echium Oil (EO)	Fish Oil (FO)	Control Diet
C16:0	7.1	22.3	10.4
C16:1	-	3.0	0.21
C18:0	3.6	6.0	2.9
C18:1*n*-9	15.5	17.9	39.6
C18:2*n*-6 (LA)	15.0	1.2	27.1
C18:3*n*-6 (GLA)	11.4	0.4	-
C18:3*n*-3 (ALA)	33.1	0.9	6.3
C18:4*n*-3 (SDA)	14.2	1.6	-
C20:0	-	0.7	-
C20:1	-	2.1	0.6
C20:2	-	3.1	-

Table 1. *Cont.*

Fatty Acid	Echium Oil (EO)	Fish Oil (FO)	Control Diet
C20:0	-	0.7	-
C20:1	-	2.1	0.6
C20:2	-	3.1	-
C20:4*n*-6 (ARA)	-	1.3	0.2
C20:5*n*-3 (EPA)	-	5.9	0.4
C22:5*n*-3 (DPA)	-	2.0	1.0
C22:6*n*-3 (DHA)	-	22.2	-

ALA, α-linolenic acid; ARA, arachidonic acid; DHA; docosahexaenoic acid; DPA, docosapentaenoic acid; EPA, eicosapentaenoic acid; GLA, γ-linolenic acid; LA, linoleic acid; SDA, stearidonic acid. Values represent the average of triplicate determinations.

2.2. *Surgical Induction of Arrhythmias*

The rodent arrhythmia model has been used extensively in this laboratory for many years [33]. In brief, rats were anaesthetised with a single intraperitoneal (i.p.) injection of sodium pentobarbitone (50 mg/kg). They were intubated using a tracheal tube to permit artificial ventilation upon the opening of the chest cavity. The right femoral artery was cannulated (polythene tubing, Boots Healthcare Pty Ltd, North Ryde, NSW 2113, Australia) for monitoring blood pressure. The chest wall was opened between the 2nd and 3rd ribs to permit the exteriorisation of the heart following the rupture of the myocardium. A loose ligature (Dynek Sutures, Hendon, SA 5014, Australia) was placed around the left descending coronary artery and the heart was returned to the chest cavity. Rats were allowed to stabilise for 5 min before the ligature was tightened creating acute myocardial ischemia. The ischemic period was maintained for a period of 30 min before release and further monitoring for 5 min. No attempts were made to terminate ventricular fibrillation. Blood pressure (DA 100C, Biopac Systems Inc., Goleta, CA, USA), and electrocardiogram (ECG100C, Biopac Systems Inc., Goleta, CA, USA) changes were monitored throughout the experimental period and recorded using a computer based data acquisition system (BioPak-MP100). Rats were killed by exsanguination and their hearts were placed in ice cold normal saline (0.9% NaCl). Zone at risk was assessed by the re-occlusion of the heart and the infusion of Evans Blue dye (0.5% in normal saline). The ventricles were removed and the stained area separated from the ischemic zone. The non-ischemic zone was used for fatty acid analysis. The ischemic zone was expressed as a percentage of the total ventricular weight. All animals included in the study had a % zone at risk of between 45% and 55%.

2.3. *Assessment of Arrhythmias*

Arrhythmias were assessed and classified into three types, ventricular ectopic beats (VEB), ventricular tachycardia (VT) and ventricular fibrillation (VF). The type and duration of each of these parameters (VEB, VT and VF) were assessed for each animal and a total of all arrhythmias occurring in the 30 min period of occlusion was made. Mortality was calculated as the number of deaths from VF within the group as a whole. A value of 124 s was allocated as the time for a fatal VF episode [33].

2.4. *Tissue Collection*

Following the completion of the coronary artery ligation, a blood sample of 10 mL was obtained from each animal at the abdominal aortic bifurcation. Blood samples were centrifuged (2000 *g*) for collection of plasma samples; the latter were stored at −80 °C until required. Heart (non-ischemic section), left kidney, and liver (frontal lobe) were removed from all treatment groups, cleared of any adhering tissue, blotted dry, and frozen in liquid nitrogen. Samples were then transferred to a −80 °C freezer and stored until required.

2.5. *Fatty Acid Composition*

Plasma and membrane phospholipids were extracted using chloroform-methanol [34]. The solvent layer was removed and dried under N_2 before reconstitution in hexane. Samples were cleaned in florisil columns and eluted with 10% diethyl ether in hexane. The dried samples were dissolved in iso-octane and injected into the gas chromatagraph (GC) (Model 6890N, Agilent Technologies Australia, Mulgrave, VIC 3170, Australia). The GC was equipped with a flame ionisation detector (FID) and a BPX70 column which was 30 m long with an internal diameter of 0.53 mm, and with a 0.5 μm film thickness (SPE Analytical Service PTY Ltd, Melrose Park, NSW 2114, Australia). The temperature program was as follows: rise from 100 °C to 180 °C at 6 °C/min, and 180 °C–230 °C at 3 °C/min. Each sample involved a split injection of 2.5 μL. The carrier gas was hydrogen (30 cm/s). Fatty acids were identified by comparing their retention time to that of their respective counterparts in a standard FAME mixture (Suppleco 37, Cat. No. 47885-U, Suppelco, Belleford, PA, USA).

2.6. Statistics

All statistics were calculated using IBM® SPSS® Statistics 20 [35]. Fatty acid data in plasma and tissue, and the parametric arrhythmia data (VEB number, (VT) duration, and (VF) duration) were analysed using the SPSS General Linear Model's Multivariate Analysis of Variance. A P-value of less than 0.05 was considered significant. For fatty acid data, oil × dose interactions were analysed in a 2 × 3 factorial omitting the Control groups. The rate of incidence of VT, VF and mortality were analysed using the Chi-Square test in SPSS. Fatty acid data were generated on a subsample of 5 animals from each group. Final number of animals per group in arrhythmia analysis ranged from 15 to 18 based on criteria for inclusion according to The Lambeth Convention [36].

3. Results

Dietary treatments had no apparent impact on growth and development. The final weights (mean ± SEM) of rats were 507 ± 12.2, 514 ± 11.5, 501 ± 14.7, 521 ± 10.1, 581 ± 9.9, 581 ± 9.6 and 506 ± 14.3 g for Control, EO-1, FO-1, EO-3, FO-3, EO-5 and FO-5, respectively. Average weight gain ranged from 2.06 to 2.56 g/day ($p > 0.05$) across oil types and doses.

3.1. Tissue Incorporations of n-3 Long-Chain Polyunsaturated Fatty Acids (LC n-3 PUFA)

Fatty acid compositions of plasma, heart, liver and kidney are presented in Tables 2–5. Plasma samples had detectable levels of ALA that showed significant positive response to increased EO supplementation. Compared to control, plasma EPA level was significantly increased by the two higher doses of EO and by all three doses of FO (Table 2). There was also significant oil–dose interaction as the three EO doses had similar values while the FO doses exhibited significant differences in plasma EPA (FO-1 < FO-3 < FO-5). Compared to the control EO-fed rats showed higher ($p < 0.05$) accumulation of DPA in plasma whilst this LC *n*-3 PUFA was absent in FO-supplemented rats. Plasma DHA was significantly affected by both oil type and dose. It was higher on FO than EO or Control groups. Plasma from FO-1 rats had a lower percentage of DHA than FO-3 and FO-5; the difference between the latter two was not significant. The change in total plasma *n*-3 PUFA as well as EPA + DHA were largely driven by plasma DHA.

The comparative changes in the fatty acids composition of heart tissues under the different dietary treatments are shown in Table 3. Across all diet groups, neither ALA nor SDA was detected in the phospholipid fatty acids of heart tissues. The level of EPA in heart tissue was significantly affected by dose, not oil type. There was no oil–dose interaction. In contrast, the level of DPA in heart tissue was significantly affected by both oil type and dose. Percentage of DPA was significantly increased by EO but not FO. EO supplementation increased DPA levels with each increased dose, while the DPA levels across FO doses remained unchanged. The reverse was true for heart DHA. Compared to control diet, both EO and FO supplementation significantly increased total *n*-3 PUFA in heart, only FO showed a significant dose response.

Liver phospholipids did not have detectable levels of ALA or SDA (Table 4). The level of EPA in liver was affected by both oil type (FO > EO) and dose (FO-1 < (FO-3 = FO-5). There was also a significant oil–dose interaction. EPA levels were similar among Control, the three doses of EO and FO-1, whereas FO-3 and FO-5 groups had greater EPA ($p < 0.05$) than the other groups. The liver

DPA concentration increased in response to EO, but not FO, supplementation. Oil type was the main determinant of liver DPA. The level of DHA in liver was significantly increased over Control by FO, but not EO, supplementation. Although there was a trend of increase in DHA with increasing dose of FO (which caused significant oil × dose interaction), the difference between FO doses was not significant. The total *n*-3 PUFA content of liver phospholipids was significantly affected by oil type and dose. Across all doses, *n*-3 PUFA levels in the liver of EO rats were similar to that of Control rats. In contrast, all FO rats had higher *n*-3 PUFA in their livers than Control or EO rats. Total *n*-3 PUFA on FO-1 was significantly lower than that observed on FO-3 and FO-5, the latter did not differ significantly. EPA + DHA values followed similar trends to that of total *n*-3 PUFA.

Kidney phospholipids did not exhibit detectable levels of ALA or SDA (Table 5). EO-3, EO-5 and all the three doses of FO had greater EPA levels than Control groups. EO-3, EO-5 and FO-1 had similar EPA levels, while FO-3 and FO-5 were the groups with the highest EPA in kidney. The level of DPA in kidney was only increased by EO, but not FO, supplementation. EO-3 and EO-5 had higher DPA than all other groups. DHA levels in kidney were similar among all EO and Control groups. In contrast, rats on the three doses of FO had significantly higher DHA in their kidney than any of the other groups. Total *n*-3 PUFA in kidney was increased by FO in a dose-related manner. Total *n*-3 PUFA in EO-1 was similar to Control groups, while EO-3 and EO-5 had higher total *n*-3 PUFA than the former.

Figure 1 presents the extent of incorporation of *n*-3 and *n*-6 PUFA (computed as total *n*-6/*n*-3 PUFA ratio) into various tissues. Except in plasma, the disparity in *n*-6/*n*-3 PUFA ratio between EO- and FO-supplemented groups increased as the oil doses increased. For example, the liver phospholipids showed virtually no change in *n*-6/*n*-3 PUFA ratio following EO whilst the FO groups showed greater incorporation of *n*-3 PUFA as the level of supplementation increased. In contrast, in the EO supplemented rats' three organs (liver, kidney and heart), the tissue uptake of *n*-3 PUFA appeared to be plateauing much earlier at the 1% supplementation level.

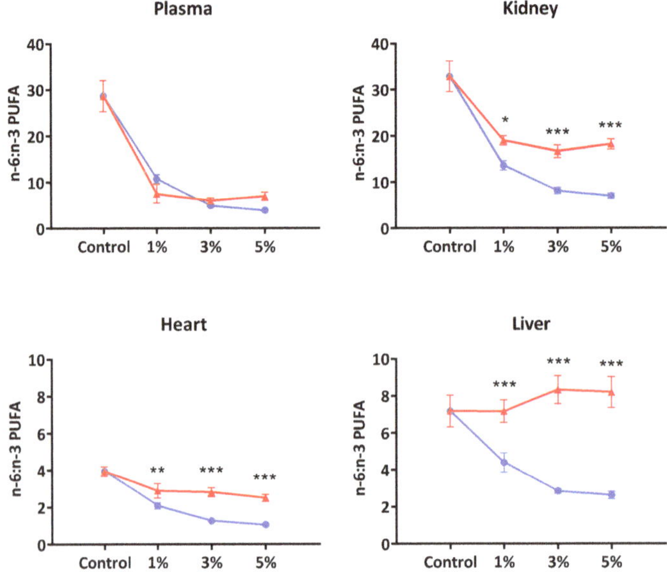

Figure 1. The ratio of total *n*-6 to total *n*-3 polyunsaturated fatty acids in tissue and plasma of rats fed standard laboratory diet (Control) or diet supplemented with Echium oil (EO, **red**) or fish oil (FO, **blue**) at 1, 3 and 5 percent (*w*/*w*). Values are mean ± SEM for *n* = 5 samples per group. Total *n*-3 PUFA = Sum (C18:3*n*-3, C18:4*n*-3, C20:5*n*-3, C22:5*n*-3 and C22:6*n*-3). Total *n*-6 PUFA = Sum (C18:2*n*-6, C20:2*n*-6, C20:3*n*-6 & C20:4*n*-6). *, **, and *** indicate significance at $p < 0.05$, $p < 0.01$ and $p < 0.001$, respectively.

Table 2. Plasma phospholipid fatty acid composition (% total fatty acids) of Sprague Dawley rats fed standard laboratory diet (Control) or diets supplemented with 1, 3 or 5% Echium oil (EO-1, EO-3 or EO-5) or Fish oil (FO-1, FO-3 or FO-5).

		Echium Oil			Fish Oil			Significant Effect		
Fatty Acids	**Control**	**EO-1**	**EO-3**	**EO-5**	**FO-1**	**FO-3**	**FO-5**	**Oil**	**Dose**	**Oil × Dose**
C16:0	19.4 ± 0.90	20.1 ± 0.91	18.77 ± 0.84	18.36 ± 0.66	19.12 ± 0.43	20.24 ± 0.38	20.37 ± 0.92	ns	ns	ns
C16:1*n*-9	1.9 ± 0.40 ^{b}	1.1 ± 0.13 ^{a}	1.2 ± 0.28 ^{a}	1.0 ± 0.18 ^{a}	1.4 ± 0.15 ^{a}	1.7 ± 0.14 ^{b}	1.90.13 ^{b}	0.003	ns	ns
C18:0	14.8 ± 0.60 ^{b}	12.5 ± 0.57 ^{a}	12.1 ± 1.04 ^{a}	13.3 ± 1.09 ^{a}	14.9 ± 0.71 ^{b}	14.6 ± 0.87 ^{b}	15.1 ± 0.72 ^{b}	0.012	ns	ns
C18:1*n*-9	17.2 ± 0.77	18.5 ± 0.29	18.0 ± 1.16	17.6 ± 0.56	18.6 ± 0.44	18.6 ± 0.57	16.9 ± 0.56	ns	ns	ns
C18:1*n*-7	5.6 ± 0.37 ^{b}	4.2 ± 0.71 ^{a}	3.2 ± 0.43 ^{a}	3.3 ± 0.18 ^{a}	5.3 ± 0.24 ^{a,b}	5.1 ± 0.39 ^{b}	4.7 ± 0.27 ^{a,b}	<0.001	ns	ns
C18:2*n*-6 (LA)	20.4 ± 0.71 ^{a,b}	21.0 ± 0.14 ^{a,b}	20.0 ± 0.62 ^{a,b}	19.2 ± 1.09 ^{a}	21.7 ± 0.54 ^{b}	19.5 ± 0.48 ^{a,b}	18.3 ± 0.42 ^{a}	ns	0.018	ns
C18:3*n*-3 (ALA)	0.0 ± 0.00 ^{a}	1.3 ± 0.29 ^{b}	2.6 ± 0.57 ^{b,c}	3.1 ± 0.41 ^{c}	0.0 ± 0.00 ^{a}	0.0 ± 0.00 ^{a}	0.0 ± 0.00 ^{a}	<0.001	ns	ns
C18:4*n*-3 (SDA)	nd	nd	nd	nd	nd	nd	nd			
C20:0	2.5 ± 0.36	1.9 ± 0.82	2.1 ± 0.64	2.7 ± 0.57	1.9 ± 0.33	2.0 ± 0.40	2.5 ± 0.38	ns	ns	ns
C20:2*n*-6	nd	nd	nd	nd	nd	nd	nd			
C20:3*n*-6	0.7 ± 0.06	0.7 ± 0.02	1.0 ± 0.07	0.9 ± 0.10	0.7 ± 0.08	0.8 ± 0.09	0.6 ± 0.07	ns	ns	ns
C20:4*n*-6 (ARA)	16.2 ± 1.66 ^{a,b}	16.0 ± 2.16 ^{a,b}	17.6 ± 2.66 ^{a,b}	17.3 ± 1.12 ^{b}	13.1 ± 0.84 ^{a,b}	11.1 ± 0.39 ^{a}	11.8 ± 1.20 ^{a,b}	0.027	ns	ns
C20:5*n*-3 (EPA)	0.2 ± 0.13 ^{a}	0.7 ± 0.06 ^{a,b}	1.3 ± 0.06 ^{b}	1.3 ± 0.07 ^{b}	0.8 ± 0.03 ^{b}	2.0 ± 0.23 ^{c}	2.7 ± 0.08 ^{d}	<0.001	<0.001	<0.001
C24:0	nd	nd	nd	nd	nd	nd	nd			
C22:5*n*-3 (DPA)	0.0 ± 0.00 ^{a}	0.5 ± 0.13 ^{b}	0.9 ± 0.13 ^{b}	0.8 ± 0.12 ^{b}	0.0 ± 0.00 ^{a}	0.0 ± 0.00 ^{a}	0.0 ± 0.00 ^{a}	<0.001	ns	ns
C22:6*n*-3 (DHA)	1.1 ± 0.09 ^{a}	1.4 ± 0.28 ^{a,b}	1.4 ± 0.11 ^{a}	1.1 ± 0.15 ^{a}	2.6 ± 0.28 ^{b}	4.5 ± 0.26 ^{c}	5.2 ± 0.53 ^{c}	<0.001	0.001	<0.001
Total *n*-3 PUFA	1.3 ± 0.10 ^{a}	2.7 ± 0.60 ^{a,b}	3.6 ± 0.22 ^{b}	3.2 ± 0.30 ^{b}	3.4 ± 0.29 ^{b}	6.5 ± 0.48 ^{c}	7.9 ± 0.52 ^{c}	<0.001	<0.001	<0.001
Total *n*-6 PUFA	37.3 ± 2.02 ^{c}	18.0 ± 1.92 ^{a}	21.2 ± 2.20 ^{a}	21.2 ± 0.95 ^{a}	35.4 ± 0.52 ^{b}	31.4 ± 1.50 ^{b}	30.7 ± 1.36 ^{b}	<0.001	ns	0.012
EPA + DHA	1.3 ± 0.10 ^{a}	2.1 ± 0.33 ^{a,b}	2.7 ± 0.09 ^{b}	2.4 ± 0.21 ^{b}	3.4 ± 0.29 ^{b}	6.5 ± 0.48 ^{c}	7.9 ± 0.52 ^{d}	<0.001	<0.001	<0.001
Total SFA	36.7 ± 0.64 ^{b}	34.6 ± 1.22 ^{a,b}	32.9 ± 1.25 ^{a}	34.4 ± 1.38 ^{a,b}	35.9 ± 0.60 ^{b}	36.9 ± 1.23 ^{b}	37.9 ± 1.98 ^{b}	0.014	ns	ns
Total MUFA	24.7 ± 1.48 ^{b}	23.8 ± 1.00 ^{a}	22.4 ± 1.62 ^{a}	22.0 ± 0.78 ^{a}	25.2 ± 0.71 ^{b}	25.3 ± 0.80 ^{b}	23.5 ± 0.27 ^{a,b}	0.027	ns	ns
Total PUFA	38.7 ± 2.00 ^{a,b}	41.6 ± 2.21 ^{a,b}	44.7 ± 1.91 ^{b}	43.7 ± 1.25 ^{a,b}	38.8 ± 0.58 ^{a,b}	37.9 ± 0.97 ^{a}	38.6 ± 1.86 ^{a,b}	0.001	ns	ns

ARA, arachidonic acid; ALA, alpha-linolenic acid; DHA, docosahexaenoic acid; DPA, docosapentaenoic acid; EPA, eicosapentaenoic acid; LA, linoleic acid; MUFA, monounsaturated fatty acids; nd, not detected; ns, not significant ($p > 0.05$); PUFA, polyunsaturated fatty acids; SDA, stearidonic acid; SFA, saturated fatty acids. Values are mean ± SEM of $n = 5$ samples per group. Means with different superscripts are significantly different ($p < 0.05$). Total *n*-3 PUFA = Sum (C18:3*n*-3, C18:4*n*-3, C20:5*n*-3, C22:5*n*-3 and C22:6*n*-3); Total *n*-6 PUFA = Sum (C18:2*n*-6, C20:2*n*-6, C20:3*n*-6 & C20:4*n*-6); Total MUFA = Sum (C16:1*n*-9, C18:1*n*-9 & C18:1*n*-7); Total PUFA = Sum (Total *n*-3 PUFA and Total *n*-6 PUFA); Total SFA = Sum (C16:0, C18:0, C20:0 and C24:0).

Table 3. Heart phospholipid fatty acid composition in rats fed diets supplemented with Echium oil or Fish oil.

		Echium Oil			Fish Oil			Significant Effect		
Fatty Acids	Control	EO-1	EO-3	EO-5	FO-1	FO-3	FO-5	Oil	Dose	Oil × Dose
C16:0	13.9 ± 0.18^{b}	$13.4 \pm 0.56^{a,b}$	$13.2 \pm 0.31^{a,b}$	12.3 ± 0.37^{a}	15.7 ± 0.57^{c}	15.5 ± 0.46^{c}	15.2 ± 0.47^{c}	<.0001	ns	ns
C16:1*n*-9	0.3 ± 0.0^{b}	0.0 ± 0.02^{a}	0.0 ± 0.0^{a}	0.0 ± 0.00^{a}	0.3 ± 0.04^{b}	0.3 ± 0.01^{b}	0.5 ± 0.09^{b}	<0.001	ns	ns
C18:0	$23.2 \pm 0.23^{a,b}$	22.7 ± 0.44^{a}	$24.0 \pm 0.47^{b,c}$	25.6 ± 0.23^{c}	$23.1 \pm 0.26^{a,b}$	24.3 ± 0.35^{c}	24.2 ± 0.36^{c}	ns	<0.001	ns
C18:1*n*-9	6.2 ± 0.14^{b}	5.2 ± 0.36^{a}	4.9 ± 0.11^{a}	4.8 ± 0.39^{a}	5.7 ± 0.16^{b}	4.7 ± 0.20^{a}	4.5 ± 0.13^{a}	ns	0.008	ns
C18:1*n*-7	5.6 ± 0.16^{c}	4.8 ± 0.22^{b}	4.4 ± 0.35^{b}	$3.7 \pm 0.29^{a,b}$	5.4 ± 0.16^{c}	4.4 ± 0.19^{b}	2.9 ± 0.54^{a}	ns	<0.001	ns
C18:2*n*-6 (LA)	21.4 ± 0.45^{d}	19.8 ± 1.05^{cd}	18.9 ± 0.48^{c}	15.7 ± 0.46^{b}	18.0 ± 0.91^{c}	$14.4 \pm 0.64^{a,b}$	13.2 ± 0.40^{a}	<0.001	<0.001	ns
C18:3*n*-3 (ALA)	nd	nd	nd	nd	nd	nd	nd			
C18:4*n*-3 (SDA)	nd	nd	nd	nd	nd	nd	nd			
C20:2*n*-6	0.2 ± 0.02^{b}	0.0 ± 0.00^{a}	0.0 ± 0.00^{a}	0.0 ± 0.00^{a}	0.2 ± 0.01^{b}	0.1 ± 0.04^{b}	0.1 ± 0.01^{b}	<0.001	ns	ns
C20:3*n*-6	0.3 ± 0.02^{a}	0.3 ± 0.03^{a}	0.5 ± 0.04^{b}	0.7 ± 0.04^{c}	0.3 ± 0.02^{a}	0.3 ± 0.03^{a}	0.3 ± 0.02^{a}	<0.001	<0.001	<0.001
C20:4*n*-6 (ARA)	18.1 ± 0.31^{c}	19.0 ± 0.53^{c}	19.5 ± 0.41^{c}	21.2 ± 0.23^{d}	14.9 ± 0.19^{b}	13.4 ± 0.38^{a}	13.4 ± 0.19^{a}	<0.001	ns	<0.001
C20:5*n*-3 (EPA)	$0.1 \pm 0.03^{a,b}$	0.0 ± 0.00^{a}	$0.2 \pm 0.01^{a,b}$	0.2 ± 0.06^{b}	$0.2 \pm 0.02^{a,b}$	0.6 ± 0.04^{c}	0.5 ± 0.02^{c}	ns	0.003	ns
C24:0	0.6 ± 0.02^{b}	0.7 ± 0.03^{b}	$0.4 \pm 0.02^{a,b}$	0.6 ± 0.16^{b}	0.4 ± 0.04^{a}	0.3 ± 0.04^{a}	0.2 ± 0.03^{a}	<0.001	ns	ns
C22:5*n*-3 (DPA)	1.6 ± 0.01^{b}	3.0 ± 0.15^{c}	4.1 ± 0.35^{d}	5.1 ± 0.15^{e}	$1.1 \pm 0.07^{a,b}$	$1.1 \pm 0.04^{a,b}$	0.9 ± 0.02^{a}	<0.001	<0.001	<0.001
C22:6*n*-3 (DHA)	8.6 ± 0.43^{a}	11.2 ± 1.22^{a}	9.8 ± 0.55^{a}	10.0 ± 0.78^{a}	14.9 ± 0.74^{b}	20.8 ± 0.67^{c}	24.1 ± 0.85^{d}	<0.001	<0.001	<0.001
Total *n*-3 PUFA	10.2 ± 0.51^{a}	14.2 ± 1.33^{b}	14.0 ± 0.68^{b}	15.3 ± 0.96^{b}	16.2 ± 0.77^{b}	22.4 ± 0.70^{c}	25.6 ± 0.86^{c}	<0.001	<0.001	0.001
Total *n*-6 PUFA	39.8 ± 0.58^{c}	39.2 ± 1.07^{c}	39.0 ± 0.77^{c}	37.7 ± 0.39^{c}	33.2 ± 0.89^{b}	28.1 ± 0.61^{a}	26.8 ± 0.58^{a}	<0.001	<0.001	0.009
EPA + DHA	8.7 ± 0.45^{a}	11.2 ± 1.22^{b}	$10.0 \pm 0.53^{a,b}$	$10.2 \pm 0.82^{a,b}$	15.1 ± 0.75^{c}	21.2 ± 0.69^{d}	24.6 ± 0.86^{e}	<0.001	<0.001	<0.001
Total SFA	$37.7 \pm 0.37^{a,b}$	36.7 ± 0.28^{a}	$37.7 \pm 0.21^{a,b}$	$38.5 \pm 0.49^{b,c}$	39.2 ± 0.61^{c}	40.1 ± 0.41^{c}	39.7 ± 0.42^{c}	<0.001	0.024	ns
Total MUFA	12.1 ± 0.26^{c}	9.9 ± 0.52^{b}	9.3 ± 0.45^{b}	$8.5 \pm 0.67^{a,b}$	11.4 ± 0.25^{c}	9.4 ± 0.35^{b}	7.3 ± 0.64^{a}	ns	0.001	ns
Total PUFA	50.2 ± 0.51^{a}	53.4 ± 0.35^{b}	53.0 ± 0.33^{b}	53.0 ± 1.16^{b}	49.5 ± 0.48^{a}	50.6 ± 0.74^{a}	52.5 ± 0.42^{b}	0.001	ns	ns

ARA, arachidonic acid; ALA, alpha-linolenic acid; DHA, docosahexaenoic acid; DPA, docosapentaenoic acid; EPA, eicosapentaenoic acid; LA, linoleic acid; MUFA, monounsaturated fatty acids; nd, not detected; ns, not significant ($p > 0.05$); PUFA, polyunsaturated fatty acids; SDA, stearidonic acid; SFA, saturated fatty acids. Values are mean ± SEM of $n = 5$ samples per group. Means with different superscripts are significantly different ($p < 0.05$). Total *n*-3 PUFA = Sum (C18:3*n*-3, C18:4*n*-3, C20:5*n*-3, C22:5*n*-3 and C22:6*n*-3); Total *n*-6 PUFA = Sum (C18:2*n*-6, C20:2*n*-6, C20:3*n*-6 & C20:4*n*-6); Total MUFA = Sum (C16:1*n*-9, C18:1*n*-9 & C18:1*n*-7); Total PUFA = Sum (Total *n*-3 PUFA and Total *n*-6 PUFA); Total SFA = Sum (C16:0, C18:0, C20:0 and C24:0).

Table 4. Liver phospholipid fatty acid composition in rats fed diets supplemented with Echium oil or Fish oil.

		Echium Oil			Fish Oil			Significant Effect		
Fatty Acids	**Control**	**EO-1**	**EO-3**	**EO-5**	**FO-1**	**FO-3**	**FO-5**	**Oil**	**Dose**	**Oil × Dose**
C16:0	17.5 ± 0.71	18.5 ± 0.73	18.6 ± 0.61	18.5 ± 0.84	18.1 ± 0.20	19.0 ± 0.69	19.0 ± 0.55	ns	ns	ns
C16:1*n*-9	0.9 ± 0.14^{b}	0.5 ± 0.09^{a}	0.4 ± 0.06^{a}	0.4 ± 0.06^{a}	0.7 ± 0.09^{b}	$0.6 \pm 0.04^{a,b}$	$0.7 \pm 0.03^{a,b}$	<0.001	ns	ns
C18:0	20.9 ± 1.42^{a}	$22.3 \pm 0.40^{a,b}$	23.4 ± 0.99^{b}	$22.4 \pm 0.42^{a,b}$	20.6 ± 0.75^{a}	21.0 ± 0.69^{a}	20.5 ± 0.42^{a}	0.001	ns	ns
C18:1*n*-9	$4.7 \pm 0.27^{a,b}$	4.4 ± 0.14^{a}	$4.7 \pm 0.14^{a,b}$	$4.5 \pm 0.30^{a,b}$	$5.0 \pm 0.38^{a,b}$	$5.3 \pm 0.26^{a,b}$	5.4 ± 0.22^{b}	0.002	ns	ns
C18:1*n*-7	5.2 ± 0.32^{c}	4.2 ± 0.11^{b}	$3.9 \pm 0.23^{a,b}$	$3.7 \pm 0.13^{a,b}$	$4.1 \pm 0.11^{a,b}$	$3.7 \pm 0.17^{a,b}$	3.4 ± 0.11^{a}	ns	0.002	ns
C18:2*n*-6 (LA)	15.0 ± 0.91^{b}	$14.5 \pm 0.32^{a,b}$	$13.2 \pm 0.44^{a,b}$	11.9 ± 0.51^{a}	16.6 ± 0.95^{b}	16.1 ± 0.75^{b}	16.2 ± 0.68^{b}	<0.001	ns	ns
C18:3*n*-3 (ALA)	nd	nd	nd	nd	nd	nd	nd	nd		
C18:4*n*-3 (SDA)	nd	nd	nd	nd	nd	nd	nd	nd		
C20:2*n*-6	$0.6 \pm 0.06^{b,c}$	0.7 ± 0.04^{c}	0.7 ± 0.02^{c}	$0.6 \pm 0.04^{b,c}$	$0.5 \pm 0.05^{a,b}$	$0.4 \pm 0.04^{a,b}$	0.4 ± 0.02^{a}	<0.001	0.006	ns
C20:3*n*-6	1.7 ± 0.15^{a}	1.4 ± 0.09^{a}	$1.9 \pm 0.08^{a,b}$	2.3 ± 0.16^{b}	1.8 ± 0.09^{a}	1.8 ± 0.06^{a}	1.6 ± 0.08^{a}	0.033	0.009	<0.001
C20:4*n*-6 (ARA)	26.9 ± 0.47^{c}	26.9 ± 1.19^{c}	27.7 ± 0.56^{d}	30.0 ± 0.81^{d}	22.6 ± 0.45^{b}	18.9 ± 0.28^{a}	18.5 ± 0.34^{a}	<0.001	ns	<0.001
C20:5*n*-3 (EPA)	0.6 ± 0.08^{a}	0.8 ± 0.16^{a}	1.1 ± 0.10^{a}	1.0 ± 0.14^{a}	1.3 ± 0.13^{a}	2.5 ± 0.36^{b}	2.8 ± 0.35^{b}	<0.001	0.002	0.028
C24:0	0.4 ± 0.02^{c}	$0.5 \pm 0.01^{b,c}$	0.4 ± 0.01^{b}	$0.3 \pm 0.09^{a,b}$	$0.4 \pm 0.03^{a,b}$	$0.3 \pm 0.02^{a,b}$	0.2 ± 0.06^{a}	0.021	0.004	ns
C22:5*n*-3 (DPA)	0.7 ± 0.04^{a}	$1.2 \pm 0.07^{b,c}$	$1.2 \pm 0.12^{b,c}$	1.4 ± 0.10^{c}	0.68 ± 0.05^{a}	$1.0 \pm 0.06^{a,b}$	0.8 ± 0.07^{a}	<0.001	ns	ns
C22:6*n*-3 (DHA)	5.0 ± 0.46^{a}	4.1 ± 0.23^{a}	3.0 ± 0.22^{a}	3.1 ± 0.29^{a}	7.8 ± 0.91^{b}	9.5 ± 0.21^{b}	10.6 ± 0.90^{b}	<0.001	ns	0.011
Total *n*-3 PUFA	6.3 ± 0.57^{a}	6.1 ± 0.30^{a}	5.3 ± 0.41^{a}	5.5 ± 0.35^{a}	9.7 ± 0.94^{b}	13.0 ± 0.39^{c}	14.2 ± 0.79^{c}	<0.001	0.014	0.001
Total *n*-6 PUFA	43.5 ± 0.74^{c}	42.8 ± 1.28^{c}	$42.8 \pm 0.73^{b,c}$	44.3 ± 1.43^{c}	$40.9 \pm 1.24^{b,c}$	$36.7 \pm 0.91^{a,b}$	36.3 ± 0.91^{a}	<0.001	ns	0.031
EPA + DHA	6.3 ± 0.53^{a}	6.1 ± 0.25^{a}	5.3 ± 0.30^{a}	5.5 ± 0.34^{a}	9.7 ± 0.91^{b}	13.0 ± 0.34^{c}	14.2 ± 0.73^{c}	<0.001	0.014	0.001
Total SFA	38.8 ± 0.76^{a}	41.3 ± 1.12^{b}	$42.3 \pm 1.08^{a,b}$	$41.1 \pm 1.26^{a,b}$	39.0 ± 0.75^{a}	40.3 ± 1.22^{a}	39.7 ± 0.47^{a}	0.029	ns	ns
Total MUFA	10.8 ± 0.53^{b}	9.8 ± 0.17^{a}	9.0 ± 0.38^{a}	8.5 ± 0.25^{a}	$9.8 \pm 0.40^{a,b}$	$9.6 \pm 0.22^{a,b}$	$9.5 \pm 0.21^{a,b}$	0.004	ns	ns
Total PUFA	50.4 ± 0.56	49.6 ± 1.18	48.7 ± 0.92	50.4 ± 1.14	51.8 ± 0.42	50.1 ± 1.00	50.8 ± 0.30	ns	ns	ns

ARA, arachidonic acid; ALA, alpha-linolenic acid; DHA, docosahexaenoic acid; DPA, docosapentaenoic acid; EPA, eicosapentaenoic acid; LA, linoleic acid; MUFA, monounsaturated fatty acids; nd, not detected; ns, not significant ($p > 0.05$); PUFA, polyunsaturated fatty acids; SDA, stearidonic acid; SFA, saturated fatty acids. Values are mean ± SEM of $n = 5$ samples per group. Means with different superscripts are significantly different ($p < 0.05$). Total *n*-3 PUFA = Sum (C18:3*n*-3, C18:4*n*-3, C20:5*n*-3, C22:5*n*-3 and C22:6*n*-3); Total *n*-6 PUFA = Sum (C18:2*n*-6, C20:2*n*-6, C20:3*n*-6 & C20:4*n*-6); Total MUFA = Sum (C16:1*n*-9, C18:1*n*-9 & C18:1*n*-7); Total PUFA = Sum (Total *n*-3 PUFA and Total *n*-6 PUFA); Total SFA = Sum (C16:0, C18:0, C20:0 and C24:0).

Table 5. Kidney phospholipid fatty acid composition in rats fed diets supplemented with Echium oil or Fish oil.

		Echium Oil			Fish Oil			Significant Effect		
Fatty Acids	Control	EO-1	EO-3	EO-5	FO-1	FO-3	FO-5	Oil	Dose	Oil × Dose
C16:0	23.4 ± 0.17^{b}	21.2 ± 0.42^{a}	21.1 ± 0.32^{a}	20.4 ± 0.36^{a}	$22.3 \pm 0.68^{a,b}$	23.4 ± 0.22^{b}	23.8 ± 0.37^{b}	<0.001	ns	0.049
C16:1n-9	0.6 ± 0.08	0.5 ± 0.08	0.6 ± 0.09	0.4 ± 0.06	0.5 ± 0.10	0.6 ± 0.09	0.7 ± 0.03	ns	ns	ns
C18:0	$21.5 \pm 0.24^{a,b}$	22.8 ± 0.50^{b}	22.7 ± 0.34^{b}	22.8 ± 0.41^{b}	$21.3 \pm 0.34^{a,b}$	21.4 ± 0.37^{a}	21.2 ± 0.24^{a}	<0.001	ns	ns
C18:1n-9	8.3 ± 0.21	8.7 ± 0.38	8.2 ± 0.67	8.6 ± 0.29	8.5 ± 0.13	8.5 ± 0.28	8.7 ± 0.16	ns	ns	ns
C18:1n-7	3.3 ± 0.21^{b}	$3.0 \pm 0.21^{a,b}$	$2.6 \pm 0.28^{a,b}$	2.2 ± 0.23^{a}	$2.5 \pm 0.34^{a,b}$	$2.5 \pm 0.21^{a,b}$	$2.7 \pm 0.17^{a,b}$	ns	ns	ns
C18:2n-6 (LA)	11.1 ± 0.34^{b}	11.7 ± 0.26^{b}	10.2 ± 0.21^{a}	10.0 ± 0.24^{a}	14.6 ± 0.28^{d}	14.0 ± 0.21^{cd}	$13.4 \pm 0.45^{b,c}$	<0.001	<0.001	ns
C18:3n-3 (ALA)	nd	nd	nd	nd	nd	nd	nd			
C18:4n-3 (SDA)	nd	nd	nd	nd	nd	nd	nd			
C20:0	nd	nd	nd	nd	nd	nd	nd			
C20:2n-6	3.0 ± 0.41^{b}	3.6 ± 0.12^{b}	3.7 ± 0.19^{b}	4.0 ± 0.15^{b}	2.0 ± 0.12^{a}	2.6 ± 0.46^{a}	2.3 ± 0.09^{a}	<0.001	ns	ns
C20:3n-6	$1.1 \pm 0.07^{a,b}$	1.2 ± 0.05^{b}	1.5 ± 0.05^{c}	1.8 ± 0.07^{d}	1.2 ± 0.12^{b}	$1.0 \pm 0.03^{a,b}$	0.9 ± 0.04^{a}	<0.001	ns	<0.001
C20:4n-6 (ARA)	24.7 ± 0.42^{b}	23.8 ± 0.95^{b}	25.6 ± 0.71^{c}	26.1 ± 0.66^{c}	22.3 ± 0.41^{b}	$19.9 \pm 0.83^{a,b}$	19.6 ± 0.40^{a}	<0.001	ns	0.003
C20:5n-3 (EPA)	0.0 ± 0.00^{a}	0.5 ± 0.04^{a}	0.6 ± 0.05^{b}	0.7 ± 0.05^{b}	1.0 ± 0.11^{b}	2.1 ± 0.26^{c}	2.5 ± 0.16^{c}	<0.001	<0.001	<0.001
C24:0	1.9 ± 0.05^{c}	$1.7 \pm 0.01^{a,b,c}$	$1.7 \pm 0.09^{a,b}$	1.6 ± 0.05^{a}	1.9 ± 0.03^{b}	1.9 ± 0.04^{b}	$1.8 \pm 0.05^{a,b,c}$	0.001	ns	ns
C22:5n-3 (DPA)	0.0 ± 0.00^{a}	0.3 ± 0.01^{b}	0.5 ± 0.03^{c}	0.4 ± 0.11^{c}	0.0 ± 0.00^{a}	0.0 ± 0.00^{a}	0.0 ± 0.00^{a}	<0.001	ns	ns
C22:6n-3 (DHA)	1.2 ± 0.12^{a}	1.2 ± 0.06^{a}	1.2 ± 0.10^{a}	1.0 ± 0.09^{a}	1.9 ± 0.13^{b}	$2.3 \pm 0.18^{b,c}$	2.5 ± 0.20^{c}	<0.001	ns	0.015
Total n-3 PUFA	1.2 ± 0.12^{a}	2.0 ± 0.10^{a}	2.3 ± 0.16^{b}	2.1 ± 0.14^{b}	2.9 ± 0.20^{b}	4.4 ± 0.34^{c}	5.0 ± 0.32^{d}	<0.001	<0.001	0.001
Total n-6 PUFA	36.8 ± 0.75^{b}	36.7 ± 0.72^{b}	37.3 ± 0.70^{b}	37.8 ± 0.42^{b}	38.1 ± 0.70^{b}	34.9 ± 0.84^{a}	33.9 ± 0.32^{a}	0.005	0.045	0.001
EPA + DHA	1.2 ± 0.12^{a}	1.7 ± 0.09^{a}	1.8 ± 0.14^{a}	1.7 ± 0.08^{a}	2.9 ± 0.20^{b}	4.4 ± 0.34^{c}	5.0 ± 0.32^{c}	<0.001	<0.001	<0.001
Total SFA	46.8 ± 0.21^{b}	$45.7 \pm 0.59^{a,b}$	$45.5 \pm 0.38^{a,b}$	44.8 ± 0.30^{a}	$45.5 \pm 0.45^{a,b}$	46.7 ± 0.62^{b}	46.8 ± 0.25^{b}	0.012	ns	ns
Total MUFA	12.2 ± 0.35	12.2 ± 0.25	11.3 ± 0.82	11.2 ± 0.45	11.5 ± 0.55	11.5 ± 0.40	12.1 ± 0.34	ns	ns	ns
Total PUFA	41.0 ± 0.46^{a}	$42.2 \pm 0.81^{a,b}$	$43.2 \pm 0.69^{a,b}$	44.0 ± 0.46^{b}	$43.0 \pm 0.76^{a,b}$	$41.8 \pm 0.66^{a,b}$	41.0 ± 0.35^{a}	0.044	ns	0.028

ARA, arachidonic acid; ALA, alpha-linolenic acid; DHA, docosahexaenoic acid; DPA, docosapentaenoic acid; EPA, eicosapentaenoic acid; LA, linoleic acid; MUFA, monounsaturated fatty acids; nd, not detected; ns, not significant ($p > 0.05$); PUFA, polyunsaturated fatty acids; SDA, stearidonic acid; SFA, saturated fatty acids. Values are mean ± SEM of $n = 5$ samples per group. Means with different superscripts are significantly different ($p < 0.05$). Total n-3 PUFA = Sum (C18:3n-3, C18:4n-3, C20:5n-3, C22:5n-3 and C22:6n-3); Total n-6 PUFA = Sum (C18:2n-6, C20:2n-6, C20:3n-6 & C20:4n-6); Total MUFA = Sum (C16:1n-9, C18:1n-9 & C18:1n-7); Total PUFA = Sum (Total n-3 PUFA and Total n-6 PUFA); Total SFA = Sum (C16:0, C18:0, C20:0 and C24:0).

3.2. *Arrhythmia Risk*

The results on various arrhythmia parameters are presented in Table 6 and Figure 2. The % incidence of VT was similar (nearly 100%) for Control, EO-1, EO-3, EO-5, FO-1 and FO-3 (Figure 2A). VT in FO-5 rats was lower than that observed under all other groups except FO-3 ($p < 0.05$). Across doses, the average % incidence under FO and EO oils were 86% and 96%, respectively ($p = 0.114$). There was a significant oil–dose interaction ($p = 0.047$) for VT incidence. There was also significant oil by dose interaction ($p = 0.031$) for VT duration. There was a gradual decline in VT duration with increasing FO supplementation. This trend was not evident across EO doses (Table 6).

There was a marked decline in % VF incidence as the dose of FO increased ($p < 0.01$; Figure 2B). Across doses, there was a significant oil type effect, with the average incidence rates under FO and EO oils being 46.3% and 71.3%, respectively ($p = 0.016$). As shown in Figure 2B, there was an oil–dose interaction ($p < 0.05$); whereas % incidence of VF remained similar across all the three doses of EO, it decreased with increasing doses of FO. The changes observed in duration of VF with increasing oil dose were markedly different between the two oils. In FO rats, duration of VF decreased with each increasing dose of FO (Table 6). The oil–dose interaction was also significant for VF duration ($p < 0.05$). FO feeding was associated with greater cardio-protection than that observed under EO feeding. Percentage of mortality in EO-3 groups was similar to that observed in FO fed rats.

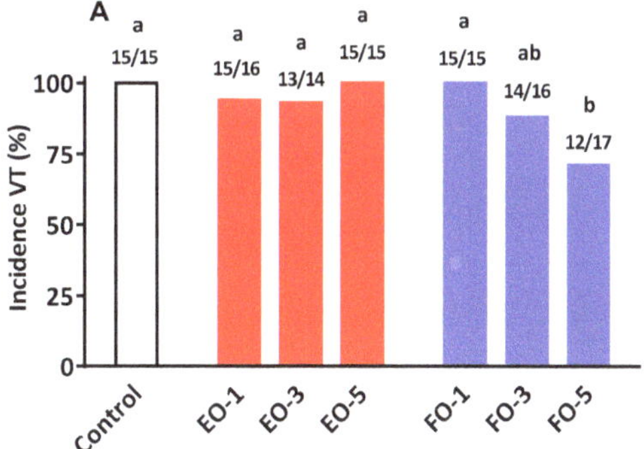

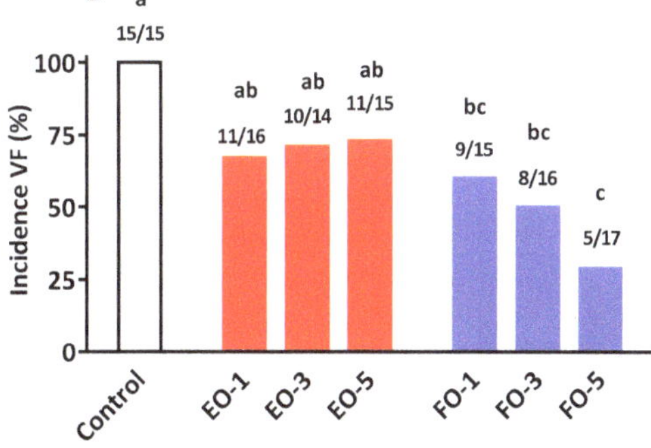

Figure 2. Percentage of incidence of (**A**) ventricular tachycardia (VT) and (**B**) ventricular fibrillation (VF) in rats fed standard laboratory diet (Control) or diet supplemented with Echium oil (EO, **red**) or Fish oil (FO, **blue**) at 1, 3 and 5 percentage (*w*/*w*). Numbers on top of the bars represent the incidence of VT or VF that occurred over the total number of animals measured. [a, b, c] Bars with different letters are significantly different ($p < 0.05$).

Table 6. The effects of oil type and dose on parameters of cardiac arrhythmia in Sprague Dawley rats fed diets supplemented with Echium oil (EO) or fish oil (FO) following coronary artery ligation.

	Dietary Groups						
	Control	EO-1	EO-3	EO-5	FO-1	FO-3	FO-5
VEB (Total, n)	821 ± 161	596 ± 197	679 ± 156	556 ± 191	723 ± 210	490 ± 137	365 ± 114
VT duration (s)	45.1 ± 10^{b}	30.4 ± 12.9^{b}	37.5 ± 12.6^{b}	33.2 ± 13.7^{b}	35.6 ± 13.2^{b}	29.0 ± 12.0^{b}	18.2 ± 9.0^{a}
VF duration (s)	94.4 ± 15.5^{c}	69.8 ± 18.7^{b}	24.2 ± 12.1^{a}	75.8 ± 17.1^{b}	51.5 ± 20.2^{b}	$33.9 \pm 12.3^{a,b}$	22.7 ± 12.0^{a}
Total mortality (%)	69 (9/15)	37.5 (6/16)	14.3 (2/14)	40 (6/15)	20 (3/15)	12.5 (2/16)	17.6 (3/17)

Values are mean ± SEM. Treatment diet groupings are similar to that described in Table 2. Sample size: number per group was 18 animals. Ischemic period maintained for 30 min. Numbers in parenthesis show actual numbers representing the % death. VEB, VT and VF defined as ventricular ectopic beats, ventricular tachycardia and ventricular fibrillation, respectively. Within row, means with different superscripts are significantly different ($p < 0.05$).

4. Discussion

The present study addressed two key questions relating to tissue fatty acid composition and cardiac arrhythmia outcomes following dietary supplementation with oils rich in *n*-3 PUFA of different origin. EO contained *n*-3 PUFA of C = 18 length (29% ALA and 14% of SDA) compared to FO which had a total LC *n*-3 PUFA, C $\geqslant$ 20 (EPA + DHA) of >30%. Both oil types resulted in marked differences in the composition of membrane phospholipids of various tissues. The previously reported [37] anti-arrhythmic actions of FO were reconfirmed in the present study. Whilst EO also led to an increased accumulation of LC *n*-3 PUFA, mainly via EPA and DPA, the extent of protection against ischemia-induced cardiac arrhythmia and sudden cardiac death was less than that observed at comparable levels of FO supplementation.

The fatty acid data from this study suggested that ALA and SDA were virtually converted to longer chain *n*-3 PUFA in heart and liver phospholipids, with no trace of 18C *n*-3 PUFA left. Previous studies have also shown very efficient conversion of both ALA and SDA to EPA and DPA in the rat liver [19]. Overall, the pattern of changes in EPA, DPA and DHA in plasma and tissue were consistent with reports from previous rat [19] and human studies [20]. The first salient feature of this study was that SDA supplementation did not yield nutritionally/physiologically meaningful DHA levels in plasma or tissue. In almost all published data, the magnitude of changes in tissue or plasma DHA as a consequence of supplementation with oils containing 18C *n*-3 PUFA were usually negligible [12]. On the contrary, SDA feeding has consistently shown significantly increased levels of EPA and DPA in plasma and tissues [19]. Our data provides further evidence that in rats there is efficient conversion of SDA up to DPA, but not DHA. In this regard, these findings also mimic the observations in humans with SDA-rich oils [20–22]. For example, James *et al.* [20] who compared the conversion of ALA, SDA to $\geqslant$20C *n*-3 PUFA (EPA, DPA and DHA) reported that dietary SDA led to an increase in EPA and DPA concentrations but not DHA levels in plasma and/or erythrocytes in a double blind, parallel group design study of six weeks' duration. The efficiency of increasing tissue EPA was 1.0, 0.3 and 0.07 for EPA, SDA and ALA, respectively. Similarly, Krul *et al.* [38] showed that the efficiency of apparent conversion of SDA to EPA in human RBC was 41%, 26% and 17% of dietary SDA for doses of 0.61, 1.89 and 5.32 g/day.

Studies using 18C *n*-3 oils have shown that the efficiency of conversion of 18C *n*-3 PUFA to $\geqslant$20C *n*-3 PUFA declines as the dose (en%) of the dietary 18C *n*-3 PUFA is increased. Gibson *et al.* [39] compared 54 different diet combinations, including various ratios of *n*-6 polyunsaturated linoleic acid (LA) to ALA (*n*-3 PUFA) to determine DHA synthesis from ALA in rats. They showed plasma phospholipid EPA, DPA and DHA increased rapidly within a narrow range—between 0 and 2 en% of dietary ALA, but suppressed to basal levels (2% total fatty acids) when the en% derived from total PUFA (LA + ALA) reached 3 en% and above.

Taken collectively, the fatty acid changes in plasma and tissues following SDA feeding had two main outcomes: increases in EPA and DPA and no change in the basal levels of DHA. These findings mirror what other studies have shown to be the case for plant-based C18 omega-3 oils in humans and different animal species (see review by Brenna *et al.* [12]). Furthermore, the present study has clearly shown that the patterns of changes in LC *n*-3 PUFA in plasma and tissues are markedly different between EO and FO. In FO-supplemented rats, EPA and DHA generally increased with greater availability of LC *n*-3 PUFA. For most parts the increased LC PUFA in plasma and tissue following supplementation with FO can be explained by way of direct incorporation of dietary EPA and DHA with some elongation and desaturation of EPA taking place. In contrast, any increase in LC *n*-3 PUFA following dietary EO would be due to further metabolism of the two C18 *n*-3 precursor fatty acids ALA and SDA since pre-formed C20 fatty acids were absent in the diet. In EO-supplemented rats, only cardiac muscle phospholipids showed a dose-related increase in DPA. In all other cases, the changes in tissue and plasma EPA and DPA beyond the first dose (EO-1) were minimal, suggesting that the linear response phase may be between 0% and 1% dietary Echium oil.

Although the tissue levels of EPA and DHA in the FO fed rats tended to show a dose-related uptake, there exist clear tissue specific differences with regard to the extent of incorporation and further metabolism of these two fatty acids. For example, compared to DHA, the EPA content of cardiac muscle showed only a minor increase amounting to <0.5% of total phospholipid fatty acids even at the 5% oil supplementation level. This differed markedly with DHA where a clear dose-related accumulation was observed (Table 3), and accounted for nearly 24% of cardiac membrane fatty acids at the highest dose tested (5% *w*/*w*). It is also evident that this increase in *n*-3 PUFAs has occurred primarily at the expense of the two major *n*-6 PUFA; LA (18:2*n*-6) and AA (20:4*n*-6). Compared to the control group, the displacement of LA by *n*-3PUFA amounted to 16%, 33% and 35% at the three dose levels of FO, respectively. AA displacement amounted to 25% at the 5% supplementation level. In contrast, the LA levels in the plasma, liver and kidney had all remained unaffected despite an increased presence of dietary *n*-3 PUFA. Similarly, the AA content of liver and kidney tended to show more resistance to be displaced by greater availability of dietary *n*-3 PUFA. Taken collectively, these observations would lend further support to the role membrane phospholipids play in maintaining the physiological functioning of specific tissues and organs. As previous publications [40–44] showed the type and amount of fatty acids in cell membranes not only influence the physical properties of the membrane bilayer (e.g., fluidity, lipid micro domains/rafts), but also modulate important biochemical functions—ion channels, transporters and enzymes. In addition, membrane and intracellular fatty acids provide substrates for the synthesis of numerous biochemical mediators including eicosanoid family of autacoids.

It is noted that in the three organs studied—liver, kidney and heart—the extent of perturbation of fatty acid composition by EO was much less, and reached saturation at the 1% level, compared to the changes observed following feeding FO rich in EPA and DHA that appeared to be dose-related (Figure 1). However, the possibility exists for the relatively high presence of *n*-6 PUFA (26%) as well as ALA (33%) in the EO to interfere with further metabolism of SDA which was present at a much lower level (14%). It is more likely that any substrate competition would be due to LA rather than ALA since the genetically modified SDA-soybean preparation which contained lower ALA than SDA levels [21] also led to similar compositional changes as observed in the present study. The LA content in SDA-soybean was 31% compared to 16.6% SDA.

The anti-arrhythmic actions of *n*-3 PUFA has been attributed to favourable changes to the heart membrane structure, favourable modulation of ion channels (e.g., Ca^{2+}) in cardiac tissue, and improved myocardial oxygen efficiency [31]. The present results conclude that while there is some anti-arrhythmic action arising from EO consumption, the efficacy is not equivalent to that achieved with FO supplementation. For example, increasing the level of dietary EO neither arrested the development of VT nor its deterioration into the more serious condition of VF (Figure 2). This differed markedly with that observed following the provision of FO, where the progression of VT to VF was reduced in a dose-related manner. At the highest supplementation level (5% *w*/*w*) FO not only reduced the incidence of VF (29% *vs.* 73% in EO group) but such episodes once occurred lasted a much shorter period of time compared to EO and/or the control group (Table 6). It is of interest to note that at the 3% supplementation level of EO displayed certain cardioprotective qualities (VF duration and % mortality) comparable to those found with FO. The reason(s) for this apparent protective actions of EO, only at this particular dose level, is difficult to explain since such benefits were not repeated at the higher supplementation level of 5%. Tissue fatty acid compositional data showed no clear differences between 3% and 5% oil incorporation levels. Furthermore, it is highly unlikely that a concentration–effect relationship for cardioprotection follows a bell-shape curve within the narrow band of EO feeding used in this study. Collectively, our findings in relation to cardio-protection and tissue fatty acid compositional alterations mirror previous studies where direct comparisons between SDA and EPA have been made with respect to several other biomarkers of cardiovascular health [20,21,25].

The data from this study and those published by others indicate that SDA containing oils lead to elevated plasma and tissue LC *n*-3 PUFA. However, the magnitude of changes reported from this study and that from the literature does not provide evidence of equivalence in potency between SDA-containing oils and fish oils. In addition, potential anti-arrhythmic action of SDA oils needs to be investigated further using other animal models as well as using pure SDA or more enriched supplements to minimise the confounding effect of ALA that is present in commercial sources of SDA oils.

In summary, evaluation of the anti-arrhythmic actions of EO and FO in a rat arrhythmia model is a novel contribution from this study. We conclude that feeding Echium oil favourably changes the *n*-3 PUFA profiles of blood and tissues in rats, especially with respect to DPA in heart tissue. Although there are emerging evidence to suggest DPA may possess unique physiological actions including anti-platelet aggregation, pancreatic lipase inhibition and potential anti-obesity effects, its efficacy in affording direct cardio-protection has not been evaluated to date using pre-formed and more pure forms of the fatty acid. The present study provides some indirect evidence for a potential role for DPA since the changes in *n*-3 PUFA profile following EO were associated with some anti-arrhythmic action, although the extent of protection did not match that achieved by FO at all three dose levels studied. Furthermore, the increased DPA may play other beneficial roles unrelated to cardiac arrhythmia. This needs to be further investigated in animal models and substantiated in relevant human cohorts.

Acknowledgments: Fish oil was kindly donated for the study by Clover Corporation, Australia.

Conflicts of Interest: The authors declare no conflict of interest.

References

1. Mozaffarian, D. Effects of dietary fats *versus* carbohydrates on coronary heart disease: A review of the evidence. *Curr. Atheroscler. Rep.* **2005**, *7*, 435–445. [CrossRef] [PubMed]
2. Mensink, R.P.; Zock, P.L.; Kester, A.D.; Katan, M.B. Effects of dietary fatty acids and carbohydrates on the ratio of serum total to HDL cholesterol and on serum lipids and apolipoproteins: A meta-analysis of 60 controlled trials. *Am. J. Clin. Nutr.* **2003**, *77*, 1146–1155. [PubMed]
3. Farvid, M.S.; Ding, M.; Pan, A.; Sun, Q.; Chiuve, S.E.; Steffen, L.M.; Willett, W.C.; Hu, F.B. Dietary linoleic acid and risk of coronary heart disease: A systematic review and meta-analysis of prospective cohort studies. *Circulation* **2014**, *130*, 1568–1578. [CrossRef] [PubMed]
4. Lichtenstein, A.H. Dietary trans fatty acids and cardiovascular disease risk: Past and present. *Curr. Atheroscler. Rep.* **2014**, *1*, 433. [CrossRef] [PubMed]
5. Michas, G.; Micha, R.; Zampelas, A. Dietary fats and cardiovascular disease: Putting together the pieces of a complicated puzzle. *Atherosclerosis* **2014**, *234*, 320–328. [CrossRef] [PubMed]
6. Mozaffarian, D.; Wu, J.H. Omega-3 fatty acids and cardiovascular disease: Effects on risk factors, molecular pathways, and clinical events. *J. Am. Coll. Cardiol.* **2011**, *58*, 2047–2067. [CrossRef] [PubMed]
7. Flock, M.R.; Harris, W.S.; Kris-Etherton, P.M. Long-chain omega-3 fatty acids: Time to establish a dietary reference intake. *Nutr. Rev.* **2013**, *71*, 692–707. [CrossRef] [PubMed]
8. Khawaja, O.A.; Gaziano, J.M.; Djoussé, L. *N*-3 fatty acids for prevention of cardiovascular disease. *Curr. Atheroscler. Rep.* **2014**, *16*, 450. [CrossRef] [PubMed]
9. Nestel, P.; Clifton, P.; Colquhoun, D.; Noakes, M.; Mori, T.A.; Sullivan, D.; Thomas, B. Indications of omega-3 long chain polyunsaturated fatty acid in the prevention and treatment of cardiovascular disease. *Heart Lung Circ.* **2015**. [CrossRef] [PubMed]
10. Fleming, J.A.; Kris-Etherton, P.M. The evidence for α-linolenic acid and cardiovascular disease benefits: Comparisons with eicosapentaenoic acid and docosahexaenoic acid. *Adv. Nutr.* **2014**, *5*, 863S–876S. [CrossRef] [PubMed]
11. Rajaram, J. Health benefits of plant-derived α-linolenic acid. *Am. J. Clin. Nutr.* **2014**, *100*, 443S–448S. [CrossRef] [PubMed]
12. Brenna, J.T.; Salem, N., Jr.; Sinclair, A.J.; Cunnane, S.C. Alpha-linolenic acid supplementation and conversion to *n*-3 long-chain polyunsaturated fatty acids in humans. *Prostaglandins Leukot. Essent. Fat. Acids* **2009**, *80*, 85–91. [CrossRef] [PubMed]

13. Burdge, G.C.; Jones, A.E.; Wootton, S.A. Eicosapentaenoic and docosapentaenoic acids are the principal products of a-linolenic acid metabolism in young men. *Br. J. Nutr.* **2002**, *88*, 355–363. [CrossRef] [PubMed]
14. Gao, F.; Kim, H.-W.; Igarashi, M.; Kiesewetter, D.; Chang, L.; Ma, K.; Rapoport, S.I. Liver conversion of docosahexaenoic and arachidonic acids from 18-carbon precursors in rats on a DHA-free but α-LNA-containing *n*-3 PUFA adequate diet. *Biochim. Biophys. Acta* **2011**, *1811*, 484–489. [CrossRef] [PubMed]
15. Yamazaki, K.; Fujikawa, M.; Hamazaki, T.; Yano, S.; Shono, T. Comparison of the conversion rates of α-linolenic acid (18:3(*n*-3)) and stearidonic acid (18:4(*n*-3)) to longer polyunsaturated fatty acids in rats. *Biochim. Biophys. Acta* **1992**, *1123*, 18–26. [CrossRef]
16. Kitessa, S.M.; Young, P. Echium oil is better than rapeseed oil in enriching poultry meat with *n*-3 polyunsaturated fatty acids, including eicosapentaenoic acid and docosapentaenoic acid. *Br. J. Nutr.* **2009**, *101*, 709–715. [CrossRef] [PubMed]
17. Elkin, R.G.; Ying, Y.; Harvatine, K.J. Feeding laying hens stearidonic acid-enriched soybean oil, as compared to flaxseed oil, more efficiently enriches eggs with very long-chain *n*-3 polyunsaturated fatty acids. *J. Agric. Food Chem.* **2015**, *63*, 2789–2797. [CrossRef] [PubMed]
18. Miller, M.R.; Nichols, P.D.; Carter, C.G. Replacement of dietary fish oil for Atlantic salmon parr (*Salmo salar* L.) with a stearidonic acid containing oil has no effect on omega-3 long-chain polyunsaturated fatty acid concentrations. *Comp. Biochem. Physiol. B Biochem. Mol. Biol.* **2007**, *146*, 197–206. [CrossRef] [PubMed]
19. Kawabata, T.; Shimoda, K.; Horiguchi, S.; Domon, M.; Hagiwara, C.; Takiyama, M.; Kagawa, Y. Influences of stearidonic acid-enriched soybean oil on the blood and organ biochemical parameters in rats. *Prostaglandins Leukot. Essent. Fat. Acids* **2013**, *88*, 179–184. [CrossRef] [PubMed]
20. James, M.J.; Ursin, V.M.; Cleland, L.G. Metabolism of stearidonic acid in human subjects: Comparison with the metabolism of other *n*-3 fatty acids. *Am. J. Clin. Nutr.* **2003**, *77*, 1140–1145. [PubMed]
21. Harris, W.S.; Lemke, S.L.; Hansen, S.N.; Goldstein, D.A.; DeRienzo, M.A.; Su, H.; Nemeth, M.A.; Taylor, M.L.; Ahmed, G.; George, C. Stearidonic acid-enriched soybean oil increased the omega-3 index, an emerging cardiovascular risk marker. *Lipids* **2008**, *43*, 805–811. [CrossRef] [PubMed]
22. Lemke, S.L.; Maki, K.C.; Hughes, G.; Taylor, M.L.; Krul, E.S.; Goldstein, D.A.; Su, H.; Tia, M.; Rains, T.M.; Mukherjea, M. Consumption of stearidonic acid_rich oil in foods increases red blood cell eicosapentaenoic acid. *J. Acad. Nutr. Diet.* **2013**, *113*, 1044–1056. [CrossRef] [PubMed]
23. Kitessa, S.M.; Nichols, P.D.; Abeywardena, M. Purple Viper's Bugloss (*Echium plantagineum*) seed oil in human health. In *Nuts and Seeds in Health and Disease Prevention*; Preedy, V.R., Watson, R.R., Eds.; Elsevier: Amsterdam, The Netherlands, 2011; pp. 951–958.
24. Surette, M.E.; Edens, M.; Chilton, F.H.; Tramposch, K.M. Dietary echium oil increases plasma and neutrophil long-chain (*n*-3) fatty acids and lowers serum triacylglycerols in hypertriglyceridemic humans. *J. Nutr.* **2004**, *134*, 1406–1411. [PubMed]
25. Khunt, K.; Fuhrmann, C.; Kohler, M.; Kiehntopf, M.; Jahreis, G. Dietary echium oil increases long-chain *n*-3 PUFAs, including docosapentaenoic acid, in blood fractions and alters biochemical markers for cardiovascular disease independently of age, sex and metabolic syndrome. *J. Nutr.* **2014**, *144*, 447–460. [CrossRef] [PubMed]
26. Pieters, D.J.; Mensink, R.P. Effects of stearidonic acid on serum triacylglycerol concentrations in overweight and obese subjects: A randomized controlled trial. *Eur. J. Clin. Nutr.* **2015**, *69*, 121–126. [CrossRef] [PubMed]
27. Zhang, P.; Boudyguina, E.; Wilson, M.D.; Gebre, A.K.; Parks, J.S. Echium oil reduces plasma lipids and hepatic lipogenic gene expression in apoB100-only LDL receptor knockout mice. *J. Nutr. Biochem.* **2008**, *19*, 655–663. [CrossRef] [PubMed]
28. Forrest, L.M.; Lough, C.M.; Chung, S.; Boudyguina, E.Y.; Gebre, A.K.; Smith, T.L.; Colvin, P.L.; Parks, J.S. Echium oil reduces plasma triglycerides by increasing intravascular lipolysis in apoB100-only low density lipoprotein (LDL) receptor knockout mice. *Nutrients* **2013**, *5*, 2629–2645. [CrossRef] [PubMed]
29. Forrest, L.M.; Boudyguina, E.; Wilson, M.D.; Parks, J.S. Echium oil reduces atherosclerosis in apoB100-only LDLrKO mice. *Atherosclerosis* **2012**, *220*, 118–121. [CrossRef] [PubMed]
30. Shewale, S.V.; Boudyguina, E.; Zhu, X.; Shen, L.; Hutchins, P.M.; Barkley, R.M.; Murphy, R.C.; Parks, J.S. Botanical oils enriched in *n*-6 and *n*-3 FADS2 products are equally effective in preventing atherosclerosis and fatty liver. *J. Lipid Res.* **2015**, *56*, 1191–1205. [CrossRef] [PubMed]

31. McLennan, P.L. Cardiac physiology and clinical efficacy of dietary fish oil clarified through cellular mechanisms of omega-3 polyunsaturated fatty acids. *Eur. J. Physiol.* **2014**, *114*, 1333–1356. [CrossRef] [PubMed]
32. Gissi-HF Investigators; Tavazzi, L.; Maggioni, A.P.; Marchioli, R.; Barlera, S.; Franzosi, M.G.; Latini, R.; Lucci, D.; Nicolosi, G.L.; Porcu, M.; *et al.* Effect of *n*-3 polyunsaturated fatty acids in patients with chronic heart failure (the GISSI-HF trial): A randomised, double-blind, placebo-controlled trial. *Lancet* **2008**, *372*, 1223–1230. [CrossRef]
33. McLennan, P.L.; Abeywardena, M.Y.; Channock, J.S. Dietary fish oil prevents ventricular fibrillation following coronary artery occlusion and reperfusion. *Am. Heart J.* **1988**, *116*, 709–717. [CrossRef]
34. Folch, J.; Lees, M.; Stanley, G.H.S. A simple method for the isolation and purification of total lipids from animal tissues. *J. Biol. Chem.* **1957**, *226*, 497–509. [PubMed]
35. IBM Corp. *Released 2011. IBM SPSS Statistics for Windows*; Version 20; IBM Corp.: Armonk, NY, USA.
36. Walker, M.J.A.; Curtis, M.J.; Hearse, D.J.; Campbell, R.W.F.; Janse, M.J.; Yellon, D.M.; Cobbe, S.M.; Coker, S.J.; Harness, J.B.; *et al.* The Lambeth Conventions: Guidelines for the study of arrhythmias in ischaemia, infarction, and reperfusion. *Cardiovasc. Res.* **1988**, *22*, 447–455. [CrossRef] [PubMed]
37. McLennan, P.L.; Abeywardena, M.Y. Membrane basis for fish oil effects on the heart: Linking natural hibernators to prevention of human sudden cardiac death. *J. Membr. Biol.* **2005**, *206*, 85–102. [CrossRef] [PubMed]
38. Krul, E.S.; Lemke, S.L.; Mukherjea, R.; Taylor, M.L.; Goldstein, D.A.; Su, H.; Liu, P.; Lawless, A.; Harris, W.S.; Maki, K.C. Effects of duration of treatment and dosage of eicosapentaenoic acid and stearidonic acid on red blood cell eicosapentaenoic acid content. *Prostaglandins Leukot. Essent. Fat. Acids* **2012**, *86*, 51–59. [CrossRef] [PubMed]
39. Gibson, R.A.; Neumann, M.A.; Lien, E.L.; Boyd, K.A.; Tu, W.C. Docosahexaenoic acid synthesis from alpha-linolenic acid is inhibited by diets high in polyunsaturated fatty acids. *Prostaglandins Leukot. Essent. Fat. Acids* **2013**, *88*, 139–146. [CrossRef] [PubMed]
40. McMurchie, E.J.; Abeywardena, M.Y.; Charnock, J.S.; Gibson, R.A. Differential modulation of rat heart mitochondrial membrane-associated enzymes of dietary lipid. *Biochim. Biophys. Acta* **1983**, *760*, 13–24. [CrossRef]
41. Abeywardena, M.Y.; McMurchie, E.J.; Russell, G.R.; Charnock, J.S. Species variation in the ouabain sensitivity of cardiac (Na^{+}+K^{+})-ATPase: A possible role for membrane lipids. *Biochem. Pharmacol.* **1984**, *33*, 3649–3654. [CrossRef]
42. Abeywardena, M.Y.; McMurchie, E.J.; Russell, G.R.; Sawyer, W.H.; Charnock, J.S. Response of rat heart membranes and associated ion-transporting ATPases to dietary lipid. *Biochim. Biophys. Acta* **1984**, *776*, 48–59. [CrossRef]
43. Abeywardena, M.Y.; Charnock, J.S. Dietary lipid modification of myocardial eicosanoids following ischaemia and reperfusion in the rat. *Lipids* **1995**, *30*, 1151–1156. [CrossRef] [PubMed]
44. Abeywardena, M.Y.; Head, R.J. Long-chain *n*-3 polyunsaturated fatty acids and blood vessel function. *Cardiovasc. Res.* **2001**, *52*, 361–371. [CrossRef]

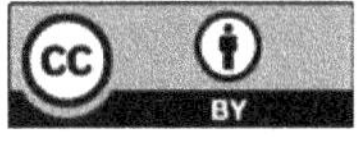

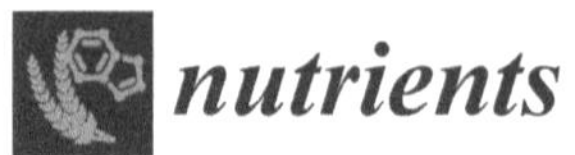

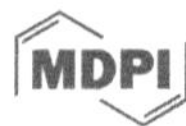

Article

Protection against Oxygen-Glucose Deprivation/Reperfusion Injury in Cortical Neurons by Combining Omega-3 Polyunsaturated Acid with *Lyciumbarbarum* Polysaccharide

Zhe Shi [1,†], Di Wu [1,†], Jian-Ping Yao [2], Xiaoli Yao [3], Zhijian Huang [1], Peng Li [1], Jian-Bo Wan [1], Chengwei He [1,*] and Huanxing Su [1,*]

1 State Key Laboratory of Quality Research in Chinese Medicine, Institute of Chinese Medical Sciences, University of Macau, Macao 999078, China; zhe.shield@gmail.com (Z.S.); dierwu@gmail.com (D.W.); hzj609@163.com (Z.H.); pengli@umac.mo (P.L.); jianbowan@umac.mo (J.-B.W.)

2 Department of Cardiac Surgery II, The First Affiliated Hospital of Sun Yat-Sen University, Guangzhou 510080, China; jianpingyao@163.com

3 Department of Neurology, National Key Clinical Department and Key Discipline of Neurology, The First Affiliated Hospital of Sun Yat-Sen University, Guangzhou 510080, China; liliyao71@163.com

* Correspondence: chengweihe@umac.mo (C.H.); huanxingsu@umac.mo (H.S.); Tel.: +853-8397-8513 (C.H.); +853-8397-8518 (H.S.); Fax: +8-532-884-1358 (C.H. & H.S.)

† These authors contributed equally to this work.

Received: 30 August 2015; Accepted: 7 December 2015; Published: 13 January 2016

Abstract: Ischemic stroke, characterized by the disturbance of the blood supply to the brain, is a severe worldwide health threat with high mortality and morbidity. However, there is no effective pharmacotherapy for ischemic injury. Currently, combined treatment is highly recommended for this devastating injury. In the present study, we investigated neuroprotective effects of the combination of omega-3 polyunsaturated fatty acids (ω-3 PUFAs) and *Lyciumbarbarum* polysaccharide (LBP) on cortical neurons using an *in vitro* ischemic model. Our study demonstrated that treatment with docosahexaenoic acid (DHA), a major component of the ω-3 PUFAs family, significantly inhibited the increase of intracellular Ca^{2+} in cultured wild type (WT) cortical neurons subjected to oxygen-glucose deprivation/reperfusion (OGD/R) injury and promoted their survival compared with the vehicle-treated control. The protective effects were further confirmed in cultured neurons with high endogenous ω-3 PUFAs that were isolated from *fat-1* mice, in that a higher survival rate was found in *fat-1* neurons compared with wild-type neurons after OGD/R injury. Our study also found that treatment with LBP (50 mg/L) activated Trk-B signaling in cortical neurons and significantly attenuated OGD/R-induced cell apoptosis compared with the control. Notably, both combining LBP treatment with ω-3 PUFAs administration to WT neurons and adding LBP to *fat-1* neurons showed enhanced effects on protecting cortical neurons against OGD/R injury via concurrently regulating the intracellular calcium overload and neurotrophic pathway. The results of the study suggest that ω-3 PUFAs and LBP are promising candidates for combined pharmacotherapy for ischemic stroke.

Keywords: Ca^{2+}; cortical neurons; DHA; LBP; OGD/R; neuroprotection; Trk-B

1. Introduction

Ischemic stroke, characterized by the disturbance of the blood supply to the brain, is a severe worldwide health threat with high mortality and morbidity [1]. However, there is no safe and effective pharmacotherapy for ischemic injury. At present, neuroprotection remains the central focus of ischemic stroke treatment after reperfusion [2]. Despite considerable research effort, the development of a suitable neuroprotective agent to treat ischemic stroke usually failed when transitioned to the clinical utilization [3]. Therefore, combined treatment is highly recommended for this devastating injury [4].

Omega-3 polyunsaturated fatty acids (ω-3 PUFAs) have been demonstrated to elicit therapeutic effects in a variety of neurological disorders including ischemic stroke [5–10]. They are essential fatty acids for human beings, which can maintain cellular membrane structural and functional integrity. Several lines of evidence have suggested that the anti-inflammation and anti-apoptosis action may account for the neuroprotective effects of ω-3 PUFAs [11–15]. It is evident that mammals cannot synthesize ω-3 PUFAs due to the lack of a fatty acid desaturase [16]. Kang *et al.* engineered a transgenic mouse carrying a *fat-1* gene from *Caenorhabditiselegans* [17], which encodes the enzyme to convert ω-6 into ω-3 PUFAs and enable the animal to maintain a steady ω-3 PUFAs level. Thus, the use of the *fat-1* transgenic mouse provides a unique chance to study the beneficial effects of endogenous ω-3 PUFAs. Moreover, abundant studies have reported that *Lyciumbarbarum* polysaccharide (LBP), a major active ingredient of *Lyciumbarbarum*, has anti-apoptotic effects in resisting ischemic cerebral injury both *in vitro* and *in vivo* [18,19]. Although the anti-apoptotic effects of LBP have been extensively demonstrated [18,20,21], no clear evidence has been provided to illustrate how LBP triggers the intracellular anti-apoptotic signal cascade. Therefore, we infer that LBP may exert its neuroprotection through a unique way different from ω-3 PUFAs. Thus, the combined therapies with ω-3 PUFAs and LBP could display a better curative effect in ischemia treatment.

Oxygen-glucose deprivation/reperfusion (OGD/R) is an *in vitro* model that mimics the *in vivo* ischemia/reperfusion injury. The reperfusion after transient deprivation of oxygen and glucose disrupts the permeability of cell membrane and eventually leads to neuronal cell death. Various interventions have been used to protect cells after OGD/R injury such as maintaining intracellular Ca^{2+} level and activating Trk receptor tyrosine kinases [22,23], since Ca^{2+} overloading is a main event which results into increased cell vulnerability and oxidative stress in the progress of apoptosis and Trk receptor tyrosine kinases, a family of transmembrane-receptor signaling systems, can subsequently trigger downstream signal pathways to induce pro-survival effects.

In the present study, we investigated the neuroprotective effects of ω-3 PUFAs, LBP and the combination of ω-3 PUFAs and LBP on rescuing cortical neurons from OGD/R and determined their distinguishing mechanisms of action through particularly activating Trk B receptor and reducing intracellular Ca^{2+} overload.

2. Materials and Method

2.1. Animals

Experimental mice were obtained by mating male *fat-1* mice (C57BL/6 background obtained from Dr. Jing X. Kang, Harvard Medical School, MA, USA) and female C57BL/6 wild type (WT) mice. Mice were fed a modified diet containing 10% corn oil (TROPHIC Animal Feed High-tech Co., Ltd, Nantong, China), with a fatty acid profile rich in ω-6 (mainly linoleic acid) and low in ω-3 PUFAs (~0.1% of the total fat supplied). Food and water were given freely until the desired age for primary neuron cultures (E16-18). All animal experiments were carried out in strict accordance with the ethical guidelines of Institute of Chinese Medical Science (ICMS), University of Macau.

2.2. Primary Cortical Neuron Cultures and Oxygen-Glucose Deprivation/Reperfusion (OGD/R)

Cortical cultures were obtained from E16.5 WT or *fat-1* embryos. The presence of the *fat-1* gene was confirmed by genotyping on each embryo. Cerebral cortices were removed, and stripped of meninges. Tissues were digested in 0.05% trypsin, and triturated. Cells were seeded in 6- or 24-well plates pre-treated with poly-L-lysine and laminin (Sigma-Aldrich, Saint Louis, MS, USA). Cultures were maintained in Neurobasal medium containing 2% B27 supplement and 0.5 mM GlutaMAX™-I (Life Technologies, Carlsbad, CA, USA). Cultures were kept at 37 °C, 100% humidity and in a 95% air/5% CO_2 atmosphere. Unless indicated, experiments were performed after 7 days *in vitro* (DIV 7).

For OGD/R, cultures were placed in a hypoxia chamber containing an atmosphere of <0.2% O_2, 5% CO_2, 95% N_2, >90% humidity, and 37 °C. Within the chamber, the medium was removed and replaced with oxygen/glucose-free balanced salt solution (BSS, in mmol/L: 116 mM NaCl, 5.4 mM KCl, 0.8 mM $MgSO_4$, 1 mM $NaH_2PO_4 \cdot 2H_2O$, 262 mM $NaHCO_3$, 1.8 mM $CaCl_2$, pH 7.2, <0.1% O_2), which was previously saturated with 95% N_2/5% CO_2 at 37 °C. Still within the chamber, cells were washed twice with oxygen/glucose-free BSS. Cultures were taken out of the chamber after 4 h and transferred to the regular cell culture incubator. Sham-treated cultures were always handled in parallel and received similar wash steps as OGD/R-treated cultures with the difference in that BSS contains 4.5 g/L glucose and regular oxygen.

2.3. *Drugs*

The preparation for LBP extracts was the same as reported previously [24]. LBP (50 mg/L) was dissolved into primary neuron culture medium immediately before use.

DHA was dissolved into 100% ethanol and stored at −20 °C in the dark as described in previous study [25]. A concentration of 10 μM was selected based on our previous finding [26]. Immediately before use, the DHA stock solution was diluted in the bath solution and adjusted to the final concentrations needed.

2.4. *Antibodies*

Rabbit anti-GFAP monoclonal antibody and mouse anti-β-tubulin III monoclonal antibody were supplied by Sigma-Aldrich (Sigma-Aldrich). Goat anti-mouse 488 and goat anti-rabbit 568 secondary antibody were obtained from Life Technologies.

Primary antibodies of goat anti-Trk-B, rabbit anti-Bcl-2 andrabbit anti-GADPH were purchased from Cell Signaling Technology (Cell Signaling Technology, Boston, MD, USA). Horseradish peroxidase secondary antibodies were from Beyotime (Beyotime, Jiangsu, China).

2.5. *Immunocytochemistry*

Cell types were characterized by immunocytochemistry. Tuj-1 was used as marker for neurons while GFAP for astrocytes. Briefly, neurons were fixed by 4% paraformaldehyde, blocked with 10% goat serum. Primary antibodies of Tuj-1 (1:500) and GFAP (1:500) diluted in blocking buffer were incubated with cells at 4 °C overnight. After PBS washing, appropriate secondary antibodies were added at room temperature in the dark, followed with DAPI counterstaining. Immunostaining was analyzed using a fluorescence microscope (Leica DM6000 B) interfaced with a digital camera and an image analysis system.

2.6. *Genomic DNA Extractions and PCR Amplification*

The *fat-1* phenotypes of each animal were characterized using isolated genomic DNA. Genomic DNA was prepared from collections of embryo brain tissues using DNA Isolation Kits. The DNA was used running polymerase chain reactions (PCR) using oligonucleotide primers that are specific for the transgene. Primer pair sets for the fat-1 gene were constructed from Invitrogen (Genewiz, Beijing, China) as follows: *Fat-1* forward: 5′-TGTTCATGCCTTCTTCTTTTTCC-3′; reverse: 5′-GCGACCATACCTCAAACTTGGA-3′. PCR was carried out using rTaq with the following conditions: 95 °C 60 s (1 cycle); 95 °C 20 s, 58 °C 30 s, 72 °C 40 s (34 cycles). Amplified fragments were separated by 1.5% agarose gel electrophoresis.

2.7. *Fatty Acid Analysis*

To examine whether the expression of the *fat-1* gene altered the PUFA composition in the primary cultured cortical neurons of the *fat-1* and WT groups, fatty acid analysis were processed by using gas chromatography-mass spectrometry (GC-MS), as described previously [27]. Briefly, cell samples were ground to powder under liquid nitrogen and subjected to fatty acid methylation by 14% boron trifluoride-methanol reagent at 100 °C for 1 h. Fatty acid methyl esters were analyzed by an Agilent GC-MS system (Agilent Technologies, Palo Alto, CA, USA) consisting of an Agilent 6890 gas chromatography and an Agilent 5973 mass spectrometer. Fatty acids were identified in forms of their methyl esters by three means: (i) searching potential compounds from NIST MS Search 2.0 database; (ii) comparing retention time with those of reference compounds (Nu-Chek Prep, Elysian, MN, USA) eluted under the identical chromatographic condition; and (iii) comparing their mass spectra plots with those of authentic standards. Quantification was performed by normalizing individual peak area as the percentage of total fatty acids.

2.8. Cell Viability Assay

Cell viability was assessed using a Cell Counting Kit-8 (CCK-8) dye (Dojindo Laboratories, Japan) according to the manufacturer's instructions. Briefly, after 10 μL of CCK-8 solution was add to each well, cells were incubated at 37 °C for 30 min and the absorbance was finally determined at 450 nm using a microplate reader. The results were expressed as relative cell viability (%).

2.9. TUNEL Staining

To identify apoptotic neurons, TUNEL assays were performed using an *in situ* cell death detection kit (Roche, No. 11 684 795 9101). After washed three times by ice-cold PBS, the cell samples were fixed with a freshly prepared fixation solution for 1h and incubated in permeabilization solution for 2 min on ice. Then, 50 μL TUNEL reaction mixture was added on each sample. Slides were incubated in a humidified atmosphere for 60 min at 37 °C in the dark, followed by counterstaining with DAPI. The number of TUNEL-positive cells was counted in 10 randomized fields per well under a fluorescence microscope. Results were the average ± SEM of data from 5 experiments unless stated otherwise in the legends.

2.10. Intracellular Calcium (Ca^{2+}) Measurements

Intracellular Ca^{2+} imaging was conducted using a Fluo4-AM dye (Dojindo Laboratories), which has strong ability to combine with free calcium ions inside living cells.

After washing 3 times with HBSS, cells prepared in 96-well plates were incubated with Fluo 4-AM working solution at 37 °C for 60 min. Washed 3 times to clean up the remains of Fluo 4-AM, cells were covered by HBSS for another 30 min at 37 °C to make deesterification of AM completely. At last, cells were analyzed under a fluorescence microscope (Leica DM6000 B) interfaced with a digital camera and an image analysis system. Images were taken under same aperture and speed. Ten pictures of each group were randomly selected and software Image Pro plus 6.0 was used to measure the intensity of each photo.

2.11. Western Blotting Analysis

Cortical neurons in 6cm dishes were washed with ice-cold PBS for 3 times and lysed with a lysis buffer containing protease inhibitors (Beyotime, Jiangsu, China) at 24 h after OGD/R treatments. The protein concentration was determined using a BCA protein assay kit. Then, protein extracts were separated by electrophoresis on 12% SEMS-polyacrylamide gel electrophoresis (SEMS-PAGE) gels and transferred onto polyvinylidene fluoride (PVDF) membranes. The membranes were sequentially incubated with primary antibodies and secondary antibodies, and enhanced chemiluminescence (ECL) solution and followed by autoradiography. The intensity of the blots was analyzed using Image Pro plus 6.0.

2.12. Statistical Analysis

The results were expressed as the mean ± SEM of triplicate measurements representative of three independent experiments. Multiple group comparisons were made by one-way ANOVA followed with Tukey *post hoc* test. Statistical significance was defined as $p < 0.05$.

3. Results

3.1. Identification, Genotyping and Fatty Acid Profiles of Primary Cortical Neurons

Primary cortical neurons were derived from E16.5 mice embryos (Figure 1A). Figure 1B shows the genotyping results of each embryo tissues. PCR analysis demonstrated the high expression of *fat-1* gene (lanes 1, 2, 4 and 5) in *fat-1* embryo tissues while no expression was found in WT embryo tissues (lanes 3, 6 and 7). As shown in Figure 1C,D, the neurons showed distinct cell bodies with synaptic connections. No obvious morphologic difference was observed between WT and *fat-1* derived neurons. Before OGD/R, immunocytochemistry was conducted using β-III tubulin and GFAP antibodies. The majority of cells were β-III tubulin-positive (>95%) and only a very small proportion were GFAP-positive in both *fat-1* neurons (Figure 1E) and WT neurons (Figure 1F). Fatty acid analyses of cultured primary neurons were performed using GC-MS. As shown in Table 1, *fat-1* neurons exhibited increased expression of ω-3 PUFAs including DPA and DHA (** $p < 0.01$ compared with WT neurons) with a significant decrease in overall ω-6/ω-3 PUFA ratio compared with WT neurons.

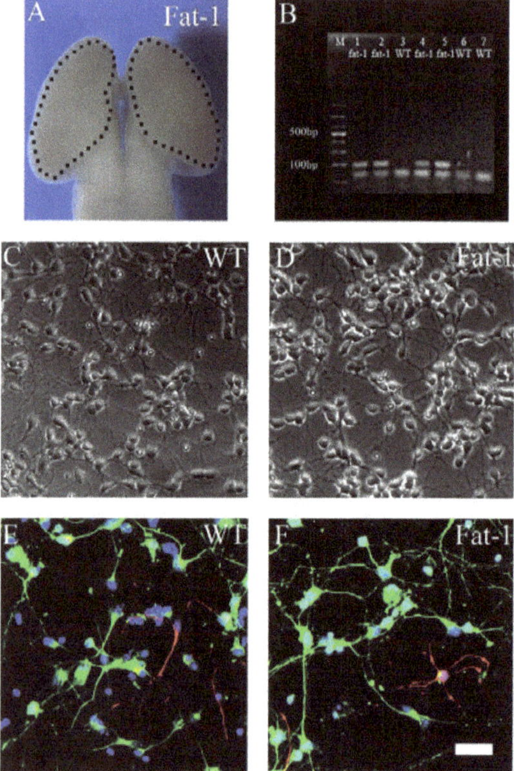

Figure 1. Identification of primary cultured neurons. Cultures were prepared from the cortex of E16.5 *fat-1* and WT embryos and examined at 7 DIV. (**A**) An image showing the cortical tissue in the embryonic brain; (**B**) gel electrophoresis of PCR products using primers for *fat-1* gene. Wild-type controls (lanes 3, 6 and 7) and positive fat-1 specimens (lanes 1, 2, 4 and 5); (**C**,**D**) examples of phase contrast images of cultured primary neurons; and (**E**,**F**) images showing immunostainning on WT and *fat-1* neurons respectively (**Green**, β-III tubulin; **Red**, GFAP; **Blue**, DAPI). Scale bar: 50 μm.

Table 1. Profiles of polyunsaturated fatty acid of primary cortical neurons derived from *fat-1* transgenic embryos and their WT littermates.

Fatty Acid	WT	*fat-1*
C14:0	3.01 ± 0.25	1.77 ± 0.33 *
C16:0	25.22 ± 0.27	24.20 ± 0.46
C16:1,9	8.65 ± 0.23	5.32 ± 0.57 **
C18:0	13.12 ± 0.85	16.11 ± 0.21 *
C18:1,9	33.12 ± 0.34	28.97 ± 0.12 **
C18:2,6	0.78 ± 0.23	0.77 ± 0.02
C18:3,3 (ALA)	0.11 ± 0.06	0.47 ± 0.11 **
C20:0	0.30 ± 0.05	0.27 ± 0.02
C20:1,9	1.22 ± 0.03	1.14 ± 0.02
C20:2,6	4.661 ± 0.24	2.88 ± 0.41 *
C20:4,6 (AA)	5.11 ± 0.18	0.88 ± 0.09 **
C20:5,3 (EPA)	0.33 ± 0.00	3.79 ± 0.73 **
C22:0	0.20 ± 0.03	0.54 ± 0.09 *
C22:1,9	3.56 ± 0.70	3.95 ± 0.63
C22:5,3 (DPA)	0.99 ± 0.03	4.37 ± 0.31 **
C22:6,3 (DHA)	1.02 ± 0.14	2.90 ± 0.03 **
C24:1	0.92 ± 0.12	1.32 ± 0.17
SFA	41.85 ± 0.34	42.89 ± 1.09
MUFA	47.47 ± 1.25	40.70 ± 1.09 **
PUFA	13.00 ± 1.05	16.06 ± 1.72 *
ω-6/ω-3	4.31 ± 4.03	0.39 ± 0.26 **

Data expressed as mol % of total fatty acids ± SEM (* $p < 0.05$ compared with WT; ** $p < 0.01$ compared with WT). Abbreviations: AA, arachidonic acid; ALA, alpha linolenic acid; DHA, docosahexaenoic acid; DPA, docosapentaenoic acid; EPA, eicosapentaenoic acid; LA, linoleic acid; MUFA, monounsaturated fatty acids (the value is given as follows: C16:1 + C18:1 + C20:1 + C22:1 + C24:1); SFA, saturated fatty acids (the value is given as follows: C14:0 + C16:0 + C18:0 + C20:0 + C22:0); PUFA, polyunsaturated fatty acids.

3.2. LBP Either Together with DHA or Endogenous ω-3 PUFAs Rescues Cortical Neurons from OGD/R Insults

To examine whether the combination of ω-3 PUFAs and LBP can promote neuronal survival under ischemia/reperfusion conditions, we induced OGD/R injury on cultured neurons at 7 DIV. The cultured neurons were exposed to a hypoxic and glucose-free environment for 3 h, followed by normal culture for 24 h to mimic ischemia/reperfusion injury. As shown in Figure 2, cortical neurons exhibited typical cell shrinkage and neurite blebbing, and a marked decrease in the cell number at 24 h after OGD/R injury. The bright hollows on the phase contrast images indicated an injury status of neurons after reperfusion, in which the most severe situation goes to WT OGD/R group. Conversely, neurons in all treatment groups showed intact cell bodies with elaborate networks of neuritis and remarkably attenuated OGD/R-induced morphological abnormalities compared with WT OGD/R neurons.

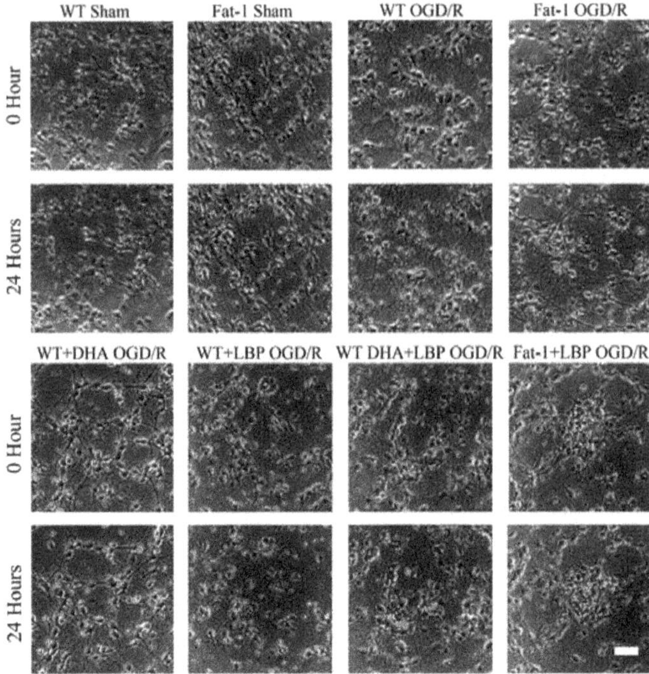

Figure 2. Primary cortical neurons were protected against OGD/R injury after LBP and ω-3 PUFAs treatment. Phase contrast images showing the morphological changes of the primary cultured neurons prior or post OGD/R injury. Scale bar: 50 μm.

3.3. LBP Either Together with DHA or Endogenous ω-3 PUFAs Significantly Prevents OGD/R-Induced Neuronal Apoptosis via Intracellular Ca^{2+} Handling or Neurotrophic Pathway Activation

The neuroprotective effects of combination of exogenous DHA and LBP were determined first. Cell viability was determined using a CCK-8 assay. OGD/R insults resulted in severe cell death in WT model group (approximately 45%). All the single treatment groups displayed a significant reduced neuronal death after OGD/R insults in that neuronal death was reduced to 34.7% in DHA-treated group and 36.6% in LBP-treated group. Notably, LBP combined with DHA further reduced neuronal cell death to 27.6% (Figure 3C). As shown in Figs. 3A and D, OGD/R induced approximately 50% TUNEL-positive cells in WT neurons. Cells in green fluorescence indicated TUNEL-positive and represented the apoptotic cells. Nuclei were labeled in blue with DAPI stands for the total number of cells in the present vision field. The ratio of apoptotic neurons was remarkably decreased in the culture of LBP- and DHA-treated WT neurons in which less TUNEL-positive cells were found after OGD/R injury (23.6% in LBP-treated group and 22.4% in DHA-treated group). Interestingly, LBP combined with DHA further reduced apoptosis after OGD/R insults (16.4%), indicating that a combined treatment exerts the maximal effect on protecting neurons against OGD/R injury among all the treatment groups. Moreover, Ca^{2+} ion plays an important role in maintaining the normal function of neurons. The concentration of Calcium ion remains a significant difference between the cell membranes and while injured, will be elevated from extracellular environment or the release of mitochondrion. Therefore, a constant rise in intracellular Ca^{2+} reflects the impaired situation of cells. Figure 3B illustrated the effect of different treatment on intracellular Ca^{2+} concentration. The results showed that WT OGD/R group displayed significant higher fluorescence intensity. Although the concentration of Ca^{2+} was slightly lower in single LBP treated group compared with WT OGD/R group, no significant statistics difference was observed between these two groups under the present experimental conditions. Furthermore, consistent with previous reports, the Fluo-4 fluorescence intensity was decreased by exogenous DHA treatment compared with WT OGD/R neurons. Intriguingly, our data demonstrated that combined use of LBP with exogenous DHA could further reduce Ca^{2+} levels, which implied a better effect on preventing Ca^{2+} overloading even compared with either single DHA treated group. Then, the expression levels of Trk-B receptor as well as Bcl-2 were determined by western blot assay. As shown in Figure 3F, the expression of Trk-B receptor and Bcl-2 were significantly decreased in WT OGD/R group. Both LBP and DHA treatment could remarkably reverse the reduction of Trk-B and Bcl-2 expression. Our data indicated that LBP might possibly exert its neuroprotection by activating Trk-B receptor and consequently initiate the pro-survival cascade. In addition, combined use of LBP together with exogenous DHA displayed an enhanced effect on activating Trk-B expression.

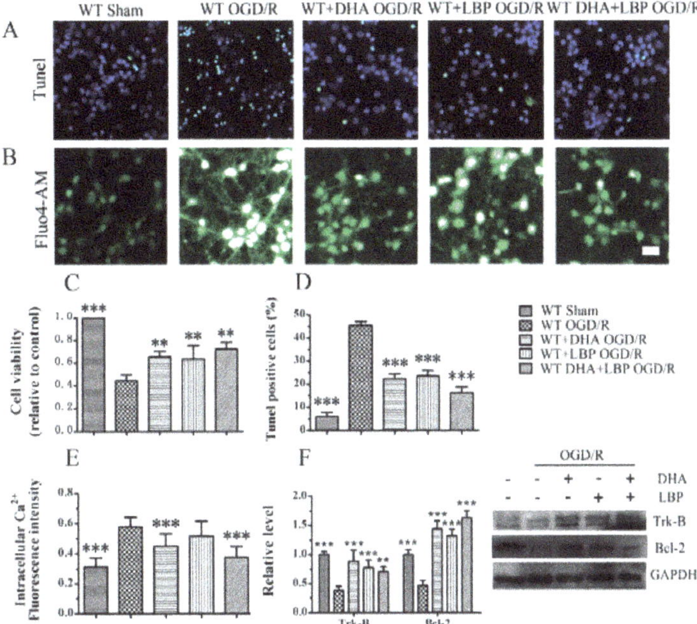

Figure 3. LBP and exogenous DHA (10 μM) significantly prevent OGD/R-induced neuronal apoptosis respectively via intracellular Ca^{2+} handling or neurotrophic pathway activation: (**A**) TUNEL staining; (**B**) fluorescent micrographs showing intracellular Ca^{2+} levels as stained by the Fluo4-AM dye; (**C**) statistic of cell viability; (**D**) statistic of TUNEL positive cells; (**E**) results of relative fluorescence intensity analysis of intracellular Ca^{2+}; and (**F**) expression levels of Trk-B and Bcl-2 measured by Western blot. Data are presented as mean ± SEM, ** $p < 0.01$, *** $p < 0.001$ indicate significant difference compared with the WT OGD group; $p < 0.05$ indicates significant difference compared with the WT DHA + LBP group (*t*-test). Scale bar: 50 μm.

Afterward, the protective effects were further confirmed in cultured neurons with high endogenous ω-3 PUFAs, which were isolated from *fat-1* mice, in that a higher survival rate was found in *fat-1* neurons compared with wild-type neurons after OGD/R injury. As shown in Figure 4C, all the single treatment groups displayed a significantly reduced neuronal death after OGD/R insults in that neuronal death was reduced to 35.5% in LBP-treated group and 33.9% in *fat-1* group. LBP combined with endogenous ω-3 PUFAs further reduced neuronal cell death to 26.3%. As shown in Figure 4A,D, the ratio of apoptotic neurons was remarkably decreased in the culture of LBP-treated WT neurons in which less TUNEL-positive cells were found after OGD/R injury (approximately 24%).

The ration of apoptotic neurons in *fat-1* neurons (19.2%) was significantly decreased compared with WT neurons, suggesting that endogenous ω-3 PUFAs have protective effects against OGD/R injury. Interestingly, LBP combined with endogenous ω-3 PUFAs further reduced apoptosis after OGD/R insults (14.0%), which confirmed the enhanced nruroprotective effects of the combined treatment on protecting neurons against OGD/R injury. Furthermore, the results in Figure 4B,E showed that the Fluo-4 fluorescence intensity was decreased by endogenous ω-3 PUFAs treatment compared with WT OGD/R neurons. Our data demonstrated that combined use of LBP with endogenous ω-3 PUFAs could further reduce Ca^{2+} levels as well. Finally, as shown in Figure 4F, the expression of Trk-B receptor and Bcl-2 were significantly decreased in WT OGD/R group. Both LBP and endogenous ω-3 PUFAs could remarkably reverse the reduction of Trk-B and Bcl-2 expression in treated groups. The results further confirmed that combined use of LBP together with endogenous ω-3 PUFAs could enhance their neroprotective effects via activating Trk-B expression.

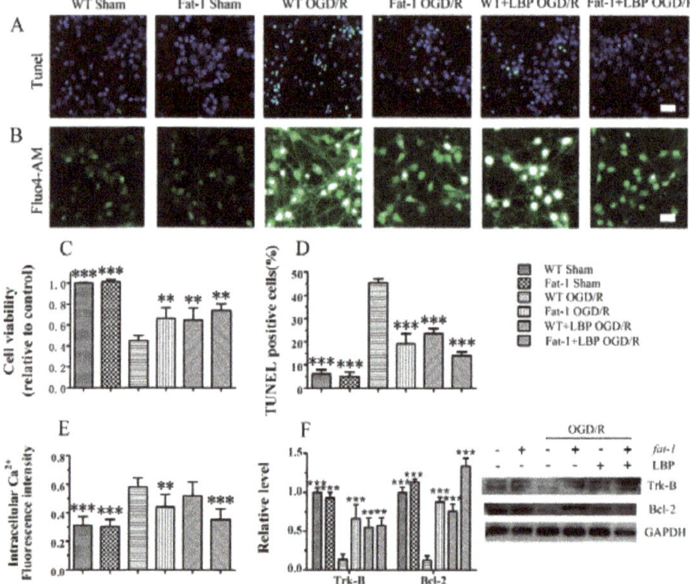

Figure 4. LBP and endogenous ω-3 PUFAs significantly prevent OGD/R-induced neuronal apoptosis respectively via intracellular Ca^{2+} handling or neurotrophic pathway activation: (**A**) TUNEL staining; (**B**) fluorescent micrographs showing intracellular Ca^{2+} levels as stained by the Fluo4-AM dye; (**C**) statistic of cell viability; (**D**) statistic of TUNEL positive cells; (**E**) results of relative fluorescence intensity analysis of intracellular Ca^{2+}; and (**F**) expression levels of Trk-B and Bcl-2 measured by Western blot. Data are presented as mean ± SEM, ** $p < 0.01$, *** $p < 0.001$ indicate significant difference compared with the WT OGD group; $p < 0.05$, $p < 0.01$ indicates significant difference compared with the WT DHA + LBP group (*t*-test). Scale bar: 50 μm.

4. Discussion

In the present study, we firstly determined the neuroprotective effect of docosahexaenoic acid (DHA), a major component of the ω-3 PUFA family, together with LBP in primary cortical neurons against OGD/R insult. The deprivation of oxygen and glucose results in the initiation of the depicted ischemic cascade that eventually leads to neuronal death [28]. Because of the loss of nutrients and oxygen, neurons are injured and a lot of devastating cascades are initiated, such as excessive excitatory amino acid release, generation of reactive oxygen species (ROS), expression of pro-apoptotic factors, mitochondrial dysfunction, as well as inflammation [29]. The OGD/R model provides a chance to dissect cellular events that occur after withdrawal of oxygen and glucose and mimic the key pathophysiological events of ischemia *in vivo*. Consistent with previous findings, both substances as well as the combined treatment significantly rescued cortical neurons from OGD/R insults [19,30].

Alterations in Ca^{2+} homeostasis, including mitochondrial Ca^{2+} overload, lead to increased cell vulnerability and oxidative stress [22]. Excessive Ca^{2+} entry ultimately induces acute or delayed neuronal death [31]. It has been reported that ω-3 PUFAs inhibited endoplasmic reticulum (ER) Ca^{2+} release in astrocyte after *in vitro* ischemia [32] and delayed Ca^{2+}-induced mitochondrial permeability transition pore opening in myocardium [33]. These findings suggest that ω-3 PUFAs have a potential to reduce intracellular Ca^{2+} overloading. Although LBP was observed to reduce 6-OHDA -induced elevation of intracellular Ca^{2+} in PC12 cells [20], no clear description on the location where Ca^{2+} accumulated was recorded. In the present research, we observed that DHA significantly inhibited the increase of intracellular Ca^{2+}, whereas single LBP treatment had limited influence on intracellular Ca^{2+} handling. The mitochondrial apoptosis pathway is controlled by pro- and anti-apoptotic Bcl-2 family proteins and either overexpression of anti-apoptotic Bcl-2, or gene deficiency in the proapoptotic bax gene to prevent excitotoxic apoptosis [34,35]. It is established that increasing the expression level of Bcl-2 can obviously reduce the impact of stroke in neuroprotective treatments [36–38]. Consistently, our observations demonstrated that both LBP and ω-3 PUFAs exert their neuroprotection via activating Bcl-2 anti-apoptotic cascade. Additionally, several lines of evidences have demonstrated that modulating Bcl-2 family proteins can only contribute to maintaining Ca^{2+} homeostasis in the ER [39,40]. It can be inferred that the confined alteration in Ca^{2+} contents has limited contribution to the entirety intracellular Ca^{2+} homeostasis. Therefore, this notion may possibly account for the limited impact of LBP on intracellular Ca^{2+} handling observed in our research.

To further determine how LBP and ω-3 PUFAs trigger intracellular pro-survival signaling, we examined the alterations of Trk-B receptors. The Trk receptor tyrosine kinases is a family of transmembrane-receptor signaling systems which promote the development and survival of neurons [41]. Trk-B receptor can be activated by specifically binding with BDNF. The activated Trk-B receptor subsequently triggers downstream signal pathway to induce pro-survival effects [23]. Enriched dietary ω-3 PUFAs has been reported to increase Trk-B mRNA expression in the cerebral cortex [42]. We noticed that both LBP and DHA treatment significantly increased the expression of Trk-B receptors in primary cultured cortical neurons suffered OGD/R insults. In the present study, we reported for the first time that LBP possibly protected neuron from OGD/R-induced apoptosis via modulating neurotrophin pathway, which initiated from the cell membrane. Notably, combined treatment of DHA and LBP showed the maximal effect on protecting cortical neurons against OGD/R injury via concurrently regulating the intracellular calcium accumulation and neurotrophic pathway.

In addition, the protective effects were further confirmed in neurons with high content of endogenous ω-3 PUFAs that were isolated from *fat-1* mice embryos. Dietary supplementation is a conventional approach to increase tissue content of ω-3 PUFAs in animal studies. However, inconsistent results were occasionally observed either due to the variance in the component of dietary supplement or the neglected relevance of the ω-3/ω-6 PUFAs ratio. Kang *et al.* engineered a transgenic mouse carrying a *fat-1* gene from *Caenorhabditiselegans* [17]. The *fat-1* gene encodes a fatty acid desaturase not normally present in mammals, which can convert ω-6 into ω-3 PUFAs. The highly expression of the *fat-1* gene leads to enrichment in endogenous ω-3 PUFAs levels and concomitantly decreased ω-6 PUFAs levels [43]. The use of *fat-1* mice embryos provides a strictly controlled model to investigate the biological properties of ω-3 PUFAs with stable content [44]. The present findings indicated that endogenous ω-3 PUFAs, combining with LBP treatment, exerted a better neuroprotective effect on OGD/R insulted neurons.

In conclusion, we observed the protective effect of ω-3 PUFAs or LBP on enhancing the survival of cultured cortical neurons using an *in vitro* OGD/R model and further demonstrated that a combined treatment of ω-3 PUFAs and LBP exerted the maximal effect on protecting neurons against OGD/R injury. The results of the study suggest that ω-3 PUFAs and LBP are promising candidates for combined pharmacotherapy for ischemic stroke.

Acknowledgments: This study was supported by Macao Science and Technology Development Fund (018/2013/A1), matching grant project MRG003/SHX/2014/ICMS, and multi-year research grant, university of Macau, MYRG122 (Y1-L3)-ICMS12-SHX and MYRG110 (Y1-L2)-ICMS13-SHX.

Author Contributions: H.S. and C.H. designed the study; Z.S., D.W., J.Y., and X.Y. performed the experiment; Z.H., P.L., J.W. and H.S. analyzed the data; Z.S., D.W., and H.S. wrote the manuscript together.

Conflicts of Interest: The authors declare no conflict of interest.

References

1. Rothwell, P.M.; Algra, A.; Amarenco, P. Medical treatment in acute and long-term secondary prevention after transient ischaemic attack and ischaemic stroke. *Lancet* **2011**, *377*, 1681–1692. [CrossRef]
2. O'Collins, V.E.; Macleod, M.R.; Donnan, G.A.; Horky, L.L.; van der Worp, B.H.; Howells, D.W. 1026 experimental treatments in acute stroke. *Ann. Neurol.* **2006**, *59*, 467–477. [PubMed]
3. Stankowski, J.N.; Gupta, R. Therapeutic targets for neuroprotection in acute ischemic stroke: Lost in translation? *Antioxid. Redox Signal.* **2011**, *14*, 1841–1851. [CrossRef] [PubMed]
4. George, P.M.; Steinberg, G.K. Novel stroke therapeutics: Unraveling stroke pathophysiology and its impact on clinical treatments. *Neuron* **2015**, *87*, 297–309. [CrossRef] [PubMed]
5. Belayev, L.; Khoutorova, L.; Atkins, K.D.; Bazan, N.G. Robust docosahexaenoic acid-mediated neuroprotection in a rat model of transient, focal cerebral ischemia. *Stroke* **2009**, *40*, 3121–3126. [CrossRef] [PubMed]
6. Zhang, W.T.; Hu, X.M.; Yang, W.; Gao, Y.Q.; Chen, J. Omega-3 polyunsaturated fatty acid supplementation confers long-term neuroprotection against neonatal hypoxic-ischemic brain injury through anti-inflammatory actions. *Stroke* **2010**, *41*, 2341–2347. [CrossRef] [PubMed]
7. Belayev, L.; Khoutorova, L.; Atkins, K.D.; Eady, T.N.; Hong, S.; Lu, Y.; Obenaus, A.; Bazan, N.G. Docosahexaenoic acid therapy of experimental ischemic stroke. *Transl. Stroke Res.* **2011**, *2*, 33–41. [CrossRef] [PubMed]
8. Oudin, A.; Wennberg, M. Fish consumption and ischemic stroke in southern sweden. *Nutr. J.* **2011**, *10*, 109. [CrossRef] [PubMed]
9. Hu, X.; Zhang, F.; Leak, R.K.; Zhang, W.; Iwai, M.; Stetler, R.A.; Dai, Y.; Zhao, A.; Gao, Y.; Chen, J. Transgenic overproduction of omega-3 polyunsaturated fatty acids provides neuroprotection and enhances endogenous neurogenesis after stroke. *Curr. Mol. Med.* **2013**, *13*, 1465–1473. [CrossRef] [PubMed]
10. Zhang, M.; Wang, S.; Mao, L.; Leak, R.K.; Shi, Y.; Zhang, W.; Hu, X.; Sun, B.; Cao, G.; Gao, Y.; *et al.* Omega-3 fatty acids protect the brain against ischemic injury by activating Nrf2 and upregulating heme oxygenase 1. *J. Neurosci.* **2014**, *34*, 1903–1915. [CrossRef] [PubMed]
11. Kichev, A.; Rousset, C.I.; Baburamani, A.A.; Levison, S.W.; Wood, T.L.; Gressens, P.; Thornton, C.; Hagberg, H. Tnf-related apoptosis-inducing ligand (TRAIL) signaling and cell death in the immature central nervous system after hypoxia-ischemia and inflammation. *J. Biol. Chem.* **2014**, *289*, 9430–9439. [CrossRef] [PubMed]
12. Zhang, M.J.; Spite, M. Resolvins: Anti-inflammatory and proresolving mediators derived from omega-3 polyunsaturated fatty acids. *Annu. Rev. Nutr.* **2012**, *32*, 203–227. [CrossRef] [PubMed]
13. Luo, C.; Ren, H.; Wan, J.B.; Yao, X.; Zhang, X.; He, C.; So, K.F.; Kang, J.X.; Pei, Z.; Su, H. Enriched endogenous omega-3 fatty acids in mice protect against global ischemia injury. *J. Lipid Res.* **2014**, *55*, 1288–1297. [CrossRef] [PubMed]
14. Cao, D.H.; Xu, J.F.; Xue, R.H.; Zheng, W.F.; Liu, Z.L. Protective effect of chronic ethyl docosahexaenoate administration on brain injury in ischemic gerbils. *Pharmacol. Biochem. Behav.* **2004**, *79*, 651–659. [CrossRef] [PubMed]
15. Siwek, M.; Sowa-Kucma, M.; Dudek, D.; Styczen, K.; Szewczyk, B.; Kotarska, K.; Misztakk, P.; Pilc, A.; Wolak, M.; Nowak, G. Oxidative stress markers in affective disorders. *Pharmacol. Rep.* **2013**, *65*, 1558–1571. [CrossRef]
16. Simopoulos, A.P. Evolutionary aspects of diet, the omega-6/omega-3 ratio and genetic variation: Nutritional implications for chronic diseases. *Biomed. Pharmacother.* **2006**, *60*, 502–507. [CrossRef] [PubMed]

17. Kang, J.X.; Wang, J.; Wu, L.; Kang, Z.B. Transgenic mice: Fat-1 mice convert *n*-6 to ω-3 fatty acids. *Nature* **2004**, *427*, 504. [CrossRef] [PubMed]
18. Wang, T.; Li, Y.; Wang, Y.; Zhou, R.; Ma, L.; Hao, Y.; Jin, S.; Du, J.; Zhao, C.; Sun, T.; *et al.* Lycium barbarum polysaccharide prevents focal cerebral ischemic injury by inhibiting neuronal apoptosis in mice. *PLoS ONE* **2014**, *9*, e90780. [CrossRef] [PubMed]
19. Rui, C.; Yuxiang, L.; Yinju, H.; Qingluan, Z.; Yang, W.; Qipeng, Z.; Hao, W.; Lin, M.; Juan, L.; Chengjun, Z.; *et al.* Protective effects of lycium barbarum polysaccharide on neonatal rat primary cultured hippocampal neurons injured by oxygen-glucose deprivation and reperfusion. *J. Mol. Histol.* **2012**, *43*, 535–542. [CrossRef] [PubMed]
20. Gao, K.; Liu, M.; Cao, J.; Yao, M.; Lu, Y.; Li, J.; Zhu, X.; Yang, Z.; Wen, A. Protective effects of lycium barbarum polysaccharide on 6-OHDA-induced apoptosis in PC12 cells through the ROS-NO pathway. *Molecules* **2015**, *20*, 293–308. [CrossRef] [PubMed]
21. Wang, H.B.; Li, Y.X.; Hao, Y.J.; Wang, T.F.; Lei, Z.; Wu, Y.; Zhao, Q.P.; Ang, H.; Ma, L.; Liu, J.; *et al.* Neuroprotective effects of LBP on brain ischemic reperfusion neurodegeneration. *Eur. Rev. Med. Pharmacol. Sci.* **2013**, *17*, 2760–2765. [PubMed]
22. Ureshino, R.P.; Rocha, K.K.; Lopes, G.S.; Bincoletto, C.; Smaili, S.S. Calcium signaling alterations, oxidative stress, and autophagy in aging. *Antioxid. Redox Signal.* **2014**, *21*, 123–137. [CrossRef] [PubMed]
23. Gupta, V.K.; You, Y.; Gupta, V.B.; Klistorner, A.; Graham, S.L. Trkb receptor signalling: Implications in neurodegenerative, psychiatric and proliferative disorders. *Int. J. Mol. Sci.* **2013**, *14*, 10122–10142. [CrossRef] [PubMed]
24. Yu, M.S.; Leung, S.K.; Lai, S.W.; Che, C.M.; Zee, S.Y.; So, K.F.; Yuen, W.H.; Chang, R.C. Neuroprotective effects of anti-aging oriental medicine lycium barbarum against beta-amyloid peptide neurotoxicity. *Exp. Gerontol.* **2005**, *40*, 716–727. [CrossRef] [PubMed]
25. He, C.; Qu, X.; Cui, L.; Wang, J.; Kang, J.X. Improved spatial learning performance of fat-1 mice is associated with enhanced neurogenesis and neuritogenesis by docosahexaenoic acid. *Proc. Natl. Acad. Sci. USA* **2009**, *106*, 11370–11375. [CrossRef] [PubMed]
26. Liu, Q.; Wu, D.; Ni, N.; Ren, H.; Luo, C.; He, C.; Kang, J.X.; Wan, J.B.; Su, H. Omega-3 polyunsaturated fatty acids protect neural progenitor cells against oxidative injury. *Mar. Drugs* **2014**, *12*, 2341–2356. [CrossRef] [PubMed]
27. Wan, J.B.; Huang, L.L.; Rong, R.; Tan, R.; Wang, J.; Kang, J.X. Endogenously decreasing tissue *n*-6/ω-3 fatty acid ratio reduces atherosclerotic lesions in apolipoprotein e-deficient mice by inhibiting systemic and vascular inflammation. *Arterioscler. Thromb. Vasc. Biol.* **2010**, *30*, 2487–2494. [CrossRef] [PubMed]
28. Doyle, K.P.; Simon, R.P.; Stenzel-Poore, M.P. Mechanisms of ischemic brain damage. *Neuropharmacology* **2008**, *55*, 310–318. [CrossRef] [PubMed]
29. Bazan, N.G.; Marcheselli, V.L.; Cole-Edwards, K. Brain response to injury and neurodegeneration: Endogenous neuroprotective signaling. *Ann. N. Y. Acad. Sci.* **2005**, *1053*, 137–147. [CrossRef] [PubMed]
30. Kim, H.Y.; Akbar, M.; Kim, K.Y. Inhibition of neuronal apoptosis by polyunsaturated fatty acids. *J. Mol. Neurosci.* **2001**, *16*, 223–227. [CrossRef]
31. D'Orsi, B.; Kilbride, S.M.; Chen, G.; Perez Alvarez, S.; Bonner, H.P.; Pfeiffer, S.; Plesnila, N.; Engel, T.; Henshall, D.C.; Dussmann, H.; *et al.* Bax regulates neuronal Ca^{2+} homeostasis. *J. Neurosci.* **2015**, *35*, 1706–1722. [CrossRef] [PubMed]
32. Begum, G.; Kintner, D.; Liu, Y.; Cramer, S.W.; Sun, D. Dha inhibits er Ca^{2+} release and er stress in astrocytes following *in vitro* ischemia. *J. Neurochem.* **2012**, *120*, 622–630. [CrossRef] [PubMed]
33. Khairallah, R.J.; O'Shea, K.M.; Brown, B.H.; Khanna, N.; des Rosiers, C.; Stanley, W.C. Treatment with docosahexaenoic acid, but not eicosapentaenoic acid, delays Ca^{2+}-induced mitochondria permeability transition in normal and hypertrophied myocardium. *J. Pharmacol. Exp. Ther.* **2010**, *335*, 155–162. [CrossRef] [PubMed]
34. Malagelada, C.; Xifro, X.; Minano, A.; Sabria, J.; Rodriguez-Alvarez, J. Contribution of caspase-mediated apoptosis to the cell death caused by oxygen-glucose deprivation in cortical cell cultures. *Neurobiol. Dis.* **2005**, *20*, 27–37. [CrossRef] [PubMed]
35. Broughton, B.R.; Reutens, D.C.; Sobey, C.G. Apoptotic mechanisms after cerebral ischemia. *Stroke* **2009**, *40*, e331–e339. [CrossRef] [PubMed]

36. Yin, W.; Cao, G.; Johnnides, M.J.; Signore, A.P.; Luo, Y.; Hickey, R.W.; Chen, J. TAT-mediated delivery of Bcl-xL protein is neuroprotective against neonatal hypoxic-ischemic brain injury via inhibition of caspases and AIF. *Neurobiol. Dis.* **2006**, *21*, 358–371. [CrossRef] [PubMed]
37. Zhao, H.; Yenari, M.A.; Cheng, D.; Sapolsky, R.M.; Steinberg, G.K. Bcl-2 overexpression protects against neuron loss within the ischemic margin following experimental stroke and inhibits cytochrome C translocation and caspase-3 activity. *J. Neurochem.* **2003**, *85*, 1026–1036. [CrossRef] [PubMed]
38. Cao, G.; Pei, W.; Ge, H.; Liang, Q.; Luo, Y.; Sharp, F.R.; Lu, A.; Ran, R.; Graham, S.H.; Chen, J. *In vivo* delivery of a Bcl-xL fusion protein containing the TAT protein transduction domain protects against ischemic brain injury and neuronal apoptosis. *J. Neurosci.* **2002**, *22*, 5423–5431. [PubMed]
39. Rong, Y.P.; Bultynck, G.; Aromolaran, A.S.; Zhong, F.; Parys, J.B.; de Smedt, H.; Mignery, G.A.; Roderick, H.L.; Bootman, M.D.; Distelhorst, C.W. The BH4 domain of Bcl-2 inhibits er calcium release and apoptosis by binding the regulatory and coupling domain of the IP3 receptor. *Proc. Natl. Acad. Sci. USA* **2009**, *106*, 14397–14402. [CrossRef] [PubMed]
40. Pinton, P.; Rizzuto, R. Bcl-2 and Ca^{2+} homeostasis in the endoplasmic reticulum. *Cell Death Differ.* **2006**, *13*, 1409–1418. [CrossRef] [PubMed]
41. Huang, E.J.; Reichardt, L.F. Trk receptors: Roles in neuronal signal transemuction. *Annu. Rev. Biochem.* **2003**, *72*, 609–642. [CrossRef] [PubMed]
42. Balogun, K.A.; Cheema, S.K. The expression of neurotrophins is differentially regulated by omega-3 polyunsaturated fatty acids at weaning and postweaning in C57BL/6 mice cerebral cortex. *Neurochem. Int.* **2014**, *66*, 33–42. [CrossRef] [PubMed]
43. Gladman, S.J.; Huang, W.; Lim, S.N.; Dyall, S.C.; Boddy, S.; Kang, J.X.; Knight, M.M.; Priestley, J.V.; Michael-Titus, A.T. Improved outcome after peripheral nerve injury in mice with increased levels of endogenous omega-3 polyunsaturated fatty acids. *J. Neurosci.* **2012**, *32*, 563–571. [CrossRef] [PubMed]
44. Kang, J.X. Fat-1 transgenic mice: A new model for omega-3 research. *Prostaglandins Leukot. Essent. Fat. Acids* **2007**, *77*, 263–267. [CrossRef] [PubMed]

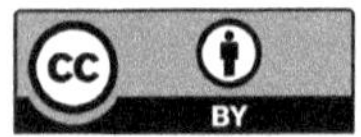

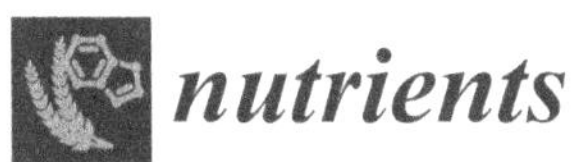
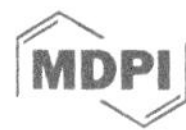

Article

Docosahexaenoic Acid Ameliorates Fructose-Induced Hepatic Steatosis Involving ER Stress Response in Primary Mouse Hepatocytes

Jinying Zheng [1], Chuan Peng [2], Yanbiao Ai [1], Heng Wang [2], Xiaoqiu Xiao [2,*] and Jibin Li [1,*]

1 School of Public Health and Management, Chongqing Medical University, Research Center for Medicine and Social Development, Innovation Center for Social Risk Governance in Health, Chongqing 400016, China; jinyingzheng1988@163.com (J.Z.); aiyanbiao1992@163.com (Y.A.)
2 Laboratory of Lipid & Glucose Metabolism, The First Affiliated Hospital of Chongqing Medical University, Chongqing 400016, China; 13527441813@163.com (C.P.); hengyy663@163.com (H.W.)
* Correspondence: xiaoxq@cqmu.edu.cn (X.X.); ljb21st@126.com (J.L.); Tel.: +86-23-8901-1866 (X.X. & J.L.); Fax: +86-23-8901-1865 (X.X. & J.L.)

Received: 5 December 2015; Accepted: 14 January 2016; Published: 20 January 2016

Abstract: The increase in fructose consumption is considered to be a risk factor for developing nonalcoholic fatty liver disease (NAFLD). We investigated the effects of docosahexaenoic acid (DHA) on hepatic lipid metabolism in fructose-treated primary mouse hepatocytes, and the changes of Endoplasmic reticulum (ER) stress pathways in response to DHA treatment. The hepatocytes were treated with fructose, DHA, fructose plus DHA, tunicamycin (TM) or fructose plus 4-phenylbutyric acid (PBA) for 24 h. Intracellular triglyceride (TG) accumulation was assessed by Oil Red O staining. The mRNA expression levels and protein levels related to lipid metabolism and ER stress response were determined by real-time PCR and Western blot. Fructose treatment led to obvious TG accumulation in primary hepatocytes through increasing expression of fatty acid synthase (FAS) and acetyl-CoA carboxylase (ACC), two key enzymes in hepatic *de novo* lipogenesis. DHA ameliorates fructose-induced TG accumulation by upregulating the expression of carnitine palmitoyltransferase 1A (CPT-1α) and acyl-CoA oxidase 1 (ACOX1). DHA treatment or pretreatment with the ER stress inhibitor PBA significantly decreased TG accumulation and reduced the expression of glucose-regulated protein 78 (GRP78), total inositol-requiring kinase 1 (IRE1α) and p-IRE1α. The present results suggest that DHA protects against high fructose-induced hepatocellular lipid accumulation. The current findings also suggest that alleviating the ER stress response seems to play a role in the prevention of fructose-induced hepatic steatosis by DHA.

Keywords: docosahexaenoic acid; fructose; ER stress; NAFLD

1. Introduction

Nonalcoholic fatty liver disease (NAFLD) has become the most common liver disease globally. It is estimated that 24% to 42% of the population in Western countries and 5% to 42% in Asian countries are affected [1,2]. NAFLD, a hepatic manifestation of metabolic syndrome, is characterized by an increase in intrahepatic triglyceride (*i.e.*, steatosis) in the absence of excessive alcohol intake. It can progress to nonalcoholic steatohepatitis (NASH) when hepatocellular injury and inflammation are present, and may lead to liver fibrosis and cirrhosis [3,4]. It is frequently associated with obesity and dyslipidemia, type 2 diabetes, insulin resistance and some dietary factors, such as high energy, fat and excess sugar intakes [5–7].

The consumption of sweetened foods and beverages, which contain high concentrations of fructose, has increased in the last few decades [8,9]. Increasing evidence indicates that high fructose intakes might be an important risk factor in the development of NAFLD [10–12]. Studies in both animals and humans have shown that high fructose consumption was associated with increased *de novo* lipogenesis, triglycerides synthesis and secretion of very low density lipoproteins, and decreased fatty acid oxidation and impaired insulin signaling [13–17].

Docosahexaenoic acid (22:6 *n*-3, DHA) and eicosapentaenoic acid (EPA), the major polyunsaturated fatty acids (PUFA) of *n*-3 series found in marine fish oil, are essential for mammals because they cannot be produced in the body and must be obtained from food. Some studies in humans and rodents demonstrated that dietary PUFA influenced hepatic triglyceride levels, insulin resistance and inflammation [18–20]. The beneficial effects of EPA and DHA supplementation on lipogenesis, fatty acid oxidation and hepatic lipid metabolism have been reported in numerous studies [20–22]. Some authors have recently demonstrated that the supplementation of *n*-3 fatty acids had potential therapeutic effects in human NAFLD as well as other metabolic disorders, such as insulin resistance, dyslipidemia, and impaired cognitive functions [11,23–25]. In addition, DHA and EPA can alter metabolic pathways, improve insulin sensitivity by modulating related gene expression and ameliorate hepatic triglycerides accumulation in rats fed a high-fructose diet [20]. These findings suggest that dietary supplements of PUFA may be beneficial for the patients with NAFLD. Nevertheless, the molecular mechanism that PUFA ameliorates NAFLD is not entirely clear.

Endoplasmic reticulum (ER) stress has long been proposed to play a crucial role in the development of NAFLD [26,27]. Interestingly, recent studies showed that the activation of ER stress pathways in high fructose-fed mice mediated *de novo* lipogenesis and then altered hepatic steatosis and insulin resistance [28]. It has been demonstrated that supplementation of *n*-3 fatty acids attenuated hepatic steatosis [11,23]. However, it remains unclear whether DHA prevents fructose-induce NAFLD by regulating ER stress pathways. In this study, we investigated the effects of DHA on hepatic lipid metabolism in fructose-treated primary mouse hepatocytes, and the changes of ER stress pathways in response to DHA treatment.

2. Materials and Methods

2.1. Materials and Reagents

DHA (purity ⩾ 98%), Oil Red O, tunicamycin, insulin, dexamethasone, rat-tail collagen and type IV collagenase were purchased from Sigma-Aldrich (Sigma-Aldrich, St. Louis, MO, USA). Briefly, the stock solution of DHA was dissolved in 95% ethanol at a concentration of 200 mM, and the working solution was prepared by adding the stock to the culture medium to achieve a final concentration of 25 μM. Epidermal growth factor was a product from Peprotech (Peprotech, Rocky Hill, NJ, USA). The primary antibodies applied in this study were anti-GRP78 (Cell Signaling Technology, Danvers, MA, USA), anti-ACC (Cell Signaling Technology, Danvers, MA, USA), anti-IRE (Santa Cruz Biotechnology, Santa Cruz, CA, USA), anti-ACOX1 (Abcam, Cambridge, UK), anti-p-IRE1α (Abcam, Cambridge, UK) and anti-β-actin (Beyotime, Shanghai, China).

2.2. Primary Mouse Hepatocytes Culture

Hepatocytes were prepared from male C57/6J mice referred to a modification of the two-step perfusion method as described previously [29]. The animals were anesthetized by intraperitoneal injection chloral hydrate (10 mL/kg, 4%). The abdominal cavity was opened, and the hepatic portal vein exposed. First, the liver was perfused with perfusion buffer 1 (calcium-free P1 medium) through a portal vein until the liver became pale in color; then perfusion buffer 2 supplemented with 0.035% type IV collagenase (P2 digestion medium) was used, keeping at a flow rate of 5 mL/min for about 6 min. The P1 and P2 medium should be warmed for 30 min in the water bath at 37 °C before use. After digestion, the hepatocytes were collected and washed with suspension medium, and then centrifuged at 50× *g* for 3 min at 4 °C twice. A cell count and cell viability assessment by trypan blue exclusion using a hemocytometer were performed. Freshly prepared hepatocytes were seeded at a final density of 1.5×10^6 cells in collagen-coated 25 cm^2 culture vessels, which were kept in tissue culture incubator set at 37 °C in a humidified atmosphere of 5% CO_2 and 95% air. The cells were maintained in 10% FBS (Gibco®, South Melbourne, Victoria, Australia) DMEM/F12 medium (Gibco®, Shanghai, China) supplemented with 1 mL penicillin-streptomycin, then the medium was replaced with serum-free DMEM/F12 medium (supplement 100 units/mL penicillin, 100 µg/mL streptomycin, 10 µg/mL insulin, 0.1 µmol/L dexamethasone, 5 ng/mL epidermal growth factor) after 4 h.

2.3. Oil Red O Staining

The cells grown on glass coverslips were washed with phosphate buffered saline (PBS) three times and then fixed with 4% paraformaldehyde for 30 min at room temperature. The fixed cells were washed with PBS and stained with freshly diluted Oil Red O working solution (0.5% Oil Red O in isopropanol: H_2O = 3:2) for 1 h, and counterstained with haematoxylin for 3 min. The primary mouse hepatocytes were observed using a microscope.

2.4. RNA Extraction and Real-Time PCR Assays

Total RNA was isolated from treated primary hepatocytes using Tripure Isolation Reagent (Roche, Mannheim, Germany) according to the manufacturer's instructions. cDNA was synthesized with a Reverse Transcription Kit (TaKaRa, Otsu, Japan). Real-time PCR analysis was performed with SYBR Green in a thermal Cycler Dice Real Time System (TaKaRa, Otsu, Japan). The relative mRNA levels of target genes were assessed by using the $2^{-\Delta\Delta Ct}$ method. Each experiment was repeated three times. The sequences for the primers pairs were as follows (forward and reverse, respectively): *GADPH*: 5′-TGCTGTCCCTGTATGCCTCTG-3′ and 5′-TCTTTGATGTCACGCACGATTT-3′, *FAS*: 5′-GGCACTGACTGTCTGTTTTCCA-3′ and 5′-GTAAAAATGACACAGTCCAGACACTTC-3′, *ACC1α*: 5′-GTTTCAGAACGGCCACTACGA-3′ and 5′-CATTGTCACCAGGAGATTCTTTTTG-3′, *CPT1a*: 5′-TCTCTGGATGCGGTAGAAAAGG-3′ and 5′-CTCTATATCCCTGTTCCGATTCGT-3′, *Acox1*: 5′-GC CAATGCTGGTATCGAAGAA-3′ and 5′-AATCCCACTGCTGTGAGAATAGC-3′, *GRP78*: 5′-CAGGG CAACCGCATCAC-3′ and 5′-CAATCAGACGCTCCCCTTCA-3′, *XBP1*: 5′-AGTTAAGAACACGCTT GGGAT-3′ and 5′-AAGATGTTCTGGGGAGGTGAC-3′, *LXR*: 5′-AGGAGTGTGTGCTGTCAGAAGAA C-3′ and 5′-TCCTCTTCTTGCCGCTTCA-3′, *ChREBP*: 5′-CCCTCAGACACCCACATCTT-3′ and 5′-CAGAGCTCAGAAAGGGGTTG-3′, *SREBP1c*: , *CHOP*: 5′-GCATGAAGGAGAAGGAGCAG-3′ and 5′-CTTCCGGAGAGACAGACAGG-3′, *C/EBP1a*: 5′-CGCAAGAGCCGAGATAAAGC-3′ and 5′- CGGTCATTGTCACTGGTCAACT-3′.

2.5. Western Blot

Hepatocytes were lysed in RIPA buffer. Aliquots of 40 µg protein were loaded onto 8% sodium dodecyl sulfate-polyacrylamide gel electrophoresis (SDS-PAGE) gel, transferred to polyvinylidene difluoride (PVDF) membranes, and subsequently blocked with 5% nonfat milk for 1 h. The membranes were incubated with primary antibodies overnight, and then the secondary antibodies for 1 h. The protein bands were visualized with enhanced chemiluminiscence (ECL) detection system. The expression levels of protein were quantified with Fusion software.

2.6. Statistical Analysis

All experimental data were expressed as the mean ± SEM. Statistical differences were analyzed by one-way ANOVA, followed by Fisher's least significant difference (LSD's) multiple comparison test using SPSS 18.0 analysis software (SPSS, Chicago, IL, USA). Statistical significance was shown as * $p < 0.05$, ** $p < 0.015$, and *** $p < 0.001$.

3. Results

3.1. DHA Prevents Fructose-Induced Lipid Accumulation in Primary Mouse Hepatocytes

To examine the effect of DHA on fructose treated primary mouse hepatocytes, cells were incubated for 24 h in DMEM/F12 medium containing 12.5 mM fructose (F), 12.5 mM fructose plus 25 μM DHA (F + DHA), or 25 μM DHA (DHA); control (CT) incubations only had vehicle. Then the cells were subjected to Oil Red O staining. After 24 h of incubation with fructose, the volume and numbers of lipid droplets were significantly increased indicating fructose treatment enhanced hepatic steatosis. In contrast, there was less triglyceride accumulation in DHA and F + DHA groups (Figure 1). Our data indicates that fructose treatment can cause TG accumulation and DHA may ameliorate this adverse effect.

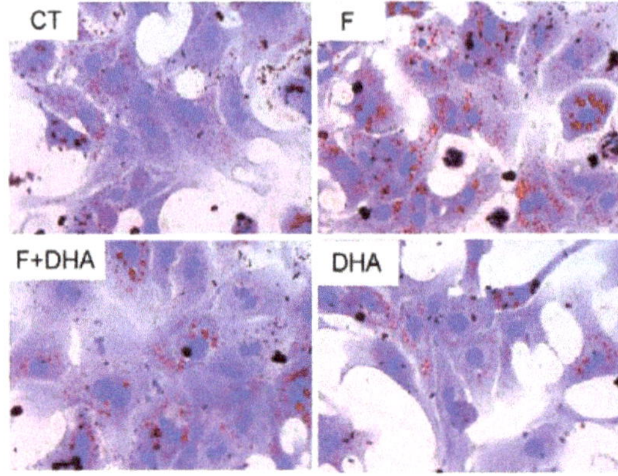

Figure 1. DHA ameliorates fructose induced TG accumulation in primary mouse hepatocytes Oil Red O staining. Original magnification: ×400; CT: control; F: fructose; F + DHA: fructose plus DHA.

3.2. DHA Attenuates Fructose-Induced Hepatic Steatosis Involving Changes in Expressions of Genes Related to Lipid Metabolism

To investigate the molecular basis for DHA preventing fructose-induced hepatic steatosis, we examined the expression of several genes involved in hepatic lipid metabolism using quantitative Real-Time PCR. The genes responsible for *de novo* lipogenesis, including *FAS* and *ACC*, were significantly up-regulated in the fructose treatment group (Figure 2A,B). Meanwhile, the other genes related to fatty acid oxidation, such as *CPT-1α* and *ACOX1* remained unchanged compared with control (Figure 2C,D). However, the DHA treatment group showed no significant increase of *FAS* and *ACC* expression compared with control (Figure 2A,B). In contrast, an upregulation of *CPT-1α* and *ACOX1* was observed in the DHA treatment groups (Figure 2C,D). These findings suggest that the ameliorating effect of DHA on fructose-induced hepatic steatosis was attributed to the increase in fatty acid oxidation and decrease in *de novo* lipogenesis.

3.3. ER Stress Pathways Mediates Fructose-Induced Lipid Accumulation

To test whether fructose triggered ER stress in hepatocytes, cells were treated with 2 μg/mL tunicamycin (TM), or pretreated with 2 mM 4-phenylbutyric acid for 1 h, and then incubated with 12.5 mM fructose (F + PBA) for 24 h respectively. Oil Red O staining showed increased TG accumulation in hepatocytes with treatment of fructose or the ER stress inducer TM. Interestingly, pretreatment with the ER stress inhibitor significantly decreased TG accumulation (Figure 3). Next, we investigated changes of mRNA levels of lipid homeostasis-related genes in response to ER stress. As illustrated in Figure 4A,B, compared with the control group, fructose and TM treatment increased the mRNA levels of *FAS* and *ACC*. However, pretreatment with the ER stress inhibitor PBA prevented these changes (Figure 4A,B). TM treatment significantly up-regulated *CPT-1α* and *ACOX1* expressions, but no changes were seen in the fructose treatment group and PBA pretreatment group (Figure 4C,D). Together, these findings suggest that fructose-induced hepatic steatosis is mediated by triggering the ER stress response.

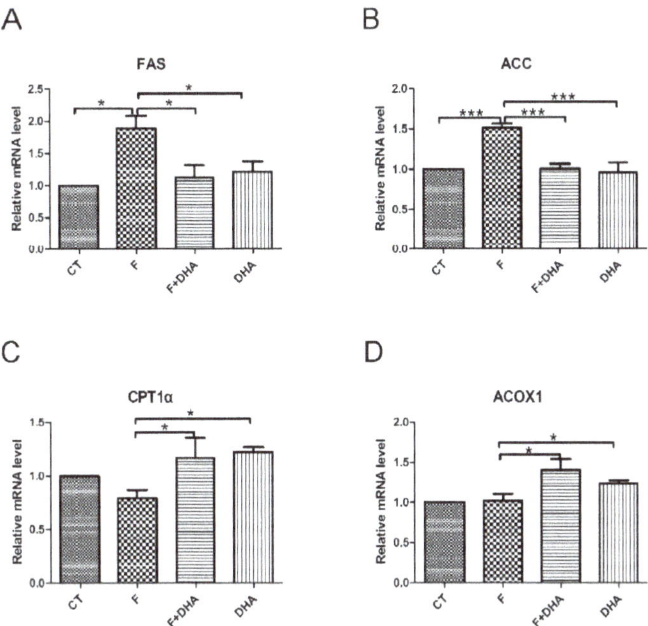

Figure 2. DHA regulates the expressions of genes involved in hepatic lipid metabolism. CT: control; F: fructose; F + DHA: fructose plus DHA. Expression values were normalized to control group. Data are expressed as mean ± SEM (n = 4). Data of the four groups were compared by ANOVA with LSD's test (* $p < 0.05$).

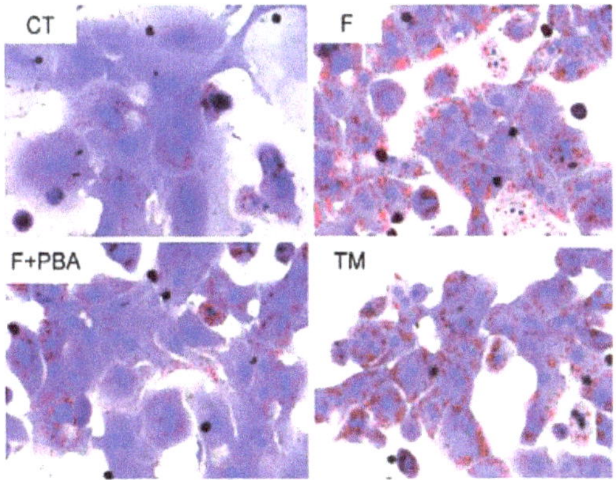

Figure 3. Effect of ER stress response on TG accumulation in primary mouse hepatocytes by treatment with ER stress inhibitor PBA or ER stress inducer TM. Oil Red O staining. Original magnification: ×400; CT: control; F: fructose; F + PBA: fructose plus PBA pretreatment; TM: tunicamycin.

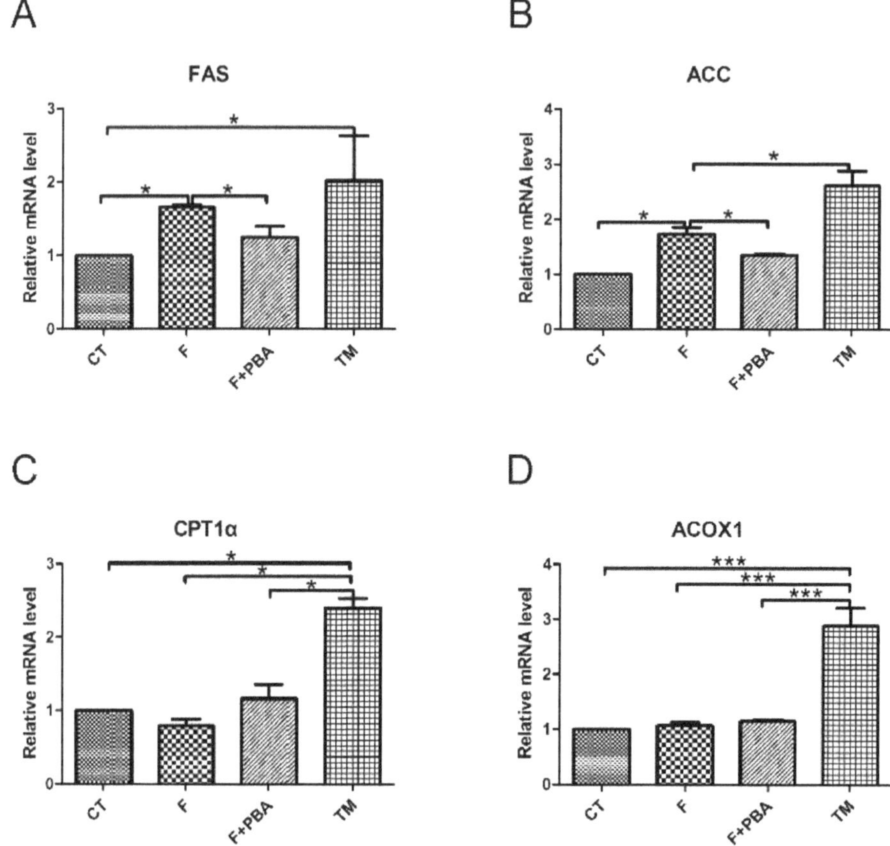

Figure 4. ER stress response mediated hepatic steatosis. CT: control; F: fructose; F + PBA: fructose plus PBA pretreatment; TM: tunicamycin. Expression values were normalized to control group. Data are expressed as mean ± SEM (n = 4). Data of the four groups were compared by ANOVA with LSD's test (* $p < 0.05$, *** $p < 0.001$).

3.4. ER Stress Response Is Involved in the Protective Effects of DHA against Fructose-Induced Hepatic Steatosis

To further delineate the protective role of DHA in fructose-induced ER stress response and hepatic steatosis, we examined the changes of markers in the ER stress-activated unfolded protein response (UPR) pathways. Firstly, we examined the effects of DHA on chaperone expression using real-time PCR. The results indicated that DHA or PBA treatment significantly decreased fructose-induced upregulation of GRP78 in primary hepatocytes (Figure 5A). The reduction of GRP78 expression was further confirmed by Western blot (Figure 5B,C). Additionally, one of the markers of ER membrane protein IRE1α and its phosphorylated form p-IRE1α were drastically increased by fructose or TM treatment. However, both DHA and PBA prevented these changes (Figure 5B,D,E). The mRNA levels of X-box binding protein 1 (*XBP-1*) and C/EBP homologous protein (*CHOP*) were significantly elevated by fructose and TM treatment, whereas transcription factor *C/EBPα* mRNA level was not significantly up-regulated compared with DHA or PBA treatment (Figure 5F–H). These results suggest that DHA may alleviate the fructose-induced ER stress response in primary hepatocytes.

Next, we investigated whether DHA could affect the expression levels of hepatic lipid-homeostasis regulators using Western blot analysis or quantitative real-time PCR. First, we detected expression levels of some nuclear transcription factors which control hepatic *de novo* lipogenesis. As shown in Figure 6, the fructose-induced upregulation of liver X receptor (LXR) was suppressed by DHA treatment (Figure 6C). Both DHA and PBA treatment significantly decreased fructose-induced sterol-regulatory element-binding protein 1 (SREBP-1c) and carbohydrate responsive element binding protein (ChREBP) expression (Figure 6A,B,G). We next assessed the levels of ACC and ACOX1 which receive regulation from the above mentioned nuclear transcription factors. A decrease in ACC protein level was observed in cells treated with DHA or PBA (Figure 6E); however, ACOX1 levels were elevated in these groups (Figure 6F). Taken together, these findings indicate that DHA ameliorates fructose-induced hepatic steatosis by alleviating the ER stress response.

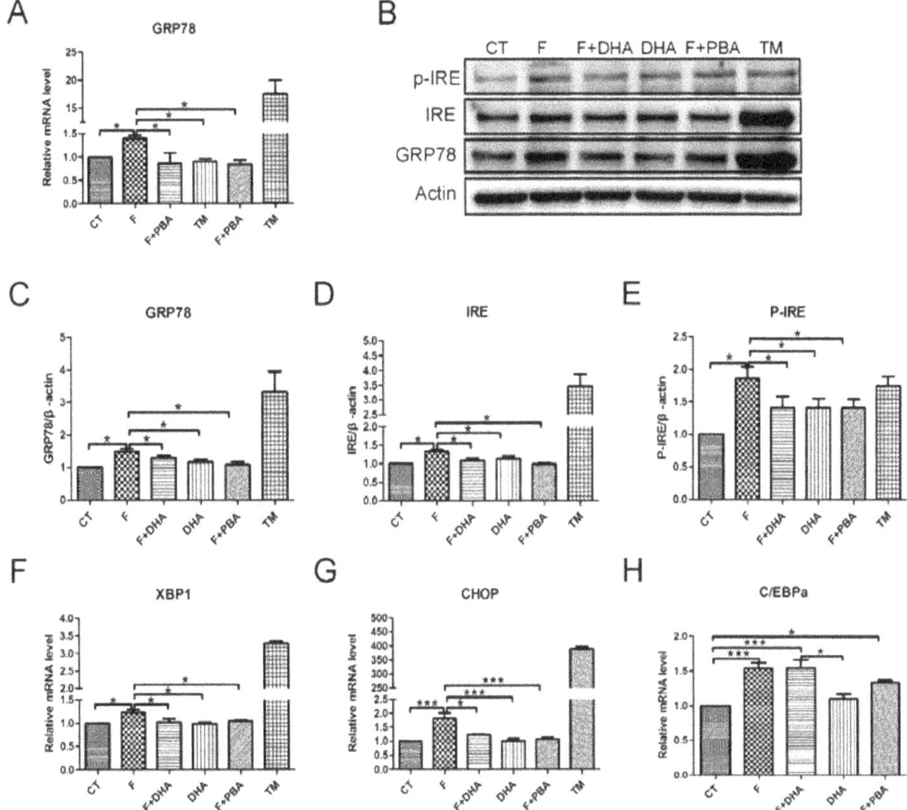

Figure 5. DHA alleviated fructose-induced ER stress response in primary mouse hepatocytes. CT: control; F: fructose; F + DHA: fructose plus DHA; F + PBA: fructose plus PBA pretreatment; TM: tunicamycin. Data are expressed as mean ± SEM (n = 4). Data of five groups were compared by ANOVA with LSD's test (* $p < 0.05$, *** $p < 0.001$).

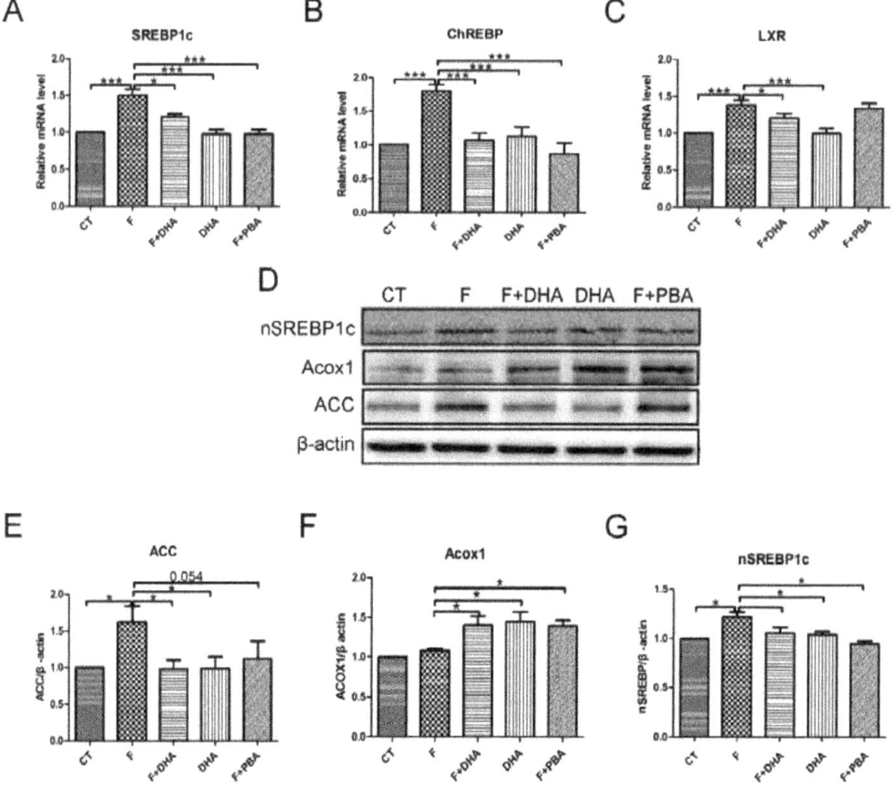

Figure 6. DHA selectively regulated gene expression related to lipid-homeostasis in primary mouse hepatocytes. CT: control; F: fructose; F + DHA: fructose plus DHA; F + PBA: fructose plus PBA pretreatment. Data are expressed as mean ± SEM (n = 4). Data of five groups were compared by ANOVA with LSD's test (* $p < 0.05$, *** $p < 0.001$).

4. Discussion

Recent epidemiological and animals studies have strongly certified that the overconsumption of fructose is involved in the development of NAFLD [10–12]. Due to the relatively slow rate of progression from mild nonalcoholic fatty liver to more severe hepatitis or fibrosis and lack of approved pharmacotherapy for NAFLD [30], we have the opportunity to take some measurements to prevent the progression of NAFLD. Previous studies have shown that supplementation of DHA and EPA-rich fish oil has a beneficial effect on hepatic lipid metabolism [20,21]. Therefore, we speculate that DHA may have a therapeutic effect on fructose-induced hepatic steatosis.

In the present study, we demonstrated that fructose treatment of primary mouse hepatocytes induced an obvious hepatic steatosis observed by Oil Red O staining. This effect is attributable in part to its upregulation of lipid-related genes such as ACC and stearoyl-CoA desaturase (SCD) causing the ER stress response. The supplementation of DHA can prevent the adverse metabolic effects caused by fructose treatment. In addition, the fructose-provoked ER stress response was also inhibited by DHA. Taking together, these findings support the notion that DHA can ameliorate fructose-induced hepatic lipid accumulation through alleviating ER stress response.

NAFLD is characterized by increased triglyceride in the liver. The accumulation of hepatic lipid is attributed to increased *de novo* lipogenesis, increased fatty acid uptake, or reduced fatty acid oxidation [31]. In the current study, primary hepatocytes treated with fructose shown enhanced *de novo* lipogenesis, which is consistent with previous reports [10–12]. Some studies suggested that the lipogenic enzymes such as FAS and ACC were significantly up-regulated in fructose solution fed mice, which play important roles during hepatic *de novo* lipogenesis [17,32]. Moreover, fructose feeding increases the binding of LXR to the SREBP-1c promoter [33]. LXR is highly expressed in the liver, which induces SREBP-1c, FAS, ACC and SCD-1 transcription. Interestingly, ChREBP is also a direct target of LXR, which was found to be elevated in fructose treated hepatocytes. In the present study, DHA significantly reduced the expression levels of these key transcription factors and target enzymes in primary mouse hepatocytes, which is consistent with previous studies with fructose or fish oil feeding [20,34]. Another important finding was that DHA might ameliorate fructose-induced TG accumulation through increasing fatty acid oxidation. Hepatic *de novo* lipogenesis is considered to have an indirect effect on the increased levels of malonyl-CoA, which decreases the amount of fatty acid entering the mitochondria via restraining carnitine palmitoyltransferase 1 (CPT1) [35]. CPT1 is a rate-limiting enzyme of β-oxidation in the liver, which is necessary for long chain fatty acid entry into mitochondria for β-oxidation [36]. The current study found that the expression of CPT1 was significantly increased upon DHA treatment. Similarly, DHA elevates the expression of acyl-CoA oxidase 1 (ACOX1), an enzyme responsible for catalyzing peroxisomal β-oxidation of fatty acids. It seems that these results are due to the nuclear transcription factor activation by DHA as a PPARα ligand [37]. This findings further support the idea that DHA exerts its protective effects on fructose-induced hepatic steatosis through reducing key lipogenic enzymes expression and increasing fatty acid oxidation in hepatocytes.

Recently, ER stress response signaling has been tightly linked to hepatic lipid metabolism, insulin action, inflammation and apoptosis [26,27,38–40]. Previous studies showed that liver-specific IRE1α deletion and ATF6 knockout mice developed serious hepatic steatosis upon pharmacological ER stress [39,40]. Transcription factor XBP1 is a key regulator of the mammalian ER stress response as a downstream target of phosphorylated IRE1α. Moreover, it is implicated that XBP1 regulates hepatic lipogenesis unrelated to its role in the ER stress response [38]. Here, we found that fructose treatment caused the ER stress response in primary hepatocytes as evidenced by improved expression of ER membrane chaperone GRP78. One of the three ER-localized proteins IRE1α, and its activated form p-IRE1α were increased in fructose-treated hepatocytes. We found that DHA can alleviate the fructose-induced ER stress response as evidenced by down-regulation of the ER stress marker GRP78 and total IREα or p-IREα. This preventive effect of DHA was further proven by using ER stress inhibiter PBA and inducer TM. It has been demonstrated that TM induced pharmacological ER stress rapidly caused hepatic steatosis [41]; However, PBA alleviates ER stress in obese ob/ob mice and prevents hepatic TG accumulation [42,43]. This study confirms that DHA serves as an important dietary factor for NAFLD prevention and treatment. The protective effects are attributable, at least in part, to its roles of ER stress alleviation. All three unfolded protein response sensors, IRE1α, PERK and ATF6 are considered to play roles in lipid storage in the liver. In the current study, we found total IRE1α or p-IRE1α were upregulated by fructose. Activation of p-IRE1α promotes the splicing of *XBP-1* mRNA and subsequently produces a potent transcriptional activator. The current study was unable to evaluate the formation of XBP-1s, however, we indeed found that the XBP-1 mRNA level was upregulated upon fructose treatment. It is therefore likely that a sustained ER stress response exists, since the spliced form of XBP-1 can keep activating transcription by autoregulating its own transcription as far as IRE1α is activated [44]. The level changes of another downstream protein—CHOP, are similar to that of XBP-1. CHOP is a member of C/EBP family of transcriptional factors, and has been proposed to be a dominant-negative regulator of their function. Previous study suggests unresolved ER stress response will lead to suppression of *C/EBPα* partially through CHOP [27]. One limitation of this current investigation lies in the fact that we did not analyze the causative effects of DHA on ER stress response signaling pathways, and specifically what is the signal involved in DHA ameliorating fructose-induced hepatic steatosis. The results of this study do not explain the hierarchy of genetic regulation downstream of DHA treatment. Further studies on the current topic are therefore recommended.

In summary, the present study contributed to the existing knowledge that DHA prevents fructose-induced hepatic lipogenesis and accelerates fatty acid oxidation. The protective effect appears to be mediated through alleviating fructose-evoked ER stress response.

5. Conclusions

Increasing sugar consumption leads to higher fructose intakes, which is considered to be a risk factor for developing NAFLD. Therefore, life style changes and optimal dietary intervention beneficial to NAFLD are necessary. The present study confirms previous findings and contributes additional evidence that DHA ameliorates fructose-induced TG accumulation by preventing hepatic lipogenesis and enhancing fatty acid oxidation. More research is needed for better understanding the ER stress response signaling involved in these process. As a major ingredient in fish oil, DHA may have a therapeutic potential in the prevention and treatment of NAFLD.

Acknowledgments: This study was supported by grants from National Natural Science Foundation of China (Grant number: 81270947 and 81570763) and National Key Basic Research Development program (Grant number: 2012CB517505) to Xiaoqiu Xiao We also thank Richa Goswami for her careful reading and editorial corrections for this manuscript.

Author Contributions: Jinying Zheng, Chuan Peng, Xiaoqiu Xiao and Jibin Li conceived and designed the experiments; Jinying Zheng, Yanbiao Ai and Heng Wang performed the experiments; Jinying Zheng, Chuan Peng, Xiaoqiu Xiao and Jibin Li analyzed the data; Jinying Zheng, Xiaoqiu Xiao and Jibin Li wrote the paper. All authors read and approved the final manuscript.

Conflicts of Interest: The authors declare no conflict of interest.

References

1. Amarapurkar, D.N.; Hashimoto, E.; Lesmana, L.A.; Sollano, J.D.; Chen, P.J.; Goh, K.L. How common is non-alcoholic fatty liver disease in the Asia-Pacific region and are there local differences? *J. Gastroenterol. Hepatol.* **2007**, *22*, 788–793. [CrossRef] [PubMed]
2. Fung, J.; Lee, C.K.; Chan, M.; Seto, W.K.; Lai, C.L.; Yuen, M.F. High prevalence of non-alcoholic fatty liver disease in the Chinese—Results from the Hong Kong liver health census. *Liver Int.* **2015**, *35*, 542–549. [CrossRef] [PubMed]
3. Farrell, G.C.; Larter, C.Z. Nonalcoholic fatty liver disease: From steatosis to cirrhosis. *Hepatology* **2006**, *43*, S99–S112. [CrossRef] [PubMed]
4. Moschen, A.R.; Kaser, S.; Tilg, H. Non-alcoholic steatohepatitis: A microbiota-driven disease. *Trends Endocrinol. Metab.* **2013**, *24*, 537–545. [CrossRef] [PubMed]
5. Fabbrini, E.; Sullivan, S.; Klein, S. Obesity and nonalcoholic fatty liver disease: Biochemical, metabolic, and clinical implications. *Hepatology* **2010**, *51*, 679–689. [CrossRef] [PubMed]
6. Postic, C.; Girard, J. Contribution of de novo fatty acid synthesis to hepatic steatosis and insulin resistance: Lessons from genetically engineered mice. *J. Clin. Investig.* **2008**, *118*, 829–838. [CrossRef] [PubMed]
7. Fan, J.G.; Saibara, T.; Chitturi, S.; Kim, B.I.; Sung, J.J.; Chutaputti, A. What are the risk factors and settings for non-alcoholic fatty liver disease in Asia-Pacific? *J. Gastroenterol. Hepatol.* **2007**, *22*, 794–800. [CrossRef] [PubMed]
8. Basaranoglu, M.; Basaranoglu, G.; Sabuncu, T.; Senturk, H. Fructose as a key player in the development of fatty liver disease. *World J. Gastroenterol.* **2013**, *19*, 1166–1172. [CrossRef] [PubMed]
9. Kelishadi, R.; Mansourian, M.; Heidari-Beni, M. Association of fructose consumption and components of metabolic syndrome in human studies: A systematic review and meta-analysis. *Nutrition* **2014**, *30*, 503–510. [CrossRef] [PubMed]
10. Ouyang, X.; Cirillo, P.; Sautin, Y.; McCall, S.; Bruchette, J.L.; Diehl, A.M.; Johnson, R.J.; Abdelmalek, M.F. Fructose consumption as a risk factor for non-alcoholic fatty liver disease. *J. Hepatol.* **2008**, *48*, 993–999. [CrossRef] [PubMed]

11. Zelber-Sagi, S.; Nitzan-Kaluski, D.; Goldsmith, R.; Webb, M.; Blendis, L.; Halpern, Z.; Oren, R. Long term nutritional intake and the risk for non-alcoholic fatty liver disease (NAFLD): A population based study. *J. Hepatol.* **2007**, *47*, 711–717. [CrossRef] [PubMed]
12. Abdelmalek, M.F.; Suzuki, A.; Guy, C.; Unalp-Arida, A.; Colvin, R.; Johnson, R.J.; Diehl, A.M. Increased fructose consumption is associated with fibrosis severity in patients with nonalcoholic fatty liver disease. *Hepatology* **2010**, *51*, 1961–1971. [CrossRef] [PubMed]
13. Stanhope, K.L.; Schwarz, J.M.; Keim, N.L.; Griffen, S.C.; Bremer, A.A.; Graham, J.L.; Hatcher, B.; Cox, C.L.; Dyachenko, A.; Zhang, W.; *et al.* Consuming fructose-sweetened, not glucose-sweetened, beverages increases visceral adiposity and lipids and decreases insulin sensitivity in overweight/obese humans. *J. Clin. Investig.* **2009**, *119*, 1322–1334. [CrossRef] [PubMed]
14. Parks, E.J.; Skokan, L.E.; Timlin, M.T.; Dingfelder, C.S. Dietary sugars stimulate fatty acid synthesis in adults. *J. Nutr.* **2008**, *138*, 1039–1046. [PubMed]
15. Chong, M.F.; Fielding, B.A.; Frayn, K.N. Mechanisms for the acute effect of fructose on postprandial lipemia. *Am. J. Clin. Nutr.* **2007**, *85*, 1511–1520. [PubMed]
16. Kawasaki, T.; Igarashi, K.; Koeda, T.; Sugimoto, K.; Nakagawa, K.; Hayashi, S.; Yamaji, R.; Inui, H.; Fukusato, T.; Yamanouchi, T. Rats fed fructose-enriched diets have characteristics of nonalcoholic hepatic steatosis. *J. Nutr.* **2009**, *139*, 2067–2071. [CrossRef] [PubMed]
17. Nomura, K.; Yamanouchi, T. The role of fructose-enriched diets in mechanisms of nonalcoholic fatty liver disease. *J. Nutr. Biochem.* **2012**, *23*, 203–208. [CrossRef] [PubMed]
18. Rossmeisl, M.; Jilkova, Z.M.; Kuda, O.; Jelenik, T.; Medrikova, D.; Stankova, B.; Kristinsson, B.; Haraldsson, G.G.; Svensen, H.; Stoknes, I.; *et al.* Metabolic effects of *n*-3 PUFA as phospholipids are superior to triglycerides in mice fed a high-fat diet: Possible role of endocannabinoids. *PLoS ONE* **2012**, *7*, e38834. [CrossRef] [PubMed]
19. Itariu, B.K.; Zeyda, M.; Hochbrugger, E.E.; Neuhofer, A.; Prager, G.; Schindler, K.; Bohdjalian, A.; Mascher, D.; Vangala, S.; Schranz, M.; *et al.* Long-chain *n*-3 PUFAs reduce adipose tissue and systemic inflammation in severely obese nondiabetic patients: A randomized controlled trial. *Am. J. Clin. Nutr.* **2012**, *96*, 1137–1149. [CrossRef] [PubMed]
20. De Castro, G.S.; Deminice, R.; Simoes-Ambrosio, L.M.; Calder, P.C.; Jordao, A.A.; Vannucchi, H. Dietary docosahexaenoic acid and eicosapentaenoic acid influence liver triacylglycerol and insulin resistance in rats fed a high-fructose diet. *Mar. Drugs* **2015**, *13*, 1864–1881. [CrossRef] [PubMed]
21. Devarshi, P.P.; Jangale, N.M.; Ghule, A.E.; Bodhankar, S.L.; Harsulkar, A.M. Beneficial effects of flaxseed oil and fish oil diet are through modulation of different hepatic genes involved in lipid metabolism in streptozotocin-nicotinamide induced diabetic rats. *Genes Nutr.* **2013**, *8*, 329–342. [CrossRef] [PubMed]
22. Sekiya, M.; Yahagi, N.; Matsuzaka, T.; Najima, Y.; Nakakuki, M.; Nagai, R.; Ishibashi, S.; Osuga, J.; Yamada, N.; Shimano, H. Polyunsaturated fatty acids ameliorate hepatic steatosis in obese mice by SREBP-1 suppression. *Hepatology* **2003**, *38*, 1529–1539. [CrossRef] [PubMed]
23. Shapiro, H.; Tehilla, M.; Attal-Singer, J.; Bruck, R.; Luzzatti, R.; Singer, P. The therapeutic potential of long-chain omega-3 fatty acids in nonalcoholic fatty liver disease. *Clin. Nutr.* **2011**, *30*, 6–19. [CrossRef] [PubMed]
24. Agrawal, R.; Gomez-Pinilla, F. "Metabolic syndrome" in the brain: Deficiency in omega-3 fatty acid exacerbates dysfunctions in insulin receptor signalling and cognition. *J. Physiol.* **2012**, *590*, 2485–2499. [CrossRef] [PubMed]
25. Gonzalez-Periz, A.; Horrillo, R.; Ferre, N.; Gronert, K.; Dong, B.; Moran-Salvador, E.; Titos, E.; Martinez-Clemente, M.; Lopez-Parra, M.; Arroyo, V.; *et al.* Obesity-induced insulin resistance and hepatic steatosis are alleviated by omega-3 fatty acids: A role for resolvins and protectins. *FASEB J.* **2009**, *23*, 1946–1957. [CrossRef] [PubMed]
26. Oyadomari, S.; Harding, H.P.; Zhang, Y.; Oyadomari, M.; Ron, D. Dephosphorylation of translation initiation factor 2α enhances glucose tolerance and attenuates hepatosteatosis in mice. *Cell Metab.* **2008**, *7*, 520–532. [CrossRef] [PubMed]
27. Rutkowski, D.T.; Wu, J.; Back, S.H.; Callaghan, M.U.; Ferris, S.P.; Iqbal, J.; Clark, R.; Miao, H.; Hassler, J.R.; Fornek, J.; *et al.* UPR pathways combine to prevent hepatic steatosis caused by ER stress-mediated suppression of transcriptional master regulators. *Dev. Cell* **2008**, *15*, 829–840. [CrossRef] [PubMed]

28. Ren, L.P.; Chan, S.M.; Zeng, X.Y.; Laybutt, D.R.; Iseli, T.J.; Sun, R.Q.; Kraegen, E.W.; Cooney, G.J.; Turner, N.; Ye, J.M. Differing endoplasmic reticulum stress response to excess lipogenesis *versus* lipid oversupply in relation to hepatic steatosis and insulin resistance. *PLoS ONE* **2012**, *7*, e30816. [CrossRef] [PubMed]
29. Severgnini, M.; Sherman, J.; Sehgal, A.; Jayaprakash, N.K.; Aubin, J.; Wang, G.; Zhang, L.; Peng, C.G.; Yucius, K.; Butler, J.; *et al.* A rapid two-step method for isolation of functional primary mouse hepatocytes: Cell characterization and asialoglycoprotein receptor based assay development. *Cytotechnology* **2012**, *64*, 187–195. [CrossRef] [PubMed]
30. Ahmed, M.H.; Abu, E.O.; Byrne, C.D. Non-Alcoholic Fatty Liver Disease (NAFLD): New challenge for general practitioners and important burden for health authorities? *Prim. Care Diabetes* **2010**, *4*, 129–137. [CrossRef] [PubMed]
31. Koo, S.H. Nonalcoholic fatty liver disease: Molecular mechanisms for the hepatic steatosis. *Clin. Mol. Hepatol.* **2013**, *19*, 210–215. [CrossRef] [PubMed]
32. Rodriguez-Calvo, R.; Barroso, E.; Serrano, L.; Coll, T.; Sanchez, R.M.; Merlos, M.; Palomer, X.; Laguna, J.C.; Vazquez-Carrera, M. Atorvastatin prevents carbohydrate response element binding protein activation in the fructose-fed rat by activating protein kinase A. *Hepatology* **2009**, *49*, 106–115. [CrossRef] [PubMed]
33. Nagai, Y.; Yonemitsu, S.; Erion, D.M.; Iwasaki, T.; Stark, R.; Weismann, D.; Dong, J.; Zhang, D.; Jurczak, M.J.; Loffler, M.G.; *et al.* The role of peroxisome proliferator-activated receptor gamma coactivator-1 beta in the pathogenesis of fructose-induced insulin resistance. *Cell Metab.* **2009**, *9*, 252–264. [CrossRef] [PubMed]
34. Nakatani, T.; Katsumata, A.; Miura, S.; Kamei, Y.; Ezaki, O. Effects of fish oil feeding and fasting on LXRalpha/RXRalpha binding to LXRE in the SREBP-1c promoter in mouse liver. *Biochim. Biophys. Acta* **2005**, *1736*, 77–86. [PubMed]
35. McGarry, J.D. Malonyl-CoA and carnitine palmitoyltransferase I: An expanding partnership. *Biochem. Soc. Trans.* **1995**, *23*, 481–485. [CrossRef] [PubMed]
36. Brown, N.F.; Weis, B.C.; Husti, J.E.; Foster, D.W.; McGarry, J.D. Mitochondrial carnitine palmitoyltransferase I isoform switching in the developing rat heart. *J. Biol. Chem.* **1995**, *270*, 8952–8957. [CrossRef] [PubMed]
37. Pan, D.A.; Mater, M.K.; Thelen, A.P.; Peters, J.M.; Gonzalez, F.J.; Jump, D.B. Evidence against the peroxisome proliferator-activated receptor alpha (PPARalpha) as the mediator for polyunsaturated fatty acid suppression of hepatic L-pyruvate kinase gene transcription. *J. Lipid Res.* **2000**, *41*, 742–751. [PubMed]
38. Lee, A.H.; Scapa, E.F.; Cohen, D.E.; Glimcher, L.H. Regulation of hepatic lipogenesis by the transcription factor XBP1. *Science* **2008**, *320*, 1492–1496. [CrossRef] [PubMed]
39. Zhang, K.; Wang, S.; Malhotra, J.; Hassler, J.R.; Back, S.H.; Wang, G.; Chang, L.; Xu, W.; Miao, H.; Leonardi, R.; *et al.* The unfolded protein response transducer IRE1alpha prevents ER stress-induced hepatic steatosis. *EMBO J.* **2011**, *30*, 1357–1375. [CrossRef] [PubMed]
40. Yamamoto, K.; Takahara, K.; Oyadomari, S.; Okada, T.; Sato, T.; Harada, A.; Mori, K. Induction of liver steatosis and lipid droplet formation in ATF6alpha-knockout mice burdened with pharmacological endoplasmic reticulum stress. *Mol. Biol. Cell* **2010**, *21*, 2975–2986. [CrossRef] [PubMed]
41. Lee, J.S.; Zheng, Z.; Mendez, R.; Ha, S.W.; Xie, Y.; Zhang, K. Pharmacologic ER stress induces non-alcoholic steatohepatitis in an animal model. *Toxicol. Lett.* **2012**, *211*, 29–38. [CrossRef] [PubMed]
42. Ozcan, L.; Ergin, A.S.; Lu, A.; Chung, J.; Sarkar, S.; Nie, D.; Myers, M.G., Jr.; Ozcan, U. Endoplasmic reticulum stress plays a central role in development of leptin resistance. *Cell Metab.* **2009**, *9*, 35–51. [CrossRef] [PubMed]
43. Zhang, C.; Chen, X.; Zhu, R.M.; Zhang, Y.; Yu, T.; Wang, H.; Zhao, H.; Zhao, M.; Ji, Y.L.; Chen, Y.H.; *et al.* Endoplasmic reticulum stress is involved in hepatic SREBP-1c activation and lipid accumulation in fructose-fed mice. *Toxicol. Lett.* **2012**, *212*, 229–240. [CrossRef] [PubMed]
44. Yoshida, H.; Matsui, T.; Yamamoto, A.; Okada, T.; Mori, K. XBP1 mRNA is induced by ATF6 and spliced by IRE1 in response to ER stress to produce a highly active transcription factor. *Cell* **2001**, *107*, 881–891. [CrossRef]

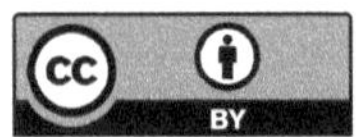

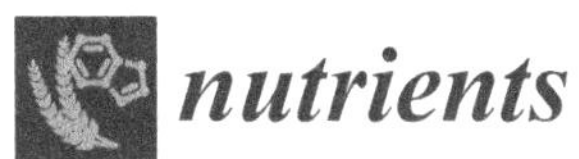

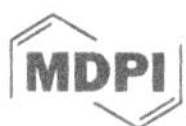

Article

Fish, Long-Chain *n*-3 PUFA and Incidence of Elevated Blood Pressure: A Meta-Analysis of Prospective Cohort Studies

Bo Yang [1], Mei-Qi Shi [2], Zi-Hao Li [1], Jian-Jun Yang [2] and Duo Li [1,*]

[1] Department of Food Science and Nutrition, Zhejiang University, Hangzhou 310058, China; ybzju@zju.edu.cn (B.Y.); 21513038@zju.edu.cn (Z.-H.L.)

[2] School of Public Health, Ningxia Medical University, Yinchuan 750004, China; shimeiqi@zju.edu.cn (M.-Q.S.); yangjianjun_1970@163.com (J.-J.Y.)

* Correspondence: duoli@zju.edu.cn; Tel.: +86-571-8898-2024

Received: 11 November 2015; Accepted: 24 December 2015; Published: 21 January 2016

Abstract: Results from prospective cohort studies on fish or long-chain (LC) *n*-3 polyunsaturated fatty acid (PUFA) intake and elevated blood pressure (EBP) are inconsistent. We aimed to investigate the summary effects. Pertinent studies were identified from PubMed and EMBASE database through October 2015. Multivariate-adjusted risk ratios (RRs) for incidence of EBP in the highest verses the bottom category of baseline intake of fish or LC *n*-3 PUFA were pooled using a random-effects meta-analysis. Over the follow-up ranging from 3 to 20 years, 20,497 EBP events occurred among 56,204 adults from eight prospective cohort studies. The summary RR (SRR) was 0.96 (95% CI: 0.81, 1.14; I^2 = 44.70%) for fish in four studies, and 0.73 (95% CI: 0.60, 0.89; I^2 = 75.00%) for LC *n*-3 PUFA in six studies (three studies for biomarker vs. three studies for diet). Circulating LC *n*-3 PUFA as biomarker was inversely associated with incidence of EBP (SRR: 0.67; 95% CI: 0.55, 0.83), especially docosahexaenoic acid (SRR: 0.64; 95% CI: 0.45, 0.88), whereas no significant association was found for dietary intake (SRR: 0.80; 95% CI: 0.58, 1.10). The present finding suggests that increased intake of docosahexaenoic acid to improve its circulating levels may benefit primary prevention of EBP.

Keywords: fish; *n*-3 PUFA; blood pressure; meta-analysis

1. Introduction

Elevated blood pressure (BP) has been known to be a strong modifiable risk factor for stroke, coronary heart disease (CHD), and early mortality worldwide [1,2]. Fish consumption plays an important role in the modulation of BP in hypertensive and normotensive adults [3–5]. Long-chain (LC) *n*-3 polyunsaturated fatty acid (PUFA), including 20:5*n*-3 (eicosapentaenoic acid, EPA), 22:5*n*-3 (docosapentaenoic acid, DPA) and 22:6*n*-3 (docosahexaenoic acid, DHA), are mainly found in fish and other marine products. Four previous meta-analyses of clinical trials showed that fish oil or LC *n*-3 PUFA supplements can dose-dependently lower BP in hypertensive patients but not in normotensive individuals [6–9]. However, investigations using animal models have shown that diets enriched in *n*-3 PUFA can protect against induced BP elevations [10,11], and dietary deficiency of *n*-3 PUFA in young rats was associated with development of hypertension in later life [12]. Some observational studies have reported that an inverse association between fish or LC *n*-3 PUFA consumption and BP elevations in normotensive participants [13–15], while others found no association [16,17]. Most observational studies use dietary questionnaires to estimate intake, which is generally a poor reflection of the usual intake of an individual. Typical fish consumption in the US and Europe is relatively low and makes it difficult to identify associations. In addition, hypertensive individuals who changed their dietary habit after the diagnosis may not have been excluded from study populations, which may also bias benefit for BP towards null.

Circulating levels of 20:5n-3 and 22:6n-3 were strongly correlated with fish or fish oil consumption, whereas 22:5n-3 was elongated from and retroconverted to 20:5n-3. In contrast to dietary estimations, circulating levels of LC n-3 PUFA as biomarker can objectively reflect both dietary consumption and biologically relevant processes. Numerous studies on diet or biomarkers of LC n-3 PUFA and BP have been cross-sectional or case-control designs, rather than prospective cohort studies. The potential for dietary change secondary to the diagnosis of high BP can be minimized in prospective cohort studies, due to exclusion of individuals with known hypertension at baseline. Nevertheless, results from prospective cohort studies of fish or LC n-3 PUFA consumption in relation to elevated BP remain inconsistent [16,18–20]. Thus, whether fish or LC n-3 PUFA intake is associated with reduced risk of elevated BP in normotensive populations is still unclear. The aim of the present systematic review and meta-analysis was to quantitatively evaluate associations between fish or LC n-3 PUFA intake (diet *vs.* biomarker) and incidence of elevated BP with available data from prospective cohort studies. We hypothesized that LC n-3 PUFA intake is inversely associated with incidence of EBP, especially 22:6n-3.

2. Methods

2.1. Literature Research

Systematic literature searches were conducted to identify prospective cohort studies of fish or LC n-3 PUFA with risk of elevated BP from EMBASE, the Cochrane Library and PubMed up to October 2015, respectively. The full details are presented in the supplementary online-data. Our search was restricted to human studies that were published in English, and duplicated studies were excluded. Authors were not contacted for the detailed information of primary studies and unpublished studies. We searched systematic reviews from the above-mentioned database, and checked the reference lists to identify publications that might have been missed.

2.2. Eligibility Criteria

The relevant studies were included if they met the following inclusion criteria: (1) Participants: Adults of any age located in different countries; (2) Exposure of interest: Assessment of fish or LC n-3 PUFA intake, and quantitative determination of total or individual (20:5n-3, 22:5n-3 and 22:6n-3) in circulating blood (serum/plasma/whole blood/erythrocytes); (3) Outcomes: Evaluation of elevated BP based on a BP cutoff value (systolic BP (SBP) $\geqslant$ 130 mm Hg and (or) diastolic BP (DBP) $\geqslant$ 85 mm Hg) or hypertension (SBP $\geqslant$ 140 mm Hg and (or) DBP $\geqslant$ 90 mm Hg), and reporting multivariate-adjusted relative risk (RR) with 95% confidence intervals (CI); and (4) Study design: prospective cohort study (cohort, nested case-control, and case-cohort study).

2.3. Data Extraction

Data extraction was completed independently and performed twice by two investigators, and disagreements were reconciled by consensus. The following data was extracted from each publication: participant characteristics (baseline age range, gender and countries), duration of follow-up, baseline fish consumption or LC n-3 PUFA intake as exposure of interest, exposure measurement (dietary estimations or laboratory analyses), exposure source (diet or biomarker) and multivariate-adjusted RR with 95% CI for all categories of fish or LC n-3 PUFA (diet or biomarker) and multiple adjustment for potential covariates.

Odds ratios (OR) in nested case-control studies were regarded as RR directly. If eligible studies reported hazard ratio (HR) with 95% CI, each HR was assumed to approximate RR. To standardize units of fish intake, we first converted frequency into grams per day (g/day). The amount of fish consumption (g/day) was estimated by multiplying the frequency of consumption (servings per day) by the corresponding portion size (grams per serving). If a publication reported servings per day as unit of measure in fish consumption, we transferred the fish amount to grams according to descriptions of the publication. If no description of portion size was reported, we deemed it to be 105 grams per serving [21]. We also defined LC n-3 PUFA as the sum of 22:6n-3, 22:5n-3, and 20:5n-3. If a publication reported individual LC n-3 PUFA as interest exposure only, RR for individual LC n-3 PUFA can be combined to approximately represent RR for total LC n-3 PUFA in the publication using a fixed effect model. In addition, if the individual study only reported RR based on gender (male *vs.* female), age (middle *vs.* elderly), or ethnic classifications (white *vs.* black), the RRs for the subgroups were combined to represent a RR for the whole sample of population.

2.4. Statistic Analysis

Statistical analyses of the combined data were performed by STATA version 11.0 (Stata CORP, College Station, TX, USA). We firstly performed a meta-analysis for the highest verses the bottom category of baseline fish consumption, LC n-3 PUFA intake and biomarker, respectively. Each multivariate-adjusted RR for the highest compared with the bottom category was firstly transformed to their logarithm (logRR), and the corresponding 95% CI was used to calculate the standard error (selogRR). Summary RR (SRR) with corresponding 95% CI as the overall risk estimate for eligible prospective cohort studies was calculated by using a random-effects model described by DerSimonian and Laird [22], which considers both within-study and between-study variability. Heterogeneity across studies was evaluated with the Q test and I^2 statistic [23]. An I^2 value greater than 50% was regarded as indicative of heterogeneity according to Cochrane Handbook. Sensitivity analysis was performed to evaluate the possible influence of individual study on summary results. Begg's test and Egger's test were conducted to test the possibility of publication bias [24].

Dose-response analyses were conducted to determine a potential curvilinear (nonlinear) or linear association of fish and LC n-3 PUFA intake with risk of elevated BP, respectively. Individual studies with three or more categories were included in the dose-response analysis. We assigned median intake of fish or LC n-3 PUFA for each category as previously described [25]. Restricted cubic splines with three knots (two spline transformations) at fixed percentiles (25%, 50%, and 75%) was firstly created [26,27], and then a P for nonlinearity was calculated to detect potential departure from a simpler linear trend by testing the coefficient of the second spline equal to zero [28]. A linear trend was estimated to achieve the associations of each 20-g/day (first quartile) increment of fish and each 150-mg/day (first quartile) increment of LC n-3 PUFA consumption with risk of elevated BP using a generalized least-squares regression model (two-stage GLST in Stata) [27], respectively. Two-tailed $p < 0.05$ was considered statistically significant.

3. Results

3.1. Literature Search

In total, 3508 unique citations were identified from electronic searches plus one additional article was retrieved from reference lists (Figure 1). After the titles and abstracts were screened, 23 articles were eligible for further full-text review. Eight relevant articles were available for the present meta-analysis and 15 articles were excluded for other reasons as described in Supplementary Table S1.

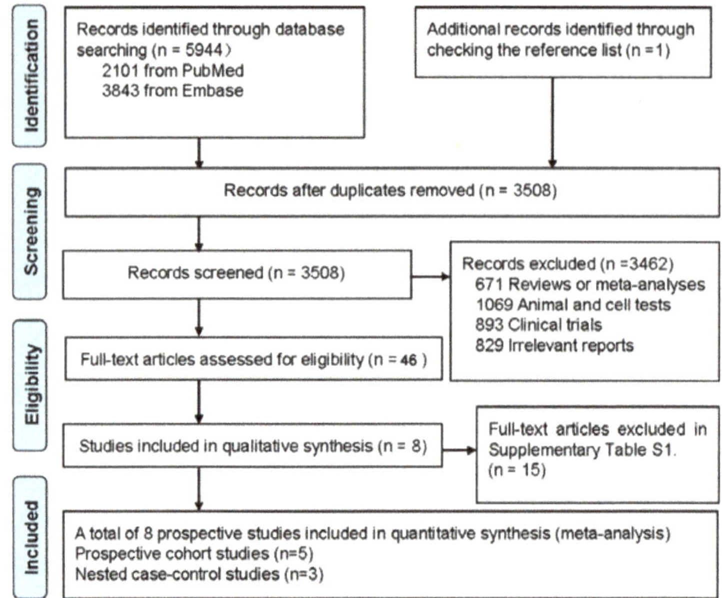

Figure 1. Preferred Reporting Items for Systematic Reviews and Meta-Analyses (PRISMA) Flow Diagram for included prospective cohort studies.

3.2. Baseline Characteristics

Overall, eight relevant prospective studies (five cohort [16–18,29,30] and three nested case-control studies [19,20,31]) were included in the present study (Table 1). Over the duration of follow up, which ranged from 3 to 20 years, a total of 20,497 EBP events occurred among 56,204 individuals aged 18–79 years from US (five studies) [16–19,29], Europe (one study) [31] and Asia (two studies) [20,30], respectively. Among the eight included studies, four studies evaluated EBP based on hypertension (SBP $\geqslant$ 140 mm Hg and (or) DBP $\geqslant$ 90 mm Hg) [16,18,19,29], whereas four studies evaluated EBP based on a BP cutoff value (SBP $\geqslant$ 130 mm Hg and (or) DBP $\geqslant$ 85 mm Hg) [17,20,30,31]. Both fish consumption and LC *n*-3 PUFA intake were investigated in 2 studies [18,30], fish consumption in two studies only [17,29], and dietary intake of LC *n*-3 PUFA in one study only [16]. Dietary data was collected by interviewer-administered FFQ, using servings/week (fish) and grams/day (LC *n*-3 PUFA) as unit of measure. Serum/plasma proportion of LC *n*-3 PUFA as a biomarker was determined in two studies [20,31], and erythrocytes in one study only [19]. Fatty acid (FA)composition in blood samples was quantified by gas liquid chromatography (GLC). Two studies separately included males and females [29,30], two studies only females [16,19], one study only males [31], and three studies included both males and females [17,18,20].

Table 1. Baseline characteristics of individual prospective cohort study.

Ref.	No. of Case/Participants	Age Range, Gender	Follow-Up Duration (Median)	Baseline Measurement		Outcomes RR (95% CI)	Multiple Adjustments
				Exposure Assessment	Exposure Range (H *vs.* L)		
[18]	999/4508	18–30 years, Both	20 years	LC *n*-3 (g/day), Fish (servings/day); FFQ	20:5*n*-3: ⩾0.078 *vs.*< 0.020	0.80 (0.66–0.96)	Age, gender, ethnicity, BMI, physical activity, education, smoking, alcohol consumption, family history of hypertension, dietary intakes of total energy, sodium, and fried fish intake.
					22:6*n*-3: ⩾0.096 *vs.*< 0.023	0.45 (0.37–0.55)	
					LC *n*-3: ⩾0.201 *vs.* < 0.060	0.65 (0.53–0.79)	
					Fish: ⩾1.258 *vs.*< 0.305	0.85 (0.70–1.03)	
[19]	516/1032	⩾39 years, Female	12.9 years	Erythrocyte PL (%), GLC	20:5*n*-3: Q_4 *vs.* Q_1 22:5*n*-3: Q_4 *vs.* Q_1 22:6*n*-3: Q_4 *vs.* Q_1 LC *n*-3: Q_4 *vs.* Q_1	0.69 (0.41–0.73) 0.59 (0.34–0.90) 0.70 (0.42–1.18) 0.65 (0.48–0.96)	Age, race, total energy intake, smoking, alcohol use, exercise, menopause status, postmenopausal hormone use, BMI, history of diabetes, and history of hypercholesterolemia.
[20]	1000/1986	55 ± 10 years, Both	3 years	Plasma PL (%), GLC	20:5*n*-3: ⩾0.76 *vs.*< 0.28	0.51 (0.33–0.80)	Age, gender, BMI, smoking, drinking, exercise, LDL cholesterol, systolic and diastolic BP, uric acid, fasting glucose levels and total fat in plasma.
					22:6n-3: ⩾3.56 *vs.*<1.97	0.59 (0.38–0.92)	
[16]	13,633/28,100	⩾39 years, Female	12.9 years	LC *n*-3 (g/day); FFQ	20:5*n*-3: Q_5 *vs.* Q_1	1.01 (0.93–1.08)	Age, race, total energy intake, drug treatment, smoking, alcohol intake, physical activity, postmenopausal status, hormone use, dietary sodium, potassium, calcium, fiber, BMI, history of diabetes, and history of hypercholesterolemia.
					22:6*n*-3: Q_5 *vs.* Q_1	1.07 (1.01–1.13)	
[30]	613/3504	40–69 years, Male and Female.	3.5 years	LC *n*-3 (g/day), fish (servings/week); FFQ	LC *n*-3: Q_4 *vs.* Q_1	0.79 (0.51–1.23)	Age, BMI, income, occupation, marital status, education level, smoking, alcohol intake, physical activity, daily intake of energy, fat, fiber, red meat, dairy products, sweetened carbonated beverages, use of multivitamin supplements, and diabetes or hypertension.
					Fish: 5–6 *vs.*<1	1.25 (0.77–2.03)	
[31]	146/880	50–70 years, Male	20 years	Serum (%), GLC	LC *n*-3: mean (SD) in noncases (1.45 (0.81))	0.74 (0.62–0.89)	BMI, smoking, and exercise.
[17]	997/4304	18–30 years, Both	15 years	Fish (times/week); dietary questionnaires	Fish: >2.5 *vs.*<0.6	1.11 (0.90, 1.38)	Age, sex, race, center, energy intake, education, physical activity, alcohol intake, smoking, and vitamin supplement.
[29]	981/5394	25–74 years, Both	10 years	Fish (times/week), FFQ	Fish: ⩾1 *vs.* <1	0.84 (0.66, 1.08)	Age, smoking, history of diabetes, education, systolic BP, serum cholesterol, BMI, pulse rate, alcohol intake, and physical activity.

Ref., reference; No., number; H, the highest exposure category; L, the lowest exposure category; RR, risk ratio; LC *n*-3 PUFA, long-chain *n*-3 polyunsaturated fatty acid; g/day, gram per day; FFQ, food frequency questionnaire; 20:5*n*-3, eicosapentaenoic acid (EPA); 22:5*n*-3, docosapentaenoic acid (DPA); 22:6*n*-3, docosahexaenoic acid (DHA); BMI, body mass index; BP, blood pressure; PL, phospholipids; GLC, gas-liquid chromatography.

3.3. Fish Consumption and Elevated BP

In total, four independent cohort studies of fish consumption in relation to elevated BP were available for meta-analysis comparing the highest to the lowest category, with 3590 elevated BP events and 17,710 participants. Fish consumption was not significantly associated with reduced risk of elevated BP (SRR = 0.96; 95% CI: 0.81, 1.14), with a moderate heterogeneity (I^2 = 44.70%) (Figure 2). In addition, three studies were eligible for dose-response trend estimations. No evidence of a nonlinear association was found between fish consumption and elevated BP (p = 0.15 for non-linearity) (Supplementary Figure S1). Each 20-g/day increment of fish consumption was not significantly associated with reduced risk of elevated BP (pooled RR = 0.98; 95% CI: 0.94, 1.03; p for trend = 0.23). A sensitivity analysis which tested the influence of any individual study on the overall results suggested no significant change in pooled association estimates (Supplementary Figure S2). No possibility of publication bias was observed by visual inspection of Begg's funnel plot (p for bias = 0.54) and Egger's regression test (p for bias = 0.34) (Supplementary Figure S3).

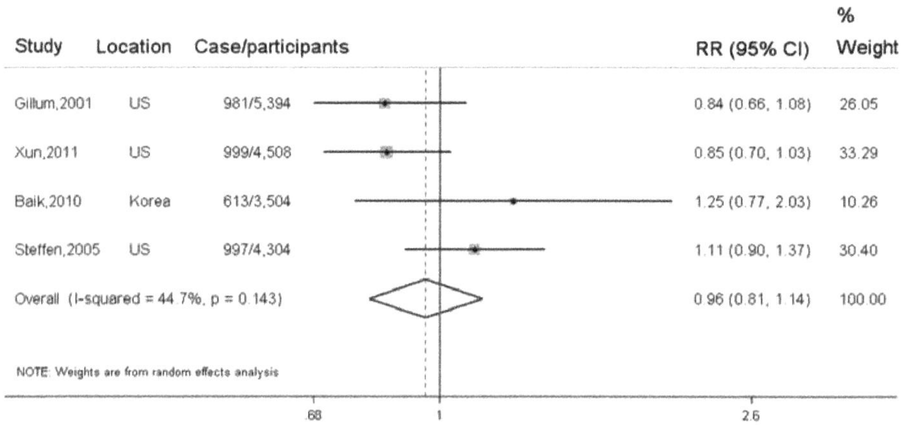

Figure 2. Associations between fish consumption and incidence of elevated BP in the highest verse the lowest exposure category.

All relevant cohort studies are referred to by first author, year of publication, locations, and the number of elevated BP events among participants. Squares represent study-specific risk ratio (RR), and horizontal lines represent 95% confidence interval (CI). The pooled RR estimated by a random-effect model in the highest compared with the bottom category of fish consumption is represented by the black squares. The degree of heterogeneity between individual study was indicated by I square statistic.

3.4. LC n-3 PUFA and Elevated BP

In total, six independent prospective cohort studies (three studies for biomarker vs. three studies for diet) were eligible to evaluate association between LC n-3 PUFA and incidence of elevated BP, with 16,907 elevated BP events and 38,494 participants. LC n-3 PUFA was inversely associated with incidence of EBP when comparing the highest with the lowest category (SRR = 0.73; 95% CI: 0.60, 0.89; I^2 = 75.00%) (Figure 3). The pooled association was not significantly changed in the sensitivity analysis (Supplementary Figure S4). Publication bias was not observed from Begg's funnel plot (p for bias = 0.73) and Egger's test (p for bias= 0.66) (Supplementary Figure S5).

Three cohort studies estimated dietary intake of LC n-3 PUFA, with 15,245 EBP events and 36,112 participants. The SRR was 0.80 (95% CI: 0.58, 1.10) for dietary intake of LC n-3 PUFA, with a high between-study heterogeneity (I^2 = 79.30%). The three studies were available for trend estimation. Evidence of a nonlinear association cannot be observed between dietary intake of LC n-3 PUFA and incidence of EBP (p = 0. 57 for non-linearity) (Supplementary Figure S6). There was also no linear association between per 150 mg/day increment of LC n-3 PUFA intake and risk of EBP (SRR = 0.94; 95% CI: 0.84, 1.05; p for trend = 0.25). Two eligible studies assessed dietary intake of individual LC n-3 PUFA, the SRR was 0.91 (95% CI: 0.73, 1.15; I^2 = 80.00%) for 20:5n-3, and 0.70 (95% CI: 0.30, 1.63; I^2 = 98.40%) for 22:6n-3, respectively.

Three prospective nested case-control studies evaluated circulating levels of LC n-3 PUFA as biomarker, with 1662 cases and 2382 participants. Circulating LC n-3 PUFA was significantly associated with reduced incidence of EBP in the highest verse lowest category (SRR = 0.67; 95% CI: 0.55, 0.83; I^2 = 47.40%) (Figure 3). For biomarker of individual LC n-3 PUFA, the SRR was 0.53 (95% CI: 0.35, 0.78; I^2 = 0.00%) for 20:5n-3 in two studies, 0.57 (95% CI: 0.36, 0.90; I^2 = 0.00%) for 22:5n-3 in one study, and 0.64 (95% CI: 0.45, 0.89; I^2 = 0.00%) for 22:6n-3 in two studies, respectively.

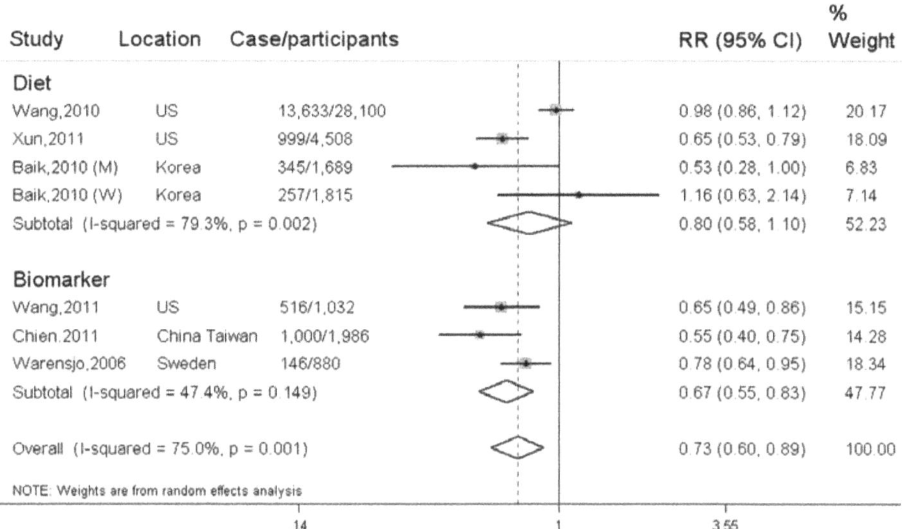

Figure 3. Associations between LC n-3 PUFA and incidence of elevated BP in the highest verse the lowest exposure category.

Included studies are subgrouped by dietary intake and biomarker of LC n-3 PUFA. All relevant cohort studies are referred to by first author, year of publication, locations, and the number of elevated BP events among participants. Squares represent study-specific risk ratio (RR); horizontal lines represent 95% confidence interval (CI); diamonds represent pooled RR from prospective cohort study. The degree of heterogeneity between individual studies was indicated by I square statistic.

4. Discussion

In the present meta-analysis, which included 20,497 EBP events and 56,204 individuals from eight prospective cohort studies, we cannot provide a strong evidence to support increased dietary consumption of fish or LC n-3 PUFA to be associated with reduced incidence of elevated BP. However, circulating LC n-3 PUFA as biomarker of food n-3 PUFA intake was significantly associated with a lower risk of elevated BP, especially 20:5n-3 and 22:6n-3, which can further build and extend on prior meta-analyses of LC n-3 PUFA in relation to BP.

Fish can be regarded as a package of LC n-3 PUFA, other nutrients and contaminants. Thus, the integrative effects of fish consumption may be reflected by the interactions between LC n-3 PUFA and other constituents in fish. A meta-analysis of observational studies found that fish consumption or LC *n*-3 PUFA intake was weakly associated with reduced risk of metabolic syndrome (MS) in two prospective cohort studies, but not in seven cross-sectional studies [32]. Consistent with the results from pooled analysis of seven cross-sectional studies, our findings also indicated that fish or LC *n*-3 PUFA intake was not significantly related to EBP as a component of MS. Most observational studies were primarily designed to focus on total fish rather than different species of fish or different preparation methods. Fish preparation methods may alter the relationship between fish intake and EBP by changing the lipid profile and by generating unexpected chemicals with the use of certain cooking methods. Frying fish, especially deep-frying, was found to generate oxidized lipids, considerably reduce the amount of LC *n*-3 PUFA but increase trans-fatty acids [33], which may modify the lowing-BP effects of total fish consumption [16]. Salted fish possibly added intake of salt, which could have substantially attenuated or masked a beneficial effect of fresh fish, due to high-salt intake being positively associated with BP [34]. In addition, the protective effect of fish intake might be attenuated or even reversed by other contaminants in fish, such as mercury and pesticides. Taken together, these limitations might contribute to the null association of fish intake with EBP in our meta-analysis.

The substantial BP reductions by LC *n*-3 PUFA supplementation usually occurred at relatively high doses (⩾3 g/day). Nevertheless, compared with the previous evidence, our findings do not support LC *n*-3 PUFA estimated by dietary questionnaires to be associated with primary prevention of EBP. Dietary data was usually estimated by dietary questionnaires, thus underestimation of effect size may still persist due to dietary measurement errors or bias with consequent limited ability to classify dietary intake of individuals accurately. In addition, most participants included in the present meta-analysis were from US and Europe, of which typical fish intake is relatively low. Thus, the average amount of LC *n*-3 PUFA intake in study populations was insufficient to strongly affect the risk of elevated BP in initially normotensive individuals. Finally, a significant relationship could also have remained undetected if most individuals were to have an adequate fish intake. However, this perhaps happened in our study, considering that less than 18% of individuals ate no or little fish in the present study. We therefore could have missed or underestimated a pronounced association due to a small range of fish or LC *n*-3 PUFA intake.

Circulating levels of LC *n*-3 PUFA as biomarkers, compared with dietary assessment, might provide a more reliable estimation of intake. In the present study, we found that circulating LC *n*-3 PUFA was inversely associated with incidence of EBP, which can further support increased intake of fish or LC *n*-3 PUFA to be beneficial for EBP. Convincing evidence from numerous studies have indicated that circulating level of LC *n*-3 PUFA was closely correlated with increased consumption of fish, especially 20:5*n*-3 and 22:6n-3 [35,36]. Recently, a cross-sectional study suggested that plasma concentration of LC *n*-3 PUFA was positively associated with marine food intake, independent of habitual exercise, alcohol intake, and smoking habit [37]. A clinical trial compared the effects of fish (2 servings/week, 16 weeks) and fish-oil capsules (1–2 capsules/day, 16 weeks) on *n*-3 PUFA content in erythrocyte and plasma phospholipids, suggesting that consumption of equal amounts of 20:5*n*-3 and 22:6*n*-3 from fish on a weekly basis or from fish-oil capsules on a daily basis is equally effective at enriching blood lipids with *n*-3 FAs [38]. Thus, LC *n*-3 PUFA derived from fish intake rather than supplements can also be incorporated into serum/plasma, platelets, and tissue lipids to change biomembrane fluidity, increase the production of vasodilators [39], reduce cardiac adrenergic activity [40], and lower BP. The lowering-BP effects may be attributable to 22:6*n*-3 but not 20:5*n*-3, which has been supported by most previous studies. A meta-analysis of clinical studies [6] showed 22:6*n*-3 had a slightly greater dose-response effect on BP levels than 20:5*n*-3 (−1.5/−0.77 mmHg *versus* −0.93/−0.53 mmHg per gram). Mori, *et al.* found that 22:6*n*-3, but not 20:5*n*-3 supplementation, reduced the 24-h and daytime ambulatory BP in mildly hyperlipidemic men [41]. However, we did not find 22:6*n*-3 to be superior to 20:5*n*-3 with respect to EBP prevention in the present study, which may be explained by insufficient statistical power due to the small sample size. Several possible mechanisms can explain the anti-hypertensive property of 22:6*n*-3. Firstly, the 22:6*n*-3 can be more preferentially incorporated into the biomembrane than 20:5*n*-3 [42]. The incorporation of 22:6*n*-3 into cardiomyocyte membranes can inhibit the beta-adrenergic system [43], which may help to explain its anti-arrhythmic and BP-lowing effects. Furthermore, calcium/calmodulin-dependent kinase 4 (CaMK4) gene deletion can impair CaMK-mediated activation of eNOS, which induces hypertension in the mice null for CaMK4 [44]. The 22:6*n*-3 can be incorporated into endothelial membranes to stimulate ATP release from the endothelium, which leads to vasodilatation mediated by nitric oxide (NO) release [45]. The induction of NO release, together with the decrease in noradrenaline levels, is likely to be responsible for BP-lowering effect of 22:6*n*-3.

Our meta-analysis has several merits. Firstly, prospective study design minimized the possibility of selection bias, and allowed inference on temporality of associations. Secondly, the included cohort studies comprised 56,204 (men and women) with a wide age range and long-term follow-up. Thirdly, biomarker of LC *n*-3 PUFA can provide objective measures of individual *n*-3 PUFA intake, independent of dietary assessment errors and bias. Fourthly, intervention trials might be impractical for prolonged compliance to the assigned amount of fish intake, thus meta-analyses of prospective cohort studies are considered to be a powerful tool in evaluating the long-term association. Finally, food LC-PUFA is directly calculated from fish consumption in all included studies, thus the consistent results between fish and LC-PUFA perhaps strengthened our ultimate findings.

Nevertheless, the potential limitations should also be considered for this study. Firstly, our search was limited to English publications, and thus a potential bias caused by the exclusion of non-English or unpublished reports may exist; Secondly, the different exposure measurement scale across included studies were not detailed enough to allow standardization of fish consumption, thus our analysis primarily considered the highest versus the lowest exposure category; Thirdly, the diet measurement errors or misclassification in dietary estimations were likely to bias the summary results towards null. However, the use of biomarkers of dietary intake may counterbalance this point; Fourthly, in spite of comprehensive adjustments in each included study, the possibility of residual confounding caused by imprecisely measured or unmeasured factors cannot be excluded; Fifthly, the possibility of measurement bias may be inevitable, because circulating levels of *n*-3 PUFA may be subject to laboratory and biological variation during follow-up. Finally, we cannot perform a stratified analysis to determine if the pooled association estimation may be modified by strata factors, due to a limited number of studies within each subgroup.

In summary, our meta-analysis of all relevant cohort studies indicated there is no association between fish or dietary LC *n*-3 PUFA consumption and incidence of elevated BP. However, our findings show that circulating LC *n*-3 PUFA as biomarkers of dietary intake are inversely associated with incidence of EBP, especially 20:5*n*-3 and 22:6*n*-3, which suggests important public health implications for primary prevention of EBP. Stressing the consumption of food rich in LC *n*-3 PUFA to ultimately improve their circulating levels is still recommended. Nevertheless, the specific biologic mechanisms behind these conclusions remain partially unclear, and thus a replication of well-designed prospective cohort studies and further experimental work in understanding the underlying biologic mechanisms is necessary.

Supplementary Materials: Supplementary Materials: Supplementary materials are available online at www.mdpi.com/2072-6643/ 8/1/58/s1.

Acknowledgments: This study was funded by the National Basic Research Program of China (973 Program: 2015CB553604); and by the Ph.D. Programs Foundation of Ministry of Education of China (J20130084). The funders have no role in study design, data collection and analysis, decision to publish, or preparation of the manuscript.

Author Contributions: B.Y. and D.L. contributed to the concept and data design. M.-Q.S. and Z.-H.L. collected data. B.Y. and M.-Q.S. analyzed and interpreted data. B.Y. drafted the article. D.L. critically revised the article and approved articles. All authors read and approved the final manuscript.

Conflicts of Interest: The authors declare no conflict of interest.

References

1. Van den Born, B.J. Blood Pressure Lowering and Cardiovascular Risk. *Lancet* **2014**, *384*, 1746. [CrossRef]

2. Muntner, P.; Whittle, J.; Lynch, A.I.; Colantonio, L.D.; Simpson, L.M.; Einhorn, P.T.; Levitan, E.B.; Whelton, P.K.; Cushman, W.C.; Louis, G.T.; *et al.* Visit-to-Visit Variability of Blood Pressure and Coronary Heart Disease, Stroke, Heart Failure, and Mortality: A Cohort Study. *Ann. Intern. Med.* **2015**, *163*, 329–338. [CrossRef] [PubMed]
3. Del Brutto, O.H.; Mera, R.M.; Gillman, J.; Castillo, P.R.; Zambrano, M.; Ha, J.E. Dietary Oily Fish Intake and Blood Pressure Levels: A Population-Based Study. *J. Clin. Hypertens.* **2015**. [CrossRef] [PubMed]
4. Colussi, G.; Catena, C.; Dialti, V.; Pezzutto, F.; Mos, L.; Sechi, L.A. Fish Meal Supplementation and Ambulatory Blood Pressure in Patients with Hypertension: Relevance of Baseline Membrane Fatty Acid Composition. *Am. J. Hypertens.* **2014**, *27*, 471–481. [CrossRef] [PubMed]
5. Cabo, J.; Alonso, R.; Mata, P. Omega-3 Fatty Acids and Blood Pressure. *Br. J. Nutr.* **2012**, *107*, S195–S200. [CrossRef] [PubMed]
6. Morris, M.C.; Sacks, F.; Rosner, B. Does Fish Oil Lower Blood Pressure? A Meta-Analysis of Controlled Trials. *Circulation* **1993**, *88*, 523–533. [CrossRef] [PubMed]
7. Miller, P.E.; van Elswyk, M.; Alexander, D.D. Long-Chain Omega-3 Fatty Acids Eicosapentaenoic Acid and Docosahexaenoic Acid and Blood Pressure: A Meta-Analysis of Randomized Controlled Trials. *Am. J. Hypertens.* **2014**, *27*, 885–896. [CrossRef] [PubMed]
8. Geleijnse, J.M.; Giltay, E.J.; Grobbee, D.E.; Donders, A.R.; Kok, F.J. Blood Pressure Response to Fish Oil Supplementation: Metaregression Analysis of Randomized Trials. *J. Hypertens* **2002**, *20*, 1493–1499. [CrossRef] [PubMed]
9. Campbell, F.; Dickinson, H.O.; Critchley, J.A.; Ford, G.A.; Bradburn, M. A Systematic Review of Fish-Oil Supplements for the Prevention and Treatment of Hypertension. *Eur. J. Prev. Cardiol.* **2013**, *20*, 107–120. [CrossRef] [PubMed]
10. Van Den Elsen, L.W.; Spijkers, L.J.; van Den Akker, R.F.; van Winssen, A.M.; Balvers, M.; Wijesinghe, D.S.; Chalfant, C.E.; Garssen, J.; Willemsen, L.E.; Alewijnse, A.E.; *et al.* Dietary Fish Oil Improves Endothelial Function and Lowers Blood Pressure Via Suppression of Sphingolipid-Mediated Contractions in Spontaneously Hypertensive Rats. *J. Hypertens.* **2014**, *32*, 1050–1058. [CrossRef] [PubMed]
11. Ogawa, A.; Suzuki, Y.; Aoyama, T.; Takeuchi, H. Dietary Alpha-Linolenic Acid Inhibits Angiotensin-Converting Enzyme Activity and Mrna Expression Levels in the Aorta of Spontaneously Hypertensive Rats. *J. Oleo Sci.* **2009**, *58*, 355–360. [CrossRef] [PubMed]
12. Begg, D.P.; Puskas, L.G.; Kitajka, K.; Menesi, D.; Allen, A.M.; Li, D.; Mathai, M.L.; Shi, J.R.; Sinclair, A.J.; Weisinger, R.S. Hypothalamic Gene Expression in Omega-3 Pufa-Deficient Male Rats Before, and Following, Development of Hypertension. *Hypertens. Res.* **2012**, *35*, 381–387. [CrossRef] [PubMed]
13. Pauletto, P.; Puato, M.; Caroli, M.G.; Casiglia, E.; Munhambo, A.E.; Cazzolato, G.; Bittolo Bon, G.; Angeli, M.T.; Galli, C.; Pessina, A.C. Blood Pressure and Atherogenic Lipoprotein Profiles of Fish-Diet and Vegetarian Villagers in Tanzania: The Lugalawa Study. *Lancet* **1996**, *348*, 784–788. [CrossRef]
14. Bountziouka, V.; Polychronopoulos, E.; Zeimbekis, A.; Papavenetiou, E.; Ladoukaki, E.; Papairakleous, N.; Gotsis, E.; Metallinos, G.; Lionis, C.; Panagiotakos, D. Long-Term Fish Intake Is Associated with Less Severe Depressive Symptoms among Elderly Men and Women: The Medis (Mediterranean Islands Elderly) Epidemiological Study. *J. Aging Health* **2009**, *21*, 864–880. [CrossRef] [PubMed]
15. Ke, L.; Ho, J.; Feng, J.; Mpofu, E.; Dibley, M.J.; Feng, X.; van, F.; Leong, S.; Lau, W.; Lueng, P.; *et al.* Modifiable Risk Factors Including Sunlight Exposure and Fish Consumption Are Associated with Risk of Hypertension in a Large Representative Population from Macau. *J. Steroid Biochem. Mol. Biol.* **2014**, *144*, 152–155. [CrossRef] [PubMed]
16. Wang, L.; Manson, J.E.; Forman, J.P.; Gaziano, J.M.; Buring, J.E.; Sesso, H.D. Dietary Fatty Acids and the Risk of Hypertension in Middle-Aged and Older Women. *Hypertension* **2010**, *56*, 598–604. [CrossRef] [PubMed]
17. Steffen, L.M.; Kroenke, C.H.; Yu, X.; Pereira, M.A.; Slattery, M.L.; van Horn, L.; Gross, M.D.; Jacobs, D.R., Jr. Associations of Plant Food, Dairy Product, and Meat Intakes with 15-Y Incidence of Elevated Blood Pressure in Young Black and White Adults: The Coronary Artery Risk Development in Young Adults (Cardia) Study. *Am. J. Clin. Nutr.* **2005**, *82*, 1169–1177. [PubMed]
18. Xun, P.; Hou, N.; Daviglus, M.; Liu, K.; Morris, J.S.; Shikany, J.M.; Sidney, S.; Jacobs, D.R.; He, K. Fish Oil, Selenium and Mercury in Relation to Incidence of Hypertension: A 20-Year Follow-Up Study. *J. Intern. Med.* **2011**, *270*, 175–186. [CrossRef] [PubMed]

19. Wang, L.; Tsai, M.; Manson, J.E.; Djousse, L.; Gaziano, J.M.; Buring, J.E.; Sesso, H.D. Erythrocyte Fatty Acid Composition Is Associated with the Risk of Hypertension in Middle-Aged and Older Women. *J. Nutr.* **2011**, *141*, 1691–1697. [CrossRef] [PubMed]
20. Chien, K.L.; Chao, C.L.; Kuo, C.H.; Lin, H.J.; Liu, P.H.; Chen, P.R.; Hsu, H.C.; Lee, B.C.; Lee, Y.T.; Chen, M.F. Plasma Fatty Acids and The Risk of Metabolic Syndrome in Ethnic Chinese Adults in Taiwan. *Lipids Health Dis.* **2011**, *10*, 33. [CrossRef] [PubMed]
21. He, K.; Song, Y.; Daviglus, M.L.; Liu, K.; van Horn, L.; Dyer, A.R.; Goldbourt, U.; Greenland, P. Fish Consumption and Incidence of Stroke: A Meta-Analysis of Cohort Studies. *Stroke* **2004**, *35*, 1538–1542. [CrossRef] [PubMed]
22. Dersimonian, R.; Laird, N. Meta-Analysis in Clinical Trials. *Control Clin. Trials* **1986**, *7*, 177–188. [CrossRef]
23. Higgins, J.P.; Thompson, S.G.; Deeks, J.J.; Altman, D.G. Measuring Inconsistency in Meta-Analyses. *BMJ* **2003**, *327*, 557–560. [CrossRef] [PubMed]
24. Egger, M.; Davey Smith, G.; Schneider, M.; Minder, C. Bias in Meta-Analysis Detected by a Simple, Graphical Test. *BMJ* **1997**, *315*, 629–634. [CrossRef] [PubMed]
25. Zheng, J.; Huang, T.; Yu, Y.; Hu, X.; Yang, B.; Li, D. Fish Consumption and CHD Mortality: An Updated Meta-Analysis of Seventeen Cohort Studies. *Public Health Nutr.* **2012**, *15*, 725–737. [CrossRef] [PubMed]
26. Jackson, D.; White, I.R.; Thompson, S.G. Extending Dersimonian and Laird's Methodology to Perform Multivariate Random Effects Meta-Analyses. *Stat. Med.* **2010**, *29*, 1282–1297. [CrossRef] [PubMed]
27. Orsini, N.; Bellocco, R.; Greenland, S. Generalized Least Squares for Trend Estimation of Summarized Dose-Response Data. *Stata J.* **2006**, *6*, 40–57.
28. Orsini, N.; Li, R.; Wolk, A.; Khudyakov, P.; Spiegelman, D. Meta-Analysis For Linear and Nonlinear Dose-Response Relations: Examples, an Evaluation of Approximations, and Software. *Am. J. Epidemiol.* **2012**, *175*, 66–73. [CrossRef] [PubMed]
29. Gillum, R.F.; Mussolino, M.E.; Madans, J.H. Fish Consumption and Hypertension Incidence in African Americans and Whites: The Nhanes I Epidemiologic Follow-Up Study. *J. Natl. Med. Assoc.* **2001**, *93*, 124–128. [PubMed]
30. Baik, I.; Abbott, R.D.; Curb, J.D.; Shin, C. Intake of Fish and *N*-3 Fatty Acids and Future Risk of Metabolic Syndrome. *J. Am. Diet. Assoc.* **2010**, *110*, 1018–1026. [CrossRef] [PubMed]
31. Warensjo, E.; Sundstrom, J.; Lind, L.; Vessby, B. Factor Analysis of Fatty Acids in Serum Lipids as a Measure of Dietary Fat Quality in Relation to the Metabolic Syndrome in Men. *Am. J. Clin. Nutr.* **2006**, *84*, 442–448. [PubMed]
32. Kim, Y.S.; Xun, P.; He, K. Fish Consumption, Long-Chain Omega-3 Polyunsaturated Fatty Acid Intake and Risk of Metabolic Syndrome: A Meta-Analysis. *Nutrients* **2015**, *7*, 2085–2100. [CrossRef] [PubMed]
33. Skog, K. Cooking Procedures and Food Mutagens—A Literature-Review. *Food Chem. Toxicol.* **1993**, *31*, 655–675. [CrossRef]
34. Kupferschmidt, K. Epidemiology. Report Reignites Battle over Low-Salt Diets. *Science* **2013**, *340*, 908. [CrossRef] [PubMed]
35. Andersen, L.F.; Solvoll, K.; Drevon, C.A. Very-Long-Chain *N*-3 Fatty Acids as Biomarkers for Intake of Fish and *N*-3 Fatty Acid Concentrates. *Am. J. Clin. Nutr.* **1996**, *64*, 305–311. [PubMed]
36. Hjartaker, A.; Lund, E.; Bjerve, K.S. Serum Phospholipid Fatty Acid Composition and Habitual Intake of Marine Foods Registered by A Semi-Quantitative Food Frequency Questionnaire. *Eur. J. Clin. Nutr.* **1997**, *51*, 736–742. [CrossRef] [PubMed]
37. Kuriki, K.; Nagaya, T.; Tokudome, Y.; Imaeda, N.; Fujiwara, N.; Sato, J.; Goto, C.; Ikeda, M.; Maki, S.; Tajima, K.; *et al.* Plasma Concentrations of (*N*-3) Highly Unsaturated Fatty Acids Are Good Biomarkers of Relative Dietary Fatty Acid Intakes: A Cross-Sectional Study. *J. Nutr.* **2003**, *133*, 3643–3650. [PubMed]
38. Harris, W.S.; Pottala, J.V.; Sands, S.A.; Jones, P.G. Comparison of the Effects of Fish and Fish-Oil Capsules on the n 3 Fatty Acid Content of Blood Cells and Plasma Phospholipids. *Am. J. Clin. Nutr.* **2007**, *86*, 1621–1625. [PubMed]
39. Mori, T.A.; Watts, G.F.; Burke, V.; Hilme, E.; Puddey, I.B.; Beilin, L.J. Differential Effects of Eicosapentaenoic Acid and Docosahexaenoic Acid on Vascular Reactivity of the Forearm Microcirculation in Hyperlipidemic, Overweight Men. *Circulation* **2000**, *102*, 1264–1269. [CrossRef] [PubMed]

40. Leaf, A.; Kang, J.X.; Xiao, Y.F.; Billman, G.E. Clinical Prevention Of Sudden Cardiac Death by *N*-3 Polyunsaturated Fatty Acids and Mechanism of Prevention of Arrhythmias by *N*-3 Fish Oils. *Circulation* **2003**, *107*, 2646–2652. [CrossRef] [PubMed]
41. Mori, T.A.; Bao, D.Q.; Burke, V.; Puddey, I.B.; Beilin, L.J. Docosahexaenoic Acid But Not Eicosapentaenoic Acid Lowers Ambulatory Blood Pressure and Heart Rate in Humans. *Hypertension* **1999**, *34*, 253–260. [CrossRef] [PubMed]
42. Mclennan, P.L. Myocardial Membrane Fatty Acids and the Antiarrhythmic Actions of Dietary Fish Oil in Animal Models. *Lipids* **2001**, *36*, S111–S114. [CrossRef] [PubMed]
43. Grynberg, A.; Fournier, A.; Sergiel, J.P.; Athias, P. Effect of Docosahexaenoic Acid and Eicosapentaenoic Acid in the Phospholipids of Rat Heart Muscle Cells on Adrenoceptor Responsiveness and Mechanism. *J. Mol. Cell. Cardiol.* **1995**, *27*, 2507–2520. [CrossRef] [PubMed]
44. Santulli, G.; Cipolletta, E.; Sorriento, D.; del Giudice, C.; Anastasio, A.; Monaco, S.; Maione, A.S.; Condorelli, G.; Puca, A.; Trimarco, B.; *et al.* Camk4 Gene Deletion Induces Hypertension. *J. Am. Heart Assoc.* **2012**, *1*, E001081. [CrossRef] [PubMed]
45. Hashimoto, M.; Shinozuka, K.; Gamoh, S.; Tanabe, Y.; Hossain, M.S.; Kwon, Y.M.; Hata, N.; Misawa, Y.; Kunitomo, M.; Masumura, S. The Hypotensive Effect of Docosahexaenoic Acid Is Associated with the Enhanced Release of Atp from the Caudal Artery of Aged Rats. *J. Nutr.* **1999**, *129*, 70–76. [PubMed]

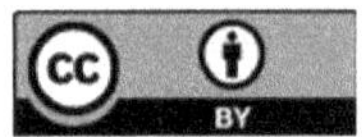

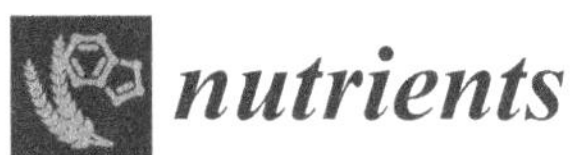

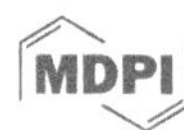

Review

Docosahexaenoic Acid and Cognition throughout the Lifespan

Michael J. Weiser [1,*], Christopher M. Butt [1] and M. Hasan Mohajeri [2]

1 DSM Nutritional Products, R&D Human Nutrition and Health, Boulder, CO, USA; Chris.Butt@DSM.com
2 DSM Nutritional Products, R&D Human Nutrition and Health, Basel, Switzerland; hasan.mohajeri@dsm.com
* Correspondence: michael.weiser@dsm.com; Tel.: +1-303-305-0488

Received: 29 December 2015; Accepted: 28 January 2016; Published: 17 February 2016

Abstract: Docosahexaenoic acid (DHA) is the predominant omega-3 (*n*-3) polyunsaturated fatty acid (PUFA) found in the brain and can affect neurological function by modulating signal transduction pathways, neurotransmission, neurogenesis, myelination, membrane receptor function, synaptic plasticity, neuroinflammation, membrane integrity and membrane organization. DHA is rapidly accumulated in the brain during gestation and early infancy, and the availability of DHA via transfer from maternal stores impacts the degree of DHA incorporation into neural tissues. The consumption of DHA leads to many positive physiological and behavioral effects, including those on cognition. Advanced cognitive function is uniquely human, and the optimal development and aging of cognitive abilities has profound impacts on quality of life, productivity, and advancement of society in general. However, the modern diet typically lacks appreciable amounts of DHA. Therefore, in modern populations, maintaining optimal levels of DHA in the brain throughout the lifespan likely requires obtaining preformed DHA via dietary or supplemental sources. In this review, we examine the role of DHA in optimal cognition during development, adulthood, and aging with a focus on human evidence and putative mechanisms of action.

Keywords: brain lipids; omega-3 polyunsaturated fatty acids; nutrition; learning; memory; comprehension; development; aging; neurodegeneration

---

1. Introduction

The cognitive ability of humans is arguably the most advanced in the entire animal kingdom. Such advancement is believed to be conferred by an expanded cerebral cortex and a highly developed prefrontal cortex, both of which are brain regions important for cognition. There are many different domains to the clinical construct of cognition. These include attention, memory (working and long-term), perception, language, problem solving, comprehension, reasoning, computation, reading and speech. Cognition changes throughout the lifespan matching the development, maturation and aging of the brain. The brain is a lipid-rich organ that consumes 20% of the body's energy, but it only comprises 2% of the body's mass. Over half of the brain's dry weight is comprised of lipids, and it is especially enriched in long-chain omega-3 (*n*-3) polyunsaturated fatty acids (PUFAs), suggesting a key role for these molecules in the optimal development, maturation and aging of neural structures and networks. A substantial amount of literature exists that highlights the crucial role of nutrition in brain development, and thus on brain function and mental performance in humans. Ultimately, the proper functioning of the brain has significant dependence upon maintaining its optimal lipid composition [1].

Quantitatively, docosahexaenoic acid (DHA; 22:6*n*-3) is the most significant *n*-3 PUFA in the brain as both eicosapentaenoic acid (EPA; 20:5*n*-3) and α-linolenic acid (ALA; 18:3*n*-3) are present in only very small quantities. DHA makes up over 90% of the *n*-3 PUFAs in the brain and 10%–20% of its total lipids. DHA is especially concentrated in the gray matter [2]. It is stored primarily in phosphatidylethanolamine (PE) and phosphatidylserine (PS) membrane phospholipids, with smaller amounts also found in phosphatidylcholine (PC; [3]), where it plays an important role in the biosynthesis of PS (DHA-PS) in the brain [4]. DHA is enriched in membranes structures found at synaptic terminals, mitochondria and endoplasmic reticulum [5], and it can ultimately affect cellular characteristics and physiological processes including membrane fluidity, lipid raft function, neurotransmitter release, transmembrane receptor function, gene expression, signal transduction, myelination, neuroinflammation, and neuronal differentiation and growth [6–8].

The brain's frontal lobes are particularly responsive to the supply of DHA during development [9]. Decades of work have clearly established the responsibilities of the frontal lobes for executive and higher-order cognitive activities including sustained attention, planning and problem solving [10], and the prefrontal lobe in particular for social, emotional and behavioral development [11]. Therefore, maintaining optimal lipid composition in these brain regions, and specifically DHA levels, is not only important during the development and maturation of the brain from gestation through childhood and adolescence [12,13], but such maintenance is also critical for successful aging of the adult brain [1,14–16]. In this review, we will discuss the importance of DHA for optimal neurological health throughout the lifespan, with a particular emphasis on cognitive function.

2. DHA Delivery to the Brain

DHA synthesized *de novo* originates from ALA via a series of desaturations and elongations primarily within the endoplasmic reticulum (ER), with the exception of the last step, a β-oxidation from tetracosahexaenoic acid (24:6*n*-3) that occurs in peroxisomes [17]. ALA is considered an essential nutrient because humans lack the *n*-3 desaturase enzyme required for its production. However, it could be argued that DHA is also an essential nutrient due to inefficiencies of the 5-desaturase and 6-desaturase enzymes (FADS1/2) needed for its biosynthesis, and the competition for these enzymes by the omega-6 (*n*-6) PUFA linoleic acid (LA; 18:2*n*-6). LA is typically consumed in high amounts in modern diets, which exacerbates the increase of *n*-6 PUFAs, as well as the decrease of *n*-3 PUFAs, that are incorporated in peripheral and neural tissues [18]. Therefore, many researchers conclude that preformed DHA consumption is required for reaching and maintaining ideal brain DHA concentrations and related neurological functions [19–21].

There is a general consensus on the recommended daily average intake requirements for infants. This consensus is driven by data from randomized control trials (RCTs) that suggest a minimum level of DHA at 0.32% of total fatty acids in formula [22–24], which is towards the lower half of the global concentration range found in human milk (0.06% to 1.4% of total fatty acids) [25,26]. The evidence for daily intake requirements for children and adults is still emerging. Nonetheless, current guidelines are in the range of 250 to 500 mg EPA + DHA per day [27–29]. However, most people do not consume enough *n*-3 PUFAs, as indicated by average modern daily dietary DHA intakes that are closer to 100 mg per day [21,30,31].

The shift in modern diets towards reduced *n*-3 PUFA intake, increased *n*-6 PUFA consumption, combined with less physical activity has had a detrimental impact on development and aging, especially with regard to cognitive function. The optimal dietary *n*-6 to *n*-3 PUFA ratio is 2:1 and below, while the current Western diet is typically in the range of 10:1 to 25:1 [32]. DHA likely played an important role in the evolution of the human brain, as significant structural changes in the encephalon and gains in cognitive abilities coincided with the use of aquaculture as a substantial portion of the human diet [33,34]. Habitats near aquatic food sources, such as lakes, rivers, and the sea provided rich dietary sources of DHA. It therefore follows that sources of preformed DHA include oils from microalgae, fatty fish (especially salmon, mackerel, sardines, and herring), and fish oil.

The human brain metabolizes approximately 4 mg of DHA per day, resulting in an estimated half-life of brain DHA of 2.5 years [35], much longer than that of DHA in peripheral tissues (e.g., two minutes in plasma; [35]). Importantly, although EPA does have significant acute anti-inflammatory actions in neural tissue [36,37] and the absorbance of EPA and DHA to the brain are similar [38,39], EPA levels are extremely low in brain tissue. This circumstance occurs because EPA is rapidly oxidized and removed from the brain, or it is elongated to the *n*-3 PUFA docosapentaenoic acid (DPAn3; 22:5*n*-3), which acts as a precursor for DHA [40]. However, EPA conversion is not a significant source of DHA [41–43]. The rapid β-oxidation of EPA may be the result of increased uptake of EPA by peroxisomes, where long chain fatty acids are initially catabolized before undergoing mitochondrial oxidation [44,45]. Such energetically costly mechanisms suggest a unique requirement for DHA. Therefore, for the purposes of this review we will consider the effects of combined *n*-3 PUFA (DHA + EPA) consumption or supplementation on brain function and cognition as being significantly dependent on DHA.

DHA is acquired during development through gestational placental transfer and from mother's milk during infancy. The levels of DHA in mother's milk can be as high as 1.4% of total fatty acids with a worldwide average of 0.32% of total fatty acids, depending on the mother's diet and number of pregnancies [25,46]. *De novo* DHA synthesis can occur in the liver, however the DHA precursor ALA does not increase plasma DHA in humans (<0.1% conversion efficiency in humans; [47–49]). In fact, neither ALA nor EPA is an effective dietary source of DHA due to the minimal *in vivo* production of DHA from these precursors in humans, indicating that preformed DHA is most effective in maintaining sufficient tissue stores [20]. On the other hand, DHA supplementation adds to the peripheral tissue pool of EPA, likely due to retroconversion [50].

DHA accretion in the brain accelerates during the middle of gestation, slows down in infancy, and reaches a plateau in early adulthood [51,52]. Half of the brain's DHA is accumulated during gestation, and the infant brain acquires five-times the level of lipids on a daily basis as the adult brain [53,54]. In adults, accretion is slower, and individuals with red blood cell DHA concentrations on par with the average European or American (~4% of total fatty acids) require 4–6 months of oral DHA supplementation to reach a steady state concentration that is dependent on DHA dose (8%–9% for 1000 mg per day; 5%–6% for 200 mg per day) [41]. Local *de novo* DHA synthesis in the brain is very low, thus DHA levels are maintained via delivery from the blood [55,56]. Circulating levels of DHA in the blood can reach as high as ~5% of that which is ingested orally [57] and ~0.5% of the circulating level is delivered to the central nervous system (CNS; [35]). After oral ingestion of DHA, lipases in the gut deliver unesterified free fatty acid (DHA-FFA) to the small intestine, and processing by the small intestine and liver results in circulating versions of DHA as DHA-triacylglycerides (DHA-TAGs), DHA-PC and DHA-FFA bound to low density lipoprotein (LDL) and albumin. These various forms are dissociated at the blood-brain barrier (BBB) through both active and passive processes that are mediated by endothelial lipases, fatty acid binding proteins (FABPs), and apolipoprotein E (ApoE) [58–61]. Unesterified DHA freely passes the BBB [39,61], and it appears that the brain derives most of its DHA from the unesterified FFA pool in blood [55]. Within the central nervous system, DHA is transported primarily via FABPs [59,60] and ApoE produced by astrocytes [61]. Membrane-incorporated DHA cycles in and out of the membrane from the phospholipids to the intracellular FFA pool via actions of DHA-coenzyme A (DHA-CoA) [62,63], providing a mechanism to respond to dynamic cellular events and to challenges during development and aging.

3. DHA and Cognition in Development

3.1. DHA during Gestation and Infancy

DHA is necessary for the growth and maturation of an infant's brain and retina [26,64,65], and as outlined earlier, DHA is conditionally essential for humans since it cannot be synthesized efficiently. This particular point needs to be stressed in that when DHA is needed in large amounts, such as during rapid phases of brain growth, it needs to be consumed via external sources. Furthermore, synthesis of DHA from its precursors in the fetus and placenta is insufficient to meet the demand of rapidly developing neural tissues [26,66–68], requiring the delivery of maternal DHA stores via placental transfer and mother's milk during pregnancy and after birth, respectively [66,67]. Therefore, the adequate supply of DHA to the developing brain is largely dependent on the dietary intake of the mother [69], and this supply is very important to the cognitive development of the progeny [70,71].

The observations above have led to the recommendation that pregnant and nursing women should consume at least 200 mg of DHA daily [26,72]. Supplementation with DHA during pregnancy may also benefit both the mother and baby by extending the length of gestation. A Cochrane review in 2006 concluded that maternal *n*-3 PUFA supplementation during pregnancy increased the gestational age by 2.5 days resulting in an average increase of birth weight by 50 g and birth length by 0.5 cm [73]. In alignment with this finding, a meta-analysis revealed that maternal *n*-3 PUFA supplementation was associated with pregnancies averaging 1.6 to 2.6 days closer to term [74]. A further meta-analysis of six RCTs found a 31% and 61% overall reduction of the risk of preterm births (defined as delivery before the 34th week of gestation) in all pregnancies and high-risk pregnancies, respectively, when mothers supplemented with *n*-3 PUFAs [75]. Lastly, maternal supplementation of 400 mg DHA per day in the second half of gestation was beneficial to children's growth tested at 18 months of age. This effect was only seen in children born to first time mothers [76]. These effects on growth and development of the fetus likely have a profound impact on cognitive abilities later in life.

Epidemiological studies have shown the importance of DHA during pregnancy for neuronal development. A large study (N = 11,875) showed that a lower intake of seafood, a rich source of DHA, during pregnancy was associated with risk of suboptimal development. In contrast, children born to mothers with a high intake of seafood during pregnancy exhibited greater pro-social behavior, better fine motor and social development scores, and higher verbal intelligence at eight years of age [77]. RCT trials have also provided evidence for a positive effect of DHA supplementation during pregnancy. For instance, taking 200 mg DHA orally per day for four months during pregnancy improved cognitive abilities of children tested at five years of age [78]. In a more recent multicenter RCT, 2399 pregnant women, who were <21 weeks into gestation with singleton pregnancies, were supplemented with 800 mg DHA and 100 mg EPA until delivery. While there was no effect of supplementation on overall mean cognitive scores in the offspring when measured at 18 months, the resulting data indicated that *n*-3 PUFA supplementation lowered the number of preterm births and low birth weights, resulted in fewer admissions to neonatal intensive care units, and reduced the number of children with cognitive scores indicative of delayed cognitive development [79].

Postnatally, the importance of DHA obtained from mother's milk for neuronal development has been reported repeatedly [80–84]. High DHA concentrations in breast milk have been associated with several brain-related positive health benefits in infants. These associations include a better ability to adjust to changes in surrounding [85], better mental development [86,87], improved hand-eye coordination [82], better attention scores [78] and memory performance later in life [88]. Nevertheless, some studies report neutral effects of DHA supplementation of lactating mothers on neurodevelopmental outcomes, results which likely depend on length and timing of DHA supplementation as well as the developmental time points assessed [82].

The DHA content of mother's milk is directly dependent on the mother's diet [26,89,90]. Dietary intake of DHA leads to a dose-dependent increase in DHA levels of breast milk [64,91]. Typically, DHA levels in tissues are higher in breastfed infants when compared to formula-fed infants [92]. Thus, it is not surprising that breastfeeding in the first six months of life is recommended for the optimal development of the baby, provided that the mother's nutritional status is favorable [81,93]. This is an important recommendation, and is corroborated by many studies that attest to superior neuronal development of breastfed infants in comparison to infants fed with formula (for a review, see [90]). For example, the Western Australian Pregnancy Cohort (Raine) Study recruited 2900 pregnant women and followed the live births for 14 years. This long-term study provided evidence that a shorter duration of breastfeeding may be a predictor of adverse developmental mental health outcomes throughout childhood and early adolescence [94].

PUFA supplementation of infant formula is an effective means to realize the benefits of breast milk in infants who are not able to be breastfed. For example, a 2007 meta-study summarized several RCTs that had examined PUFA supplementation of term infants and found a consistent association of DHA (and ARA) supplementation with beneficial effects on visual development in the first year of life [95]. For example, in a prospective, double-blind RCT (the DIAMOND study), 181 infants were enrolled at 1–9 days of age and assigned randomly to receive one of four term infant formulas with one of four levels of DHA: Control (0% DHA, 0% ARA), 0.32% DHA, 0.64% DHA, or 0.96% DHA for 12 months. All DHA-supplemented formulas contained 0.64% ARA. At 18 months of age, children who received DHA-supplemented formulas showed a significantly higher MDI score [96]. In another trial, 420 healthy term infants were randomized to receive a DHA-enriched fish oil supplement (containing at least 250 mg DHA and 60 mg EPA per day) or a placebo from birth to six months. Developmental assessment occurred at 18 months via the Bayley Scales of Infant and Toddler Development and the Child Behavior Checklist. Language assessment occurred at 12 and 18 months via the Macarthur–Bates Communicative Development Inventory. When compared to placebo, the fish oil group had significantly higher erythrocyte and plasma phospholipid DHA levels at six months of age. In a small subset analysis (about 40% of the total population), children in the DHA-enriched fish oil group had significantly higher percentile ranks of both later developing gestures at 12 and 18 months and the total number of gestures [97]. Supplementation of infant formula with DHA and ARA (0.32% and 0.72% of total fatty acids, respectively) provided for the first 17 weeks of life resulted in visual acuity scores similar to breastfed infants who performed better than control formula fed children at four years of age [98]. However, linolenic acid (precursor to DHA) provided via formula was ineffective in a separate trial in a similar measure of visual acuity at 16 and 34 weeks of age [99]. These results suggest that dietary supplementation of DHA during the first year of life likely leads to enhanced cognitive performance.

The studies cited above highlight the importance of maintaining sufficient intake of DHA during both pregnancy and nursing. For example, Helland *et al.* found that the supplementation of pregnant women with *n*-3 PUFAs from Week 18 of pregnancy through lactation conferred a cognitive benefit to their children on an intelligence test at four years of age, and the cognitive benefits in the children correlated significantly with maternal intake of DHA [87]. Furthermore, mathematical modelling revealed that a 100 mg/day increase in maternal DHA intake resulted in a small but significant increase in the intelligence quotient (IQ) of infants between 10 and 39 months of age [100]. Systematic review of maternal DHA supplementation indicated that DHA supported mental development and longer-term cognitive functioning of the child. When DHA was given to pregnant and lactating women, an increase in maternal intake of 1 g per day of DHA increased the child's IQ by 0.8 to 1.8 points [100]. However, when pregnant mothers were supplemented with 4 g of fish oil daily for a shorter period (only during late gestation) no effects were observed on overall mental or psychomotor development when measured at 10 months of age, but did positively affect hand and eye coordination at 2.5 years [101,102]. Similarly, supplementation of infant formula with DHA (0.2% of total fatty acids) for the first four months of infancy had no effect on Bayley Mental Index scores at 12 months of age [103]. These data suggest that the best neurodevelopmental effects of DHA, including those on cognitive performance, might be best achieved by exposure during both pregnancy and lactation [87]. Such findings emphasize the urgency of adequate intake of dietary DHA by pregnant and lactating women to ensure the healthy development of the brain and visual system in their offspring.

3.2. Preterm Infants and DHA

As alluded to above, the rapid growth of the brain during the last trimester of pregnancy requires a relatively high amount of DHA for proper brain development. Due to this circumstance, infants born prematurely are uniquely susceptible to the effects of DHA deficiency. Moreover, the ability of preterm infants to synthesize DHA *de novo* via elongation and desaturation of precursor fatty acids is insufficient to make up for their substantial deficits in DHA tissue levels [104]. Beneficial effects of PUFA supplementation in preterm babies for cognitive [105] and psychomotor development are well-established [106]. For example, Henriksen and colleagues showed that supplementation of expressed mother milk with 32 mg DHA and 31 mg of the *n*-6 PUFA arachidonic acid (ARA; 20:4*n*-6) per day resulted in better cognitive performance of premature infants weighing 1500 g or less at birth when examined six months later [107].

PUFA supplementation of infant formula for preterm infants has consistently demonstrated positive effects on aspects of neurobehavioral development [108]. High-DHA (approximately 1% total fatty acids) formula was compared to standard DHA (approximately 0.3% total fatty acids) from Day 2 to 4 of life until term-corrected age in an RCT of preterm infants. At 18 months of age, infants born at less than 1250 g in the high DHA group had a 50% lower likelihood of showing mental delay, as measured by the Bayley Mental Delay Index (MDI), when compared to infants in the standard DHA group [109]. In addition, an overall positive effect of DHA on MDI measured at 18 months of age was only observed among girls, who had less than half the risk of mild mental delay and less than a fifth of the risk of severe mental delay after high DHA supplementation compared to the standard DHA group. This effect was strongest among infants of mothers with low level of education, while no significant effect on mental development was seen among infants of mothers with higher education. However, when the same group was studied seven years later no differences between high-DHA and standard-DHA groups were evident in measures of weight, height, head circumference, or visual function [110,111]. Overall, current data suggest that infants fed formula benefit greatly from standard DHA supplementation and that this is especially important for preterm infants.

3.3. DHA during Infancy and the Relationship to Socioeconomic Conditions

The effect sizes associated with *n*-3 PUFA supplementation on postnatal growth and neurodevelopment in infants are relatively small. This circumstance is likely due to study populations that have been limited to formula-fed infants in high-income countries. Well-designed studies examining the effect of postnatal PUFA supplementation on infant growth in low-income countries are scarce, but some emerging data exist. For instance, a trial in rural Gambia that randomized 183 infants to receive fish oil or olive oil placebo from 3 to 9 months of age resulted in significant increases of growth parameters, such as mid-upper arm circumference and skin thickness in the fish oil group [112]. Interestingly, a recent Cochrane review came to the conclusion that, in high-income countries, "there is inconclusive evidence to support or refute the practice of giving PUFA supplementation to breastfeeding mothers in order to improve neurodevelopment," a similar conclusion to that of Scholtz *et al.* in a review highlighting the need for better study designs in future studies [113]. Nonetheless, the Cochrane review reported moderate positive evidence for measures obtained beyond 24 months related to language development and body weight in children. However, the authors also reported neutral findings for outcomes related to child length, intelligence and problem-solving, psychomotor development, motor development, and visual acuity among other measures. Most positive effects were dependent upon a specific developmental stage (with some realized short-term at birth to 12 months, and/or medium term at 12 to 24 months, and/or long term beyond 24 months). Lastly, no side effects were reportedly associated with *n*-3 PUFA supplementation [114].

The financial resources of the family can impact maternal consumption of DHA via dietary or supplementary means, ultimately affecting the DHA content of breast milk [115]. Studies of children aged 3–5 years reveal a low intake of ALA, DHA, as well as total fat in low-income countries [116,117]. The intake of fatty acids, especially DHA, of pregnant or lactating women and their young children do not meet the recommendations in many low-income countries [117,118]. Conversely, intake of the *n*-3 PUFA precursor ALA during pregnancy generally meets the recommendation in Mexico and the USA, but does not in Chile, Bangladesh, and India [76,117,119,120]. In studies examining the intake of DHA during pregnancy, none of the women in Mexico, Bangladesh or India met recommendations [76,117,120]. Postnatally, a decline in fat intake from 50% to 25% of energy between birth and 18 months is also observed in children in developing countries, which is primarily driven by a decline in intake of mother's milk. This decline intensifies further to about 15% of energy from fat by 2–3 years of age [112]. Importantly, the decline in breast milk intake leads to rapid reduction of dietary *n*-3 PUFA intake whereas the *n*-6 PUFA intake remains relatively stable. Since *n*-6 and *n*-3 PUFA precursors compete for the same elongation and desaturation enzymes, this increase in the *n*-6:*n*-3 ratio results in further decreases in *n*-3 PUFAs beyond what is attributable to total ingested levels. These data highlight the need for DHA supplementation in poorer communities in order to promote optimal cognitive development and possibly socioeconomic development.

3.4. DHA and Cognition in Children

The effect of DHA supplementation on cognition during childhood is controversial, with studies reporting no effects [121] or suggesting an improvement in verbal learning and memory [122]. Lower total plasma *n*-3 PUFA concentrations in boys of 6–12 years are correlated with a greater number of learning and behavior problems [123]. Children, 7–9 years of age, who were given an *n*-3 PUFA enriched diet for six months exhibited significantly higher plasma and red blood cell DHA and EPA levels, and these PUFA levels correlated with superior verbal learning, spelling and reading abilities [122]. Moreover, activation of the prefrontal cortex, a brain region critical for executive function, during a cognitive challenge was enhanced in 8–10-year-old normal boys who were supplemented daily for eight weeks with 1.2 g DHA compared to placebo [124].

In the DHA Oxford Learning and Behavior (DOLAB) study, Richardson *et al.* performed an RCT in 362 healthy school children aged 7–9 years from mainstream primary schools in The United Kingdom that initially underperformed in reading ability (bottom tertile). The children received either 600 mg of algal DHA each day for 16 weeks or a corn or soybean oil placebo designed to match both taste and color. Reading ability, working memory and behavior were measured using British Ability Scales (BAS II) assessments and parent/teacher observations using the Conners' Rating Scales. The results showed subtle reading improvements across the sample, but significant results were observed in the poorest-reading subgroup (lowest quintile). This subgroup experienced an eight-month improvement in reading age after DHA supplementation. Moreover, parent-rated behavior problems (ADHD-type symptoms) were significantly reduced by DHA supplementation. These data are valuable because, in contrast to the well-known critical period for the beneficial actions of DHA on brain function during prenatal development and early life, the DOLAB study showed that DHA can affect brain function well beyond early development in healthy children [125].

In a recent Australian RCT, the question was asked whether supplementation of *n*-3 PUFAs or *n*-6 PUFAs could improve cognitive performance in children [126]. A total of 616 term infants were randomized to receive tuna fish oil (high in *n*-3 PUFAs) or sunflower oil (high in *n*-6 PUFAs) from the time breastfeeding ceased or at the age of six months until the age of five years. Academic performance was measured by the National Assessment Program Literacy and Numeracy (NAPLAN) in school years 3, 5, 7 and 9. Plasma *n*-3 PUFA levels were measured at regular intervals until eight years of age. No significant differences in NAPLAN scores were observed between active and control groups. However, at eight years, *n*-3 PUFA levels in plasma were positively associated with the NAPLAN score measured at five years of age. These data are encouraging, because the observed correlation between the academic performance and *n*-3 PUFA levels was evident even though the supplementation had stopped three years earlier. Furthermore, there are a few issues that may explain the lack of overall effect in NAPLAN scale. First, the attrition of the test cohort was extremely high, and less than half of the original study population completed the final assessment. This situation rendered the final test size of the cohort too small to reveal statistical significance. Secondly, a relatively low amount of *n*-3 PUFAs were supplemented (135 mg of DHA and 32 mg of EPA), making it less likely to find significant effects when assessing cognitive performance. Lastly, the authors acknowledged that the parents of the children in the NAPLAN cohort were slightly older and more likely to be tertiary educated. Moreover, the mothers were more likely to have fully breastfed than the mothers of those who did not consent to or provide NAPLAN data, making it very likely that background intake of *n*-3 and *n*-6 PUFAs would also confound the results in this relatively prosperous group [126].

The positive effects of a diet rich in DHA on cognitive abilities may also have select sex differences. A large cohort of USA children aged 6–16 years of age, who were part of the third National Health and Nutrition Examination Survey (NHANES III), revealed cognitive benefits of higher *n*-3 PUFA consumption in both boys and girls, but the effects were twice as prominent in girls [127]. The authors speculated that the sex differences were due to a greater need for DHA in girls, since they need it not only for their own growth and development, but also in order to accrue peripheral stores destined to provide DHA for the neurodevelopment of their offspring. Indeed, recent animal work indicates greater peripheral synthesis of DHA from its precursor ALA in females as compared to males, an effect that emerges at the time of sexual maturity [128]. Interestingly, while the peripheral levels of DHA (plasma and liver phospholipids) were higher, the brain levels were similar, leading the authors to conclude similarly to Lassek *et al.* [127] that "the additional production of DHA in the liver of sexually mature females was not particularly intended for the brain, but probably for storage and mobilization upon future pregnancy."

There is a fair amount of inconsistency between studies examining the effects *n*-3 PUFA supplementation on cognitive performance in children or infants. Thus, there are several potential reasons for varying results including genetic factors, study design and methodological flaws, *etc.* It is also conceivable that genetic variation in fatty acid metabolism affects PUFA status. Potential genetic and environmental factors are not typically considered when recruiting for a study, and they likely contribute to some of the discrepancies between studies. Several study design considerations may help to reduce data variability. For example, stratification of the study population based on baseline DHA levels may help to avoid ceiling effects. It is also worthwhile to specify whether supplements should be taken on an empty stomach or with food, since certain food matrices can affect the bioavailability of *n*-3 PUFAs [129]. Using sensitive, standardized and validated analytical methods and cognitive tests as well as sufficient statistical power, dose and supplementation duration might also help resolve some supplementation effects. Importantly, the source of DHA (the particular type of fish flesh or oil, organ meat, oils derived from algae or crustaceans such as krill, *etc.*) as well as the ratio of EPA to DHA may affect the overall bioavailability of the *n*-3 PUFAs [130–132]. Assessment of tissue levels of DHA is also critically dependent upon the sample assayed, where erythrocytes are preferred over plasma fractions since their DHA content correlates better with peripheral and central concentrations of DHA rather than being heavily influenced by recent dietary intake as is the case for plasma [133]. Furthermore, the consumption and tissue levels of other nutrients should be considered. Very recent research published by Jernerén *et al.*, [134] suggests that homocysteine (Hcy) status, which is affected by B-vitamin status, may also determine the effects of *n*-3 PUFAs on cognitive decline and dementia (discussed in a subsequent section). Thus, B-vitamin status may explain some more of the inconsistent data across *n*-3 PUFAs supplementation trials. Last, but not least: it is important that the supplemented materials are of high quality, the source is completely defined, and the dosages are clearly defined and validated. In summary, assessments of dietary intakes of DHA suggest that pregnant and lactating women and young children often do not meet recommendations. Improving the dietary habits of mothers-to-be, pregnant and lactating women, and infants and children, with a particular focus on consuming high-quality sources of DHA, may be feasible strategies to enhance tissue levels and reap the corresponding developmental and cognitive benefits.

3.5. Mechanisms of DHA Actions during Development

As already outlined, DHA is accumulated in the brain tissue mainly during the second half of pregnancy and during the first two years of life [135]. Currently the consumption of one to two portions of fish per week, including oily fish, which is a rich source of DHA, is recommended. The challenging question is: What are DHA's actions in the developing brain that lead to gains in cognitive function? This question is far from being answered, but several pathways can be identified, many of which overlap with those occurring during adulthood and aging (described in a subsequent section).

DHA, as the most abundant *n*-3 PUFA in the brain and retina, contributes to the structure of brain cell membranes. DHA is also implicated in neurogenesis, neurotransmission, and cell survival within the CNS [136,137]. DHA contributes to cell membrane fluidity [138] and to signal transduction within the CNS by activating cell membrane receptors [135]. DHA also alters gene expression in mammalian brain tissue [139,140] that influences neurite outgrowth and learning and memory [141,142]. The process of neurite outgrowth in hippocampal neurons is enhanced by DHA, which may in turn promote learning [141]. Growth of neurites requires the accumulation of lipids in new membranes, and DHA helps to organize lipid raft domains in the membrane by pushing cholesterol into these structures important for neurite extension, myelination, and membrane-mediated signaling [143–146]. Also important for neurite outgrowth, DHA enhances protein kinase B (PKB; also known as Akt) signaling and in turn the mTOR (mechanistic target of rapamycin) complex, which promotes neuronal growth [147,148]. DHA improves learning and memory by facilitating the formation of pre- and postsynaptic proteins that enable synaptic transmission and long-term potentiation (LTP) [149]. Under oxidative stress, DHA can promote repair and growth of neurons by activating peroxisome proliferator-activated receptor gamma (PPAR) and through its activating effect on syntaxin-3 (STX-3) [150].

DHA is deposited within the cerebral cortex at an accelerated rate during the last trimester of gestation and during the first two years after birth, rendering this phase of neuronal development particularly vulnerable to nutritional insufficiencies [151]. This early accelerated rate of DHA deposition coincides with the onset of myelination, a process that is sensitive to DHA accumulation and stores [54,152]. Notably, animal data show that it is physiologically difficult to reverse the effects of early brain DHA depletion [153] and that reduction of *n*-3 PUFAs in the diet negatively affects DHA concentrations within the brain [154–156]. Studies in non-human primates show that low DHA levels are associated with deficits in the visual system, in brain functions [157], and in motor capabilities [158]. Furthermore, animal models provide solid evidence that the consequences of dietary DHA deficiency are a high *n*-6 to *n*-3 PUFA ratio in brain fatty acid composition and deficiencies in learning and memory behaviors [142,159], possibly due, in part, to negative impacts on neurite outgrowth and myelination [160].

4. DHA and Cognition in Adulthood and Aging

4.1. DHA during Adulthood

Cognitive function reaches its peak during middle adulthood. Thus, the detection of measurable effects of DHA consumption requires lengthy observational or treatment periods, and measurable effects are most effectively observed in cases of DHA-insufficiency or cognitive impairment. Indeed, a recent meta-analysis by Abubakari *et al.* [161] of 12 RCTs in adults found no effect of *n*-3 PUFAs on cognitive measures. However, the authors selected trials with subjects exhibiting a multitude of baseline cognitive conditions and/or subjects diagnosed with psychiatric conditions such as depression and schizophrenia, in addition to cognitive test parameters that likely clouded any measurable effect of *n*-3 PUFAs. Another recent meta-analysis of 34 RCTs found no effect of *n*-3 PUFA supplementation on cognitive performance, but the investigators combined trials performed with children, adults and elderly without performing any subgroup analyses that considered age or dose [162]. This limited their conclusions greatly since assessment of cognitive function is highly dependent on developmental timeline and age. Conversely, a well-designed meta-analysis by Yurko-Mauro and colleagues revealed that DHA + EPA supplementation improves episodic memory outcomes in adults with mild memory complaints, an effect primarily attributable to daily DHA doses above 580 mg [163].

Observational studies suggest a correlation between blood levels of DHA and cognition in healthy adults. For example, higher serum DHA levels were associated with better non-verbal reasoning, mental flexibility, working memory and vocabulary in 35 to 54 year-olds with no neuropsychiatric disorders and no supplemental fish oil use [164]. In an extension of this study, Leckie *et al.* [165] found that a higher ratio of DHA to ARA in serum counteracted the negative effect of low physical activity on both working memory and the trail marking task. This is important since physical activity can increase gray matter volumes and reduce the overall risk for Alzheimer's disease [166,167].

RCTs performed with adults report mixed results for DHA and *n*-3 PUFA supplementation on cognition. Supplementation of healthy adults from 18 to 70 years of age with 850 mg DHA and 630 mg EPA daily for 12 weeks had no appreciable effect on cognition [168]. Likewise, supplementation of young adults (18 to 35 year-olds) with 1000 mg DHA and 200 mg EPA for 12 weeks had no significant cognitive effects [169]. Furthermore, daily supplementation with 250 mg DHA and 1740 mg EPA in a college-age cohort for four weeks had no effect on attention, memory, or inhibitory responses [170]. In contrast, another study performed with college-age students and a higher daily DHA dose (480 mg DHA and 720 mg EPA) for four weeks found improvements in verbal learning and memory in the supplemented group despite the very short treatment interval [171]. Similarly, Stonehouse *et al.* (2013) reported improvement of episodic and working memory in 18 to 35 year-olds provided a high-DHA supplement containing 1160 mg DHA and 170 mg EPA daily for six months compared to placebo controls [172]. Interestingly, the effect on episodic memory was driven primarily by the women in the study, whereas the men were largely responsible for the effect on working memory. This is not completely surprising given the existence of sex differences in particular cognitive domains, including spatial working memory [173,174]. Recently, it was also shown that deficits in episodic memory observed in lonely individuals was prevented by *n*-3 PUFA supplementation for four months [175]. These data suggest that detecting cognitive effects in adults likely requires substantial levels of DHA provided for extended treatment periods in an experimental cohort with a relatively narrow age range.

4.2. DHA during Normal Aging

The age demographics of the global population is shifting as lifespans increase over time due in part to advancements in medicine and positive economic development. The segment of people 65 and older is projected to triple to 1.5 billion globally by 2050 (WHO, [176]). Unfortunately, cognitive ability declines naturally with age even in the healthiest of individuals. This decline is typically subtle, but it is nonetheless undesirable and ultimately affects the quality of life. Environmental factors such as diet, exercise, and DHA consumption can positively affect the normal aging process and overall mental health and performance.

Total gray matter volume declines with age [177], matching a parallel decrease in DHA composition [178]. This drop in DHA may be partially due to changes in activities for the enzymes responsible for DHA accretion into phospholipids [179,180] or to shifts in plasma pharmacokinetics [181]. Importantly, *n*-3 PUFA intake is positively correlated with gray matter volume in adults [182] and in brain regions responsible for cognition in normal, elderly adults [183]. During normal aging there is a gradual 10%–15% loss of total neuronal synapses resulting in a cognitive decline that is typically noticed around age 65 [184], and an increasing risk of dementia that is largely negligible before age 60 [185]. However, processes leading to neuronal loss and the impairment of brain functions may be active at much younger ages [186]. For example, in susceptible young adults, an age-related reduction of neurons in the brain is reported [187]. Of note, declines in episodic memory can begin as early as 20 years of age [188].

Support of the clinical findings above can be found in preclinical animal experimentation, in which age-related neuronal loss was shown to begin at the end of adolescence in rat brains [189]. Total synaptic loss is the best correlate of cognitive decline during aging, as overall synaptic density affects cognitive ability [190]. Increases in oxidative stress and inflammation in both nervous and immune systems also occur with aging [191], leading to DNA damage and telomere shortening. DHA has proven synaptic effects that improve synapse strength and numbers, and DHA can help prevent or mitigate oxidative stress and neuroinflammation. These actions will be discussed in more detail in the section on potential DHA mechanisms during aging.

Many observational studies have linked dietary consumption of *n*-3 PUFAs, and DHA in particular, with improvements in cognitive function and/or reductions in cognitive decline in healthy, aging populations. For example, DHA intake was correlated with performance and speed in a verbal learning test performed in a cohort of 45 to 70 year-old healthy individuals [192]. Van Gelder *et al.* [193] performed a prospective study using longitudinal data that calculated EPA + DHA consumption at baseline and at five years later in 70 to 89 year-olds and found that the decline in baseline mini-mental state exam (MMSE) scores was negatively associated with dietary EPA + DHA levels. In a group of 65 to 80 year-old healthy individuals, consumption of greater than 2.1 g of *n*-3 PUFAs per day was associated with better memory and executive function [194]. Velho *et al.* [195] reported that, in a cohort of healthy elderly (over 65 years-old), those that improved their MMSE scores at 8.5 months from baseline had higher consumption of *n*-3 PUFAs than those who did not show improvements. Cross-sectional analysis of elderly Spanish residents ($N = 304$), with an average age of 75 years-old, found a positive correlation between dietary DHA consumption and MMSE scores and that lower DHA intake was a predictor of cognitive impairment [196]. In a large cohort of Chinese adults (average age of 65; part of the Singapore Longitudinal Aging Studies) the daily consumption of fish oil supplements was associated with higher baseline MMSE scores and a lower risk of decline in cognition over a 1.5-year span [197]. Titiova *et al.* [198] more recently reported a prospective observational study in a healthy elderly population where baseline dietary DHA intake levels at age 70 were positively correlated with larger gray matter volume and declarative memory test performance (seven minute screen) at age 75. In a larger prospective study using data from the China Health and Nutrition Survey, Qin *et al.* [199] examined the decline in global cognitive scores over an average of 5.3 years in a group of Chinese adults ($N = 1566$, mean age 63 years old). This study detected a positive correlation between at least one serving of fish per week and slower declines in global cognitive function, composite and verbal memory scores. Finally, most recently del Brutto *et al.* [200] reported on a cohort from a rural middle-to-low income area of Ecuador that cognitive function as measured by Montreal Cognitive Assessment (MoCA) scores was positively related to the number of fish servings per week, and the data suggested an intake of at least four fish servings per week was best.

While dietary DHA intake is a convenient measure, there are inherent flaws in the reliability and accuracy of data acquired from food frequency questionnaires [201]. Therefore, studies that measure tissue levels of DHA could provide a more appropriate measure of current and past DHA status in relation to cognitive performance. Indeed, some but not all observational studies have linked DHA concentrations in blood with overall cognition and select cognitive domains. For example, a recent study measured the cognitive function of 2157 postmenopausal women at baseline and annually for six years and found no correlation between erythrocyte DHA + EPA and cognitive performance in seven cognitive domains at baseline or over time [202]. On the other hand, the Etude du Vieillissement Arteriel (EVA) cohort of French 63 to 74 year-olds exhibited a reduced risk of overall cognitive decline over four years in those with higher erythrocyte *n*-3 PUFA content [203]. Dullemeijer *et al.* [204] performed a cross-sectional longitudinal study in a Dutch cohort (50–70 years old) and found that higher plasma concentrations of total *n*-3 PUFAs at baseline was associated with less decline in sensorimotor and complex speed-related cognitive domains three years later. However, they did not observe associations with changes in memory, information-processing speed, or word fluency. Whalley *et al.* [205] performed a battery of cognitive tests in a Scottish cohort at ages 64, 66, and 68 years old and found a positive correlation between overall cognitive performance over time and erythrocyte DHA content at baseline (64 years old). Interestingly, this effect was only apparent in the absence of the ApoE4 allele, indicating a genetic influence on the link between peripheral DHA levels and cognition. The Framingham Offspring Study performed in a large group of elderly women (mean age 67 years old) reported that the women with erythrocyte DHA levels (but not EPA) in the lowest quartile had lower brain volume and poorer scores for visual memory, executive function, and abstract thinking than those in the top three quartiles [206]. Lower serum DHA (but not EPA) was also found in a small selected case study group of elderly with reduced performance in the MMSE compared to a cognitively healthy control group [207]. In this study, DHA serum concentrations were correlated with performance on a majority of the tests (memory, attention, and mental flexibility). Recently, Otsuka *et al.* [208] reported results of a cross-sectional longitudinal study in Japanese elderly adults that revealed a link between low serum DHA levels and a greater risk for cognitive decline over a decade as measured by the MMSE. This is especially profound given that elderly Japanese have twice the circulating levels of DHA as compared to similar cohorts in England [208,209]. Overall, these reports provide a suggestive link between the tissue levels of DHA and cognition during aging.

Data from RCTs in healthy aging adults has been historically sparse, but recently more trials have been reported, with some mixed but generally positive effects of DHA and *n*-3 PUFA supplementation on cognition. Initial reports indicated no differences in overall cognition in a group of elderly individuals over 65 years of age receiving daily high or low dose fish oil for 26 weeks, however subgroup analysis did reveal improvements in attention in those with the ApoE4 genotype [210]. Similarly, Dangour *et al.* [209] found no effect of daily *n*-3 PUFA supplementation for two years on cognitive measures in a group of 70 to 79 year old healthy individuals. However, controls in this study did not have a decline in cognitive performance over the two-year span, possibly masking any potential effect of DHA. Additionally, Stough *et al.* [211] reported no effect of daily DHA (252 mg) for 90 days on cognition as measured by Cognitive Drug Research (CDR) scores, however this cohort included a wide range of ages (45 to 80) and a small sample size, making interpretations difficult. In contrast, a combined supplementation of 800 mg DHA and 12 mg lutein for four months in healthy 60 to 80 year-old women, improvements in verbal fluency, memory scores, and rate of learning were seen [212].

More recent RCTs have yielded more compelling results than the earlier work. The Memory Improvement With Docosahexaenoic Acid Study (MIDAS) study, performed by Yurko-Mauro and colleagues [213], provided 900 mg of DHA or a placebo daily for 24 weeks in 485 healthy elderly individuals (mean age of 70 years-old) who had a self-reported mild memory complaint and a MMSE score over 26 (cognitively normal). Those supplemented with DHA exhibited improved episodic and visual recognition memory, but not in executive or working memory, and plasma DHA levels were directly correlated to scores in episodic memory. Furthermore, Vakhapova *et al.* [214,215] reported benefits in an elderly population with memory complaints (non-dementia) of improved immediate recall memory and sustained attention when provided a daily 300 mg DHA-phosphatidylserine supplement for 15 weeks. In a cross-over RCT, Nilsson *et al.* [216] reported a benefit of 3 g daily *n*-3 PUFA supplementation (1050 mg DHA) for five weeks in measures of working memory and selective attention in a group of middle age to elderly subjects. It is intriguing to think that the metric used by Yurko-Mauro *et al.* and Vakhapova *et al.* of a mild subjective memory complaint might be an early correlate of age-related cognitive decline, and their findings could indicate the potential power of DHA supplementation during the long, early and undetectable phases of cognitive impairment and dementia.

Recent RCTs have also associated the cognitive benefits of DHA with neurophysiology or anatomical changes in the brain. Witte *et al.* provided *n*-3 PUFA supplementation (880 mg DHA and 1320 mg EPA) for 26 weeks in healthy subjects (age 50 to 75) and found improvements in executive function, white matter integrity, gray matter volume, and parameters of neurovascular function compared to individuals provided a placebo. Tokuda *et al.* [217] provided 55 to 64 year old Japanese men who already consumed an average of 543 mg DHA per day and had substantial plasma DHA levels (7.0% of fatty acids) a supplement containing 300 mg DHA, 100 mg EPA, and 120 mg of ARA daily for four weeks. They report that treatment prevented a decline in auditory event-related potential (ERP) latencies (a measure of cognitive processing speed) that was observed in the placebo group. Deficits in auditory ERPs are typically observed in Alzheimer's disease [218]. Finally, a very recent study reported by Strike *et al.* [219] suggests that a combined supplemental approach may be beneficial. They gave a group of postmenopausal women between the ages of 60 and 84 years-old a daily supplement containing 1000 mg DHA, 160 mg EPA, 240 mg ginkgo biloba, 60 mg phosphatidylserine, 20 mg tocopherol, 1 mg folic acid, and 20 g vitamin B12 for six months and found a shorter mean psychomotor response latency (a measure of information processing speed) and verbal recognition memory in the treatment group relative to the placebo group. They did not detect any changes in executive function or paired associate learning. In totality, data from studies reporting the effect of dietary DHA consumption, blood DHA concentrations, and supplementation with DHA on parameters of cognition in normal aging individuals provide a substantial argument for obtaining sufficient amounts of DHA via dietary or supplemental means during aging.

4.3. DHA and Cognition in Mild Cognitive Impairment and Dementia

During aging, an increasing share of the resources available for normal cellular maintenance are spent on repair mechanisms needed by the cell to cope with the cumulative effects of oxidative, inflammatory, and other environmental insults. With this shift in demand, any diminished availability of energy, as a result of poor mitochondrial function, may result in neurodegenerative processes that can lead to neuronal loss and eventually to cognitive impairment, dementia, or other neuropsychiatric maladies. Unfortunately, neurodegenerative processes and neuronal cell death occur well before clinical signs of cognitive deficits are confirmed [186]. Dementia is not a disease itself, but rather a group of chronic symptoms that are common to several neuropsychiatric disorders (Alzheimer's disease (AD), Lewy body dementia, Parkinson's disease, *etc.*). Dementia symptoms, such as deficits in memory, language and executive function, lead to poor cognitive function in these individuals [186]. Dementia often results in poor self-care that can lead to inadequate nutrition, which could potentially exacerbate the cognitive deficits. In the most severe cases of dementia there is a loss of functional independence that results in institutionalization. Worst-case scenarios occur in low- and middle-income, developing countries where access to nutrient-dense foods and the ability to afford medical and functional care are leading to exponential growth in dementia prevalence rates [220].

There is a normal degradation in cognitive ability and brain atrophy with age [221,222]. However, the rate of atrophy is markedly higher in mild cognitive impairment (MCI) and dementia. The atrophy rate is especially high in the subgroup of MCI subjects that eventually develop clinically diagnosed AD [223], the most prevalent neurodegenerative disease. Approximately half of all individuals with MCI progress into AD within five years. Furthermore, brain glucose metabolism decreases 10%–15% during normal aging, and the extent of cognitive decline in MCI and AD is associated with the degree of glucose metabolism loss (nearly 35% in some brain regions; [224–226]). Preclinical animal studies have convincingly shown that DHA provided over a substantial amount of time can reduce neuronal loss and improve learning and memory as the animals age (For meta-analysis, see [227]). However, studying the effects of DHA on the risk of dementia is very challenging given the low incidence rates in cognitively healthy individuals. Some estimates have called for nearly 50,000 participants at baseline for proper statistical power [228], whereas the rate of cognitive decline during dementia is a more accessible measure. In addition, changes in cognitive domains are dependent upon the specific type of dementia. For example, early changes in AD are seen in episodic memory, whereas in vascular dementia early deficits in executive function are seen. Later stages of dementia and AD involve a multitude of cognitive domains.

Observational studies have linked the consumption of *n*-3 PUFAs with a lower prevalence of dementia [229] and lower overall risk of developing dementia [230]. Albanese *et al.* found a significant dose-dependent decrease in dementia relative to fish intake in a large group of subjects (14,960) residing in middle-to-low income areas [229]. The Three-City cohort study of 8085 French residents over the age of 65 found an inverse relationship between fish consumption and overall risk of dementia over a four-year timeframe in ApoE4 non-carriers (80% of subjects) [230]. Blood levels of DHA have also been tied inversely to mild cognitive impairment (MCI) and dementia. For instance, in the Framingham study, plasma phosphatidylcholine fatty acid content was measured in 899 subjects with an average age of 76 and no dementia at baseline. When re-assessed for cognitive ability nine years later, individuals in the top quartile for baseline plasma PC-DHA levels had a 47% lower risk of all-dementia (grouped with AD) *versus* the other three quartiles combined. No other fatty acid was significantly correlated (including EPA), and food intake surveys revealed that this quartile had an average DHA intake of 180 mg per day [231,232]. Cherubini *et al.* [233] also reported higher levels of plasma DHA in cognitively normal subjects as compared to those with dementia in an aging Italian cohort. With regards to MCI, Milte *et al.* [234] detected higher levels of the *n*-6 PUFA docosapentaenoic acid (DPA*n*-6; 22:5(*n*-6)) in the erythrocytes of MCI patients relative to healthy controls. More recently, Yin *et al.* [235] reported lower blood levels of DHA in amnestic and multi-domain MCI patients as compared to normal control subjects. These are intriguing findings since the DPA*n*-6 replaces DHA in the brain during DHA deficiency in an inefficient attempt to retain function.

Combinations with other nutrients are likely also important. Interesting results from the homocysteine and B vitamins in cognitive impairment (VITACOG) trial were very recently published in which 168 patients with MCI ($\geqslant$70 years of age) were given placebo or high dose Hcy-lowering B vitamins (folic acid, B6, B12) and assessed for brain atrophy via MRI at baseline and at a two-year follow-up [134]. B vitamin treatment reduced the brain atrophy rates by 40%, an effect only observed in the subgroup with the highest tertile of baseline plasma *n*-3 PUFA levels. Baseline plasma DHA, but not EPA, was a significant predictor of reduced yearly brain atrophy rate in those who took B vitamins, but not in placebo controls. Thus, the DHA status of the MCI patient affected the correlation between vitamin B supplementation and brain atrophy, and possibly cognitive decline by extension. It would be interesting to determine whether the Hcy and DHA status of the MCI subject affects or predicts the rate of conversion from MCI to dementia (about 5%–10% per year). If so, perhaps supplementation with B vitamins in combination with DHA in MCI patients would be an effective prophylactic treatment aimed at reducing the risk of further cognitive decline and the development of dementia.

RCTs have provided evidence indicating largely positive effects of *n*-3 PUFA supplementation on cognitive measures in subjects with MCI or dementia. Early evidence from Terano *et al.* [236] indicated improved dementia scores in patients with moderately severe dementia caused by thrombotic cerebrovascular disorder who received 720 mg of DHA daily for 12 months. Combined supplementation with DHA (240 mg) and ARA (240 mg) daily for 90 days was shown to improve attention and immediate memory in patients with mild cognitive dysfunction [237]. Furthermore, supplementation with 720 mg DHA and 1080 mg EPA daily for 24 weeks in MCI patients improved their scores in the Clinician's Global Impression of Change (CIBC)-plus and Alzheimer's Disease Assessment Scale (ADAS)-cog [238]. Sinn *et al.* [239] administered several doses of *n*-3 PUFAs, including high EPA (1670 mg), high DHA (1550 mg), or high LA (2200 mg) daily for six months in MCI patients and detected improvements only in the high DHA group particularly for Initial Letter Fluency, a measure of fluid thinking ability. The other cognitive measures did not show any differences, but the baseline erythrocyte DHA levels in this study were higher than those of Chiu *et al.* (5% *vs.* 4.2%). In a small, preliminary trial of 25 MCI patients, administration of a high-DHA (1440 mg) supplement also containing small amounts of EPA, tryptophan, phospholipids, and melatonin daily for three months improved MMSE scores, semantic verbal fluency and olfactory sensitivity [240]. The benefits of DHA on cognition in MCI may be dose-dependent since a recent report found no effect of daily supplementation with 180 mg DHA plus 120 mg EPA for 180 days in mild to moderate MCI patients on scores in the MMSE and Abbreviated Mental Test (AMT) [241]. Overall, optimal tissue levels of DHA are important in reducing the likelihood of developing, and improving the symptoms of, MCI and dementia.

4.4. DHA and Cognition in Alzheimer's Disease

AD is a uniquely human, progressive neurological disease resulting in hallmark neuropathology consisting of senile plaques, neurofibrillary tangles, neuronal atrophy, and abnormal brain glucose metabolism. AD accounts for more than 70% of dementia cases and has an estimated worldwide prevalence of about 4.4% of the population over 65 years old [242]. This prevalence is expected to grow from 5.2 million Americans in 2014 to 13.8 million Americans and to 115 million people globally by 2050 (Alzheimer's Association 2014 report [243], WHO 2012 Dementia Report [244]). Deaths from AD rose by 66% in a recent eight-year span, highlighting the lack of efficacious therapeutic options currently available, aging societal demographics, and shifting environmental impacts such as nutrition and physical activity [186]. A recent study in Medicare fee-for-service beneficiaries in the US found that the average total cost for a patient with dementia during the final five years of life was nearly $300,000. The out-of-pocket expenses during the final five years of life were approximately 80 times more for dementia patients when compared to those with heart disease or cancer [245]. Caretaking costs associated with dementia and Alzheimer's in the US is not generally reimbursed by Medicare, and these costs often completely deplete the household wealth of the patient and/or family member caretakers. Unfortunately, no therapeutic cure is currently available, and few investigational new drugs are currently being tested as pharmaceutical companies have traditionally experienced frequent failures in attempts to find efficacy [186,246].

Late onset sporadic AD (LOAD) is the most prevalent form of AD and has the lowest identifiable link to genetics. Therefore, LOAD may be most sensitive to environmental factors, such as diet and DHA intake. This is especially true given that neuropathological changes occur decades before clinically identifiable cognitive deficits, providing a long window of time for the cumulative effects of environmental factors to affect the manifestation of the disease. Traditionally, clinical studies have focused on later stages of the disease, when the disease neuropathology appears to be intractable and resistant to therapeutic approaches. AD affects 32% of people over 85 years old [247], and age is the single greatest risk factor, suggesting that even AD can be considered normal physiological aging.

Brain DHA composition likely plays a role in AD. The brains of non-DHA supplemented Alzheimer's patients have 65–95 nmol/g of unesterified DHA, much less than normal controls (110 nmol/g; [248,249]). Furthermore, deficient liver biosynthesis of DHA has been observed in AD patients, where it appears that DHA biosynthesis halts at the last β-oxidation step from tetracosahexaenoic acid (24:6*n*-3) to DHA [248]. However, this is likely a minimal source of DHA (*vs.* preformed via diet). Recent data also suggests that AD patients have problems processing DHA [61], therefore the magnitude of DHA's effects may be less in later stages of the disease [250]. Phospholipids PC and PE from various brain regions (particularly hippocampus) in the AD brain have reduced DHA content compared to control brains, further implicating DHA in the etiology of the disease [251,252].

Observational studies are generally supportive of a preventative role of dietary *n*-3 PUFAs and DHA with regards to risk and incidence of AD. Morris *et al.* [253] found that one or more servings of fish per week (or about 200 mg of DHA) was associated with a 60% lower risk of developing AD and that total intake of DHA (but not EPA) was also a determinant of lower AD risk. Furthermore, patients with early stage AD reportedly have lower dietary intakes of *n*-3 PUFAs as compared to healthy individuals [254]. Very recently, the AD Neuroimaging Initiative trial reported results in 229 normal, 397 MCI, and 193 AD patients assessed frequently over a two-year period. They found significant correlations between fish oil supplement use and lower brain atrophy in the hippocampus and cortical gray matter areas across all subjects [255]. There is some inconsistency in the reports of blood DHA levels in AD patients likely due to altered DHA pharmacology and bioavailability and the particular tissue or lipid fraction analyzed. One of the earlier reports indicated that total PL, PC and PE isolated from the plasma of subjects with AD, dementia, or cognitive impairment no dementia (CIND) contained less DHA than found in healthy elderly controls [256]. Furthermore, Tully *et al.* [257] reported that community-living elderly with AD had approximately half the serum concentrations of cholesteryl ester-DHA in comparison to non-dementia controls. These data also indicated that DHA and total saturated fatty acid levels were determinants of the clinical dementia rating. Wang *et al.* [258] found that lower scores on the MMSE in mild and moderate AD patients were associated with lower erythrocyte DHA content. More recently, Lopez *et al.* [259] evaluated an elderly cohort with an average age of 80 years-old for dementia and blood DHA levels. They reported that plasma DHA levels in the highest tertile had 65% reduced odds of all-cause dementia and a 60% reduced chance of AD, an effect that was recapitulated with dietary intake questionnaire data (highest tertile of DHA intake had 72% reduced odds of developing AD). Phillips *et al.* [260] also found positive correlations between composite memory scores (verbal reasoning, contextual, visual, and verbal memory) and overall cognitive status with plasma PC-DHA content across a cohort of normal elderly, cognitive impairment no dementia, and AD subjects.

RCTs investigating the therapeutic potential of DHA in improving the symptoms of AD are scarce and have mixed results at best. One of the first studies was performed by Kotani and colleagues [237], where they supplemented AD patients for 90 days with a daily dose of 240 mg DHA plus 240 mg ARA. This study found no significant changes in the repeatable battery for assessment of neuropsychological status test (RBANS; test five main cognitive domains). It would have been intriguing if Kotani *et al.* had a DHA-alone group to assess any potential counteractive effects of ARA in the combination administration. Subsequently, initial results from the OmegAD study in 174 mild-to-moderate AD patients (mean age 74) provided 1720 mg DHA plus 600 mg EPA daily for six months found no changes in ADAS-cog, MMSE, or Alzheimer's Prevention Initiative (API) tests [261,262]. However, in this early report of the OmegAD study, they did discover that a small subset of AD patients with milder cognitive dysfunction had lower declines in MMSE scores after supplementation. The next reported study was a small preliminary RCT that dosed AD patients for 24 weeks with a daily supplement containing 720 mg of DHA and 1080 mg of EPA. It reported improvements in the Clinician's Interview-Based Impression of Change Scale (CIBIC-plus), but not the ADAS-cog score [238]. Subsequently a large (N = 295), multi-center (51) study was reported by Quinn and colleagues [250], where they provided approximately 1000 mg of algal DHA daily for 18 months to patients with mild to moderate AD. They did not detect any differences in ADAS-cog or clinical dementia rating, suggesting that DHA is likely more effective as a prophylactic rather than a therapeutic treatment for AD. Interestingly, DHA-treated subjects in the ApoE4 negative subgroup had less decline in ADAS-cog and MMSE over time *versus* placebo, indicating a potential genotype dependence for DHA's effects in AD. Most recently, updated results have been described by the investigators of the OmegAD study where they have analyzed the levels of n-3 PUFAs present in the plasma acquired at baseline and after six months of the high-DHA supplement [263]. They report that increasing plasma levels of DHA in these AD patients was tied to preservation of cognition as measured by ADAS-cog scores. Higher concentrations of plasma DHA resulted in a lower rate of cognitive decline, an effect that was similar across genders. Cerebrospinal fluid (CSF) measures were also obtained in a small group of patients (N = 33) from the OmegAD study [264]. The patients in the treatment group had significant increases in the concentration of DHA in the CSF, and these concentrations were inversely correlated to CSF levels of tau (total and phosphorylated) and directly proportional to CSF levels of interleukin (IL)-1 receptor type II (anti-inflammatory effect). Tau levels are elevated during the prodromal phase (total tau) and clinical phase (phosphorylated tau) of AD, and these intriguing results suggest that DHA may be able to mitigate this increase to some extent.

The role of DHA in aging and dementia continues to be an emerging area of research, and more clinical work is certainly warranted given the limited, yet promising results thus far. The later stages of AD are largely intractable, so emphasis should be placed on prophylactic and early-stage therapeutic uses of DHA. Recent negative RCTs in AD patients have been focused on symptomatic effects in already diseased individuals, where significant and irreversible neuronal loss has occurred. DHA effects may be best determined with the disease-modifying effects of DHA focused upon in a large secondary population with mild cognitive complaints (much like the MIDAS study), along with several risk factors for dementia and AD (e.g., ApoE4, cardiovascular disease, low n-3 PUFA levels, early plasma AD biomarkers, *etc*). Pre-planned analysis of DHA effects within specific subgroups (dementia, genotype, baseline indicators, *etc.*) on repeated measures of cognitive function over a substantial amount of time is preferable, but this approach would certainly be costly and time-consuming. Nonetheless, these types of trials are needed to determine the prophylactic effects of DHA and the population subgroups that may benefit the most. In this regard, the ability of DHA to save neurons, and ultimately cognitive capacity, from a seemingly predestined fate could be determined. Considering that the aging of the brain occurs over decades, a general recommendation for maintaining DHA consumption throughout adulthood seems appropriate given the substantial data in aging populations, regardless of cognitive ability or disability.

4.5. Mechanisms of DHA Actions during Aging

Many of the effects of DHA during aging likely occur via several of the same pathways utilized during development. These include those important for neuron growth and survival, maintenance of myelination, reduction or resolution of inflammation, synaptic plasticity, membrane receptor function and lipid raft organization. There is certainly overlap with mechanisms of DHA action between normal and pathological aging. For example, the human brain contains extensive myelination that requires resource-demanding maintenance and repair, and oligodendrocytes, the primary myelinating cell of the CNS, require 2–3 times more energy other brain cell types [265]. It is this homeostatic maintenance and repair of myelin that some researchers consider the weakest link in maintaining brain health in the face of environmental insults and undesirable genetic factors. Myelin sheath abnormalities and defects are observed in normal aging, and white matter is affected in the initial stages of neurodegeneration [266]. Additionally, brain regions myelinated last in development are first to be affected in AD [267], suggesting a unique susceptibility of these late-myelinated areas to white matter defects and degeneration [268]. These observations have led to the hypothesis that amyloidogenesis and hyperphosphorylation of tau might be byproducts of pathological strain on myelin homeostatic processes, rather than causes [269]. The brain sacrifices axonal transport mechanisms for the sake of saving myelin and/or as a result of poor glucose uptake and overwhelmed anti-oxidative capacity of the neuron. These circumstances often result in synaptic loss and axonal degeneration [269,270]. Interestingly, Virtanen *et al.* [271] found that, in a large cohort of elderly subjects (N = 3660; ⩾65 years old), higher plasma DHA was associated with a better white matter grade as measured by MRI as well as a lower risk of subclinical brain infarcts. White matter intensities are a predictor of AD conversion in MCI subjects, and silent brain infarcts are associated with more precipitous declines in cognitive functions over time [272].

DHA also likely has cardiovascular benefits throughout adulthood leading to better perfusion of the brain. These benefits include lower blood pressure, improved vasoreactivity, dampened hepatic triglyceride synthesis, and reduced platelet aggregation. The brain is decidedly the most perfused organ of the human body [273], and cardiovascular diseases (common with aging) increase the risk of developing dementia [274]. Vascular dementia is the second most common form of dementia behind AD, and cerebral blood flow reductions and vascular pathologies are often reported in AD [275,276]. Jackson and colleagues [277] provided young adults (mean age of 22 years old) DHA-rich oil, EPA-rich oil, or placebo daily for 12 weeks and reported increased cerebral blood flow as measured by concentration of oxygenated hemoglobin in the DHA group as compared to placebo controls. There was no effect of high-EPA oil treatment on blood flow. This is in line with results from Beydoun *et al.* [278], who observed a positive correlation between *n*-3 PUFAs levels in plasma and cognitive performance in hypertensive and dyslipidemic middle-aged people. Moreover, this correlation was stronger than what was observed in healthy individuals. In addition, Baierle *et al.* [207] found that both increased blood Hcy levels (a risk factor for cardiovascular disease) and reduced serum DHA levels were associated with decreased cognitive performance in healthy elderly. DHA can alter the expression of genes encoding enzymes important for Hcy metabolism, methionine adenosyltransferase (MAT) and methylenetetrahydrofolate reductase (MTHFR) [279], and plasma Hcy and MTHFR polymorphisms are risk factors for dementia [280].

DHA can also affect processes involved in neural plasticity and LTP, which are essential for proper learning and memory function. DHA increases brain-derived neurotrophic factor (BDNF) and both DHA and BDNF affect AkT and ERK/MAPK/CREB signaling pathways to ultimately promote neural plasticity and LTP, which require synaptic modifications that are critical to learning and memory [281–283]. Calcium/calmodulin-dependent kinase II (CaMKII) and *N*-methyl-D-aspartate (NMDA) receptor function are essential for the maintenance of LTP and are positively modulated by DHA [284,285]. DHA also mitigates loss of the intracellular scaffold in neurodegeneration models, helping to maintain healthy axons and synaptic structures integral to cognitive function [284,286]. Furthermore, DHA supplementation may improve cognition by enhancing neurogenesis via the retinoid X receptor (RXR) and retinoic acid receptor (RAR), which decrease in expression with age in animal models [287].

The aging of the brain, and especially pathological aging, is also considered to be a consequence of sustained chronic inflammation. Alzheimer patients replete with amyloid plaques who do not exhibit signs of dementia (high pathology controls) have very few signs of neuroinflammation and neurodegeneration [288–290], suggesting that an inflammatory component to AD is at minimum partially responsible for the neurodegeneration and dementia. Brains from AD patients exhibit high levels of activated microglia [291], and the degree of cognitive impairment is inversely correlated with the extent of microglial activation [292,293]. Cytokines from these activated microglia break down neural membranes and release pro-inflammatory ARA metabolites, and anti-inflammatory DHA metabolites. Elevated pro-inflammatory cytokines have been identified in the CSF of AD patients [294–296], and amyloid beta (Aβ) itself has been shown to induce pro-inflammatory cytokines via activation of inflammasomes [297,298]. DHA can potentially counteract the effects of Aβ since recent data indicates that DHA enhances phagocytosis of Aβ42 by human microglia [299]. Further implicating inflammation in neurodegeneration, gestational immune insult via a viral mimetic, followed by a second similar insult in adulthood, leads to an AD-like phenotype in mice that includes CNS protein aggregates and deficits in cognition [300]. Interestingly, our recent work in this maternal immune activation model has shown that DHA provided throughout development and adulthood significantly dampens subsequent immune stimulation by a second insult with a viral mimetic in adulthood [301].

Important to the resolving process of inflammation, specialized pro-resolving mediators (SPMs) are derivatives of *n*-3 PUFAs and are reduced in AD where brain inflammation is increased [302]. SPMs have anti-inflammatory and pro-resolving characteristics and include protectins, D-series resolvins, and maresins derived from DHA via cyclooxygenase (COX) and lipoxygenase (LOX) pathways [303]. Recent results from the OmegAD trial found that cultured peripheral blood mononuclear cells (PBMCs) from AD patients who received the *n*-3 PUFA supplementation maintained levels of SPMs lipoxin A4 and resolvin D1 in culture over time, even when insulted with Aβ40, whereas PBMCs from control AD patients did not [302]. Furthermore, the effect on SPMs was positively correlated with cognitive changes and changes in transthyretin (prealbumin), which has been shown to inhibit the toxic effects of A. DHA and its metabolites can affect inflammation via several pathways including activation of PPARs, inhibition of nuclear factor kappa-B (NFκB), and activation of the transmembrane receptor GPR120. This is confirmed by observational studies showing that blood levels of *n*-3 PUFAs are associated with lower cytokine levels [304,305], and supplementation with fish oil for 26 weeks changes over 1000 genes in the PBMCs of an elderly cohort, resulting in a more anti-inflammatory gene expression profile [306]. Furthermore, daily supplementation with high-DHA (1700 mg DHA and 600 mg EPA) for six months in AD patients (OmegAD study) reduced the levels of lipopolysaccharide (LPS)-induced cytokines (IL-1B, IL-6) released from isolated PBMCs relative to within-patient baseline levels [307].

During pathological aging of the brain (and even in some cognitively normal elderly), inflammation results in neurofibrillary tangles made of abnormal forms of tau protein that cause alterations in cytoskeletal stability, axonal transport, and loss of synaptic contacts [269,300]. This can affect protein extrusion mechanisms and axonal energy metabolism, resulting in even more phosphorylated tau (p-tau), axonal blockage and leakage, and ultimately cell death. DHA can reduce p-tau levels likely by inhibition of the phosphorylation of tau via c-Jun *N*-terminal kinase 1

(JNK1) [308,309] or Akt through glycogen synthase kinase-3β (GSK3β) [308,310], and help to stabilize white matter [311]. Activation of the Akt pathway promotes cell survival via inhibition of caspase-3, potentially saving neurons during metabolic stress in neurodegeneration. These effects are similar to those seen in developmental reelin-signaling pathways that affect neuronal migration and cortical structure [312,313]. Reelin expression decreases with age and increases with sufficient DHA, and reelin is thought to be involved in the pathogenesis of AD [314]. Both reelin and DHA increase phosphoinositide 3-kinase (PI3K) activity, which activates AkT, which in turn inhibits GSK3β. GSK3β inhibits glycogen production and phosphorylates tau, and ultimately it is this poor glucose uptake and storage in combination with tau hyperphosphorylation that likely precipitates AD pathology [315]. This is in line with emerging data that suggest AD pathophysiology is at least partially mediated by impairments in brain insulin sensitivity, and in glucose metabolism and utilization, that lead to oxidative stress and inflammation [316]. Accordingly, diabetes patients are more likely to develop dementia [317]. Interestingly, animal and *in vitro* studies identify positive effects of DHA on endothelial and glial GLUT1 levels and brain glucose uptake [318–321].

In AD, extraneuronal Aβ aggregates to form senile plaques that limit plasticity and spine formation, promote loss of memory, increase inflammation via activated microglia, and increase pro-inflammatory cytokines. DHA can inhibit the activity of β-secretase, thereby inhibiting the formation of aggregates [322], and stimulate microglia to phagocytose Aβ peptides *in vitro* [299]. The production of Aβ from amyloid precursor protein (APP) via β-secretase is impacted by the integrity of lipid rafts, which can act to separate APP from the enzyme. Interestingly, there is a decrease in the DHA content of lipid rafts in cortex of AD patients [323], and this decrease in DHA enhances interactions between APP and β-secretase, thereby promoting amyloidogenesis in these subjects [324]. Furthermore, Aβ42 interacts with caveolin-1 containing membranes of erythrocytes in a stronger fashion in DHA-enriched erythrocytes, suggesting that DHA might help with the clearance of Aβ via lipid-raft mediated degradation [325]. These data are corroborated by a cross-sectional study that measured plasma Aβ40 and Aβ42 in 1,219 normal elderly over 65 years of age and found a strong inverse correlation between *n*-3 PUFA intake and plasma Aβ40 and Aβ42 levels [326].

5. General Considerations and Conclusions

There is substantial evidence regarding DHA's importance during pregnancy and infancy on the development of the brain and resulting cognitive function of the child. These effects on learning ability are dependent upon accumulation of DHA during gestation and nursing, and they highlight the need for maternal consumption of dietary or supplemental sources of DHA. Beyond development, a greater understanding of the impact of DHA across decades of life may require piecing together several well-designed longitudinal epidemiological studies. However, epidemiological studies may underestimate the effect of DHA on cognition due to other long-term factors that impact mortality and therefore those potentially helped most by DHA do not reach the age at which cognitive decline or dementia occurs. Nutrition and diet can also be affected by education and socioeconomic factors that can influence cognitive abilities, not to mention a propensity for a healthier lifestyle in general. Such long-term effects on overall health, and in particular on the cardiovascular and neurological systems, will clearly play into an individual's cognitive abilities.

Regarding intervention trials, inter-individual and day-to-day intra-individual variability in DHA consumption likely contributes to an under-estimation of the effect of DHA supplementation on cognition in RCTs. The interventions are comparably much shorter than long-term dietary habits, and RCTs are often not focused on a subject pool that is likely to benefit the most from interventions, such as those with insufficient DHA levels. Accordingly, basal DHA levels must be taken into consideration, as an effect of DHA is likely to be inconsequential in those with adequate tissue levels of DHA. Linking familial risks with early plasma indicators of AD and dementia (C-reactive protein, interleukin-6 and α1-antichymotrypsin, for example) with plasma DHA status may also help to identify those with the most potential for benefit from supplementation. In observational trials, caution must be exercised when examining dietary DHA intake levels and blood concentrations of DHA. Dietary intake only accounts for 66% of the variance in erythrocyte *n*-3 PUFAs concentrations, indicating that age, sex, BMI, physical activity, micronutrient status and other factors are also involved [327]. Similarly, due to the long half-life of brain DHA (2–3 years), fatty acid content of blood compartments may not accurately depict brain lipid composition, especially in the cases of subjects with cognitive impairment or AD and their likely associations with altered DHA processing [61,328]. Even if peripheral levels are comparable between subjects, the availability of DHA for various tissues and cell types may very well be different. This is highlighted by some recent studies utilizing isotopically labeled DHA indicating changes in DHA dynamics within the body as we age. DHA dynamics may also be dependent on genetic factors such as ApoE4 allele carrier status. For example, a single oral 50 mg dose of ^{13}C-DHA took significantly longer to clear from the blood of elderly subjects than young subjects [181]. Furthermore, the half-life of ^{13}C-DHA has been measured as 32 days in ApoE4 carriers, and 140 days in non-carriers [329].

Another consideration is the use of other supplements in boosting the effects of DHA, or acting in synergy, especially with regards to aging. For example, curcumin can boost DHA levels in the brain of animals [330], and it is intriguing to speculate that curcumin could help mitigate the losses in DHA that are associated with the heightened β-oxidation that is observed in AD. As previously mentioned, B vitamins and DHA work in tandem to reduce brain atrophy in MCI patients [134]. B vitamins lower Hcy, an intermediate in some oxidative stress-related pathways that are a risk factor for vascular disease as well as dementia. Hcy can also serve as notification that pathological neurodegenerative processes are occurring. Additionally, B vitamins may promote DHA incorporation into phospholipids, and likely have synergistic anti-inflammatory effects. In support of a combinatorial approach, Scheltens *et al.* [331] observed improvements in memory after daily supplementation with DHA, EPA, phospholipids, choline, uridine monophosphate, vitamin E, vitamin C, selenium, folic acid, vitamin B6, and vitamin B12 for 24 weeks in subjects with mild AD.

The non-steroidal anti-inflammatory drug (NSAID) aspirin might be another potential synergistic agent. Acetylation by aspirin enables COX-2 to initiate the biosynthetic pathway that produces resolvins (D1–D6) from DHA [332,333]. Aspirin-dependent resolvins are potent DHA-derived pro-resolving immune mediators [334]. Resolvin D3 has been shown to be especially effective in the late-resolving phase of inflammation (catabasis), the completion of which is critical to prevent an acute inflammatory response from becoming chronic activation [335]. The use of NSAIDs has been associated with a reduced risk for AD, especially in long-time users [336,337]. However, these effects are not realized in currently diagnosed AD, highlighting the likely importance of preventative supplementation [338].

Overall, DHA appears to have the ability to influence many different signaling pathways, receptor systems, enzyme activities, membrane structures and dynamics that ultimately lead to overall better development, maintenance and aging of the CNS, resulting in optimal cognition throughout the lifespan. These benefits likely require a sustained supply of DHA across development, adolescence and adulthood to build and maintain sufficient pools and/or to replenish depleted neural stores. For those unable to obtain sufficient amounts of DHA via dietary means, supplemental DHA from fish oil or vegetarian (algal oil) sources is ideal. DHA-containing supplements are taken daily by millions of people worldwide and have been shown to be safe and well tolerated even at high doses [339].

Acknowledgments: Literature search and review, and manuscript composition was made possible via internal support by DSM Nutritional Products Ltd.

Author Contributions: Michael J. Weiser and M. Hasan Mohajeri wrote the manuscript. Christopher M. Butt provided content and reviewed the manuscript.

Conflicts of Interest: Michael J. Weiser, Christopher M. Butt and M. Hasan Mohajeri are employees of DSM Nutritional Products Ltd.

Abbreviations

The following abbreviations are used in this manuscript:

Aβ	amyloid beta
AD	Alzheimer's disease
ADAS	Alzheimer's disease assessment scale
Akt	protein kinase B (also PKB)
ALA	α-linolenic acid
AMT	abbreviated mental test
API	Alzheimer's prevention initiative
ApoE	apolipoprotein E
APP	amyloid precursor protein
BBB	blood brain barrier
BDNF	brain-derived neurotrophic factor
CaMKII	calcium/calmodulin-dependent kinase II
CDR	cognitive drug research
CIBC	clinician's global impression of change
CIND	cognitive impairment no dementia
COX	cyclooxygenase
CNS	central nervous system
CSF	cerebrospinal fluid
DHA	docosahexaenoic acid
DHA-CoA	docosahexaenoic acid coenzyme A
DPAn3	omega-3 docosapentaenoic acid
DPAn6	omega-6 docosapentaenoic acid
EPA	eicosapentaenoic acid
ER	endoplasmic reticulum
ERP	event-related potential
FABP	fatty acid binding protein
FFA	free fatty acid
GSK3β	glycogen synthase kinase 3-β
Hcy	homocysteine
IL	interleukin
IQ	intelligence quotient
JNK1	c-Jun *N*-terminal kinase 1
LA	linoleic acid
LDL	low density lipoprotein
LOX	lipoxygenase
LPS	lipopolysaccharide
LTP	long-term potentiation
MAT	methionine adenosyltransferase
MCI	mild cognitive impairment
MMSE	mini-mental state exam
MoCA	montreal cognitive assessment
MTHFR	methylenetetrahydrofolate reductase
mTOR	mechanistic target of rapamycin
n-3	omega-3
NFκB	nuclear factor kappa-B
NMDA	*N*-methyl-D-aspartate
NSAID	non-steroidal anti-inflammatory drug

PBMC	peripheral blood mononuclear cells
PC	phosphatidylcholine
PE	phosphatidylethanolamine
PI3K	phosphoinositide 3-kinase
PL	phospholipid
PPAR	peroxisome proliferator-activated receptor gamma
PUFA	polyunsaturated fatty acid
PS	phosphatidylserine
RAR	retinoic acid receptor
RBANS	repeatable battery for assessment of neuropsychological status test
RCT	randomized control trials
RXR	retinoid X receptor
SPM	specialized proresolving mediators
STX-3	syntaxin-3
TAG	triacylglyceride

References

1. Bryan, J.; Osendarp, S.; Hughes, D.; Calvaresi, E.; Baghurst, K.; van Klinken, J.W. Nutrients for cognitive development in school-aged children. *Nutr. Rev.* **2004**, *62*, 295–306. [CrossRef] [PubMed]
2. Brenna, J.T.; Diau, G.Y. The influence of dietary docosahexaenoic acid and arachidonic acid on central nervous system polyunsaturated fatty acid composition. *Prostaglandins Leukot. Essent. Fat. Acids* **2007**, *77*, 247–250. [CrossRef] [PubMed]
3. Rapoport, S.I. *In vivo* fatty acid incorporation into brain phospholipids in relation to signal transduction and membrane remodeling. *Neurochem. Res.* **1999**, *24*, 1403–1415. [CrossRef] [PubMed]
4. Garcia, M.C.; Ward, G.; Ma, Y.C.; Salem, N., Jr.; Kim, H.Y. Effect of docosahexaenoic acid on the synthesis of phosphatidylserine in rat brain in microsomes and C6 glioma cells. *J. Neurochem.* **1998**, *70*, 24–30. [CrossRef] [PubMed]
5. Suzuki, H.; Manabe, S.; Wada, O.; Crawford, M.A. Rapid incorporation of docosahexaenoic acid from dietary sources into brain microsomal, synaptosomal and mitochondrial membranes in adult mice. *Int. J. Vitam. Nutr. Res.* **1997**, *67*, 272–278. [PubMed]
6. Uauy, R.; Dangour, A.D. Nutrition in brain development and aging: Role of essential fatty acids. *Nutr. Rev.* **2006**, *64*, S24–S33. [CrossRef] [PubMed]
7. Haubner, L.; Sullivan, J.; Ashmeade, T.; Saste, M.; Wiener, D.; Carver, J. The effects of maternal dietary docosahexaenoic acid intake on rat pup myelin and the auditory startle response. *Dev. Neurosci.* **2007**, *29*, 460–467. [CrossRef] [PubMed]
8. Orr, S.K.; Bazinet, R.P. The emerging role of docosahexaenoic acid in neuroinflammation. *Curr. Opin. Investig. Drugs* **2008**, *9*, 735–743. [PubMed]
9. Goustard-Langelier, B.; Guesnet, P.; Durand, G.; Antoine, J.M.; Alessandri, J.M. *n*-3 and *n*-6 fatty acid enrichment by dietary fish oil and phospholipid sources in brain cortical areas and nonneural tissues of formula-fed piglets. *Lipids* **1999**, *34*, 5–16. [CrossRef] [PubMed]
10. Anderson, V.; Fenwick, T.; Manly, T.; Robertson, I. Attentional skills following traumatic brain injury in childhood: A componential analysis. *Brain Inj.* **1998**, *12*, 937–949. [CrossRef] [PubMed]
11. Barkley, R.A. The executive functions and self-regulation: An evolutionary neuropsychological perspective. *Neuropsychol. Rev.* **2001**, *11*, 1–29. [CrossRef] [PubMed]
12. Kuratko, C.N.; Barrett, E.C.; Nelson, E.B.; Salem, N. The relationship of docosahexaenoic acid (DHA) with learning and behavior in healthy children: A review. *Nutrients* **2013**, *5*, 2777–2810. [CrossRef] [PubMed]
13. Stonehouse, W. Does consumption of LC omega-3 PUFA enhance cognitive performance in healthy school-aged children and throughout adulthood? Evidence from clinical trials. *Nutrients* **2014**, *6*, 2730–2758. [CrossRef] [PubMed]

14. Cederholm, T.; Salem, N., Jr.; Palmblad, J. Omega-3 fatty acids in the prevention of cognitive decline in humans. *Adv. Nutr.* **2013**, *4*, 672–676. [CrossRef] [PubMed]
15. Joffre, C.; Nadjar, A.; Lebbadi, M.; Calon, F.; Laye, S. *n*-3 LCPUFA improves cognition: The young, the old and the sick. *Prostaglandins Leukot. Essent. Fat. Acids* **2014**, *91*, 1–20. [CrossRef] [PubMed]
16. Salem, N.; Vandal, M.; Calon, F. The benefit of docosahexaenoic acid for the adult brain in aging and dementia. *Prostaglandins Leukot. Essent. Fat. Acids* **2015**, *92*, 15–22. [CrossRef] [PubMed]
17. Sprecher, H.; Luthria, D.L.; Mohammed, B.S.; Baykousheva, S.P. Reevaluation of the pathways for the biosynthesis of polyunsaturated fatty acids. *J. Lipid Res.* **1995**, *36*, 2471–2477. [PubMed]
18. Emken, E.A.; Adlof, R.O.; Gulley, R.M. Dietary linoleic acid influences desaturation and acylation of deuterium-labeled linoleic and linolenic acids in young adult males. *Biochim. Biophys. Acta* **1994**, *1213*, 277–288. [CrossRef]
19. Barcelo-Coblijn, G.; Murphy, E.J. Alpha-linolenic acid and its conversion to longer chain *n*-3 fatty acids: Benefits for human health and a role in maintaining tissue *n*-3 fatty acid levels. *Prog. Lipid Res.* **2009**, *48*, 355–374. [CrossRef] [PubMed]
20. Brenna, J.T.; Salem, N., Jr.; Sinclair, A.J.; Cunnane, S.C. Alpha-linolenic acid supplementation and conversion to *n*-3 long-chain polyunsaturated fatty acids in humans. *Prostaglandins Leukot. Essent. Fat. Acids* **2009**, *80*, 85–91. [CrossRef] [PubMed]
21. Salem, N.; Eggersdorfer, M. Is the world supply of omega-3 fatty acids adequate for optimal human nutrition? *Curr. Opin. Clin. Nutr. Metab. Care* **2015**, *18*, 147–154. [CrossRef] [PubMed]
22. Birch, E.E.; Carlson, S.E.; Hoffman, D.R.; Fitzgerald-Gustafson, K.M.; Fu, V.L.; Drover, J.R.; Castaneda, Y.S.; Minns, L.; Wheaton, D.K.; Mundy, D.; *et al.* The diamond (DHA intake and measurement of neural development) study: A double-masked, randomized controlled clinical trial of the maturation of infant visual acuity as a function of the dietary level of docosahexaenoic acid. *Am. J. Clin. Nutr.* **2010**, *91*, 848–859. [CrossRef] [PubMed]
23. Hoffman, D.R.; Boettcher, J.A.; Diersen-Schade, D.A. Toward optimizing vision and cognition in term infants by dietary docosahexaenoic and arachidonic acid supplementation: A review of randomized controlled trials. *Prostaglandins Leukot. Essent. Fat. Acids* **2009**, *81*, 151–158. [CrossRef] [PubMed]
24. Makrides, M. Is there a dietary requirement for DHA in pregnancy? *Prostaglandins Leukot. Essent. Fat. Acids* **2009**, *81*, 171–174. [CrossRef] [PubMed]
25. Brenna, J.T.; Varamini, B.; Jensen, R.G.; Diersen-Schade, D.A.; Boettcher, J.A.; Arterburn, L.M. Docosahexaenoic and arachidonic acid concentrations in human breast milk worldwide. *Am. J. Clin. Nutr.* **2007**, *85*, 1457–1464. [PubMed]
26. Koletzko, B.; Lien, E.; Agostoni, C.; Bohles, H.; Campoy, C.; Cetin, I.; Decsi, T.; Dudenhausen, J.W.; Dupont, C.; Forsyth, S.; *et al.* The roles of long-chain polyunsaturated fatty acids in pregnancy, lactation and infancy: Review of current knowledge and consensus recommendations. *J. Perinat. Med.* **2008**, *36*, 5–14. [CrossRef] [PubMed]
27. Aranceta, J.; Pérez-Rodrigo, C. Recommended dietary reference intakes, nutritional goals and dietary guidelines for fat and fatty acids: A systematic review. *Br. J. Nutr.* **2012**, *107*, S8–S22. [CrossRef] [PubMed]
28. Mosca, L.; Benjamin, E.J.; Berra, K.; Bezanson, J.L.; Dolor, R.J.; Lloyd-Jones, D.M.; Newby, L.K.; Pina, I.L.; Roger, V.L.; Shaw, L.J.; *et al.* Effectiveness-based guidelines for the prevention of cardiovascular disease in women—2011 update: A guideline from the American Heart Association. *Circulation* **2011**, *123*, 1243–1262. [CrossRef] [PubMed]
29. World Health Organization; Food and Agriculture Organization of the United Nations. *Report of the Joint FAO/WHO Expert Consultation on the Risks and Benefits of Fish Consumption*; FAO Fisheries and Aquaculture Report No. 978; WHO: Geneva, Switzerland; FAO: Rome, Italy, 2010; Volume 978, pp. 25–29.
30. Blasbalg, T.L.; Hibbeln, J.R.; Ramsden, C.E.; Majchrzak, S.F.; Rawlings, R.R. Changes in consumption of omega-3 and omega-6 fatty acids in the United States during the 20th century. *Am. J. Clin. Nutr.* **2011**, *93*, 950–962. [CrossRef] [PubMed]
31. Meyer, B.J. Are we consuming enough long chain omega-3 polyunsaturated fatty acids for optimal health? *Prostaglandins Leukot. Essent. Fat. Acids* **2011**, *85*, 275–280. [CrossRef] [PubMed]
32. Simopoulos, A.P. Evolutionary aspects of diet: The omega-6/omega-3 ratio and the brain. *Mol. Neurobiol.* **2011**, *44*, 203–215. [CrossRef] [PubMed]

33. Broadhurst, C.L.; Cunnane, S.C.; Crawford, M.A. Rift valley lake fish and shellfish provided brain-specific nutrition for early homo. *Br. J. Nutr.* **1998**, *79*, 3–21. [CrossRef] [PubMed]
34. Crawford, M.A.; Bloom, M.; Broadhurst, C.L.; Schmidt, W.F.; Cunnane, S.C.; Galli, C.; Gehbremeskel, K.; Linseisen, F.; Lloyd-Smith, J.; Parkington, J. Evidence for the unique function of docosahexaenoic acid during the evolution of the modern hominid brain. *Lipids* **1999**, *34*, S39–S47. [CrossRef] [PubMed]
35. Umhau, J.C.; Zhou, W.; Carson, R.E.; Rapoport, S.I.; Polozova, A.; Demar, J.; Hussein, N.; Bhattacharjee, A.K.; Ma, K.; Esposito, G.; *et al.* Imaging incorporation of circulating docosahexaenoic acid into the human brain using positron emission tomography. *J. Lipid Res.* **2009**, *50*, 1259–1268. [CrossRef] [PubMed]
36. Kawashima, A.; Harada, T.; Imada, K.; Yano, T.; Mizuguchi, K. Eicosapentaenoic acid inhibits interleukin-6 production in interleukin-1beta-stimulated C6 glioma cells through peroxisome proliferator-activated receptor-gamma. *Prostaglandins Leukot. Essent. Fat. Acids* **2008**, *79*, 59–65. [CrossRef] [PubMed]
37. Orr, S.K.; Trepanier, M.O.; Bazinet, R.P. *n*-3 polyunsaturated fatty acids in animal models with neuroinflammation. *Prostaglandins Leukot. Essent. Fat. Acids* **2013**, *88*, 97–103. [CrossRef] [PubMed]
38. Chen, C.T.; Liu, Z.; Ouellet, M.; Calon, F.; Bazinet, R.P. Rapid beta-oxidation of eicosapentaenoic acid in mouse brain: An *in situ* study. *Prostaglandins Leukot. Essent. Fat. Acids* **2009**, *80*, 157–163. [CrossRef] [PubMed]
39. Ouellet, M.; Emond, V.; Chen, C.T.; Julien, C.; Bourasset, F.; Oddo, S.; LaFerla, F.; Bazinet, R.P.; Calon, F. Diffusion of docosahexaenoic and eicosapentaenoic acids through the blood-brain barrier: An *in situ* cerebral perfusion study. *Neurochem. Int.* **2009**, *55*, 476–482. [CrossRef] [PubMed]
40. Chen, C.T.; Bazinet, R.P. Beta-oxidation and rapid metabolism, but not uptake regulate brain eicosapentaenoic acid levels. *Prostaglandins Leukot. Essent. Fat. Acids* **2015**, *92*, 33–40. [CrossRef] [PubMed]
41. Arterburn, L.M.; Hall, E.B.; Oken, H. Distribution, interconversion, and dose response of *n*-3 fatty acids in humans. *Am. J. Clin. Nutr.* **2006**, *83*, 1467S–1476S. [PubMed]
42. Chen, C.T.; Domenichiello, A.F.; Trépanier, M.O.; Liu, Z.; Masoodi, M.; Bazinet, R.P. The low levels of eicosapentaenoic acid in rat brain phospholipids are maintained via multiple redundant mechanisms. *J. Lipid Res.* **2013**, *54*, 2410–2422. [CrossRef] [PubMed]
43. Kaur, G.; Molero, J.C.; Weisinger, H.S.; Sinclair, A.J. Orally administered [14C] DPA and [14C] DHA are metabolised differently to [14C] EPA in rats. *Br. J. Nutr.* **2013**, *109*, 441–448. [CrossRef] [PubMed]
44. Eaton, S.; Bartlett, K.; Pourfarzam, M. Mammalian mitochondrial beta-oxidation. *Biochem. J.* **1996**, *320*, 345–357. [CrossRef] [PubMed]
45. Reddy, J.K.; Hashimoto, T. Peroxisomal beta-oxidation and peroxisome proliferator-activated receptor alpha: An adaptive metabolic system. *Annu. Rev. Nutr.* **2001**, *21*, 193–230. [CrossRef] [PubMed]
46. Morse, N.L. Benefits of docosahexaenoic acid, folic acid, vitamin D and iodine on foetal and infant brain development and function following maternal supplementation during pregnancy and lactation. *Nutrients* **2012**, *4*, 799–840. [CrossRef] [PubMed]
47. Lin, Y.H.; Llanos, A.; Mena, P.; Uauy, R.; Salem, N., Jr.; Pawlosky, R.J. Compartmental analyses of 2H5-alpha-linolenic acid and CU-eicosapentaenoic acid toward synthesis of plasma labeled 22:6*n*-3 in newborn term infants. *Am. J. Clin. Nutr.* **2010**, *92*, 284–293. [CrossRef] [PubMed]
48. Pawlosky, R.J.; Salem, N., Jr. Perspectives on alcohol consumption: Liver polyunsaturated fatty acids and essential fatty acid metabolism. *Alcohol* **2004**, *34*, 27–33. [CrossRef] [PubMed]
49. Plourde, M.; Cunnane, S.C. Extremely limited synthesis of long chain polyunsaturates in adults: Implications for their dietary essentiality and use as supplements. *Appl. Physiol. Nutr. Metab.* **2007**, *32*, 619–634. [CrossRef] [PubMed]
50. Egert, S.; Lindenmeier, M.; Harnack, K.; Krome, K.; Erbersdobler, H.F.; Wahrburg, U.; Somoza, V. Margarines fortified with alpha-linolenic acid, eicosapentaenoic acid, or docosahexaenoic acid alter the fatty acid composition of erythrocytes but do not affect the antioxidant status of healthy adults. *J. Nutr.* **2012**, *142*, 1638–1644. [CrossRef] [PubMed]
51. Carver, J.; Benford, V.; Han, B.; Cantor, A. The relationship between age and the fatty acid composition of cerebral cortex and erythrocytes in human subjects. *Brain Res. Bull.* **2001**, *56*, 79–85. [CrossRef]
52. Martinez, M. Tissue levels of polyunsaturated fatty acids during early human development. *J. Pediatr.* **1992**, *120*, S129–S138. [CrossRef]
53. Bourre, J.M. Effects of nutrients (in food) on the structure and function of the nervous system: Update on dietary requirements for brain. Part 1: Micronutrients. *J. Nutr. Health Aging* **2006**, *10*, 377–385. [PubMed]

54. McNamara, R.K.; Carlson, S.E. Role of omega-3 fatty acids in brain development and function: Potential implications for the pathogenesis and prevention of psychopathology. *Prostaglandins Leukot. Essent. Fat. Acids* **2006**, *75*, 329–349. [CrossRef] [PubMed]
55. Chen, C.T.; Kitson, A.P.; Hopperton, K.E.; Domenichiello, A.F.; Trepanier, M.O.; Lin, L.E.; Ermini, L.; Post, M.; Thies, F.; Bazinet, R.P. Plasma non-esterified docosahexaenoic acid is the major pool supplying the brain. *Sci. Rep.* **2015**, *5*, 15791. [CrossRef] [PubMed]
56. DeMar, J.C., Jr.; Ma, K.; Chang, L.; Bell, J.M.; Rapoport, S.I. Alpha-linolenic acid does not contribute appreciably to docosahexaenoic acid within brain phospholipids of adult rats fed a diet enriched in docosahexaenoic acid. *J. Neurochem.* **2005**, *94*, 1063–1076. [CrossRef] [PubMed]
57. Lemaitre-Delaunay, D.; Pachiaudi, C.; Laville, M.; Pousin, J.; Armstrong, M.; Lagarde, M. Blood compartmental metabolism of docosahexaenoic acid (DHA) in humans after ingestion of a single dose of [13C] DHA in phosphatidylcholine. *J. Lipid Res.* **1999**, *40*, 1867–1874. [PubMed]
58. Chen, S.; Subbaiah, P.V. Regioisomers of phosphatidylcholine containing DHA and their potential to deliver DHA to the brain: Role of phospholipase specificities. *Lipids* **2013**, *48*, 675–686. [CrossRef] [PubMed]
59. Liu, R.Z.; Mita, R.; Beaulieu, M.; Gao, Z.; Godbout, R. Fatty acid binding proteins in brain development and disease. *Int. J. Dev. Biol.* **2010**, *54*, 1229–1239. [CrossRef] [PubMed]
60. Pan, Y.; Scanlon, M.J.; Owada, Y.; Yamamoto, Y.; Porter, C.J.H.; Nicolazzo, J.A. Fatty acid-binding protein 5 facilitates the blood-brain barrier transport of docosahexaenoic acid. *Mol. Pharm.* **2015**, *12*, 4375–4385. [CrossRef] [PubMed]
61. Vandal, M.; Alata, W.; Tremblay, C.; Rioux-Perreault, C.; Salem, N.; Calon, F.; Plourde, M. Reduction in DHA transport to the brain of mice expressing human APOE4 compared to APOE 2. *J. Neurochem.* **2014**, *129*, 516–526. [CrossRef] [PubMed]
62. Chen, C.T.; Green, J.T.; Orr, S.K.; Bazinet, R.P. Regulation of brain polyunsaturated fatty acid uptake and turnover. *Prostaglandins Leukot. Essent. Fat. Acids* **2008**, *79*, 85–91. [CrossRef] [PubMed]
63. Kennedy, E.P.; Weiss, S.B. The function of cytidine coenzymes in the biosynthesis of phospholipides. *J. Biol. Chem.* **1956**, *222*, 193–214. [PubMed]
64. Jensen, C.L.; Lapillonne, A. Docosahexaenoic acid and lactation. *Prostaglandins Leukot. Essent. Fat. Acids* **2009**, *81*, 175–178. [CrossRef] [PubMed]
65. Simmer, K.; Patole, S.K.; Rao, S.C. Long-chain polyunsaturated fatty acid supplementation in infants born at term. *Cochrane Database Syst. Rev.* **2011**. [CrossRef]
66. Chambaz, J.; Ravel, D.; Manier, M.C.; Pepin, D.; Mulliez, N.; Bereziat, G. Essential fatty acids interconversion in the human fetal liver. *Biol. Neonate* **1985**, *47*, 136–140. [CrossRef] [PubMed]
67. Innis, S.M. Essential fatty acid transfer and fetal development. *Placenta* **2005**, *26*, S70–S75. [CrossRef] [PubMed]
68. Uauy, R.; Mena, P.; Rojas, C. Essential fatty acids in early life: Structural and functional role. *Proc. Nutr. Soc.* **2000**, *59*, 3–15. [CrossRef] [PubMed]
69. Grantham-McGregor, S.; Cheung, Y.B.; Cueto, S.; Glewwe, P.; Richter, L.; Strupp, B. Developmental potential in the first 5 years for children in developing countries. *Lancet* **2007**, *369*, 60–70. [CrossRef]
70. Farquharson, J.; Cockburn, F.; Patrick, W.A.; Jamieson, E.C.; Logan, R.W. Infant cerebral cortex phospholipid fatty-acid composition and diet. *Lancet* **1992**, *340*, 810–813. [CrossRef]
71. Makrides, M.; Neumann, M.; Simmer, K.; Pater, J.; Gibson, R. Are long-chain polyunsaturated fatty acids essential nutrients in infancy? *Lancet* **1995**, *345*, 1463–1468. [CrossRef]
72. European Food Safety Authority. Scientific opinion on dietary reference values for fats, including saturated fatty acids, polyunsaturated fatty acids, monounsaturated fatty acids, trans fatty acids, and cholesterol. *EFSA J.* **2010**, *8*, 1461.
73. Makrides, M.; Duley, L.; Olsen, S.F. Marine oil, and other prostaglandin precursor, supplementation for pregnancy uncomplicated by pre-eclampsia or intrauterine growth restriction. *Cochrane Database Syst Rev.* **2006**, *3*. [CrossRef]
74. Szajewska, H.; Horvath, A.; Koletzko, B. Effect of *n*-3 long-chain polyunsaturated fatty acid supplementation of women with low-risk pregnancies on pregnancy outcomes and growth measures at birth: A meta-analysis of randomized controlled trials. *Am. J. Clin. Nutr.* **2006**, *83*, 1337–1344. [PubMed]

75. Horvath, A.; Koletzko, B.; Szajewska, H. Effect of supplementation of women in high-risk pregnancies with long-chain polyunsaturated fatty acids on pregnancy outcomes and growth measures at birth: A meta-analysis of randomized controlled trials. *Br. J. Nutr.* **2007**, *98*, 253–259. [CrossRef] [PubMed]
76. Ramakrishnan, U.; Stein, A.D.; Parra-Cabrera, S.; Wang, M.; Imhoff-Kunsch, B.; Juarez-Marquez, S.; Rivera, J.; Martorell, R. Effects of docosahexaenoic acid supplementation during pregnancy on gestational age and size at birth: Randomized, double-blind, placebo-controlled trial in Mexico. *Food Nutr. Bull.* **2010**, *31*, S108–S116. [CrossRef] [PubMed]
77. Hibbeln, J.R.; Davis, J.M.; Steer, C.; Emmett, P.; Rogers, I.; Williams, C.; Golding, J. Maternal seafood consumption in pregnancy and neurodevelopmental outcomes in childhood (ALSPAC study): An observational cohort study. *Lancet* **2007**, *369*, 578–585. [CrossRef]
78. Jensen, C.L.; Voigt, R.G.; Llorente, A.M.; Peters, S.U.; Prager, T.C.; Zou, Y.L.; Rozelle, J.C.; Turcich, M.R.; Fraley, J.K.; Anderson, R.E.; *et al.* Effects of early maternal docosahexaenoic acid intake on neuropsychological status and visual acuity at five years of age of breast-fed term infants. *J. Pediatr.* **2010**, *157*, 900–905. [CrossRef] [PubMed]
79. Makrides, M.; Gibson, R.A.; McPhee, A.J.; Yelland, L.; Quinlivan, J.; Ryan, P. Effect of DHA supplementation during pregnancy on maternal depression and neurodevelopment of young children: A randomized controlled trial. *JAMA* **2010**, *304*, 1675–1683. [CrossRef] [PubMed]
80. Belfort, M.B.; Rifas-Shiman, S.L.; Kleinman, K.P.; Guthrie, L.B.; Bellinger, D.C.; Taveras, E.M.; Gillman, M.W.; Oken, E. Infant feeding and childhood cognition at ages 3 and 7 years: Effects of breastfeeding duration and exclusivity. *JAMA Pediatr.* **2013**, *167*, 836–844. [CrossRef] [PubMed]
81. Hoddinott, P.; Tappin, D.; Wright, C. Breast feeding. *BMJ* **2008**, *336*, 881–887. [CrossRef] [PubMed]
82. Jensen, C.L.; Voigt, R.G.; Prager, T.C.; Zou, Y.L.; Fraley, J.K.; Rozelle, J.C.; Turcich, M.R.; Llorente, A.M.; Anderson, R.E.; Heird, W.C. Effects of maternal docosahexaenoic acid intake on visual function and neurodevelopment in breastfed term infants. *Am. J. Clin. Nutr.* **2005**, *82*, 125–132. [PubMed]
83. Uauy, R.; Hoffman, D.R.; Mena, P.; Llanos, A.; Birch, E.E. Term infant studies of DHA and ara supplementation on neurodevelopment: Results of randomized controlled trials. *J. Pediatr.* **2003**, *143*, S17–S25. [CrossRef]
84. Walker, S.P.; Wachs, T.D.; Gardner, J.M.; Lozoff, B.; Wasserman, G.A.; Pollitt, E.; Carter, J.A.; the International Child Development Steering Group. Child development: Risk factors for adverse outcomes in developing countries. *Lancet* **2007**, *369*, 145–157. [CrossRef]
85. Hart, S.L.; Boylan, L.M.; Carroll, S.R.; Musick, Y.A.; Kuratko, C.; Border, B.G.; Lampe, R.M. Brief report: Newborn behavior differs with decosahexaenoic acid levels in breast milk. *J. Pediatr. Psychol.* **2006**, *31*, 221–226. [CrossRef] [PubMed]
86. Decsi, T.; Campoy, C.; Koletzko, B. Effect of *n*-3 polyunsaturated fatty acid supplementation in pregnancy: The nuheal trial. *Adv. Exp. Med. Biol.* **2005**, *569*, 109–113. [PubMed]
87. Helland, I.B.; Smith, L.; Saarem, K.; Saugstad, O.D.; Drevon, C.A. Maternal supplementation with very-long-chain *n*-3 fatty acids during pregnancy and lactation augments children's IQ at 4 years of age. *Pediatrics* **2003**, *111*, e39–e44. [CrossRef] [PubMed]
88. Boucher, O.; Burden, M.J.; Muckle, G.; Saint-Amour, D.; Ayotte, P.; Dewailly, E.; Nelson, C.A.; Jacobson, S.W.; Jacobson, J.L. Neurophysiologic and neurobehavioral evidence of beneficial effects of prenatal omega-3 fatty acid intake on memory function at school age. *Am. J. Clin. Nutr.* **2011**, *93*, 1025–1037. [CrossRef] [PubMed]
89. Innis, S.M. Impact of maternal diet on human milk composition and neurological development of infants. *Am. J. Clin. Nutr.* **2014**, *99*, 734S–741S. [CrossRef] [PubMed]
90. Agostoni, C.; Brunetti, I.; Marco, A.D. Polyunsaturated fatty acids in development in breastfed infants human and neurological. *Curr. Pediatr. Rev.* **2005**, 25–30. [CrossRef]
91. Gibson, R.A.; Neumann, M.A.; Makrides, M. Effect of increasing breast milk docosahexaenoic acid on plasma and erythrocyte phospholipid fatty acids and neural indices of exclusively breast fed infants. *Eur. J. Clin. Nutr.* **1997**, *51*, 578–584. [CrossRef] [PubMed]
92. Innis, S.M. Dietary (*n*-3) fatty acids and brain development. *J. Nutr.* **2007**, *137*, 855–859. [PubMed]
93. Horta, B.; Bahl, R.; Martines, J.; Victora, C. *Evidence on the Long-Term Effects of Breastfeeding*; WHO: Geneva, Switzerland, 2007; pp. 1–52.

94. Oddy, W.H.; Kendall, G.E.; Li, J.; Jacoby, P.; Robinson, M.; de Klerk, N.H.; Silburn, S.R.; Zubrick, S.R.; Landau, L.I.; Stanley, F.J. The long-term effects of breastfeeding on child and adolescent mental health: A pregnancy cohort study followed for 14 years. *J. Pediatr.* **2010**, *156*, 568–574. [CrossRef] [PubMed]
95. Eilander, A.; Hundscheid, D.C.; Osendarp, S.J.; Transler, C.; Zock, P.L. Effects of *n*-3 long chain polyunsaturated fatty acid supplementation on visual and cognitive development throughout childhood: A review of human studies. *Prostaglandins Leukot. Essent. Fat. Acids* **2007**, *76*, 189–203. [CrossRef] [PubMed]
96. Drover, J.R.; Hoffman, D.R.; Castañeda, Y.S.; Morale, S.E.; Garfield, S.; Wheaton, D.H.; Birch, E.E. Cognitive function in 18-month-old term infants of the diamond study: A randomized, controlled clinical trial with multiple dietary levels of docosahexaenoic acid. *Early Hum. Dev.* **2011**, *87*, 223–230. [CrossRef] [PubMed]
97. Meldrum, S.J.; D'Vaz, N.; Simmer, K.; Dunstan, J.A.; Hird, K.; Prescott, S.L. Effects of high-dose fish oil supplementation during early infancy on neurodevelopment and language: A randomised controlled trial. *Br. J. Nutr.* **2012**, *108*, 1443–1454. [CrossRef] [PubMed]
98. Birch, E.E.; Garfield, S.; Castañeda, Y.; Hughbanks-Wheaton, D.; Uauy, R.; Hoffman, D. Visual acuity and cognitive outcomes at 4 years of age in a double-blind, randomized trial of long-chain polyunsaturated fatty acid-supplemented infant formula. *Early Hum. Dev.* **2007**, *83*, 279–284. [CrossRef] [PubMed]
99. Makrides, M.; Neumann, M.A.; Jeffrey, B.; Lien, E.L.; Gibson, R.A. A randomized trial of different ratios of linoleic to alpha-linolenic acid in the diet of term infants: Effects on visual function and growth. *Am. J. Clin. Nutr.* **2000**, *71*, 120–129. [PubMed]
100. Cohen, J.T.; Bellinger, D.C.; Connor, W.E.; Shaywitz, B.A. A quantitative analysis of prenatal intake of *n*-3 polyunsaturated fatty acids and cognitive development. *Am. J. Prev. Med.* **2005**, *29*, 366–374. [CrossRef] [PubMed]
101. Tofail, F.; Kabir, I.; Hamadani, J.D.; Chowdhury, F.; Yesmin, S.; Mehreen, F.; Huda, S.N. Supplementation of fish-oil and soy-oil during pregnancy and psychomotor development of infants. *J. Health Popul. Nutr.* **2006**, *24*, 48–56. [PubMed]
102. Dunstan, J.A.; Simmer, K.; Dixon, G.; Prescott, S.L. Cognitive assessment of children at age 2 (1/2) years after maternal fish oil supplementation in pregnancy: A randomised controlled trial. *Arch. Dis. Child. Fetal Neonatal Ed.* **2008**, *93*, F45–F50. [CrossRef] [PubMed]
103. Scott, D.T.; Janowsky, J.S.; Carroll, R.E.; Taylor, J.A.; Auestad, N.; Montalto, M.B. Formula supplementation with long-chain polyunsaturated fatty acids: Are there developmental benefits? *Pediatrics* **1998**, *102*, E59. [CrossRef] [PubMed]
104. Hoffman, D.R.; Uauy, R. Essentiality of dietary omega 3 fatty acids for premature infants: Plasma and red blood cell fatty acid composition. *Lipids* **1992**, *27*, 886–895. [CrossRef] [PubMed]
105. Fewtrell, M.S.; Abbott, R.A.; Kennedy, K.; Singhal, A.; Morley, R.; Caine, E.; Jamieson, C.; Cockburn, F.; Lucas, A. Randomized, double-blind trial of long-chain polyunsaturated fatty acid supplementation with fish oil and borage oil in preterm infants. *J. Pediatr.* **2004**, *144*, 471–479. [CrossRef] [PubMed]
106. Clandinin, M.T.; van Aerde, J.E.; Merkel, K.L.; Harris, C.L.; Springer, M.A.; Hansen, J.W.; Diersen-Schade, D.A. Growth and development of preterm infants fed infant formulas containing docosahexaenoic acid and arachidonic acid. *J. Pediatr.* **2005**, *146*, 461–468. [CrossRef] [PubMed]
107. Henriksen, C.; Haugholt, K.; Lindgren, M.; Aurvåg, A.K.; Rønnestad, A.; Grønn, M.; Solberg, R.; Moen, A.; Nakstad, B.; Berge, R.K.; *et al.* Improved cognitive development among preterm infants attributable to early supplementation of human milk with docosahexaenoic acid and arachidonic acid. *Pediatrics* **2008**, *121*, 1137–1145. [CrossRef] [PubMed]
108. Makrides, M.; Collins, C.T.; Gibson, R.A. Impact of fatty acid status on growth and neurobehavioural development in humans. *Mater. Child Nutr.* **2011**, *7* (Suppl. 2), 80–88. [CrossRef] [PubMed]
109. Makrides, M.; Gibson, R.A.; McPhee, A.J.; Collins, C.T.; Davis, P.G.; Doyle, L.W.; Simmer, K.; Colditz, P.B.; Morris, S.; Smithers, L.G.; *et al.* Neurodevelopmental outcomes of preterm infants fed high-dose docosahexaenoic acid: A randomized controlled trial. *JAMA* **2009**, *301*, 175–182. [CrossRef] [PubMed]
110. Collins, C.T.; Gibson, R.A.; Anderson, P.J.; McPhee, A.J.; Sullivan, T.R.; Gould, J.F.; Ryan, P.; Doyle, L.W.; Davis, P.G.; McMichael, J.E.; *et al.* Neurodevelopmental outcomes at 7 years' corrected age in preterm infants who were fed high-dose docosahexaenoic acid to term equivalent: A follow-up of a randomised controlled trial. *BMJ Open* **2015**, *5*. [CrossRef] [PubMed]

111. Molloy, C.S.; Stokes, S.; Makrides, M.; Collins, C.T.; Anderson, P.J.; Doyle, L.W. Long-term effect of high-dose supplementation with DHA on visual function at school age in children born at <33 wk gestational age: Results from a follow-up of a randomized controlled trial. *Am. J. Clin. Nutr.* **2016**, *103*, 268–275. [PubMed]
112. Prentice, A.M.; van der Merwe, L. Impact of fatty acid status on immune function of children in low-income countries. *Mater. Child Nutr.* **2011**, *7* (Suppl. S2), 89–98. [CrossRef] [PubMed]
113. Scholtz, S.A.; Colombo, J.; Carlson, S.E. Clinical overview of effects of dietary long-chain polyunsaturated fatty acids during the perinatal period. *Nestle Nutr. Inst. Workshop Ser.* **2013**, *77*, 145–154. [PubMed]
114. Delgado-Noguera, M.F.; Calvache, J.A.; Bonfill Cosp, X.; Kotanidou, E.P.; Galli-Tsinopoulou, A. Supplementation with long chain polyunsaturated fatty acids (LCPUFA) to breastfeeding mothers for improving child growth and development. *Cochrane Database Syst. Rev.* **2015**, *7*. [CrossRef]
115. Michaelsen, K.F.; Dewey, K.G.; Perez-Exposito, A.B.; Nurhasan, M.; Lauritzen, L.; Roos, N. Food sources and intake of *n*-6 and *n*-3 fatty acids in low-income countries with emphasis on infants, young children (6–24 months), and pregnant and lactating women. *Mater. Child Nutr.* **2011**, *7* (Suppl. 2), 124–140. [CrossRef] [PubMed]
116. Barbarich, B.N.; Willows, N.D.; Wang, L.; Clandinin, M.T. Polyunsaturated fatty acids and anthropometric indices of children in rural China. *Eur. J. Clin. Nutr.* **2006**, *60*, 1100–1107. [CrossRef] [PubMed]
117. Yakes, E.A.; Arsenault, J.E.; Islam, M.M.; Hossain, M.B.; Ahmed, T.; German, J.B.; Gillies, L.A.; Rahman, A.S.; Drake, C.; Jamil, K.M.; *et al.* Intakes and breast-milk concentrations of essential fatty acids are low among Bangladeshi women with 24–48-month-old children. *Br. J. Nutr.* **2011**, *105*, 1660–1670. [CrossRef] [PubMed]
118. Huybregts, L.F.; Roberfroid, D.A.; Kolsteren, P.W.; van Camp, J.H. Dietary behaviour, food and nutrient intake of pregnant women in a rural community in Burkina Faso. *Mater. Child Nutr.* **2009**, *5*, 211–222. [CrossRef] [PubMed]
119. Mardones, F.; Urrutia, M.T.; Villarroel, L.; Rioseco, A.; Castillo, O.; Rozowski, J.; Tapia, J.L.; Bastias, G.; Bacallao, J.; Rojas, I. Effects of a dairy product fortified with multiple micronutrients and omega-3 fatty acids on birth weight and gestation duration in pregnant Chilean women. *Public Health Nutr.* **2008**, *11*, 30–40. [CrossRef] [PubMed]
120. Muthayya, S.; Eilander, A.; Transler, C.; Thomas, T.; van der Knaap, H.C.; Srinivasan, K.; van Klinken, B.J.; Osendarp, S.J.; Kurpad, A.V. Effect of fortification with multiple micronutrients and *n*-3 fatty acids on growth and cognitive performance in Indian schoolchildren: The champion (children's health and mental performance influenced by optimal nutrition) study. *Am. J. Clin. Nutr.* **2009**, *89*, 1766–1775. [CrossRef] [PubMed]
121. Osendarp, S.J.; Baghurst, K.I.; Bryan, J.; Calvaresi, E.; Hughes, D.; Hussaini, M.; Karyadi, S.J.; van Klinken, B.J.; van der Knaap, H.C.; Lukito, W.; *et al.* Effect of a 12-mo micronutrient intervention on learning and memory in well-nourished and marginally nourished school-aged children: 2 parallel, randomized, placebo-controlled studies in Australia and Indonesia. *Am. J. Clin. Nutr.* **2007**, *86*, 1082–1093. [PubMed]
122. Dalton, A.; Wolmarans, P.; Witthuhn, R.C.; van Stuijvenberg, M.E.; Swanevelder, S.A.; Smuts, C.M. A randomised control trial in schoolchildren showed improvement in cognitive function after consuming a bread spread, containing fish flour from a marine source. *Prostaglandins Leukot. Essent. Fat. Acids* **2009**, *80*, 143–149. [CrossRef] [PubMed]
123. Stevens, L.J.; Zentall, S.S.; Abate, M.L.; Kuczek, T.; Burgess, J.R. Omega-3 fatty acids in boys with behavior, learning, and health problems. *Physiol. Behav.* **1996**, *59*, 915–920. [CrossRef]
124. McNamara, R.K.; Able, J.; Jandacek, R.; Rider, T.; Tso, P.; Eliassen, J.C.; Alfieri, D.; Weber, W.; Jarvis, K.; DelBello, M.P.; *et al.* Docosahexaenoic acid supplementation increases prefrontal cortex activation during sustained attention in healthy boys: A placebo-controlled, dose-ranging, functional magnetic resonance imaging study. *Am. J. Clin. Nutr.* **2010**, *91*, 1060–1067. [CrossRef] [PubMed]
125. Richardson, A.J.; Burton, J.R.; Sewell, R.P.; Spreckelsen, T.F.; Montgomery, P. Docosahexaenoic acid for reading, cognition and behavior in children aged 7–9 years: A randomized, controlled trial (the DOLAB study). *PLoS ONE* **2012**, *7*, e43909.
126. Brew, B.K.; Toelle, B.G.; Webb, K.L.; Almqvist, C.; Marks, G.B.; Investigators, C. Omega-3 supplementation during the first 5 years of life and later academic performance: A randomised controlled trial. *Eur. J. Clin. Nutr.* **2015**, *69*, 419–424. [CrossRef] [PubMed]
127. Lassek, W.D.; Gaulin, S.J.C. Sex differences in the relationship of dietary fatty acids to cognitive measures in American children. *Front. Evol. Neurosci.* **2011**, *3*, 5. [CrossRef] [PubMed]

128. Extier, A.; Langelier, B.; Perruchot, M.H.; Guesnet, P.; van Veldhoven, P.P.; Lavialle, M.; Alessandri, J.M. Gender affects liver desaturase expression in a rat model of *n*-3 fatty acid repletion. *J. Nutr. Biochem.* **2010**, *21*, 180–187. [CrossRef] [PubMed]
129. Schram, L.B.; Nielsen, C.J.; Porsgaard, T.; Nielsen, N.S.; Holm, R.; Mu, H. Food matrices affect the bioavailability of (*n*-3) polyunsaturated fatty acids in a single meal study in humans. *Food Res. Int.* **2007**, *40*, 1062–1068. [CrossRef]
130. Ulven, S.M.; Kirkhus, B.; Lamglait, A.; Basu, S.; Elind, E.; Haider, T.; Berge, K.; Vik, H.; Pedersen, J.I. Metabolic effects of krill oil are essentially similar to those of fish oil but at lower dose of EPA and DHA, in healthy volunteers. *Lipids* **2011**, *46*, 37–46. [CrossRef] [PubMed]
131. Elvevoll, E.O.; Barstad, H.; Breimo, E.S.; Brox, J.; Eilertsen, K.E.; Lund, T.; Olsen, J.O.; Osterud, B. Enhanced incorporation of *n*-3 fatty acids from fish compared with fish oils. *Lipids* **2006**, *41*, 1109–1114. [CrossRef] [PubMed]
132. Arterburn, L.M.; Oken, H.A.; Hoffman, J.P.; Bailey-Hall, E.; Chung, G.; Rom, D.; Hamersley, J.; McCarthy, D. Bioequivalence of docosahexaenoic acid from different algal oils in capsules and in a DHA -fortified food. *Lipids* **2007**, *42*, 1011–1024. [CrossRef] [PubMed]
133. Kuratko, C.N.; Salem, N., Jr. Biomarkers of DHA status. *Prostaglandins Leukot. Essent. Fat. Acids* **2009**, *81*, 111–118. [CrossRef] [PubMed]
134. Jernerén, F.; Elshorbagy, A.K.; Oulhaj, A.; Smith, S.M.; Refsum, H.; Smith, A.D. Brain atrophy in cognitively impaired elderly: The importance of long-chain ω-3 fatty acids and B vitamin status in a randomized controlled trial. *Am. J. Clin. Nutr.* **2015**, *102*, 215–221. [CrossRef] [PubMed]
135. McCann, J.C.; Ames, B.N. Is docosahexaenoic acid, an *n*-3 long-chain polyunsaturated fatty acid, required for development of normal brain function? An overview of evidence from cognitive and behavioral tests in humans and animals. *Am. J. Clin. Nutr.* **2005**, *82*, 281–295. [PubMed]
136. Fleith, M.; Clandinin, M.T. Dietary pufa for preterm and term infants: Review of clinical studies. *Crit. Rev. Food Sci Nutr.* **2005**, *45*, 205–229. [CrossRef] [PubMed]
137. Innis, S.M. Fatty acids and early human development. *Early Hum. Dev.* **2007**, *83*, 761–766. [CrossRef] [PubMed]
138. Youdim, K.A.; Martin, A.; Joseph, J.A. Essential fatty acids and the brain: Possible health implications. *Int. J. Dev. Neurosci.* **2000**, *18*, 383–399. [CrossRef]
139. De Urquiza, A.M.; Liu, S.; Sjoberg, M.; Zetterstrom, R.H.; Griffiths, W.; Sjovall, J.; Perlmann, T. Docosahexaenoic acid, a ligand for the retinoid X receptor in mouse brain. *Science* **2000**, *290*, 2140–2144. [CrossRef] [PubMed]
140. Kitajka, K.; Sinclair, A.J.; Weisinger, R.S.; Weisinger, H.S.; Mathai, M.; Jayasooriya, A.P.; Halver, J.E.; Puskas, L.G. Effects of dietary omega-3 polyunsaturated fatty acids on brain gene expression. *Proc. Natl. Acad. Sci. USA* **2004**, *101*, 10931–10936. [CrossRef] [PubMed]
141. Calderon, F.; Kim, H.Y. Docosahexaenoic acid promotes neurite growth in hippocampal neurons. *J. Neurochem.* **2004**, *90*, 979–988. [CrossRef] [PubMed]
142. Moriguchi, T.; Greiner, R.S.; Salem, N., Jr. Behavioral deficits associated with dietary induction of decreased brain docosahexaenoic acid concentration. *J. Neurochem.* **2000**, *75*, 2563–2573. [CrossRef] [PubMed]
143. Lingwood, B.E.; Healy, G.N.; Sullivan, S.M.; Pow, D.V.; Colditz, P.B. MAP2 provides reliable early assessment of neural injury in the newborn piglet model of birth asphyxia. *J. Neurosci. Methods* **2008**, *171*, 140–146. [CrossRef] [PubMed]
144. Shaikh, S.R.; Dumaual, A.C.; Castillo, A.; LoCascio, D.; Siddiqui, R.A.; Stillwell, W.; Wassall, S.R. Oleic and docosahexaenoic acid differentially phase separate from lipid raft molecules: A comparative NMR, DSC, AFM, and detergent extraction study. *Biophys. J.* **2004**, *87*, 1752–1766. [CrossRef] [PubMed]
145. Stillwell, W.; Shaikh, S.R.; Zerouga, M.; Siddiqui, R.; Wassall, S.R. Docosahexaenoic acid affects cell signaling by altering lipid rafts. *Reprod. Nutr. Dev.* **2005**, *45*, 559–579. [CrossRef] [PubMed]
146. Vinson, M.; Rausch, O.; Maycox, P.R.; Prinjha, R.K.; Chapman, D.; Morrow, R.; Harper, A.J.; Dingwall, C.; Walsh, F.S.; Burbidge, S.A.; *et al.* Lipid rafts mediate the interaction between myelin-associated glycoprotein (MAG) on myelin and MAG-receptors on neurons. *Mol. Cell. Neurosci.* **2003**, *22*, 344–352. [CrossRef]
147. Jaworski, J.; Sheng, M. The growing role of mtor in neuronal development and plasticity. *Mol. Neurobiol.* **2006**, *34*, 205–219. [CrossRef]

148. Jin, Y.; Sui, H.J.; Dong, Y.; Ding, Q.; Qu, W.H.; Yu, S.X.; Jin, Y.X. Atorvastatin enhances neurite outgrowth in cortical neurons *in vitro* via up-regulating the Akt/mTOR and Akt/GSK-3beta signaling pathways. *Acta Pharmacol. Sin.* **2012**, *33*, 861–872. [CrossRef] [PubMed]
149. Cao, D.; Kevala, K.; Kim, J.; Moon, H.S.; Jun, S.B.; Lovinger, D.; Kim, H.Y. Docosahexaenoic acid promotes hippocampal neuronal development and synaptic function. *J. Neurochem.* **2009**, *111*, 510–521. [CrossRef] [PubMed]
150. Darios, F.; Davletov, B. Omega-3 and omega-6 fatty acids stimulate cell membrane expansion by acting on syntaxin 3. *Nature* **2006**, *440*, 813–817. [CrossRef] [PubMed]
151. Nyaradi, A.; Li, J.; Hickling, S.; Foster, J.; Oddy, W.H. The role of nutrition in children's neurocognitive development, from pregnancy through childhood. *Front. Hum. Neurosci.* **2013**, *7*, 97. [CrossRef] [PubMed]
152. Bourre, J.M.; Pascal, G.; Durand, G.; Masson, M.; Dumont, O.; Piciotti, M. Alterations in the fatty acid composition of rat brain cells (neurons, astrocytes, and oligodendrocytes) and of subcellular fractions (myelin and synaptosomes) induced by a diet devoid of *n*-3 fatty acids. *J. Neurochem.* **1984**, *43*, 342–348. [CrossRef] [PubMed]
153. Ikemoto, A.; Ohishi, M.; Sato, Y.; Hata, N.; Misawa, Y.; Fujii, Y.; Okuyama, H. Reversibility of *n*-3 fatty acid deficiency-induced alterations of learning behavior in the rat: Level of *n*-6 fatty acids as another critical factor. *J. Lipid Res.* **2001**, *42*, 1655–1663. [PubMed]
154. Brenna, J.T. Animal studies of the functional consequences of suboptimal polyunsaturated fatty acid status during pregnancy, lactation and early post-natal life. *Mater. Child Nutr.* **2011**, *7* (Suppl. 2), 59–79. [CrossRef] [PubMed]
155. Diau, G.Y.; Hsieh, A.T.; Sarkadi-Nagy, E.A.; Wijendran, V.; Nathanielsz, P.W.; Brenna, J.T. The influence of long chain polyunsaturate supplementation on docosahexaenoic acid and arachidonic acid in baboon neonate central nervous system. *BMC Med.* **2005**, *3*, 11. [CrossRef] [PubMed]
156. Luchtman, D.W.; Song, C. Cognitive enhancement by omega-3 fatty acids from child-hood to old age: Findings from animal and clinical studies. *Neuropharmacology* **2013**, *64*, 550–565. [CrossRef] [PubMed]
157. Neuringer, M.; Connor, W.E.; Lin, D.S.; Barstad, L.; Luck, S. Biochemical and functional effects of prenatal and postnatal omega 3 fatty acid deficiency on retina and brain in rhesus monkeys. *Proc. Natl. Acad. Sci. USA* **1986**, *83*, 4021–4025. [CrossRef] [PubMed]
158. Champoux, M.; Hibbeln, J.R.; Shannon, C.; Majchrzak, S.; Suomi, S.J.; Salem, N., Jr.; Higley, J.D. Fatty acid formula supplementation and neuromotor development in rhesus monkey neonates. *Pediatr. Res.* **2002**, *51*, 273–281. [CrossRef] [PubMed]
159. Greiner, R.S.; Moriguchi, T.; Hutton, A.; Slotnick, B.M.; Salem, N., Jr. Rats with low levels of brain docosahexaenoic acid show impaired performance in olfactory-based and spatial learning tasks. *Lipids* **1999**, *34* (Suppl. 1), S239–S243. [CrossRef] [PubMed]
160. Novak, E.M.; Dyer, R.A.; Innis, S.M. High dietary omega-6 fatty acids contribute to reduced docosahexaenoic acid in the developing brain and inhibit secondary neurite growth. *Brain Res.* **2008**, *1237*, 136–145. [CrossRef] [PubMed]
161. Abubakari, A.R.; Naderali, M.M.; Naderali, E.K. Omega-3 fatty acid supplementation and cognitive function: Are smaller dosages more beneficial? *Int. J. Gen. Med.* **2014**, *7*, 463–473. [PubMed]
162. Jiao, J.; Li, Q.; Chu, J.; Zeng, W.; Yang, M.; Zhu, S. Effect of *n*-3 PUFA supplementation on cognitive function throughout the life span from infancy to old age: A systematic review and meta-analysis of randomized controlled trials. *Am. J. Clin. Nutr.* **2014**, *100*, 1422–1436. [CrossRef] [PubMed]
163. Yurko-Mauro, K.; Alexander, D.D.; van Elswyk, M.E. Docosahexaenoic acid and adult memory: A systematic review and meta-analysis. *PLoS ONE* **2015**, *10*, e0120391.
164. Muldoon, M.F.; Ryan, C.M.; Sheu, L.; Yao, J.K.; Conklin, S.M.; Manuck, S.B. Serum phospholipid docosahexaenonic acid is associated with cognitive functioning during middle adulthood. *J. Nutr.* **2010**, *140*, 848–853. [CrossRef] [PubMed]
165. Leckie, R.L.; Manuck, S.B.; Bhattacharjee, N.; Muldoon, M.F.; Flory, J.M.; Erickson, K.I. Omega-3 fatty acids moderate effects of physical activity on cognitive function. *Neuropsychologia* **2014**, *59*, 103–111. [CrossRef] [PubMed]
166. Erickson, K.I.; Voss, M.W.; Prakash, R.S.; Basak, C.; Szabo, A.; Chaddock, L.; Kim, J.S.; Heo, S.; Alves, H.; White, S.M.; *et al.* Exercise training increases size of hippocampus and improves memory. *Proc. Natl. Acad. Sci. USA* **2011**, *108*, 3017–3022. [CrossRef] [PubMed]

167. Erickson, K.I.; Weinstein, A.M.; Lopez, O.L. Physical activity, brain plasticity, and Alzheimer's disease. *Arch. Med. Res.* **2012**, *43*, 615–621. [CrossRef] [PubMed]
168. Rogers, P.J.; Appleton, K.M.; Kessler, D.; Peters, T.J.; Gunnell, D.; Hayward, R.C.; Heatherley, S.V.; Christian, L.M.; McNaughton, S.A.; Ness, A.R. No effect of *n*-3 long-chain polyunsaturated fatty acid (EPA and DHA) supplementation on depressed mood and cognitive function: A randomised controlled trial. *Br. J. Nutr.* **2008**, *99*, 421–431. [CrossRef] [PubMed]
169. Jackson, P.A.; Deary, M.E.; Reay, J.L.; Scholey, A.B.; Kennedy, D.O. No effect of 12 weeks' supplementation with 1 g DHA -rich or EPA-rich fish oil on cognitive function or mood in healthy young adults aged 18–35 years. *Br. J. Nutr.* **2012**, *107*, 1232–1243. [CrossRef] [PubMed]
170. Antypa, N.; van der Does, A.J.W.; Smelt, A.H.M.; Rogers, R.D. Omega-3 fatty acids (fish-oil) and depression-related cognition in healthy volunteers. *J. Psychopharmacol.* **2009**, *23*, 831–840. [CrossRef] [PubMed]
171. Karr, J.E.; Grindstaff, T.R.; Alexander, J.E. Omega-3 polyunsaturated fatty acids and cognition in a college-aged population. *Exp. Clin. Psychopharmacol.* **2012**, *20*, 236–242. [CrossRef] [PubMed]
172. Stonehouse, W.; Conlon, C.A.; Podd, J.; Hill, S.R.; Minihane, A.M.; Haskell, C.; Kennedy, D. DHA supplementation improved both memory and reaction time in healthy young adults: A randomized controlled trial. *Am. J. Clin. Nutr.* **2013**, *94*, 1134–1143. [CrossRef] [PubMed]
173. Duff, S.J.; Hampson, E. A sex difference on a novel spatial working memory task in humans. *Brain Cogn.* **2001**, *47*, 470–493. [CrossRef] [PubMed]
174. Halpern, D.F. Mapping cognitive processes onto the brain: Mind the gap. *Brain Cogn.* **2000**, *42*, 128–130. [CrossRef] [PubMed]
175. Jaremka, L.M.; Derry, H.M.; Bornstein, R.; Prakash, R.S.; Peng, J.; Belury, M.A.; Andridge, R.R.; Malarkey, W.B.; Kiecolt-Glaser, J.K. Omega-3 supplementation and loneliness-related memory problems. *Psychosom. Med.* **2014**, *76*, 650–658. [CrossRef] [PubMed]
176. Services, H. *Global Health and Aging*; National Institutes of Health: Bethesda, MD, USA, 2011; Volume 1, pp. 273–277.
177. Resnick, S.M.; Pham, D.L.; Kraut, M.A.; Zonderman, A.B.; Davatzikos, C. Longitudinal magnetic resonance imaging studies of older adults: A shrinking brain. *J. Neurosci.* **2003**, *23*, 3295–3301. [PubMed]
178. McNamara, R.K.; Liu, Y.; Jandacek, R.; Rider, T.; Tso, P. The aging human orbitofrontal cortex: Decreasing polyunsaturated fatty acid composition and associated increases in lipogenic gene expression and stearoyl-CoA desaturase activity. *Prostaglandins Leukot. Essent. Fat. Acids* **2008**, *78*, 293–304. [CrossRef] [PubMed]
179. Andre, A.; Juaneda, P.; Sebedio, J.L.; Chardigny, J.M. Plasmalogen metabolism-related enzymes in rat brain during aging: Influence of *n*-3 fatty acid intake. *Biochimie* **2006**, *88*, 103–111. [CrossRef] [PubMed]
180. Giusto, N.M.; Salvador, G.A.; Castagnet, P.I.; Pasquare, S.J.; de Boschero, M.G.I. Age-associated changes in central nervous system glycerolipid composition and metabolism. *Neurochem. Res.* **2002**, *27*, 1513–1523. [CrossRef] [PubMed]
181. Plourde, M.; Chouinard-Watkins, R.; Vandal, M.; Zhang, Y.; Lawrence, P.; Brenna, J.T.; Cunnane, S.C. Plasma incorporation, apparent retroconversion and beta-oxidation of 13c-docosahexaenoic acid in the elderly. *Nutr. Metab.* **2011**, *8*, 5. [CrossRef] [PubMed]
182. Conklin, S.M.; Gianaros, P.J.; Brown, S.M.; Yao, J.K.; Hariri, A.R.; Manuck, S.B.; Muldoon, M.F. Long-chain omega-3 fatty acid intake is associated positively with corticolimbic gray matter volume in healthy adults. *Neurosci. Lett.* **2007**, *421*, 209–212. [CrossRef] [PubMed]
183. Raji, C.A.; Erickson, K.I.; Lopez, O.L.; Kuller, L.H.; Gach, H.M.; Thompson, P.M.; Riverol, M.; Becker, J.T. Regular fish consumption and age-related brain gray matter loss. *Am. J. Prev. Med.* **2014**, *47*, 444–451. [CrossRef] [PubMed]
184. Masliah, E.; Crews, L.; Hansen, L. Synaptic remodeling during aging and in Alzheimer's disease. *J. Alzheimer's Dis.* **2006**, *9*, 91–99.
185. Jorm, A.F.; Jolley, D. The incidence of dementia: A meta-analysis. *Neurology* **1998**, *51*, 728–733. [CrossRef] [PubMed]
186. Mohajeri, M.H.; Troesch, B.; Weber, P. Inadequate supply of vitamins and DHA in the elderly: Implications for brain aging and Alzheimer-type dementia. *Nutrition* **2015**, *31*, 261–275. [CrossRef] [PubMed]

187. Reiman, E.M.; Quiroz, Y.T.; Fleisher, A.S.; Chen, K.; Velez-Pardo, C.; Jimenez-Del-Rio, M.; Fagan, A.M.; Shah, A.R.; Alvarez, S.; Arbelaez, A.; *et al.* Brain imaging and fluid biomarker analysis in young adults at genetic risk for autosomal dominant Alzheimer's disease in the presenilin 1 E280A kindred: A case-control study. *Lancet Neurol.* **2012**, *11*, 1048–1056. [CrossRef]
188. Ellinson, M.; Thomas, J.; Patterson, A. A critical evaluation of the relationship between serum vitamin B, folate and total homocysteine with cognitive impairment in the elderly. *J. Hum. Nutr. Diet.* **2004**, *17*, 371–383. [CrossRef] [PubMed]
189. Adunsky, A.; Arinzon, Z.; Fidelman, Z.; Krasniansky, I.; Arad, M.; Gepstein, R. Plasma homocysteine levels and cognitive status in long-term stay geriatric patients: A cross-sectional study. *Arch. Gerontol. Geriatr.* **2005**, *40*, 129–138. [CrossRef] [PubMed]
190. Terry, R.D. Cell death or synaptic loss in Alzheimer disease. *J. Neuropathol. Exp. Neurol.* **2000**, *59*, 1118–1119. [CrossRef] [PubMed]
191. Vida, C.; Gonzalez, E.M.; de la Fuente, M. Increase of oxidation and inflammation in nervous and immune systems with aging and anxiety. *Curr. Pharm. Des.* **2014**, *20*, 4656–4678. [CrossRef] [PubMed]
192. Kalmijn, S.; van Boxtel, M.P.J.; Ocke, M.; Verschuren, W.M.M.; Kromhout, D.; Launer, L.J. Dietary intake of fatty acids and fish in relation to cognitive performance at middle age. *Neurology* **2004**, *62*, 275–280. [CrossRef] [PubMed]
193. Van Gelder, B.M.; Tijhuis, M.; Kalmijn, S.; Kromhout, D. Fish consumption, *n*-3 fatty acids, and subsequent 5-y cognitive decline in elderly men: The Zutphen elderly study. *Am. J. Clin. Nutr.* **2007**, *85*, 1142–1147. [PubMed]
194. Eskelinen, M.H.; Ngandu, T.; Helkala, E.L.; Tuomilehto, J.; Nissinen, A.; Soininen, H.; Kivipelto, M. Fat intake at midlife and cognitive impairment later in life: A population-based caide study. *Int. J. Geriatr. Psychiatry* **2008**, *23*, 741–747. [CrossRef] [PubMed]
195. Velho, S.; Marques-Vidal, P.; Baptista, F.; Camilo, M.E. Dietary intake adequacy and cognitive function in free-living active elderly: A cross-sectional and short-term prospective study. *Clin. Nutr.* **2008**, *27*, 77–86. [CrossRef] [PubMed]
196. González, S.; Huerta, J.M.; Fernández, S.; Patterson, A.M.; Lasheras, C. The relationship between dietary lipids and cognitive performance in an elderly population. *Int. J. Food Sci. Nutr.* **2010**, *61*, 217–225. [CrossRef] [PubMed]
197. Gao, Q.; Niti, M.; Feng, L.; Yap, K.B.; Ng, T.P. Omega-3 polyunsaturated fatty acid supplements and cognitive decline: Singapore longitudinal aging studies. *J. Nutr. Health Aging* **2011**, *15*, 32–35. [CrossRef] [PubMed]
198. Titova, O.E.; Sjögren, P.; Brooks, S.J.; Kullberg, J.; Ax, E.; Kilander, L.; Riserus, U.; Cederholm, T.; Larsson, E.M.; Johansson, L.; *et al.* Dietary intake of eicosapentaenoic and docosahexaenoic acids is linked to gray matter volume and cognitive function in elderly. *Age* **2013**, *35*, 1495–1505. [CrossRef] [PubMed]
199. Qin, B.; Plassman, B.L.; Edwards, L.J.; Popkin, B.M.; Adair, L.S.; Mendez, M.A. Fish intake is associated with slower cognitive decline in Chinese older adults. *J. Nutr.* **2014**, *144*, 1579–1585. [CrossRef] [PubMed]
200. Del Brutto, O.H.; Mera, R.M.; Gillman, J.; Zambrano, M.; Ha, J.E. Oily fish intake and cognitive performance in community-dwelling older adults: The Atahualpa project. *J. Community Health* **2016**, *41*, 82–86. [CrossRef] [PubMed]
201. Archer, E.; Pavela, G.; Lavie, C.J. The inadmissibility of what we eat in America and nhanes dietary data in nutrition and obesity research and the scientific formulation of national dietary guidelines. *Mayo Clin. Proc.* **2015**, *90*, 911–926. [CrossRef] [PubMed]
202. Ammann, E.M.; Pottala, J.V.; Harris, W.S.; Espeland, M.A.; Wallace, R.; Denburg, N.L.; Carnahan, R.M.; Robinson, J.G. Omega-3 fatty acids and domain-specific cognitive aging: Secondary analyses of data from WHISCA. *Neurology* **2013**, *81*, 1484–1491. [CrossRef] [PubMed]
203. Heude, B.; Ducimetiere, P.; Berr, C. Cognitive decline and fatty acid composition of erythrocyte membranes—The EVA study. *Am. J. Clin. Nutr.* **2003**, *77*, 803–808. [PubMed]
204. Dullemeijer, C.; Durga, J.; Brouwer, I.A.; van de Rest, O.; Kok, F.J.; Brummer, R.J.M.; van Boxtel, M.P.; Verhoef, P. *n*-3 fatty acid proportions in plasma and cognitive performance in older adults. *Am. J. Clin. Nutr.* **2007**, *86*, 1479–1485. [PubMed]
205. Whalley, L.J.; Deary, I.J.; Starr, J.M.; Wahle, K.W.; Rance, K.A.; Bourne, V.J.; Fox, H.C. *n*-3 fatty acid erythrocyte membrane content, APOEe4, and cognitive variation: An observational follow-up study in late adulthood. *Am. J. Clin. Nutr.* **2008**, *87*, 449–454. [PubMed]

206. Tan, Z.S.; Harris, W.S.; Beiser, a.S.; Au, R.; Himali, J.J.; Debette, S.; Pikula, A.; Decarli, C.; Wolf, P.A.; Vasan, R.S.; *et al.* Red blood cell ω-3 fatty acid levels and markers of accelerated brain aging. *Neurology* **2012**, *78*, 658–664. [CrossRef] [PubMed]
207. Baierle, M.; Vencato, P.; Oldenburg, L.; Bordignon, S.; Zibetti, M.; Trentini, C.; Duarte, M.; Veit, J.; Somacal, S.; Emanuelli, T.; *et al.* Fatty acid status and its relationship to cognitive decline and homocysteine levels in the elderly. *Nutrients* **2014**, *6*, 3624–3640. [CrossRef] [PubMed]
208. Otsuka, R.; Tange, C.; Nishita, Y.; Kato, Y.; Imai, T.; Ando, F.; Shimokata, H. Serum docosahexaenoic and eicosapentaenoic acid and risk of cognitive decline over 10 years among elderly Japanese. *Eur. J. Clin. Nutr.* **2014**, *68*, 503–509. [CrossRef] [PubMed]
209. Dangour, A.D.; Allen, E.; Elbourne, D.; Fasey, N.; Fletcher, A.E.; Hardy, P.; Holder, G.E.; Knight, R.; Letley, L.; Richards, M.; *et al.* Effect of 2-y *n*-3 long-chain polyunsaturated fatty acid supplementation on cognitive function in older people: A randomized, double-blind, controlled trial. *Am. J. Clin. Nutr.* **2010**, *91*, 1725–1732. [CrossRef] [PubMed]
210. Van de Rest, O.; Geleijnse, J.M.; Kok, F.J.; van Staveren, W.A.; Dullemeijer, C.; OldeRikkert, M.G.M.; Beekman, A.T.F.; de Groot, C.P.G.M. Effect of fish oil on cognitive performance in older subjects: A randomized, controlled trial. *Neurology* **2008**, *71*, 430–438. [CrossRef] [PubMed]
211. Stough, C.; Downey, L.; Silber, B.; Lloyd, J.; Kure, C.; Wesnes, K.; Camfield, D. The effects of 90-day supplementation with the omega-3 essential fatty acid docosahexaenoic acid (DHA) on cognitive function and visual acuity in a healthy aging population. *Neurobiol. Aging* **2012**, *33*, e821–e823. [CrossRef] [PubMed]
212. Johnson, E.J.; Mcdonald, K.; Caldarella, S.M.; Chung, H.Y.; Troen, A.M.; Snodderly, D.M. Cognitive findings of an exploratory trial of docosahexaenoic acid and lutein supplementation in older women. *Nutr. Neurosci.* **2008**, *11*, 75–83. [CrossRef] [PubMed]
213. Yurko-Mauro, K.; McCarthy, D.; Rom, D.; Nelson, E.B.; Ryan, A.S.; Blackwell, A.; Salem, N.; Stedman, M. Beneficial effects of docosahexaenoic acid on cognition in age-related cognitive decline. *Alzheimer's Dement.* **2010**, *6*, 456–464. [CrossRef] [PubMed]
214. Vakhapova, V.; Cohen, T.; Richter, Y.; Herzog, Y.; Kam, Y.; Korczyn, A.D. Phosphatidylserine containing omega-3 fatty acids may improve memory abilities in nondemented elderly individuals with memory complaints: Results from an open-label extension study. *Dement. Geriatr. Cogn. Disord.* **2014**, *38*, 39–45. [CrossRef] [PubMed]
215. Vakhapova, V.; Cohen, T.; Richter, Y.; Herzog, Y.; Korczyn, A.D. Phosphatidylserine containing ω–3 fatty acids may improve memory abilities in non-demented elderly with memory complaints: A double-blind placebo-controlled trial. *Dement. Geriatr. Cogn. Disord.* **2010**, *29*, 467–474. [CrossRef] [PubMed]
216. Nilsson, A.; Radeborg, K.; Salo, I.; Bjorck, I. Effects of supplementation with *n*-3 polyunsaturated fatty acids on cognitive performance and cardiometabolic risk markers in healthy 51 to 72 years old subjects: A randomized controlled cross-over study. *Nutr. J.* **2012**, *11*, 99. [CrossRef] [PubMed]
217. Tokuda, H.; Sueyasu, T.; Kontani, M.; Kawashima, H.; Shibata, H.; Koga, Y. Low doses of long-chain polyunsaturated fatty acids affect cognitive function in elderly Japanese men: A randomized controlled trial. *J. Oleo Sci.* **2015**, *2015*, 1–12. [CrossRef] [PubMed]
218. Ito, J. Auditory event-related potentials (ERPs) in healthy subjects and patients with dementia. *Jpn. J. Clin. Path. (Rinsho Byori).* **1991**, *39*, 859–864.
219. Strike, S.C.; Carlisle, A.; Gibson, E.L.; Dyall, S.C. A high omega-3 fatty acid multinutrient supplement benefits cognition and mobility in older women: A randomized, double-blind, placebo-controlled pilot study. *J. Gerontol. Ser. A Biol. Sci. Med. Sci.* **2016**, *71*, 236–242. [CrossRef] [PubMed]
220. Maestre, G.E. Assessing dementia in resource-poor regions. *Curr. Neurol. Neurosci. Rep.* **2012**, *12*, 511–519. [CrossRef] [PubMed]
221. Deary, I.J.; Corley, J.; Gow, A.J.; Harris, S.E.; Houlihan, L.M.; Marioni, R.E.; Penke, L.; Rafnsson, S.B.; Starr, J.M. Age-associated cognitive decline. *Br. Med. Bull.* **2009**, *92*, 135–152. [CrossRef] [PubMed]
222. Scahill, R.I.; Frost, C.; Jenkins, R.; Whitwell, J.L.; Rossor, M.N.; Fox, N.C. A longitudinal study of brain volume changes in normal aging using serial registered magnetic resonance imaging. *Arch. Neurol.* **2003**, *60*, 989–994. [CrossRef] [PubMed]
223. Risacher, S.L.; Saykin, A.J.; West, J.D.; Shen, L.; Firpi, H.A.; McDonald, B.C.; Alzheimer's Disease Neuroimaging Initiative. Baseline MRI predictors of conversion from MCI to probable AD in the ADNI cohort. *Curr. Alzheimer Res.* **2009**, *6*, 347–361. [CrossRef] [PubMed]

224. Kalpouzos, G.; Eustache, F.; de la Sayette, V.; Viader, F.; Chetelat, G.; Desgranges, B. Working memory and FDG-PET dissociate early and late onset Alzheimer disease patients. *J. Neurol.* **2005**, *252*, 548–558. [CrossRef] [PubMed]
225. Landau, S.M.; Harvey, D.; Madison, C.M.; Koeppe, R.A.; Reiman, E.M.; Foster, N.L.; Weiner, M.W.; Jagust, W.J.; the Alzheimer's Disease Neuroimaging Initiative. Associations between cognitive, functional, and FDG-PET measures of decline in AD and MCI. *Neurobiol. Aging* **2011**, *32*, 1207–1218. [CrossRef] [PubMed]
226. Nugent, S.; Tremblay, S.; Chen, K.W.; Ayutyanont, N.; Roontiva, A.; Castellano, C.A.; Fortier, M.; Roy, M.; Courchesne-Loyer, A.; Bocti, C.; *et al.* Brain glucose and acetoacetate metabolism: A comparison of young and older adults. *Neurobiol. Aging* **2014**, *35*, 1386–1395. [CrossRef] [PubMed]
227. Hooijmans, C.R.; Pasker-de Jong, P.C.M.; de Vries, R.B.M.; Ritskes-Hoitinga, M. The effects of long-term omega-3 fatty acid supplementation on cognition and Alzheimer's pathology in animal models of Alzheimer's disease: A systematic review and meta-analysis. *J. Alzheimer's Dis.* **2012**, *28*, 191–209.
228. Richard, E.; Andrieu, S.; Solomon, A.; Mangialasche, F.; Ahtiluoto, S.; van Charante, E.P.M.; Coley, N.; Fratiglioni, L.; Neely, A.S.; Vellas, B.; *et al.* Methodological challenges in designing dementia prevention trials—The European dementia prevention initiative (EDPI). *J. Neurol. Sci.* **2012**, *322*, 64–70. [CrossRef] [PubMed]
229. Albanese, E.; Dangour, A.D.; Uauy, R.; Acosta, D.; Guerra, M.; Guerra, S.S.G.; Huang, Y.; Jacob, K.S.; Rodriguez, J.L.D.; Noriega, L.H.; *et al.* Dietary fish and meat intake and dementia in latin America, China, and India: A 10/66 dementia research group population-based study. *Am. J. Clin. Nutr.* **2009**, *90*, 392–400. [CrossRef] [PubMed]
230. Barberger-Gateau, P.; Raffaitin, C.; Letenneur, L.; Berr, C.; Tzourio, C.; Dartigues, J.F.; Alpe, A. Dietary patterns and risk of dementia. *Neurology* **2007**, *69*, 1921–1930. [CrossRef] [PubMed]
231. Schaefer, E.J.; Bongard, V.; Beiser, A.S.; Lamon-Fava, S.; Robins, S.J.; Au, R.; Tucker, K.L.; Kyle, D.J.; Wilson, P.W.F.; Wolf, P.A. Plasma phosphatidylcholine docosahexaenoic acid content and risk of dementia and Alzheimer disease: The Framingham heart study. *Arch. Neurol.* **2006**, *63*, 1545–1550. [CrossRef] [PubMed]
232. Wu, S.; Ding, Y.; Wu, F.; Li, R.; Hou, J.; Mao, P. Omega-3 fatty acids intake and risks of dementia and Alzheimer's disease: A meta-analysis. *Neurosci. Biobehav. Rev.* **2015**, *48*, 1–9. [CrossRef] [PubMed]
233. Cherubini, A.; Andres-Lacueva, C.; Martin, A.; Lauretani, F.; Iorio, A.D.; Bartali, B.; Corsi, A.; Bandinelli, S.; Mattson, M.P.; Ferrucci, L. Low plasma *n*-3 fatty acids and dementia in older persons: The InCHIANTI study. *J. Gerontol. Ser. A Biol. Sci. Med. Sci.* **2007**, *62*, 1120–1126. [CrossRef]
234. Milte, C.M.; Sinn, N.; Street, S.J.; Buckley, J.D.; Coates, A.M.; Howe, P.R.C. Erythrocyte polyunsaturated fatty acid status, memory, cognition and mood in older adults with mild cognitive impairment and healthy controls. *Prostaglandins Leukot. Essent. Fat. Acids* **2011**, *84*, 153–161. [CrossRef] [PubMed]
235. Yin, Y.; Fan, Y.; Lin, F.; Xu, Y.; Zhang, J. Nutrient biomarkers and vascular risk factors in subtypes of mild cognitive impairment: A cross-sectional study. *J. Nutr. Health Aging* **2015**, *19*, 39–47. [CrossRef] [PubMed]
236. Terano, T.; Fujishiro, S.; Ban, T.; Yamamoto, K.; Tanaka, T.; Noguchi, Y.; Tamura, Y.; Yazawa, K.; Hirayama, T. Docosahexaenoic acid supplementation improves the moderately severe dementia from thrombotic cerebrovascular diseases. *Lipids* **1999**, *34*, S345–S346. [CrossRef] [PubMed]
237. Kotani, S.; Sakaguchi, E.; Warashina, S.; Matsukawa, N.; Ishikura, Y.; Kiso, Y.; Sakakibara, M.; Yoshimoto, T.; Guo, J.; Yamashima, T. Dietary supplementation of arachidonic and docosahexaenoic acids improves cognitive dysfunction. *Neurosci. Res.* **2006**, *56*, 159–164. [CrossRef] [PubMed]
238. Chiu, C.C.; Su, K.P.; Cheng, T.C.; Liu, H.C.; Chang, C.J.; Dewey, M.E.; Stewart, R.; Huang, S.Y. The effects of omega-3 fatty acids monotherapy in Alzheimer's disease and mild cognitive impairment: A preliminary randomized double-blind placebo-controlled study. *Prog. Neuro Psychopharmacol. Biol. Psychiatry* **2008**, *32*, 1538–1544. [CrossRef] [PubMed]
239. Sinn, N.; Milte, C.M.; Street, S.J.; Buckley, J.D.; Coates, A.M.; Petkov, J.; Howe, P.R.C. Effects of *n*-3 fatty acids, EPA v. DHA, on depressive symptoms, quality of life, memory and executive function in older adults with mild cognitive impairment: A 6-month randomised controlled trial. *Br. J. Nutr.* **2012**, *107*, 1682–1693. [CrossRef] [PubMed]

240. Cazzola, R.; Rondanelli, M.; Faliva, M.; Cestaro, B. Effects of DHA -phospholipids, melatonin and tryptophan supplementation on erythrocyte membrane physico-chemical properties in elderly patients suffering from mild cognitive impairment. *Exp. Gerontol.* **2012**, *47*, 974–978. [CrossRef] [PubMed]
241. Mahmoudi, M.; Hedayat, M.; Sharifi, F.; Mirarefin, M.; Nazari, N.; Mehrdad, N.; Ghaderpanahi, M.; Tajalizadekhoob, Y.; Badamchizade, Z.; Larijani, B.; *et al.* Effect of low dose ω-3 poly unsaturated fatty acids on cognitive status among older people: A double-blind randomized placebo-controlled study. *J. Diabetes Metab. Disord.* **2014**, *13*, 34. [CrossRef] [PubMed]
242. Ward, A.; Crean, S.; Mercaldi, C.J.; Collins, J.M.; Boyd, D.; Cook, M.N.; Arrighi, H.M. Prevalence of apolipoprotein E4 genotype and homozygotes (APOE e4/4) among patients diagnosed with Alzheimer's disease: A systematic review and meta-analysis. *Neuroepidemiology* **2012**, *38*, 1–17. [CrossRef] [PubMed]
243. Alzheimer's Association. 2014 Alzheimer's disease facts and figures. *Alzheimer's Dement.* **2014**, *10*, e47–e92.
244. World Health Organization. Dementia: A public health priority. In *Dementia*; WHO: Geneva, Switzerland, 2012; p. 112.
245. Kelley, A.S.; McGarry, K.; Gorges, R.; Skinner, J.S. The burden of health care costs for patients with dementia in the last 5 years of life. *Ann. Intern. Med.* **2015**, *163*, 729–736. [CrossRef] [PubMed]
246. Cummings, J.L.; Zhong, K. Repackaging FDA-approved drugs for degenerative diseases: Promises and challenges. *Expert Rev. Clin. Pharmacol.* **2014**, *7*, 161–165. [CrossRef] [PubMed]
247. Hebert, L.E.; Weuve, J.; Scherr, P.A.; Evans, D.A. Alzheimer disease in the United States (2010–2050) estimated using the 2010 census. *Neurology* **2013**, *80*, 1778–1783. [CrossRef] [PubMed]
248. Astarita, G.; Jung, K.M.; Berchtold, N.C.; Nguyen, V.Q.; Gillen, D.L.; Head, E.; Cotman, C.W.; Piomelli, D. Deficient liver biosynthesis of docosahexaenoic acid correlates with cognitive impairment in Alzheimer's disease. *PLoS ONE* **2010**, *5*, e12538. [CrossRef] [PubMed]
249. Igarashi, M.; Ma, K.; Gao, F.; Kim, H.W.; Rapoport, S.I.; Rao, J.S. Disturbed choline plasmalogen and phospholipid fatty acid concentrations in Alzheimer's disease prefrontal cortex. *J. Alzheimer's Dis.* **2011**, *24*, 507–517.
250. Quinn, J.F.; Raman, R.; Thomas, R.G.; Yurko-Mauro, K.; Nelson, E.B.; van Dyck, C.; Galvin, J.E.; Emond, J.; Jack, C.R., Jr.; Weiner, M.; *et al.* Docosahexaenoic acid supplementation and cognitive decline in Alzheimer disease: A randomized trial. *JAMA* **2010**, *304*, 1903–1911. [CrossRef] [PubMed]
251. Prasad, M.R.; Lovell, M.A.; Yatin, M.; Dhillon, H.; Markesbery, W.R. Regional membrane phospholipid alterations in Alzheimer's disease. *Neurochem. Res.* **1998**, *23*, 81–88. [CrossRef] [PubMed]
252. Soderberg, M.; Edlund, C.; Kristensson, K.; Dallner, G. Fatty acid composition of brain phospholipids in aging and in Alzheimer's disease. *Lipids* **1991**, *26*, 421–425. [CrossRef] [PubMed]
253. Morris, M.C.; Evans, D.a.; Bienias, J.L.; Tangney, C.C.; Bennett, D.a.; Wilson, R.S.; Aggarwal, N.; Schneider, J. Consumption of fish and *n*-3 fatty acids and risk of incident Alzheimer disease. *Arch. Neurol.* **2003**, *60*, 940–946. [CrossRef] [PubMed]
254. Shatenstein, B.; Kergoat, M.J.; Reid, I. Poor nutrient intakes during 1-year follow-up with community-dwelling older adults with early-stage Alzheimer dementia compared to cognitively intact matched controls. *J. Am. Diet. Assoc.* **2007**, *107*, 2091–2099. [CrossRef] [PubMed]
255. Daiello, L.A.; Gongvatana, A.; Dunsiger, S.; Cohen, R.A.; Ott, B.R. Association of fish oil supplement use with preservation of brain volume and cognitive function. *Alzheimer's Dement.* **2015**, *11*, 226–235. [CrossRef] [PubMed]
256. Conquer, J.; Tierney, M.; Zecevic, J.; Bettger, W.; Fisher, R. Fatty acid analysis of blood plasma of patients with Alzheimer's disease, other types of dementia, and cognitive impairment. *Lipids* **2000**, *35*, 1305–1312. [CrossRef] [PubMed]
257. Tully, A.M.; Roche, H.M.; Doyle, R.; Fallon, C.; Bruce, I.; Lawlor, B.; Coakley, D.; Gibney, M.J. Low serum cholesteryl ester-docosahexaenoic acid levels in Alzheimer's disease: A case–control study. *Br. J. Nutr.* **2003**, *89*, 483. [CrossRef] [PubMed]
258. Wang, W.; Shinto, L.; Connor, W.E.; Quinn, J.F. Nutritional biomarkers in Alzheimer's disease: The association between carotenoids, *n*-3 fatty acids, and dementia severity. *J. Alzheimer's Dis.* **2008**, *13*, 31–38.
259. Lopez, L.B.; Kritz-Silverstein, D.; Barrett-Connor, E. High dietary and plasma levels of the omega-3 fatty acid docosahexaenoic acid are associated with decreased dementia risk: The rancho bernardo study. *J. Nutr. Health Aging* **2011**, *15*, 25–31. [CrossRef] [PubMed]

260. Phillips, M.A.; Childs, C.E.; Calder, P.C.; Rogers, P.J. Lower omega-3 fatty acid intake and status are associated with poorer cognitive function in older age: A comparison of individuals with and without cognitive impairment and Alzheimer's disease. *Nutr. Neurosci.* **2012**, *15*, 271–278. [CrossRef] [PubMed]
261. Freund-Levi, Y.; Basun, H.; Cederholm, T.; Faxen-Irving, G.; Garlind, A.; Grut, M.; Vedin, I.; Palmblad, J.; Wahlund, L.O.; Eriksdotter-Jonhagen, M. Omega-3 supplementation in mild to moderate Alzheimer's disease: Effects on neuropsychiatric symptoms. *Int. J. Geriatr. Psychiatry* **2008**, *23*, 161–169. [CrossRef] [PubMed]
262. Freund-Levi, Y.; Eriksdotter-Jonhagen, M.; Cederholm, T.; Basun, H.; Faxen-Irving, G.; Garlind, A.; Vedin, I.; Vessby, B.; Wahlund, L.O.; Palmblad, J. Omega-3 fatty acid treatment in 174 patients with mild to moderate Alzheimer disease: Omegad study: A randomized double-blind trial. *Arch. Neurol.* **2006**, *63*, 1402–1408. [CrossRef] [PubMed]
263. Eriksdotter, M.; Vedin, I.; Falahati, F.; Freund-Levi, Y.; Hjorth, E.; Faxen-Irving, G.; Wahlund, L.O.; Schultzberg, M.; Basun, H.; Cederholm, T.; *et al.* Plasma fatty acid profiles in relation to cognition and gender in Alzheimer's disease patients during oral omega-3 fatty acid supplementation: The omegad study. *J. Alzheimer's Dis.* **2015**, *48*, 805–812. [CrossRef] [PubMed]
264. Levi, Y.F.; Vedin, I.; Cederholm, T.; Basun, H.; Irving, G.F.; Eriksdotter, M.; Hjorth, E.; Schultzberg, M.; Vessby, B.; Wahlund, L.O.; *et al.* Transfer of omega-3 fatty acids across the blood-brain barrier after dietary supplementation with a docosahexaenoic acid-rich omega-3 fatty acid preparation in patients with Alzheimer's disease: The omegad study. *J. Intern. Med.* **2014**, *275*, 428–436. [CrossRef] [PubMed]
265. Connor, J.R.; Menzies, S.L. Relationship of iron to oligodendrocytes and myelination. *Glia* **1996**, *17*, 83–93. [CrossRef]
266. Peters, A. Age-related changes in oligodendrocytes in monkey cerebral cortex. *J. Comp. Neurol.* **1996**, *371*, 153–163. [CrossRef]
267. Thompson, P.M.; Hayashi, K.M.; de Zubicaray, G.; Janke, A.L.; Rose, S.E.; Semple, J.; Herman, D.; Hong, M.S.; Dittmer, S.S.; Doddrell, D.M.; *et al.* Dynamics of gray matter loss in Alzheimer's disease. *J. Neurosci.* **2003**, *23*, 994–1005. [PubMed]
268. Braak, H.; Braak, E. Development of Alzheimer-related neurofibrillary changes in the neocortex inversely recapitulates cortical myelogenesis. *Acta Neuropathol.* **1996**, *92*, 197–201. [CrossRef] [PubMed]
269. Bartzokis, G. Alzheimer's disease as homeostatic responses to age-related myelin breakdown. *Neurobiol. Aging* **2011**, *32*, 1341–1371. [CrossRef] [PubMed]
270. Beal, M.F. Oxidative damage as an early marker of Alzheimer's disease and mild cognitive impairment. *Neurobiol. Aging* **2005**, *26*, 585–586. [CrossRef] [PubMed]
271. Virtanen, J.K.; Siscovick, D.S.; Lemaitre, R.N.; Longstreth, W.T.; Spiegelman, D.; Rimm, E.B.; King, I.B.; Mozaffarian, D. Circulating omega-3 polyunsaturated fatty acids and subclinical brain abnormalities on MRI in older adults: The Cardiovascular Health Study. *J. Am. Heart Assoc.* **2013**, 2. [CrossRef] [PubMed]
272. Vermeer, S.E.; Prins, N.D.; den Heijer, T.; Hofman, A.; Koudstaal, P.J.; Breteler, M.M. Silent brain infarcts and the risk of dementia and cognitive decline. *N. Engl. J. Med.* **2003**, *348*, 1215–1222. [CrossRef] [PubMed]
273. Peters, A.; Schweiger, U.; Pellerin, L.; Hubold, C.; Oltmanns, K.M.; Conrad, M.; Schultes, B.; Born, J.; Fehm, H.L. The selfish brain: Competition for energy resources. *Neurosci. Biobehav. Rev.* **2004**, *28*, 143–180. [CrossRef] [PubMed]
274. Whitmer, R.A.; Sidney, S.; Selby, J.; Johnston, S.C.; Yaffe, K. Midlife cardiovascular risk factors and risk of dementia in late life. *Neurology* **2005**, *64*, 277–281. [CrossRef] [PubMed]
275. Kalaria, R.N.; Ballard, C. Overlap between pathology of Alzheimer disease and vascular dementia. *Alzheimer Dis. Assoc. Disord.* **1999**, *13* (Suppl. 3), S115–S123. [CrossRef] [PubMed]
276. Roher, A.E.; Debbins, J.P.; Malek-Ahmadi, M.; Chen, K.; Pipe, J.G.; Maze, S.; Belden, C.; Maarouf, C.L.; Thiyyagura, P.; Mo, H.; *et al.* Cerebral blood flow in Alzheimer's disease. *Vasc. Health Risk Manag.* **2012**, *8*, 599–611. [CrossRef] [PubMed]
277. Jackson, P.A.; Reay, J.L.; Scholey, A.B.; Kennedy, D.O. DHA -rich oil modulates the cerebral haemodynamic response to cognitive tasks in healthy young adults: A near ir spectroscopy pilot study. *Br. J. Nutr.* **2012**, *107*, 1093–1098. [CrossRef] [PubMed]
278. Beydoun, M.A.; Kaufman, J.S.; Satia, J.A.; Rosamond, W.; Folsom, A.R. Plasma *n*-3 fatty acids and the risk of cognitive decline in older adults: The atherosclerosis risk in communities study. *Am. J. Clin. Nutr.* **2007**, *85*, 1103–1111. [PubMed]

279. Huang, T.; Hu, X.; Khan, N.; Yang, J.; Li, D. Effect of polyunsaturated fatty acids on homocysteine metabolism through regulating the gene expressions involved in methionine metabolism. *Sci. World J.* **2013**, *2013*. [CrossRef] [PubMed]
280. Ford, A.H.; Flicker, L.; Alfonso, H.; Hankey, G.J.; Norman, P.E.; van Bockxmeer, F.M.; Almeida, O.P. Plasma homocysteine and MTHFRC677T polymorphism as risk factors for incident dementia. *J. Neurol. Neurosurg. Psychiatry* **2012**, *83*, 70–75. [CrossRef] [PubMed]
281. Boneva, N.B.; Yamashima, T. New insights into "GPR40-CREB interaction in adult neurogenesis" specific for primates. *Hippocampus* **2012**, *22*, 896–905. [CrossRef] [PubMed]
282. Brand, A.; Schonfeld, E.; Isharel, I.; Yavin, E. Docosahexaenoic acid-dependent iron accumulation in oligodendroglia cells protects from hydrogen peroxide-induced damage. *J. Neurochem.* **2008**, *105*, 1325–1335. [CrossRef] [PubMed]
283. Gururajan, A.; van den Buuse, M. Is the mtor-signalling cascade disrupted in schizophrenia? *J. Neurochem.* **2014**, *129*, 377–387. [CrossRef] [PubMed]
284. Calon, F.; Lim, G.P.; Morihara, T.; Yang, F.; Ubeda, O.; Salem, N.; Frautschy, S.A.; Cole, G.M. Dietary *n*-3 polyunsaturated fatty acid depletion activates caspases and decreases NMDA receptors in the brain of a transgenic mouse model of Alzheimer's disease. *Eur. J. Neurosci.* **2005**, *22*, 617–626. [CrossRef] [PubMed]
285. Nishikawa, M.; Kimura, S.; Akaike, N. Facilitatory effect of docosahexaenoic acid on *N*-methyl-D-aspartate response in pyramidal neurones of rat cerebral cortex. *J. Physiol.* **1994**, *475*, 83–93. [CrossRef] [PubMed]
286. Calon, F.; Lim, G.P.; Yang, F.; Morihara, T.; Teter, B.; Ubeda, O.; Rostaing, P.; Triller, A.; Salem, N., Jr.; Ashe, K.H.; *et al.* Docosahexaenoic acid protects from dendritic pathology in an Alzheimer's disease mouse model. *Neuron* **2004**, *43*, 633–645. [CrossRef] [PubMed]
287. Dyall, S.C.; Michael, G.J.; Michael-Titus, A.T. Omega-3 fatty acids reverse age-related decreases in nuclear receptors and increase neurogenesis in old rats. *J. Neurosci. Res.* **2010**, *88*, 2091–2102. [CrossRef] [PubMed]
288. Maarouf, C.L.; Daugs, I.D.; Kokjohn, T.A.; Walker, D.G.; Hunter, J.M.; Kruchowsky, J.C.; Woltjer, R.; Kaye, J.; Castano, E.M.; Sabbagh, M.N.; *et al.* Alzheimer's disease and non-demented high pathology control nonagenarians: Comparing and contrasting the biochemistry of cognitively successful aging. *PLoS ONE* **2011**, *6*, e27291. [CrossRef] [PubMed]
289. Morimoto, K.; Horio, J.; Satoh, H.; Sue, L.; Beach, T.; Arita, S.; Tooyama, I.; Konishi, Y. Expression profiles of cytokines in the brains of Alzheimer's disease (ad) patients compared to the brains of non-demented patients with and without increasing ad pathology. *J. Alzheimer's Dis.* **2011**, *25*, 59–76.
290. Parachikova, A.; Agadjanyan, M.G.; Cribbs, D.H.; Blurton-Jones, M.; Perreau, V.; Rogers, J.; Beach, T.G.; Cotman, C.W. Inflammatory changes parallel the early stages of Alzheimer disease. *Neurobiol. Aging* **2007**, *28*, 1821–1833. [CrossRef] [PubMed]
291. Cagnin, A.; Brooks, D.J.; Kennedy, A.M.; Gunn, R.N.; Myers, R.; Turkheimer, F.E.; Jones, T.; Banati, R.B. *In-vivo* measurement of activated microglia in dementia. *Lancet* **2001**, *358*, 461–467. [CrossRef]
292. Edison, P.; Archer, H.A.; Gerhard, A.; Hinz, R.; Pavese, N.; Turkheimer, F.E.; Hammers, A.; Tai, Y.F.; Fox, N.; Kennedy, A.; *et al.* Microglia, amyloid, and cognition in Alzheimer's disease: An [11C](R)PK11195-PET and [11C]PIB-PET study. *Neurobiol. Dis.* **2008**, *32*, 412–419. [CrossRef] [PubMed]
293. Yokokura, M.; Mori, N.; Yagi, S.; Yoshikawa, E.; Kikuchi, M.; Yoshihara, Y.; Wakuda, T.; Sugihara, G.; Takebayashi, K.; Suda, S.; *et al.* *In vivo* changes in microglial activation and amyloid deposits in brain regions with hypometabolism in Alzheimer's disease. *Eur. J. Nucl. Med. Mol. Imaging* **2011**, *38*, 343–351. [CrossRef] [PubMed]
294. Blum-Degen, D.; Muller, T.; Kuhn, W.; Gerlach, M.; Przuntek, H.; Riederer, P. Interleukin-1 beta and interleukin-6 are elevated in the cerebrospinal fluid of Alzheimer's and de novo parkinson's disease patients. *Neurosci. Lett.* **1995**, *202*, 17–20. [CrossRef]
295. Heneka, M.T.; Kummer, M.P.; Latz, E. Innate immune activation in neurodegenerative disease. *Nat. Rev. Immunol.* **2014**, *14*, 463–477. [CrossRef] [PubMed]
296. Jia, J.P.; Meng, R.; Sun, Y.X.; Sun, W.J.; Ji, X.M.; Jia, L.F. Cerebrospinal fluid tau, abeta1–42 and inflammatory cytokines in patients with Alzheimer's disease and vascular dementia. *Neurosci. Lett.* **2005**, *383*, 12–16. [CrossRef] [PubMed]
297. Halle, A.; Hornung, V.; Petzold, G.C.; Stewart, C.R.; Monks, B.G.; Reinheckel, T.; Fitzgerald, K.A.; Latz, E.; Moore, K.J.; Golenbock, D.T. The NALP3 inflammasome is involved in the innate immune response to amyloid-beta. *Nat. Immunol.* **2008**, *9*, 857–865. [CrossRef] [PubMed]

298. Salminen, A.; Ojala, J.; Suuronen, T.; Kaarniranta, K.; Kauppinen, A. Amyloid-beta oligomers set fire to inflammasomes and induce Alzheimer's pathology. *J. Cell. Mol. Med.* **2008**, *12*, 2255–2262. [CrossRef] [PubMed]
299. Hjorth, E.; Zhu, M.; Toro, V.C.; Vedin, I.; Palmblad, J.; Cederholm, T.; Freund-Levi, Y.; Faxen-Irving, G.; Wahlund, L.O.; Basun, H.; *et al.* Omega-3 fatty acids enhance phagocytosis of Alzheimer's disease-related amyloid-β42 by human microglia and decrease inflammatory markers. *J. Alzheimer's Dis.* **2013**, *35*, 697–713.
300. Krstic, D.; Knuesel, I. Deciphering the mechanism underlying late-onset Alzheimer disease. *Nat. Rev. Neurol.* **2012**, *9*, 25–34. [CrossRef] [PubMed]
301. Weiser, M.J.; Mucha, B.; Denheyer, H.; Atkinson, D.; Schanz, N.; Vassiliou, E.; Benno, R.H. Dietary docosahexaenoic acid alleviates autistic-like behaviors resulting from maternal immune activation in mice. *Prostaglandins Leukot. Essent. Fat. Acids* **2015**. [CrossRef] [PubMed]
302. Wang, X.; Hjorth, E.; Vedin, I.; Eriksdotter, M.; Freund-Levi, Y.; Wahlund, L.O.; Cederholm, T.; Palmblad, J.; Schultzberg, M. Effects of *n*-3 FA supplementation on the release of proresolving lipid mediators by blood mononuclear cells: The OmegAD study. *J. Lipid Res.* **2015**, *56*, 674–681. [CrossRef] [PubMed]
303. Serhan, C.N.; Dalli, J.; Colas, R.A.; Winkler, J.W.; Chiang, N. Protectins and maresins: New pro-resolving families of mediators in acute inflammation and resolution bioactive metabolome. *Biochim. Biophys. Acta* **2015**, *1851*, 397–413. [CrossRef] [PubMed]
304. Alfano, C.M.; Imayama, I.; Neuhouser, M.L.; Kiecolt-Glaser, J.K.; Smith, A.W.; Meeske, K.; McTiernan, A.; Bernstein, L.; Baumgartner, K.B.; Ulrich, C.M.; *et al.* Fatigue, inflammation, and omega-3 and omega-6 fatty acid intake among breast cancer survivors. *J. Clin. Oncol.* **2012**, *30*, 1280–1287. [CrossRef] [PubMed]
305. Kiecolt-Glaser, J.K.; Belury, M.A.; Andridge, R.; Malarkey, W.B.; Glaser, R. Omega-3 supplementation lowers inflammation and anxiety in medical students: A randomized controlled trial. *Brain Behav. Immun.* **2011**, *25*, 1725–1734. [CrossRef] [PubMed]
306. Bouwens, M.; Bromhaar, M.G.; Jansen, J.; Muller, M.; Afman, L.A. Postprandial dietary lipid-specific effects on human peripheral blood mononuclear cell gene expression profiles. *Am. J. Clin. Nutr.* **2010**, *91*, 208–217. [CrossRef] [PubMed]
307. Vedin, I.; Cederholm, T.; Levi, Y.F.; Basun, H.; Garlind, A.; Irving, G.F. Effects of docosahexaenoic acid-rich *n*-3 fatty acid supplementation on cytokine release from blood mononuclear leukocytes: The OmegAD study. *Am. Soc. Nutr.* **2008**, *87*, 1616–1622.
308. Green, K.N.; Martinez-Coria, H.; Khashwji, H.; Hall, E.B.; Yurko-Mauro, K.A.; Ellis, L.; LaFerla, F.M. Dietary docosahexaenoic acid and docosapentaenoic acid ameliorate amyloid-beta and tau pathology via a mechanism involving presenilin 1 levels. *J.Neurosci.* **2007**, *27*, 4385–4395. [CrossRef] [PubMed]
309. Ma, Q.L.; Yang, F.; Rosario, E.R.; Ubeda, O.J.; Beech, W.; Gant, D.J.; Chen, P.P.; Hudspeth, B.; Chen, C.; Zhao, Y.; *et al.* Beta-amyloid oligomers induce phosphorylation of tau and inactivation of insulin receptor substrate via c-Jun *N*-terminal kinase signaling: Suppression by omega-3 fatty acids and curcumin. *J. Neurosci.* **2009**, *29*, 9078–9089. [CrossRef] [PubMed]
310. Calon, F. Omega-3 polyunsaturated fatty acids in Alzheimer's disease: Key questions and partial answers. *Curr. Alzheimer Res.* **2011**, *8*, 470–478. [CrossRef] [PubMed]
311. Janssen, C.I.F.; Kiliaan, A.J. Long-chain polyunsaturated fatty acids (LCPUFA) from genesis to senescence: The influence of LCPUFA on neural development, aging, and neurodegeneration. *Prog. Lipid Res.* **2014**, *53*, 1–17. [CrossRef] [PubMed]
312. Krstic, D.; Pfister, S.; Notter, T.; Knuesel, I. Decisive role of reelin signaling during early stages of Alzheimer's disease. *Neuroscience* **2013**, *246*, 108–116. [CrossRef] [PubMed]
313. Yavin, E.; Himovichi, E.; Eilam, R. Delayed cell migration in the developing rat brain following maternal omega 3 alpha linolenic acid dietary deficiency. *Neuroscience* **2009**, *162*, 1011–1022. [CrossRef] [PubMed]
314. Botella-Lopez, A.; Burgaya, F.; Gavin, R.; Garcia-Ayllon, M.S.; Gomez-Tortosa, E.; Pena-Casanova, J.; Urena, J.M.; del Rio, J.A.; Blesa, R.; Soriano, E.; *et al.* Reelin expression and glycosylation patterns are altered in Alzheimer's disease. *Proc. Natl. Acad. Sci. USA* **2006**, *103*, 5573–5578. [CrossRef] [PubMed]
315. Medhi, B.; Chakrabarty, M. Insulin resistance: An emerging link in Alzheimer's disease. *Neurol. Sci.* **2013**, *34*, 1719–1725. [CrossRef] [PubMed]
316. De la Monte, S.M.; Tong, M. Brain metabolic dysfunction at the core of Alzheimer's disease. *Biochem. Pharmacol.* **2014**, *88*, 548–559. [CrossRef] [PubMed]

317. Velayudhan, L.; Poppe, M.; Archer, N.; Proitsi, P.; Brown, R.G.; Lovestone, S. Risk of developing dementia in people with diabetes and mild cognitive impairment. *Br. J. Psychiatry* **2010**, *196*, 36–40. [CrossRef] [PubMed]
318. Hennebelle, M.; Harbeby, E.; Tremblay, S.; Chouinard-Watkins, R.; Pifferi, F.; Plourde, M.; Guesnet, P.; Cunnane, S.C. Challenges to determining whether DHA can protect against age-related cognitive decline. *Clin. Lipidol.* **2015**, *10*, 91–102. [CrossRef]
319. Pifferi, F.; Jouin, M.; Alessandri, J.M.; Haedke, U.; Roux, F.; Perriere, N.; Denis, I.; Lavialle, M.; Guesnet, P. *n*-3 fatty acids modulate brain glucose transport in endothelial cells of the blood-brain barrier. *Prostaglandins Leukot. Essent. Fat. Acids* **2007**, *77*, 279–286. [CrossRef] [PubMed]
320. Pifferi, F.; Jouin, M.; Alessandri, J.M.; Roux, F.; Perriere, N.; Langelier, B.; Lavialle, M.; Cunnane, S.; Guesnet, P. *n*-3 long-chain fatty acids and regulation of glucose transport in two models of rat brain endothelial cells. *Neurochem. Int.* **2010**, *56*, 703–710. [CrossRef] [PubMed]
321. Pifferi, F.; Roux, F.; Langelier, B.; Alessandri, J.M.; Vancassel, S.; Jouin, M.; Lavialle, M.; Guesnet, P. (*n*-3) polyunsaturated fatty acid deficiency reduces the expression of both isoforms of the brain glucose transporter glut1 in rats. *J. Nutr.* **2005**, *135*, 2241–2246. [PubMed]
322. Grimm, M.O.; Kuchenbecker, J.; Grosgen, S.; Burg, V.K.; Hundsdorfer, B.; Rothhaar, T.L.; Friess, P.; de Wilde, M.C.; Broersen, L.M.; Penke, B.; *et al.* Docosahexaenoic acid reduces amyloid beta production via multiple pleiotropic mechanisms. *J. Biol. Chem.* **2011**, *286*, 14028–14039. [CrossRef] [PubMed]
323. Martín, V.; Fabelo, N.; Santpere, G.; Puig, B.; Marín, R.; Ferrer, I.; Díaz, M. Lipid alterations in lipid rafts from Alzheimer's disease human brain cortex. *J. Alzheimer's Dis.* **2010**, *19*, 489–502.
324. Fabelo, N.; Martin, V.; Marin, R.; Moreno, D.; Ferrer, I.; Diaz, M. Altered lipid composition in cortical lipid rafts occurs at early stages of sporadic Alzheimer's disease and facilitates APP/BACE1 interactions. *Neurobiol. Aging* **2014**, *35*, 1801–1812. [CrossRef] [PubMed]
325. Hashimoto, M.; Hossain, S.; Katakura, M.; al Mamun, A.; Shido, O. The binding of aβ1–42 to lipid rafts of rbc is enhanced by dietary docosahexaenoic acid in rats: Implicates to Alzheimer's disease. *Biochim. Biophys. Acta* **2015**, *1848*, 1402–1409. [CrossRef] [PubMed]
326. Gu, Y.; Schupf, N.; Cosentino, S.A.; Luchsinger, J.A.; Scarmeas, N. Nutrient intake and plasma beta-amyloid. *Neurology* **2012**, *78*, 1832–1840. [CrossRef] [PubMed]
327. Flock, M.R.; Skulas-Ray, A.C.; Harris, W.S.; Etherton, T.D.; Fleming, J.A.; Kris-Etherton, P.M. Determinants of erythrocyte omega-3 fatty acid content in response to fish oil supplementation: A dose-response randomized controlled trial. *J. Am. Heart Assoc.* **2013**, *2*. [CrossRef] [PubMed]
328. Cunnane, S.C.; Schneider, J.A.; Tangney, C.; Tremblay-Mercier, J.; Fortier, M.; Bennett, D.A.; Morris, M.C. Plasma and brain fatty acid profiles in mild cognitive impairment and Alzheimer's disease. *J. Alzheimer's Dis.* **2012**, *29*, 691–697.
329. Chouinard-Watkins, R.; Rioux-Perreault, C.; Fortier, M.; Tremblay-Mercier, J.; Zhang, Y.; Lawrence, P.; Vohl, M.C.; Perron, P.; Lorrain, D.; Brenna, J.T.; *et al.* Disturbance in uniformly 13c-labelled DHA metabolism in elderly human subjects carrying the apoE ε4 allele. *Br. J. Nutr.* **2013**, *110*, 1751–1759. [CrossRef] [PubMed]
330. Wu, A.; Noble, E.E.; Tyagi, E.; Ying, Z.; Zhuang, Y.; Gomez-Pinilla, F. Curcumin boosts DHA in the brain: Implications for the prevention of anxiety disorders. *Biochim. Biophys. Acta* **2015**, *1852*, 951–961. [CrossRef] [PubMed]
331. Scheltens, P.; Twisk, J.W.R.; Blesa, R.; Scarpini, E.; von Arnim, C.A.F.; Bongers, A.; Harrison, J.; Swinkels, S.H.N.; Stam, C.J.; de Waal, H.; *et al.* Efficacy of souvenaid in mild Alzheimer's disease: Results from a randomized, controlled trial. *J. Alzheimer's Dis.* **2012**, *31*, 225–236.
332. Serhan, C.N. Lipoxins and aspirin-triggered 15-epi-lipoxin biosynthesis: An update and role in anti-inflammation and pro-resolution. *Prostaglandins Other Lipid Mediat.* **2002**, *68–69*, 433–455. [CrossRef]
333. Serhan, C.N.; Gotlinger, K.; Hong, S.; Arita, M. Resolvins, docosatrienes, and neuroprotectins, novel omega-3-derived mediators, and their aspirin-triggered endogenous epimers: An overview of their protective roles in catabasis. *Prostaglandins Other Lipid Mediat.* **2004**, *73*, 155–172. [CrossRef] [PubMed]
334. Ariel, A.; Serhan, C.N. Resolvins and protectins in the termination program of acute inflammation. *Trends Immunol.* **2007**, *28*, 176–183. [CrossRef] [PubMed]
335. Dalli, J.; Winkler, J.W.; Colas, R.A.; Arnardottir, H.; Cheng, C.Y.; Chiang, N.; Petasis, N.A.; Serhan, C.N. Resolvin D3 and aspirin-triggered resolvin D3 are potent immunoresolvents. *Chem. Biol.* **2013**, *20*, 188–201. [CrossRef] [PubMed]

336. Esiri, M.M. The interplay between inflammation and neurodegeneration in CNS disease. *J. Neuroimmunol.* **2007**, *184*, 4–16. [CrossRef] [PubMed]
337. Etminan, M.; Gill, S.; Samii, A. Effect of non-steroidal anti-inflammatory drugs on risk of Alzheimer's disease: Systematic review and meta-analysis of observational studies. *BMJ* **2003**, *327*, 128. [CrossRef] [PubMed]
338. Lehrer, S. Nasal nsaids for Alzheimer's disease. *Am. J. Alzheimers Dis. Other Dement.* **2014**, *29*, 401–403. [CrossRef] [PubMed]
339. Lewis, M.D.; Bailes, J. Neuroprotection for the warrior: Dietary supplementation with omega-3 fatty acids. *Mil. Med.* **2011**, *176*, 1120–1127. [CrossRef] [PubMed]

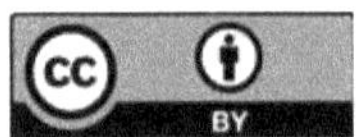

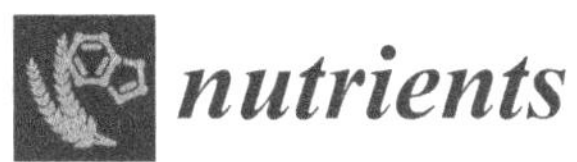

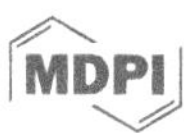

Article

Australians are not Meeting the Recommended Intakes for Omega-3 Long Chain Polyunsaturated Fatty Acids: Results of an Analysis from the 2011–2012 National Nutrition and Physical Activity Survey

Barbara J. Meyer

School of Medicine, University of Wollongong, Northfields Ave, Wollongong, NSW 2522, Australia; bmeyer@uow.edu.au; Tel.: +61-2-4221-3459

Received: 18 December 2015; Accepted: 14 February 2016; Published: 24 February 2016

Abstract: Health benefits have been attributed to omega-3 long chain polyunsaturated fatty acids (*n*-3 LCPUFA). Therefore it is important to know if Australians are currently meeting the recommended intake for *n*-3 LCPUFA and if they have increased since the last National Nutrition Survey in 1995 (NNS 1995). Dietary intake data was obtained from the recent 2011–2012 National Nutrition and Physical Activity Survey (2011–2012 NNPAS). Linoleic acid (LA) intakes have decreased whilst alpha-linolenic acid (LNA) and *n*-3 LCPUFA intakes have increased primarily due to *n*-3 LCPUFA supplements. The median *n*-3 LCPUFA intakes are less than 50% of the mean *n*-3 LCPUFA intakes which highlights the highly-skewed *n*-3 LCPUFA intakes, which shows that there are some people consuming high amounts of *n*-3 LCPUFA, but the vast majority of the population are consuming much lower amounts. Only 20% of the population meets the recommended *n*-3 LCPUFA intakes and only 10% of women of childbearing age meet the recommended docosahexaenoic acid (DHA) intake. Fish and seafood is by far the richest source of *n*-3 LCPUFA including DHA.

Keywords: *n*-3 LCPUFA; dietary intakes; Australian 2011–2012 national nutrition and physical activity survey; recommended *n*-3 LCPUFA intakes

1. Introduction

Dietary fatty acids consist of saturated, monounsaturated, and polyunsaturated fatty acids (PUFA), where the PUFA comprise of omega-6 (*n*-6) and omega-3 (*n*-3) PUFA. The major dietary *n*-6 PUFA are linoleic acid (LA) and arachidonic acid (AA), whilst the major dietary *n*-3 PUFA are alpha-linoleic acid (LNA), eicosapentaenoic acid (EPA), docosapentaenoic acid (DPA), and docosahexaenoic acid (DHA) [1]. The *n*-3 long-chain PUFA (*n*-3 LCPUFA) comprise of EPA, DPA, and DHA, and are also referred to as the marine sources of *n*-3 PUFA. This distinction between LNA and *n*-3 LCPUFA is necessary because the majority of health benefits have been attributed to the *n*-3 LCPUFA rather than to LNA.

There are numerous health benefits associated with *n*-3 LCPUFA [2–7]. The vast majority of health benefits attributed to *n*-3 LCPUFA is in cardiovascular disease. The GISSI prevenzione trial showed that supplementation of 0.85 g of EPA and DHA per day in men who had a previous myocardial infarction resulted in 20% reduction in total death, 30% reduction in cardiovascular death and 45% reduction in sudden death [5]. There is emerging evidence for the benefits of *n*-3 LCPUFA in mental health [8] with the biological plausibility explained in the review by Parletta *et al.* [9]. Given these health benefits various organisations, including government organisations, have come up with recommended *n*-3 LCPUFA intakes for optimal health.

In Australia, the National Health and Medical Research Council (NHMRC) has nutrient reference values (NRV) which include recommended intakes for macronutrients and micronutrients for various age and gender categories [10]. The NHMRC NRV includes adequate intakes (AI) which is defined as the median intakes of the population and is not a recommended intake [10]. The NHMRC NRV suggested dietary target (SDT) intakes are recommended intakes for the prevention of chronic disease [10]. The SDT for *n*-3 LCPUFA is 430 mg/day for female adults and 610 mg/day for male adults [10] and these recommendations are based on the 90th centile of intakes from the Australian National Nutrition Survey conducted in 1995 (NNS 1995) [11].

The International Society for the Study of Fatty Acids and Lipids (ISSFAL) recommends 500 mg *n*-3 LCPUFA per day for cardiovascular health [12]. ISSFAL also has a separate recommendation for pregnancy and lactating women and this recommendation is to consume at least 200 mg per day of DHA based on a position paper by Berthold *et al.* [13].

Given these recommended intakes for *n*-3 LCPUFA, it is important to know what Australians are currently consuming and if they are meeting these recommendations. Therefore, the overall aims are to describe the current PUFA intakes; to compare the *n*-3 LCPUFA intakes to recommended intakes and to compare current intakes to previous intakes. The specific aims are: (1) to report on the macronutrient intake, including *n*-3 LCPUFA, per age category as published by Howe *et al.* [11]; (2) to compare the median and mean *n*-3 LCPUFA intakes from the 2011–2012-NNPAS from food and supplements per age category; (3) to compare the *n*-3 LCPUFA intakes to recommended intakes; (4) to determine if women of childbearing age met the *n*-3 LCPUFA and DHA recommended intakes during pregnancy; (5) to compare the actual adult Australian food intake from five different food groups to the respective *n*-3 LCPUFA intakes; and (6) to compare the current 2011–2012 NNPAS PUFA intakes, including *n*-3 LCPUFA intakes, to previous PUFA intakes from the NNS 1995 [11].

2. Results

2.1. Numbers of Subjects from the 2011–2012 NNPAS and the NNS 1995 Surveys

Table 1 shows the number of people surveyed for each age and gender category from both surveys. Overall the numbers are slightly lower in the 2011–2012 NNPAS except for the 12–18 years and the 65+ years categories.

Table 1. Total number of study participants per sex and age and category.

Age Category	2011–2012 NNPAS sample			NNS 1995 Sample		
	Female	Male	Total	Female	Male	Total
All ages	6451	5702	12,153	7242	6616	13,858
2–11 years	857	854	1711	950	971	1921
12–18 years	535	566	1101	522	564	1086
19–24 years	360	326	686	575	485	1060
25–64 years	3506	3046	6552	4137	3694	7831
⩾65 years	1193	910	2103	1058	902	1960
⩾19 years	5059	4282	9341	5770	5081	10,851

2011–2012 NNPAS: the 2011–2012 National Nutrition and Physical Activity Survey; NNS 1995: the National Nutrition Survey in 1995.

2.2. The 2011–2012 NNPAS PUFA, LA, LNA, and n-3 LCPUFA Intakes per Day

Table 2 shows the PUFA, LA, LNA and the n-3 LCPUFA intakes per day (mean $\pm$ SEM) per age category and gender. Generally the PUFA intakes are higher in males than females for all age categories, except the *n*-3 LCPUFA intakes are higher in females aged 65+ years than males of the same age category. The *n*-3 LCPUFA intakes range from 133 mg per day to 494 mg per day.

Table 2. 2011–2012 NNPAS polyunsaturated fatty acids (PUFA), linoleic acid (LA), whilst alpha-linolenic acid (LNA) and the *n*-3 long-chain PUFA (*n*-3 LCPUFA) intakes per day (mean ± SEM).

Age Category and Gender	PUFA (g)	LA (g)	LNA (g)	*n*-3 LCPUFA (mg)
Total F	9.5 ± 0.1	7.8 ± 0.06	1.2 ± 0.01	335 ± 9
Total M	11.4 ± 0.1	9.4 ± 0.08	1.4 ± 0.01	346 ± 9
2–11 F	7.1 ± 0.1	5.9 ± 0.12	0.9 ± 0.02	138 ± 10
2–11 M	8.2 ± 0.2	6.8 ± 0.13	1.0 ± 0.02	158 ± 11
12–18 F	9.6 ± 0.2	8.1 ± 0.22	1.2 ± 0.03	133 ± 7
12–18 M	11.5 ± 0.3	9.6 ± 0.22	1.4 ± 0.03	213 ± 15
19–24 F	10.1 ± 0.3	8.5 ± 0.28	1.2 ± 0.04	175 ± 14
19–24 M	13.4 ± 0.5	11.2 ± 0.42	1.6 ± 0.06	346 ± 36
25–64 F	10.2 ± 0.1	8.3 ± 0.09	1.3 ± 0.02	378 ± 14
25–64 M	12.4 ± 0.1	10.2 ± 0.12	1.5 ± 0.02	395 ± 14
⩾65 F	9.1 ± 0.2	7.2 ± 0.13	1.2 ± 0.03	494 ± 26
⩾65 M	10.5 ± 0.2	8.4 ± 0.17	1.4 ± 0.03	441 ± 24
⩾19 F	9.9 ± 0.1	8.0 ± 0.07	1.2 ± 0.01	390 ± 11
⩾19 M	12.1 ± 0.1	9.9 ± 0.10	1.5 ± 0.02	401 ± 12

F—Female; M—Male.

2.3. Comparison of the Median and Mean n-3 LCPUFA Intakes from the 2011–2012 NNPAS (Figure 1)

Figure 1 compares the median and mean *n*-3 LCPUFA intakes as well as the amounts coming from food and supplement sources. The median intakes are less than 50% of the mean intakes for all age categories, except for the 12–18 years olds which is 54% of the mean intakes. For adults (19+ years) the median intake is 32% of the mean intakes, which is largely driven by the 65+ years age category where the median intake is 26% of the mean intakes. This shows that *n*-3 LCPUFA intakes are highly skewed with few people consuming high amounts of *n*-3 LCPUFA and many people consuming low amounts of *n*-3 LCPUFA. The few people consuming large amounts of *n*-3 LCPUFA are consuming *n*-3 LCPUFA supplements. The proportion of *n*-3 LCPUFA coming from supplements is 27% for 25–64 years, 40% for 65+ years, and 30% of 19+ years and, therefore, the mean intakes are much higher than the mean intakes.

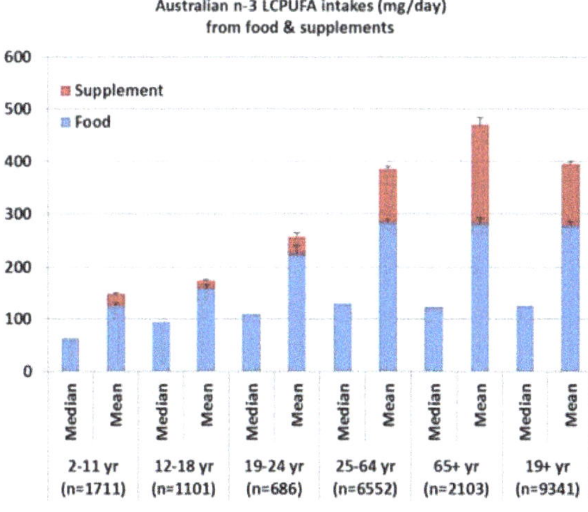

Figure 1. Comparison of the median and mean *n*-3 LCPUFA intakes from food and supplements per age category.

2.4. Comparison of n-3 LCPUFA Intakes to Recommended Intakes

2.4.1. The Proportion of Adult Female and Male (19+ Years) Meeting the Recommended Intakes (Table 3)

The NHMRC NRV for *n*-3 LCPUFA SDT are based on the 90th centile of intakes from the previous National Nutrition Survey 1995 [11]. Less than a quarter of Australian adults are meeting the *n*-3 LCPUFA recommendations for optimal health. However, those adults consuming *n*-3 LCPUFA supplements approximately 50% are meeting the recommended intakes, whilst those not consuming supplements, only approximately 10% are meeting the recommended intakes.

Table 3. Meeting the recommended intakes for *n*-3 LCPUFA with and without supplements.

Recommended Intakes for Females 19+ Years	Females 19+ Years (*n* = 5059)	No Supplements (*n* = 4054, 75%)	With Supplements (*n* = 1005, 25%)
>430 mg per day *	*n* = 1126 (22%)	*n* = 446 (11%)	*n* = 673 (67%)
>500 mg per day #	*n* = 1001 (20%)	*n* = 386 (9.5%)	*n* = 613 (61%)
Recommended Intakes for Males 19+ Years	**Males 19+ Years (*n* = 4282)**	**No supplements (*n* = 3625, 85%)**	**With supplements (*n* = 657, 15%)**
>500 mg per day #	*n* = 844 (20%)	*n* = 399 (11%)	*n* = 368 (56%)
>610 mg per day *	*n* = 702 (16%)	*n* = 326 (9%)	*n* = 302 (46%)

* National Health & Medical Research Council (NHMRC) nutrient reference values (NRV) suggested dietary target (SDT) intakes for adult females and males; # ISSFAL recommendations for cardiovascular health.

When considering the median intakes, there was no contribution from *n*-3 LCPUFA supplements (Figure 1), as only 25% of adult women and 15% of adult men consumed *n*-3 LCPUFA supplements (Table 3).

2.4.2. Adult Females of Childbearing Age (16–50 Years) n-3 LCPUFA and DHA Intakes across Centiles and Comparison to the ISSFAL Recommendations for DHA Intake (Figure 2)

There is a separate recommendation for pregnant women and the International Society for the Study of Fatty Acids and Lipids (ISSFAL) recommends at least 200 mg DHA per day during pregnancy and lactation [12,13]. Figure 2 shows the current consumption of *n*-3 LCPUFA and the respective estimated DHA intakes for women of childbearing age.

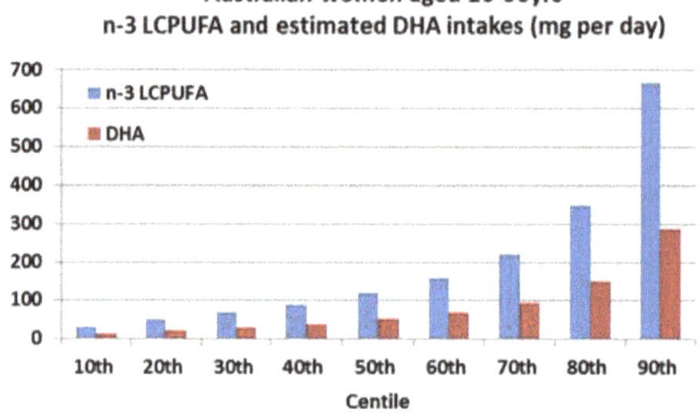

Figure 2. Australian women's consumption of *n*-3 LCPUFA and the respective estimated docosahexaenoic acid (DHA) (mg per day) per centile.

The median *n*-3 LCPUFA intake is 119 mg/day. DHA is estimated to be 43% of the total *n*-3 LCPUFA [11] and, therefore, the median DHA intake is estimated at 51 mg per day. Women in the 90th centile consume on average 287 mg DHA per day which meets the recommended DHA intake of at least 200 mg DHA per day.

2.5. Comparison of Adult Australian Intakes of food and the Respective n-3 LCPUFA in Those Foods

2.5.1. Comparison of the Amount of Food Eaten (g per Day) by Adult Australians and the Respective Amount of *n*-3 LCPUFA Intakes (mg per Day) from the 2011–2012 NNPAS (Figure 3)

Figure 3 shows the amount of food eaten as grams per day by adult Australians and the respective amount of *n*-3 LCPUFA intakes as milligram per day. Female and male adults consume on average 24 g and 28 g of fish/seafood per day, respectively. Female and male adults consume on average 117 g and 170 g of meat, poultry, and game products and dishes, respectively, which are 4.5 and six times, respectively, higher than fish/seafood. Milk products and dishes and cereal products and dishes are consumed in greater quantities but make a small contribution to overall *n*-3 LCPUFA intakes. Eggs products and dishes are consumed the least in terms of gram amounts, but provide more *n*-3 LCPUFA per gram of food compared to milk products and dishes, and cereal products and dishes.

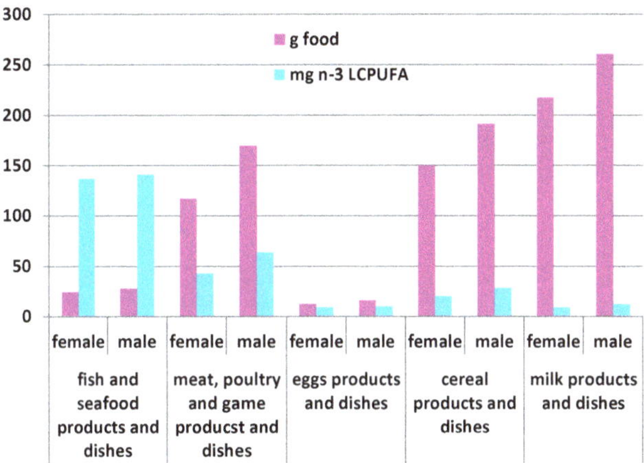

Figure 3. Comparison of the amount of food eaten (g per day) by adult Australians and the respective amount of *n*-3 LCPUFA intakes (mg per day) for five main food groups. Fish and seafood: fish, fish and chips, prawns, canned tuna, fish with pasta, paella with seafood; meat, poultry, and game: beef patty, steak, rabbit, offal, ham, lamb casserole, chicken stir-fry; egg products and dishes: eggs, omelette with cheese, spinach soufflé; cereal products and dishes: biscuits, cakes, pies (including meat pies), fried rice, pizza, *vol-au-vents*, quiche, gnocchi, lasagne, commercial hamburgers, croissants, pancakes; milk products and dishes: milk, yogurt, cream, cheese, ice cream, custard, milkshakes.

Approximately 16% of the Australian population consumes "nuts and nut products". Seven percent of the Australian population consumes "peanuts and peanut products", but peanuts do not contain *n*-3 fatty acids. Seven percent of the Australian population consumes "other nuts and nut product and dishes" and 2% consume "mixed nuts or nuts and seeds", which would contribute to LNA, but not the *n*-3 LCPUFA.

2.5.2. Comparison of the Adult Female and Male Mean Consumption *n*-3 LCPUFA Intakes (mg per g of Food) for the Various Food Groups (Figure 4)

Even though the consumption of fish and seafood is low (female and male mean intake of 24 g and 28 g, respectively), fish and seafood provide the largest amount of *n*-3 LCPUFA per gram of food (as shown in Figure 4).

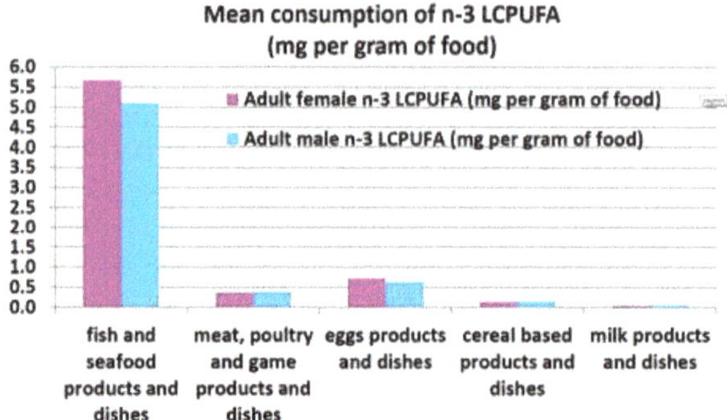

Figure 4. The actual adult female and males (19+ years) mean consumption of *n*-3 LCPUFA expressed as mg per gram of food for the various food groups.

When expressing the actual mean *n*-3 LCPUFA intakes per gram of food, fish and seafood products and dishes are 15-fold higher than meat, poultry, and game products and dishes; nine-fold higher than egg products and dishes; 38-fold higher than cereal-based products and dishes; and 114-fold higher than milk products and dishes.

2.6. Comparison of the 2011–2012 NNPAS and NNS 1995

2.6.1. Comparison of the PUFA Intakes from the Two Australian National Nutrition Surveys: NNS 1995 and 2011–2012 NNPAS (Figure 5)

As shown in Figure 5, the total PUFA and LA intakes have decreased from 1995 to 2012, but the LNA intakes have increased. For all ages, total PUFA decreased by 12%, LA decreased by 18% and LNA increased by 24%. These changes differed slightly between the different age groups but the general trend was the same.

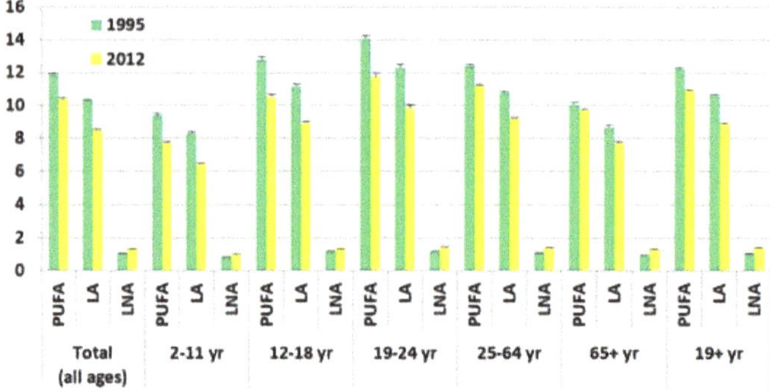

Figure 5. Comparison of the PUFA intakes (total PUFA, linoleic acid (LA), and alpha-linolenic acid (LNA)) (g per day) per age category.

2.6.2. Comparison of the *n*-3 LCPUFA Intakes from the Two Australian National Nutrition Surveys: NNS 1995 and 2011–2012 NNPAS (Figure 6)

As shown in Figure 6, for all ages the *n*-3 LCPUFA intakes have increased by 54% from 1995 to 2012, with the greatest increase of 115% in the 65+ years age category. The younger adult age group (19–24 years) has not changed and there has been a slight 11% reduction in intakes in the 12–18 years category. The 2–11 years old age group has also increased their *n*-3 LCPUFA intakes by 35%.

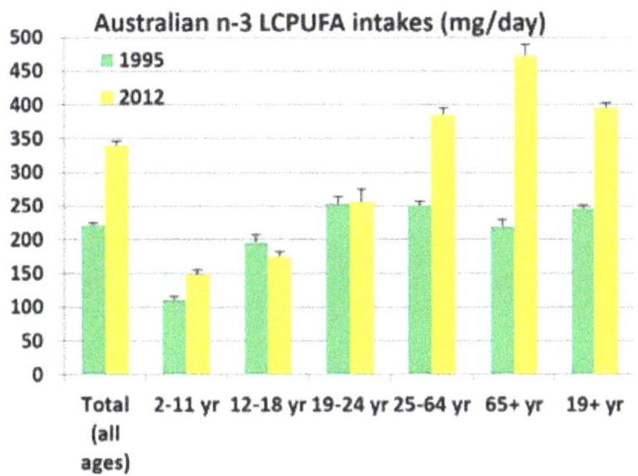

Figure 6. Comparison of the *n*-3 LCPUFA intakes per age category.

3. Discussion

This study has shown that overall the Australian PUFA intakes have decreased since 1995, but there is an increase in omega-3 PUFA, LNA, and *n*-3 LCPUFA. These differences could be explained as follows. Different databases were used for the two surveys. The NNS 1995 used a custom food composition database which was developed by FSANZ (then known as ANZFA). The 2011–2012 NNPAS used an updated database from a custom food composition database prepared by FSANZ (AUSNUT 2011–2013). Differences in the nutrient values between the two databases reflect not only changes in the composition of foods, but also changes in available data and improvements in analytical methods over the period. Furthermore, a food model booklet was produced to aid in reporting of measures in 2011–2012 NNPAS. Food groups known to have been impacted by this change in methodology include "cereals and mixed dishes", which could explain the differences in PUFA intakes in particular LA and LNA [14].

This increase, especially in *n*-3 LCPUFA is good as numerous health benefits have been associated with the consumption of *n*-3 LCPUFA [2–7]. Current mean *n*-3 LCPUFA intakes for adult Australians is 395 mg/day (277 mg/day from food and 118 mg/day from supplements), which have increased 1.6 fold since 1995, where the mean intakes were 246 mg/day. The increase can be explained by increased intakes in adults 25 years old or older, as there were no differences in *n*-3 LCPUFA intakes in the 19–24 years old category (Figure 6). The increase in *n*-3 LCPUFA can be probably explained by an increase in *n*-3 LCPUFA supplements, given that fish consumption (the major dietary sources of *n*-3 LCPUFA) has not changed from 26 g per day on average in NNS 1995 to 26 g in 2011–2012 NNPAS (24 g females and 28 g males). The NNS 1995 did not report on *n*-3 LCPUFA supplementation. However, currently the proportion of adults taking *n*-3 LCPUFA supplements is 25% for adult women and 15% for adult men (Table 3).

However, the current adult Australian *n*-3 LCPUFA median intakes of 126 mg/day (from food) and 154 mg/day (from food and supplements) are less than 50% of the mean intakes suggesting that the *n*-3 LCPUFA intakes are highly skewed and that there are some people consuming high amounts of *n*-3 LCPUFA, but the vast majority of the population are not consuming enough for optimal health. In fact when compared to recommended intakes only approximately 20% of the population met the recommendations for optimal health. A vast majority of adult Australians that were taking *n*-3 LCPUFA supplements met the recommended intakes (ranging from 46% to 67%); however, those people not taking *n*-3 LCPUFA supplements, only approximately 10% of the population met the recommended intakes. Given that approximately 20% of the population is consuming *n*-3 LCPUFA supplements, 80% of the Australian population is not meeting the recommended intake for *n*-3 LCPUFA for optimal health.

The current adult (19+ years) Australian *n*-3 LCPUFA intakes are higher than the US intakes of 113 mg *n*-3 LCPUFA intakes per day [15], but still falls far short of populations that consume high amounts of *n*-3 LCPUFA (810 mg per day, [16] and 905 mg per day [17]), such as the Japanese [16,17]. Fish and seafood is the richest source of *n*-3 LCPUFA and populations that consume fish/seafood, more so than meat and poultry, have higher intakes of *n*-3 LCPUFA. In the current Australian population the mean fish consumption is approximately six times lower than meat; yet consuming only one-sixth of the meat consumption from fish/seafood provides much more *n*-3 LCPUFA than consuming meat as shown in Figure 5. Moreover when the data is expressed as the mean consumption of *n*-3 LCPUFA as mg per gram of food (Figure 6), *n*-3 LCPUFA intakes are 15-fold higher than meat.

Fayet *et al.* [18] has conducted dietary modelling to achieve the Australian dietary recommended intakes for *n*-3 LCPUFA for all life stages [18] and the easiest way to achieve the recommended intakes is to consume fish and seafood. The most cost effective way of meeting these recommendations is to consume fish and seafood [18]. Fish may be expensive per kilogram; e.g., Atlantic salmon cost approximately $29 AUD per kilogram but this translates to 16 cents per 100 mg of *n*-3 LCPUFA, whilst meat costs $2 AUD per 100 mg *n*-3 LCPUFA (assuming meat costs approximately $25 AUD per kilogram) [18].

There appears to be a controversy about the efficacy of recent randomised controlled trials that assessed the health benefits of *n*-3 LCPUFA but there is an explanation for this. Randomised controlled trials and meta-analysis of trials up to the year 2002 demonstrated that supplementation with *n*-3 LCPUFA resulted in up to a 45% reduction in overall mortality from cardiac death [5,19]. However, reviews and meta-analyses of recent trials reported a lack of efficacy, suggesting that the *n*-3 LCPUFA are dead in the water [20,21]. Critical analyses of these recent trials have suggested that the lack of efficacy may be due to methodological problems [22]. Following the earlier successful trials, the American Heart Association issued guidelines for people with heart disease, suggesting consumption of at least two fish meals per week [23] in addition to fish oil supplements [24]. Between 2000 and 2010, the importation of fish oils into the USA escalated more than 10-fold from 2000 to 22,000 metric tonnes [25]. However, trials conducted after 2002 failed to screen people for high fish and/or fish oil supplement intake resulting in great variability of *n*-3 LCPUFA status across trial conditions [24]. Where screening did occur, the upper 50% of the control subjects and the lower 50% of the fish oil intervention subjects overlapped [26], suggesting that the two groups were not separated enough to demonstrate an effect in the test arm (*n*-3). Thus, future trials need to attenuate the possible ceiling effects created by high baseline, by taking blood samples to determine compliance and correlations between increased *n*-3 LCPUFA status and response.

It is well recognized that consumption of *n*-3 LCPUFA, especially DHA, is important for neurological development [27,28]. Previous data has shown the importance of DHA during the latter stages of pregnancy when the brain accrues its tissue mass [29]. More recently, however, it has been shown that DHA is also vital at the stage of when the neural tube closes at day 28 of gestation [30]. Due to its importance, there are specific recommendations for DHA intake for pregnant and lactating women. The Society for the Study of Fatty Acids and Lipids (ISSFAL) recommends at least 200 mg of DHA per day during pregnancy and lactation [12,13]. The current median *n*-3 LCPUFA and estimated DHA intakes in women from childbearing age are 119 mg per day and 51mg per day, respectively (Figure 4). In order to meet the recommended 200 mg DHA intake per day, only 10% of women (*i.e.*, the 90th centile, Figure 4) are consuming enough DHA. An Australian study of pregnant women

(n = 94) consumed a median DHA intake of 75 mg/day [31], which still falls short of the recommended 200 mg/day [12,13].

The main food sources of n-3 LCPUFA is from the fish and seafood category. Previous research in Australia has shown that meat and eggs also contribute to n-3 LCPUFA intakes [1,32], with meat contributing nearly 50% of the n-3 LCPUFA intakes [11]. This large contribution of n-3 LCPUFA intakes is not because meat is a rich source of n-3 LCPUFA but Australians consume at least six times more meat than fish/seafood. Yet consumption of only 26 g of fish seafood provides more than double the n-3 LCPUFA than if one was to consume approximately 150 g of meat. To really illustrate that fish/seafood is by far the richest source of n-3 LCPUFA, when the data is expressed as n-3 LCPUFA consumption as mg per gram of food, fish/seafood is 15-fold higher than meat (Figure 6).

The strengths of this study are (1) the large dataset (n = 12,153 from all ages 2+ years) that accurately reflects population intakes and (2) the ability to compare to previously published National Nutrition Survey intakes from 1995 per age/gender category to determine the changes in PUFA intakes. The weakness of this study is the use of 24-h recall data as fish/seafood consumption is not usually a frequently (daily) consumed food. However, to maximise the accuracy of the data, an average of the two 24-h recall data was used for all nutrients presented here, including n-3 LCPUFA. Furthermore, the NNS 1995 used a food frequency questionnaire (n = 8321) in addition to the 24-h recall data, and found no differences in n-3 LCPUFA intakes from 24-h recall data and the food frequency questionnaire [11]. Whilst the current 2011–2012 NNPAS did not use a food frequency questionnaire and hence the 24-h recall data cannot be checked against FFQ data, one could suggest that the use of 24-h recall data in a large population dataset assesses n-3 LCPUFA accurately, especially given that there was no difference in intakes between the 24-h recall and the FFQ in the NNS1995 [11].

4. Materials and Methods

4.1. The Australian Health Survey 2011-13 (AHS) Containing the 2011–2012 National Nutrition and Physical Activity Survey (2011–2012 NNPAS) Data from the Australian Bureau of Statistics (ABS)

In Australia, the Australian Health Survey 2011–2013 (AHS) was conducted by the Australian Bureau of Statistics (ABS) and they have released several publications on their website [32]. The AHS contains the 2011–2012 NNPAS and data was collected in 2011 and 2012 and reports made available on the ABS website [33].

Participants (n = 12,153 individuals aged two years and older) in the 2011–2012 NNPAS were interviewed by telephone and 24-h dietary recall of all food, beverages and supplements were recorded. Approximately eight days later, a second 24-h dietary recall was conducted by telephone interview. The interviewers used the automated multiple-pass method developed by the Agricultural Research Service of the United States Department of Agriculture [34]. For further detailed information on this dietary data collection, please refer to the ABS website [35].

4.2. NNS 1995 Survey Data

The NNS 1995 survey was conducted jointly by the Australian Bureau of Statistics and the then Department of Health and Family Services, with representation from rural and urban areas of all Australian states and territories [36]. Food intakes were surveyed in 13,858 individuals who were interviewed in their homes by qualified nutritionists using the 24-h dietary recall method; 8321 of them also completed a food frequency questionnaire.

4.3. Confidential Unit Record Files (CURF)

The CURF [37] contained unidentified information from each individual in the study, which included the individual's identity number and demographic descriptors (including age and gender) as well as the amounts of each encoded food consumed by the individual in the 24-h recalls. Permission was sought to use the CURF data and hence the 24-h dietary recall data was obtained from the CURF and analysed as explained below.

4.4. Analysis of 2011–2012 NNPAS 24-h Recall Data

The mean (±SEM) of the energy and macronutrient intakes were tabulated by gender using the same age categories as the NNS1995 as reported by Howe *et al.* [11] for ease of comparison. The average of the two 24-h recalls was calculated for each individual and each nutrient. The mean (±SEM) intakes for all age groups and gender were calculated and are reported as total intakes and separated into food and supplement intakes. The median *n*-3 LCPUFA intakes for all age groups and gender were also calculated.

4.5. Comparison of n-3 LCPUFA to Recommended Intakes

The NHMRC NRV for the prevention of chronic disease has postulated SDT intakes for *n*-3 LCPUFA. The SDT are based on the 90th centile of *n*-3 LCPUFA intakes per gender; 430 mg/day for women and 610 mg/day for men [10]. The ISSFAL has recommendations for *n*-3 LCPUFA for cardiovascular health; ISSFAL recommends 500 mg/day [12].

From the 2011–2012 NNPAS, the proportion of female and male adults (19+ years) meeting the recommended *n*-3 LCPUFA was calculated for the total sample, plus those not taking and taking *n*-3 LCPUFA supplements.

From the 2011–2012 NNPAS, the women of child-bearing age (16–50 years) consumption of *n*-3 LCPUFA intakes were determined per centile from 10th to 90th centile. As DHA was not available from the 2011–2012 NNPAS, DHA was estimated to be 43% of the total *n*-3 LCPUFA [11] and, hence, also determined per centile from 10th to 90th centile. These data were compared to the recommended intake of at least 200 mg/day of DHA for pregnant and lactating women [12].

4.6. Comparison of Adult Australian Mean Food Intake and the Respective n-3 LCPUFA Intakes

The actual mean amount of food intake from the five main food sources of *n*-3 LCPUFA were compared to the respective mean amount of *n*-3 LCPUFA. The mean amount of *n*-3 LCPUFA (mg) was divided by the mean amount of food (g) to get *n*-3 LCPUFA expressed as mg per gram of food.

4.7. Comparisons of NNS 1995 and 2011–2012 NNPAS

The current PUFA intakes (2011–2012 NNPAS) were compared to the NNS 1995 PUFA intakes which were published previously by Howe *et al.* [11].

5. Conclusions

Adult Australian PUFA intakes (LA intakes) may have decreased, whilst *n*-3 PUFA intakes may have increased since 1995. However approximately 80% of Australians are not meeting the *n*-3 LCPUFA recommended intakes for optimal health and 90% of childbearing women are not meeting the recommendations for DHA intakes during pregnancy and lactation.

Acknowledgments: Australian Bureau of Statistics for the 2011–2012 NNPAS and the NNS 1995 data collection.

Conflicts of Interest: The author declares no conflict of interest.

Abbreviations

The following abbreviations are used in this manuscript:

MDPI	Multidisciplinary Digital Publishing Institute
DOAJ	Directory of open access journals
TLA	Three letter acronym
LD	linear dichroism

References

1. Meyer, B.J.; Mann, N.J.; Lewis, J.L.; Milligan, G.C.; Sinclair, A.J.; Howe, P.R.C. Dietary intakes and food sources of omega-6 and omega-3 polyunsaturated fatty acids. *Lipids* **2003**, *38*, 391–398. [CrossRef] [PubMed]
2. Connor, W.E. Importance of *n*-3 fatty acids in health and disease. *Am. J. Clin. Nutr.* **2000**, *71*, 171–175.
3. Siscovick, D.S.; Raghunathan, T.E.; King, I.; Weinmann, S.; Wicklund, K.G.; Albright, J.; Bovbjerg, V.; Arbogast, P.; Smith, H.H.; Kushi, L.H.; *et al.* Dietary-intake and cell-membrane levels of long-chain *n*-3 polyunsaturated fatty-acids and the risk of primary cardiac-arrest. *J. Am. Med. Assoc.* **1995**, *274*, 1363–1367. [CrossRef]
4. De Lorgeril, M.; Salen, P.; Martin, J.L.; Monjaud, I.; Delaye, J.; Mamelle, N. Mediterranean diet, traditional risk factors and the rate of cardiovascular complications after myocardial infarction—Final report of the Lyon diet heart study. *Circulation* **1999**, *99*, 779–785. [CrossRef] [PubMed]
5. GISSI-Prevenzione Investigators. Dietary supplementation with *n*-3 polyunsaturated fatty acids and vitamin E after myocardial infarction: Results of the GISSI-Pevenzione trial. *Lancet* **1999**, *354*, 447–455.
6. Simopoulos, A.P. Essential fatty acids in health and chronic disease. *Am. J. Clin. Nutr.* **1999**, *70*, 560–569.
7. Von Schacky, C.; Angerer, P.; Kothny, W.; Theisen, K.; Mudra, H. The effect of dietary omega-3 fatty acids on coronary atherosclerosis—A randomised, double-blind, placebo-controlled trial. *Ann. Int. Med.* **1999**, *130*, 554–562. [CrossRef] [PubMed]
8. Sinn, N.; Milte, C.; Howe, P.R.C. Oiling the brain: A review of randomised controlled trials of omega-3 fatty acids in psychopathology across the lifespan. *Nutrients* **2010**, *2*, 128–170. [CrossRef] [PubMed]
9. Parletta, N.; Milte, C.M.; Meyer, B.J. Nutritional modulation of cognitive function and mental health. *J. Nutr. Biochem.* **2013**, *24*, 725–743. [CrossRef] [PubMed]
10. National Health and Medical Research Council. *Nutrient Reference Values for Australia and New Zealand including Recommended Dietary Intakes*; Australian Government Department of Health and Ageing: Canberra, Australia, 2006.
11. Howe, P.; Meyer, B.J.; Record, S.; Baghurst, K. Dietary intake of long-chain *n*-3 polyunsaturated fatty acids: Contribution of meat sources. *Nutrition* **2006**, *22*, 47–53. [CrossRef] [PubMed]
12. International Society for the Study of Fatty Acids and Lipids (ISSFAL). PUFA Recommendations. Available online: http://www.issfal.org/statements/pufa-recommendations (accessed on 15 December 2015).
13. Koletzko, B.; Cetin, I.; Brenna, J.T.; the Perinatal Lipid Intake Working Group. Consensus Statement: Dietary fat intakes for pregnant and lactating women. *Br. J. Nutr.* **2007**, *98*, 873–877. [CrossRef] [PubMed]
14. Australian Bureau of Statistics. 4363.0.55.001-Australian Health Survey: Users' Guide, 2011–2013. Comparisons with 1995 NNS. Available online: http://www.abs.gov.au/ausstats/abs@.nsf/Lookup/FB554091B09E8C05CA257CD2001E3214?opendocument (accessed on 3 February 2016).
15. Papanikolau, Y.; Brooks, J.; Reider, C.; Fulgoni, V.L. U.S. adults are not meeting recommended levels for fish and omega-3 fatty acid intake: Results of an analysis using observational data from NHANES 2003–2008. *Nutr. J.* 2014, 13, p. 31. Available online: http://www.nutritionj.com/content/13/1/31 (accessed on 15 December 2015). [CrossRef] [PubMed]
16. Nakamura, Y.; Ueshima, H.; Okuda, N.; Miura, K.; Kita, Y.; Okamura, T.; Turin, T.C.; Okayama, A.; Rodriguez, B.; Curb, J.D.; *et al.* Relation of dietary and other lifestyle traits to difference in serum adiponectin concentrations of Japanese in Japan and Hawaii: The INTERLIPID Study. *Am. J. Clin. Nutr.* **2008**, *88*, 424–430. [PubMed]
17. Hino, A.; Adachi, H.; Toyomasu, K.; Yoshida, N.; Enomoto, M.; Hiratsuka, A.; Hirai, Y.; Satoh, A.; Imaizumi, T. Very long chain *n*-3 fatty acids intake and carotid atherosclerosis. An epidemiological study evaluated by ultrasonography. *Atherosclerosis* **2004**, *176*, 145–149. [CrossRef] [PubMed]
18. Fayet-Moore, F.; Baghurst, K.; Meyer, B.J. Four models including fish, seafood, red meat and enriched foods to achieve Australian dietary recommendations for the *n*-3 LCPUFA for all life-stages. *Nutrients* **2015**, *7*, 8112–8126. [CrossRef] [PubMed]
19. Bucher, H.C.; Hengstler, P.; Schindler, C.; Meier, G. *n*-3 polyunsaturated fatty acids in coronary heart disease: A meta-analysis of randomized controlled trials. *Am. J. Med.* **2002**, *112*, 298–304. [CrossRef]
20. Wen, Y.T.; Dai, J.H.; Gao, Q. Effects of omega-3 fatty acid on major cardiovascular events and mortality with coronary heart disease: A meta-analysis of randomized controlled trials. *Nutr. Metab. Cardiovasc. Dis.* **2014**, *24*, 470–475. [CrossRef] [PubMed]

21. Nestel, P.; Clifton, P.; Colquhoun, D.; Noakes, M.; Mori, T.A.; Thomas, B. Indications for omega-3 long chain polyunsaturated fatty acid in the prevention and treatment of cardiovascular disease. *Heart Lung Circ.* **2015**, *24*, 769–779. [CrossRef] [PubMed]
22. James, M.; Sullivan, T.R.; Metcalf, R.G.; Cleland, L.G. Pitfalls in the use of randomized controlled trials for fish oil studies with cardiac patients. *Br. J. Nutr.* **2014**, *112*, 812–820. [CrossRef] [PubMed]
23. Krauss, R.M.; Eckel, R.H.; Howard, B.; Appel, L.J.; Daniels, S.R.; Deckelbaum, R.J.; Erdman, J.W., Jr.; Kris-Etherton, P.; Goldberg, I.J.; Kotchen, K.A.; *et al.* AHA dietary guidelines: Revision 2000: A statement for healthcare professionals from the Nutrition Committee of the American Heart Association. *Circulation* **2000**, *102*, 2284–2299. [CrossRef] [PubMed]
24. Kris-Etherton, P.M.; Harris, W.S.; Appel, L.J. Fish consumption, fish oil, omega-3 fatty acids, and cardiovascular disease. *Circulation* **2002**, *106*, 2747–2757. [CrossRef] [PubMed]
25. Bimbo, A.P. *The Evolution of Fish Oils to Omega 3 Fatty Acids and a Global Consumer Market of US$25 Billion*; West Virginia University Research Corporation Forum Linking Innovation, Industry, and Commercialization Dean's Open Forum on Innovation and Entrepreneurship Davis College of Agriculture, Natural Resources & Design: Morgantown, WV, USA; 25; April; 2013.
26. Farquharson, A.L.; Metcalf, R.G.; Sanders, P.; Stuklis, R.; Edwards, J.R.M.; Gibson, R.A.; Cleland, L.G.; Sullivan, T.R.; James, M.J.; Young, G.D. Effect of dietary fish oil on atrial fibrillation after cardiac surgery. *Am. J. Cardiol.* **2011**, *108*, 851–856. [CrossRef] [PubMed]
27. Makrides, M.; Gibson, R.A. Long-chain polyunsaturated fatty acid requirements during pregnancy and lactation. *Am. J. Clin. Nutr.* **2000**, *71*, 307S–311S. [PubMed]
28. Sattar, N.; Berry, C.; Greer, I.A. Essential fatty acids in relation to pregnancy complications and fetal development. *Br. J. Obstet. Gynaecol.* **1998**, *105*, 1248–1255. [CrossRef] [PubMed]
29. Innis, S.M.; Friesen, R.W. Essential *n*-3 fatty acids in pregnant women and early visual acuity maturation in term infants. *Am. J. Clin. Nutr.* **2008**, *87*, 548–557. [PubMed]
30. Meyer, B.J.; Onyiaodike, C.C.; Brown, E.A.; Jordan, F.; Murray, H.; Nibbs, R.J.B.; Sattar, N.; Lyall, H.; Nelson, S.M.; Freeman, D.J. Maternal plasma DHA levels increase prior to 29 days post-LH surge in women undergoing frozen embryo transfer: A prospective, observational study of human pregnancy. *J. Clin. Endo. Metab.* **2016**. in press. [CrossRef] [PubMed]
31. Cosatto, V.F.; Else, P.L.; Meyer, B.J. Do pregnant women and those at risk of developing post-natal depression consume lower amounts of long chain omega-3 polyunsaturated fatty acids? *Nutrients* **2010**, *2*, 198–213. [CrossRef] [PubMed]
32. Ollis, T.E.; Meyer, B.J.; Howe, P.R.C. Australian food sources and intakes of omega-6 and omega-3 polyunsaturated fatty acids. *Ann. Nutr. Metab.* **1999**, *43*, 346–355. [CrossRef] [PubMed]
33. Australian Bureau of Statistics. Australian Health Survey. Available online: http://www.abs.gov.au/australianhealthsurvey (accessed on 15 December 2015).
34. Bliss, R.M. Researchers produce innovation in dietary recall. *Agric. Res.* **2004**, *52*, 10–12.
35. Australian Bureau of Statistics. 4363.0.55.001-Australian Health Survey: Users' guide, 2011–2013. 24-h Dietary Recall. Available online: http://www.abs.gov.au/ausstats/abs@.nsf/Lookup/0D6B1FE95EAB8FF3CA257CD2001CA113?opendocument (accessed on 15 December 2015).
36. McLennan, W.; Podger, A. *National Nutrition Survey, Selected Highlights, Australia*; Government Publishing Service: Canberra, Australian, 1997.
37. Australian Bureau of Statistics. 4324.0.55.002–Microdata: Australian Health Survey: Nutrition and Physical Activity, 2011–2012. Introduction. Available online: http://abs.gov.au/AUSSTATS/abs@.nsf/Lookup/4324.0.55.002Main+Features12011-12 (accessed on 15 December 2015).

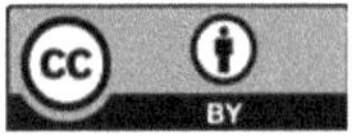

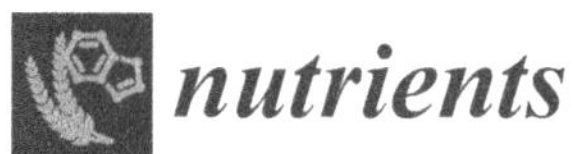

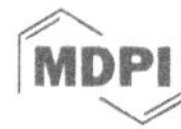

Review

Impact of Genotype on EPA and DHA Status and Responsiveness to Increased Intakes

Anne Marie Minihane

Department of Nutrition and Preventive Medicine, Norwich Medical School, BCRE, University of East Anglia (UEA), James Watson Road, Norwich NR4 7UQ, UK; a.minihane@uea.ac.uk; Tel.: +44-1603-592-389

Received: 24 January 2016; Accepted: 23 February 2016; Published: 2 March 2016

Abstract: At a population level, cardioprotective and cognitive actions of the fish oil (FO) derived long-chain *n*-3 polyunsaturated fatty acids (LC *n*-3 PUFAs) eicosapentaenoic acid (EPA) and docosahexaenoic acid (DHA) have been extensively demonstrated. In addition to dietary intake, which is limited for many individuals, EPA and DHA status is dependent on the efficiency of their biosynthesis from α-linolenic acid. Gender and common gene variants have been identified as influencing the rate-limiting desaturase and elongase enzymes. Response to a particular intake or status is also highly heterogeneous and likely influenced by genetic variants which impact on EPA and DHA metabolism and tissue partitioning, transcription factor activity, or physiological end-point regulation. Here, available literature relating genotype to tissue LC *n*-3 PUFA status and response to FO intervention is considered. It is concluded that the available evidence is relatively limited, with much of the variability unexplained, though *APOE* and *FADS* genotypes are emerging as being important. Although genotype × LC *n*-3 PUFA interactions have been described for a number of phenotypes, few have been confirmed in independent studies. A more comprehensive understanding of the genetic, physiological and behavioural modulators of EPA and DHA status and response to intervention is needed to allow refinement of current dietary LC *n*-3 PUFA recommendations and stratification of advice to "vulnerable" and responsive subgroups.

Keywords: eicosapentaenoic acid; EPA; docosahexaenoic acid; DHA; long chain *n*-3 PUFA; genotype; *APOE*; *FADS*

---

1. Introduction

Although randomised controlled trials (RCT) are inconsistent [1–4], there is a large body of cell, animal and human prospective cohort data demonstrating the cardiovascular and cognitive benefits of increased fish consumption and eicosapentaenoic acid (EPA) and docosahexaenoic acid (DHA) intake and tissue status, with underlying physiological and molecular mechanisms identified [5–9]. Such evidence has translated into typical national and international recommended intakes of >500 mg of EPA + DHA per day in the general population to improve cardiovascular health, >1 g EPA + DHA per day for the secondary prevention of CVD, with >200 mg DHA per day recommended in pregnancy [10–12]. Despite the provision of such generic recommended intakes there is a wide recognition that intake-independent EPA and DHA status and response to increased EPA and DHA intakes is highly variable, with the aetiology of this heterogeneity poorly understood.

Unlike typical nutrients, which cannot be synthesised *in vivo*, EPA and DHA can to some extent be synthesised from the precursor plant derived shorter chain *n*-3 fatty acids, α-linolenic acid (αLNA) [13,14], with gender [15] and variants [16] in the rate limiting enzymes of the biosynthetic pathway emerging as important determinants of the biosynthetic efficiency (Figure 1). Genotype is also known to be important in taste and sensory perception and therefore food preference and intake [17,18]. In many populations oily fish is poorly tolerated relative to other foods, and regularly consumed by only a minority of the population [19]. Although completely unknown it is likely that genotype is an important modulator of oily fish taste sensitivity and consumption and therefore EPA and DHA intake. Once consumed the absorption of EPA and DHA, their subsequent tissue and cellular partitioning, and their oxidation or metabolism into lipid derived bioactivities, is variable and likely genotype dependent. Finally the impact of a particular tissue/cell EPA and DHA (or their metabolite) status on cell signalling, physiological processes and ultimately health biomarkers or clinical end-points will also be modulated be numerous variants in genes encoding, fatty acid responsive transcription factors and other cell signalling molecules and their physiological targets.

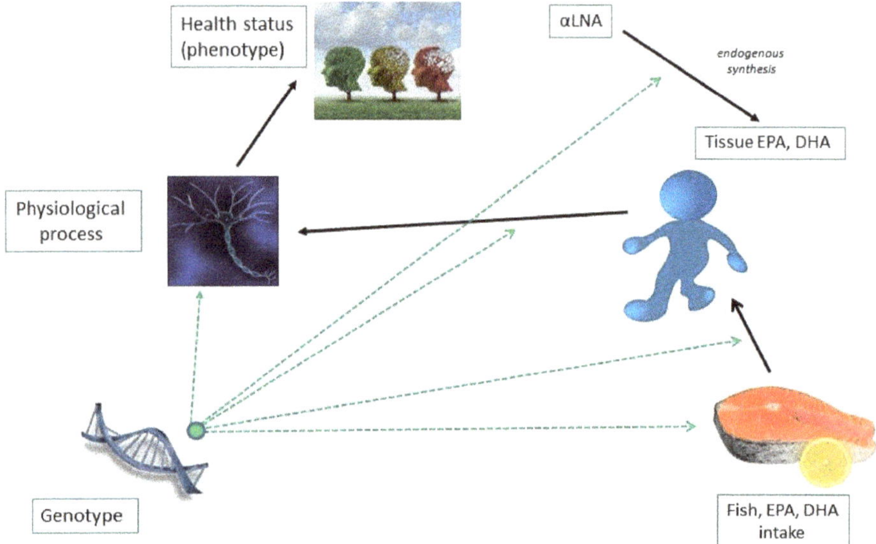

Figure 1. Overview of the potential of genotype to influence EPA and DHA status and responsiveness.

There are numerous single reports in the literature of the impact of individual gene variants on LC *n*-3 PUFA responsiveness. Rather than attempt to be exhaustive and report on all of these findings, the majority of which require confirmation in independent studies, the review will largely focus on a select number of genes and genotypes which have been relatively consistently shown to regulate EPA and DHA status or responsiveness. Such genotypes may in the future be useful in the targeting of specific EPA and DHA recommendations towards individuals likely to be deficient and responsive.

2. Genetic Determinants of EPA and DHA Biosynthesis and Status

Familial aggregation analysis indicates that 40%–70% of (red blood cell (RBC)) fatty acid status is heritable [20]. In the Framingham Heart Study, 73% of the variability in the RBC omega-3 index (EPA + DHA as a % total of total fatty acids (FA)) was explained by participant characteristics added to the regression model, which included heritability (24%), EPA + DHA intake (25%), and fish oil supplementation (15%) [21].

The endogenous synthesis of the LC PUFA, arachidonic acid (AA), and EPA/DHA occurs mainly in the liver in humans, via a common series of desaturation and elongation reactions (Figure 2), with delta-5 desaturase (D5DS) and delta-6 desaturase (D6DS) encoded by *FADS1* and *FADS2* genes representing major regulatory steps. This pathway is the main source of tissue EPA and DHA in those who consume little or no seafood or fish oil supplements. The efficiency of the pathway is inherently low in humans, with an estimated conversion of αLNA to EPA of 0.2%–6% and <0.1% for

DHA [13], and therefore any changes in bioconversion efficiency have potentially large impacts on LC PUFA status.

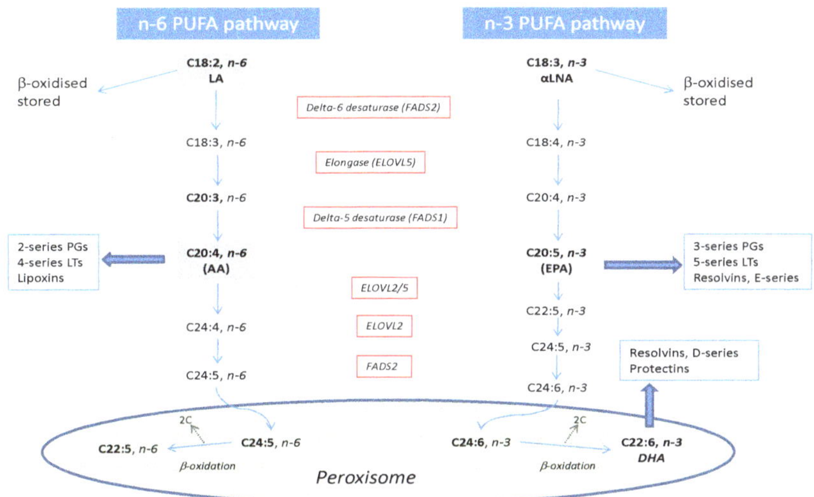

Figure 2. Long chain polyunsaturated fatty acid biosynthetic pathway.

The *FADSs* genes located as a head-to-head cluster on chromosome 11 (11q12.2-q13.1) [22] are highly polymorphic with 4391 variants, predominately single nucleotide polymorphisms (SNP), described in the *National Center for Biotechnology Information* dbSNP database [23], 217 of which are missense resulting in amino acid changes in the D5DS and D6DS proteins. In 2006, 18 SNPs in the gene cluster were genotyped in 727 adults in the *German Centre of the European Community Respiratory Health Survey* [24]. All haplotypes (grouping of variants) which included the minor alleles were associated with increases in αLNA and linoleic acid (LA) and decreases in γ-linolenic acid, AA, EPA and *n*-3 docosapentaenoic acid (DPA), with no significant impact on DHA or *n*-6 DPA evident. A 5-locus haplotype explained 27.7%, 5.2% and 1.4% of the variability in AA, EPA and DHA levels respectively. Interestingly this haplotype was associated with a greater than 50% lower incidence of the chronic inflammatory conditions atopic eczema and allergic rhinitis, which may be due to the lower availability of AA for cyclooxygenation to the strong pro-inflammatory 2-series prostaglandins and 4-series leukotrienes. Over the last decade, and taking a similar candidate gene approach, these initial observations of the association between *FADS1-FADS2* SNPs and haplotypes and D5DS and D6DS activities, plasma, tissue and breast milk fatty acid composition and the incidence of diseases with chronic inflammatory components have been confirmed in subsequent studies [25–32]. In the *Verona Heart Study*, a strong association with coronary artery disease was evident, with an incidence of 84% *versus* 66% in individuals with 6–7 *versus* 2–3 risk alleles [27].

DHA status during pregnancy influences infant growth and development, with breast feeding generally recommended till at least 6 month post-partum. Xie *et al.*, demonstrated lower breast milk ARA, EPA, *n*-3 DPA and DHA in individuals homozygous for *FADS1-FADS2* minor alleles [30]. In Danish infants the impact of breast feeding, fish intake and *FADS* genotype on RBC DHA status at 9 m and 3 years of age was assessed [33]. Collectively these variables explained 25% of the variation in status at 9 m (mean DHA of 6.6% of total FA%). Homozygous carriers of the minor allele of rs1535 had a DHA increase of 1.8 FA% whereas minor allele carriers of rs174448 and rs174575 had a decrease of 1.1 and 2.0 FA%, relative to the wild-type genotype. Interestingly further analysis indicated that about a 50 g fish intake would be needed to mitigate the impact of having only two DHA "raising" allele relative to five, highlighting the importance of *FADS* genotype on infant DHA status against a background of limited intake. In the *Koala Birth Cohort* the observation of an association between low maternal DHA intake with a reduced birth weight only in *FADS* minor allele carriers [34], again reinforces the importance of DHA intake in maternal-infant nutrition against a *FADS* genotype background associated with reduced endogenous synthesis.

Along with candidate gene approaches, untargeted unbiased genome wide association study (GWAS) has approaches have also identified the *FADS1-3* and also *elongase* (*ELOVL)* genes, as being associated with LC PUFA status [35–38]. In five population-based cohorts comprising approximately 900 individual, and consistent with the initial observation of Schaeffer *et al.*, published in 2006 [24], variant alleles of *FADS1* and *FADS2* were associated with higher levels of αLNA and lower levels of EPA and DPA, with variant alleles of *ELOVL2* associated with higher EPA and DPA and lower DHA, suggesting a decreased elongation of DPA to DHA [35]. *ELOVL2* encodes elongase 2 which is critical in the elongation of DPA to DHA [39] (Figure 2) The associations were independent of fatty fish intake, with an absence of interaction consistent with the *Koala Birth Cohort* who observed similar slopes of plasma EPA and DHA in those with 0, 1 or 2 minor *FADS1-FADS2* alleles [40].

GWAS have highlighted the physiological significance of variation in the *FADS* locus, with associations with plasma total cholesterol (TC), LDL-cholesterol (LDL-C), triglycerides (TG) and PUFA composition reported [36,41,42]. In a recent GWAS analysis to investigate genetic signatures of diet and climate adaptation in Greenland Inuits, who have a high LC *n*-3 PUFA intake, *FADS* was the strongest locus associated with height, weight, growth hormone regulation and membrane fatty acid composition [43].

In addition to observational analysis, the impact of *FADS* variants on response to EPA and DHA supplementation has been examined. In the *MARINA* RCT, the *FADS* rs174537 genotype interacted with treatment to determine D5DS activity; however no genotype × treatment interaction was evident for RBC EPA% and DHA%, which the authors suggested may be due to insufficient power [44]. In the same RCT *ELOVL2* gene SNPs did emerge as modulators of the TG response. After the 1.8 g/day dose, minor allele carriers had approximately 30% higher proportions of EPA and 9% higher DHA than non-carriers [45].

Although *FADS* and *elongase* variants have emerged as strong determinants of LC *n*-3 PUFA and some information is available as to factors which may modulate genotype-fatty acid status [46] granularity is still lacking regarding the relative effect size in various populations and the likely influences of factors such as ethnicity and habitual intake on the penetrance of genotype. Furthermore in the studies reported thus far associations between a large number of individual SNPs in *FADS* and *elongases* genes and fatty acid status and "health" outcomes have been observed many of which exist in a highly preserved linkage disequilibrium (LD) block and therefore co-inherited. The question remains as to which are the actual functional SNPs and what is the molecular aetiology of the effect of the variant on EPA and DHA status. In a recent seminal paper, Wang and co-workers conducted an analysis of the association between six *FADS* SNPs and the lipidomic profile, *FADS1-3* gene expression and protein levels in 154 human liver samples All six allele were associated with *FADS1* but not *FADS2* and 3 gene expression and also FADS1 protein levels, indicating *FADS 1* is the causal gene [38]. Furthermore they identified that among 42 highly linked SNPs, 29 were in the transcription factor (TF) binding sites of the locus. Although it is unclear exactly which SNP(s) is causal for the altered FADS1 gene function, and the exact nature of how the SNP influences TF interaction with *FADS1*, such mechanistic insights add considerable credibility to the observed association between *FADS* and EPA and DHA. Further such work will lead to the identification of the most significant variant(s) which could be used to, identify individuals at risk of compromised EPA and DHA status, and target recommendations for additional intakes.

3. Impact of *APOE* Genotype on EPA and DHA Status and the Response to Fish Oil Intervention

Apolipoprotein E, first described as a component of circulating lipoproteins and a modulator of their metabolism [47,48], has subsequently been identified as the main lipid transporter in the central nervous system (CNS). Two missense SNPs in the *APOE* gene on chromosome 19, result in three apoE protein isoforms, namely apoE2, apoE3 and apoE4 which are distinguished by cysteine to arginine substitutions at positions 112 and 158 in the protein: apo2 contains cysteine at both positions, apoE3 contains cysteine at 112 and arginine at 158, with apoE4 containing arginine at both sites [47,49]. Although not in the receptor or lipid binding regions, the amino changes influence salt bridge formation between the *N*- and *C*-terminals domains of the protein which have profound impacts on receptor biding activities, lipoprotein preference and apoE stability and ultimately tissue protein concentrations [49]. *APOE4* carriers have been inconsistently shown to be at higher risk of cardiovascular diseases [50,51], with a variable penetrance attributed to modifiers such as, saturated fat [52] and cholesterol [53] intakes, and smoking status [54]. *APOE* genotype has emerged as the strongest identified common genetic predictor of longevity [55,56]. In the Genetics of Healthy Ageing Study, the prevalence of the *APOE4* allele was 6.8% in nonagenarians (90–99 years old), compared to 12.7% in matched control (55–75 years old), with *APOE4* carriers having a 50% lower chance (odds ratio (OR) = 0.48, 95% CI, 0.42–0.55) of reaching age 90 years compared to non-*APOE4* carriers [55]. This reduced longevity reflects the effect of genotype on risk of age-related cognitive decline and Alzheimer's disease (AD), with *APOE3/E4* (20% Caucasians) and *APOE4/E4* (1%–2% Caucasians) individuals at approximately 4- and 15-fold increased risk of AD with a 10–20 years earlier age of onset [57].

Numerous potential mechanisms have been proposed to explain this association with cardiovascular and cognitive health, including an impact of *APOE* genotype on LC *n*-3 PUFA status and response of risk biomarkers to LC *n*-3 PUFA intakes. Brain tissue is highly enriched in DHA, indicating its essentiality to neuronal function. Although not investigated prospectively or as a primary study aim, a limited number of human studies have retrospectively reported that the cognitive benefits associated with DHA/fish intake were absent or lower in *APOE4* carriers [58–60]. For example in the *Cardiovascular Health Cognition Study*, Huang and co-workers reported that in the cohort as a whole consumption of oily fish more than twice per week was associated with a reduction in risk of AD by 41%, but stratification by *APOE* showed this effect to be selective to those without the *APOE4* allele [55]. Supplementation with DHA for 18 m did not slow the rate of cognitive decline in patients with mild to moderate Alzheimer disease [59]. Retrospective subgroup analysis indicated some cognitive benefits in non-*E4* carriers consistent with the epidemiological data. Variability in LC *n*-3 PUFA metabolism according to *APOE* genotype is likely to partly explain the differential cognitive response to increased DHA intake and status. In the *Three-City Cohort* of older adults, plasma EPA and DHA proportions did not differ according to *APOE* genotype but the association between fish consumption and plasma DHA was weaker in *APOE4* carriers. This is consistent with the *SATGENE* intervention, in which participants were prospectively recruited by *APOE* genotype. Following supplementation with DHA (3.5 g per day) for 8 weeks, a 21% lower plasma phospholipid DHA enrichment was observed in overweight *APOE3/E4* relative to *APOE3/E3* individuals [61]. *APOE4* carriers have lower plasma concentrations of apoE, which is in part attributed to lower hepatic apoE recycling, and apoE4 is preferentially associated with VLDL rather than HDL, with the opposite true for apoE3 [62]. Hence, although the aetiology of differential cognitive and plasma DHA responses to changes in DHA intake is currently poorly understood these *APOE* mediated differences in overall protein concentrations and lipoprotein partitioning together with a higher β-oxidation of DHA and lower brain uptake of a (14C)-DHA uptake associated with the *APOE4* allele [63,64], are likely to be involved.

Brain DHA is sourced from the systemic circulation with transport across the BBB involving a number of traditional members of the LDL-receptor family which use apoE as a ligand [65], along with the recently identified Mfsd2a [66]. The impact of *APOE* genotype on the expression and function of these transporters is currently unknown.

Although not fully consistent *APOE* genotype has also been shown to influence the plasma lipid response to EPA and DHA intervention, with indications of greater responsiveness in *APOE4* carriers, which may in part reflect the above described impact of genotype on fatty acid partitioning or the higher baseline LDL-C and TG evident in *APOE4* individuals [67–72]. In the *SATGENE* intervention a genotype × diet interaction was evident for plasma TG, with 17% and 30% decreases in *APOE3/E3* and *APOE3/E4* individuals after the high fat-high saturated fat-DHA relative to the low-fat diet [67]. A greater LC *n*-3 PUFA induced increase in adipose tissue lipoprotein lipase expression may in part explain the greater TG lowering in *APOE4* carriers [73], with endothelial associated LPL being the main enzyme responsible for the hydrolysis of circulating TG-rich lipoproteins. There is some earlier evidence of a borderline significant LDL-cholesterol raising effect of DHA in *APOE4* carriers in those with modest hypertrigylceridaemia [71] which was not evident in later studies in normolipdaemic individuals [67] or using more moderate intervention doses [68]. In a cross-sectional analysis in 137,000 individuals Harris *et al.*, observed no association between RBC omega-3 index and plasma LDL-C concentrations [69].

4. Genetic Variability and the Triglyceride Response to EPA and DHA

Elevated fasting and postprandial TGs are highly clinically significant CVD risk factors, of ever increasing prevalence, due to their strong association with adiposity and a loss if insulin sensitivity [74]. Perhaps the best described effect of EPA and DHA supplementation is its hypotrigylceridaemic actions, with the *American Heart Association* recommending intakes of 2–4 g per day as a TG lowering strategy [12]. But the TG response to increased EPA and DHA intakes is highly variable. In the *FINGEN* trial, although an overall significant impact of intervention was observed, no TG lowering was evident in 118 out of 312 participants in response to the higher dose [68,75]. As yet the genetic basis for this variable TG response is poorly understood. In addition to *APOE* and *FADS* genotype described above effects of variants in a number of genes involved in fatty acid metabolism and in LC *n*-3 responsive transcription factors have been described [27,76–80], the majority of which have not yet been confirmed in independent studies. For example in the 208 adults in the *Quebec City* Cohort, who were supplemented with ~3 g EPA + DHA per day, SNPs in two lipogenic genes, namely *ATP citrate lyase* (*ACLY*) and *acetyl-CoA carboxylase* (*ACACA*) explained 8% of the TG response [76]. In the same cohort and using an untargeted GWAS approach, SNP frequencies were compared in responders and non-responders. Although no SNP were identified using the calculated threshold for statistical significance ($p < 1.87 \times 10^{-8}$), 13 variants emerged using a more lenient statistically suggestive *p* value ($p < 1 \times 10^{-5}$). A genetic risk score (GRS) constructed using these SNPs explained 22% of the variation in the TG response to supplementation, with this GRS explaining a much more modest proportion of variation in the TG response in the confirmatory *FINGEN* cohort [81].

5. Closing Remarks

Dietary recommendations typically suggest an intake of EPA plus DHA of at least 500 mg per day. It is likely that higher intakes are needed to meaningfully modify many of the responsive CVD risk factors, providing some justification for increasing the current recommended intakes. However EPA and DHA supply and sustainability is an issue, with current sources, almost exclusively derived from fish, providing only 40% of what is needed in order for individuals globally to consume 500 mg per day [82]. The heterogeneity in response and this issue of supply provides a rationale to stratify advice to responsive individuals. But current understanding of the determinants of response is incomplete, with only a proportion of the genetic contribution identified and fully substantiated, and the mechanistic basis of identified genotype × LC *n*-3 PUFA interactions poorly understood. Such information must be gained from adequately powered "fit-for-purpose" studies, avoiding under-powered investigations which may be associated with spurious conclusions. Research to date has largely employed a candidate gene type approaches, with a future wider use of untargeted approaches such as GWAS or sequencing, in combination with a sensitive capture of EPA and DHA intake or status, needed to identify novel genetic modulators of EPA and DHA responses.

6. Conclusions

Common gene variants are likely to be an important determinant of EPA and DHA status and associated physiological impacts. In the future, and with a more robust knowledge base, it is hoped that genotype could contribute to the targeting of dietary advice with for example increased intakes recommended in pregnancy to those with a *FADS-elongase* genetic profile indicative of a compromised EPA and DHA endogenous biosynthesis, or to *APOE4* individuals who may be likely to particularly benefit from the cognitive or TG lowering benefits.

Acknowledgments: The author's research in the area of EPA, DHA and "health" is part funded by a BBSRC Institute Strategic Program grant (BB/J004545/1).

Conflicts of Interest: The author declare no conflict of interest.

References

1. GISSI-Prevenzione Investigators. Dietary supplementation with *n*-3 polyunsaturated fatty acids and vitamin E after myocardial infarction: Results of the gissi-prevenzione trial. Gruppo italiano per lo studio della sopravvivenza nell'infarto miocardico. *Lancet* **1999**, *354*, 447–455.
2. Points, E. *n*-3 fatty acids in patients with multiple cardiovascular risk factors. *N. Engl. J. Med.* **2013**, *368*, 1800–1808.
3. Von Schacky, C. Omega-3 fatty acids in cardiovascular disease—An uphill battle. *Prostaglandins Leukot. Essent. Fat. Acids* **2015**, *92*, 41–47. [CrossRef] [PubMed]
4. Bosch, J.; Gerstein, H.C.; Dagenais, G.R.; Diaz, R.; Dyal, L.; Jung, H.; Maggiono, A.P.; Probstfield, J.; Ramachandran, A.; Riddle, M.C.; *et al.* *n*-3 fatty acids and cardiovascular outcomes in patients with dysglycemia. *N. Engl. J. Med.* **2012**, *367*, 309–318. [PubMed]
5. Cederholm, T.; Salem, N., Jr.; Palmblad, J. Omega-3 fatty acids in the prevention of cognitive decline in humans. *Adv. Nutr.* **2013**, *4*, 672–676. [CrossRef] [PubMed]
6. Hu, F.B.; Bronner, L.; Willett, W.C.; Stampfer, M.J.; Rexrode, K.M.; Albert, C.M.; Hunter, D.; Manson, J.E. Fish and omega-3 fatty acid intake and risk of coronary heart disease in women. *JAMA* **2002**, *287*, 1815–1821. [CrossRef] [PubMed]
7. Janssen, C.I.; Kiliaan, A.J. Long-chain polyunsaturated fatty acids (LCPUFA) from genesis to senescence: The influence of LCPUFA on neural development, aging, and neurodegeneration. *Prog. Lipid Res.* **2014**, *53*, 1–17. [CrossRef] [PubMed]
8. Mozaffarian, D.; Wu, J.H. Omega-3 fatty acids and cardiovascular disease: Effects on risk factors, molecular pathways, and clinical events. *J. Am. Coll. Cardiol.* **2011**, *58*, 2047–2067. [CrossRef] [PubMed]
9. Saravanan, P.; Davidson, N.C.; Schmidt, E.B.; Calder, P.C. Cardiovascular effects of marine omega-3 fatty acids. *Lancet* **2010**, *376*, 540–550. [CrossRef]
10. TSO (The Stationary Office). *Scientific Advisory Committee on Nutrition (Sacn) and Committee on Toxicology (Cot), Advice on Fish Consumption: Benefits and Risks*; TSO (The Stationary Office): Norwich, UK, 2004.
11. Global Organisation for EPA and DHA (GOED). Global Recommendations for EPA and DHA Intake. Available online: http://www.goedomega3.com/index.php/files/download/304 (accessed on 25 February 2016).
12. Kris-Etherton, P.M.; Harris, W.S.; Appel, L.J. Fish consumption, fish oil, omega-3 fatty acids, and cardiovascular disease. *Circulation* **2002**, *106*, 2747–2757. [CrossRef] [PubMed]
13. Burdge, G.C. Metabolism of α-linolenic acid in humans. *Prostaglandins Leukot. Essent. Fat. Acids* **2006**, *75*, 161–168. [CrossRef] [PubMed]
14. Burdge, G.C.; Finnegan, Y.E.; Minihane, A.M.; Williams, C.M.; Wootton, S.A. Effect of altered dietary *n*-3 fatty acid intake upon plasma lipid fatty acid composition, conversion of [13C]α-linolenic acid to longer-chain fatty acids and partitioning towards β-oxidation in older men. *Br. J. Nutr.* **2003**, *90*, 311–321. [CrossRef] [PubMed]
15. Childs, C.E.; Kew, S.; Finnegan, Y.E.; Minihane, A.M.; Leigh-Firbank, E.C.; Williams, C.M.; Calder, P.C. Increased dietary α-linolenic acid has sex-specific effects upon eicosapentaenoic acid status in humans: Re-examination of data from a randomised, placebo-controlled, parallel study. *Nutr. J.* **2014**, *13*. [CrossRef] [PubMed]

16. Gillingham, L.G.; Harding, S.V.; Rideout, T.C.; Yurkova, N.; Cunnane, S.C.; Eck, P.K.; Jones, P.J. Dietary oils and FADS1-FADS2 genetic variants modulate (13C)α-linolenic acid metabolism and plasma fatty acid composition. *Am. J. Clin. Nutr.* **2013**, *97*, 195–207. [CrossRef] [PubMed]
17. Feeney, E.; O'Brien, S.; Scannell, A.; Markey, A.; Gibney, E.R. Genetic variation in taste perception: Does it have a role in healthy eating? *Proc. Nutr. Soc.* **2011**, *70*, 135–143. [CrossRef] [PubMed]
18. Mennella, J.A.; Bobowski, N.K. The sweetness and bitterness of childhood: Insights from basic research on taste preferences. *Physiol. Behavior* **2015**, *152*, 502–507. [CrossRef] [PubMed]
19. Ian Givens, D.; Gibbs, R.A. Current intakes of EPA and DHA in European populations and the potential of animal-derived foods to increase them. *Proc. Nutr. Soc.* **2008**, *67*, 273–280. [CrossRef] [PubMed]
20. Lemaitre, R.N.; Siscovick, D.S.; Berry, E.M.; Kark, J.D.; Friedlander, Y. Familial aggregation of red blood cell membrane fatty acid composition: The kibbutzim family study. *Metab. Clin. Exp.* **2008**, *57*, 662–668. [CrossRef] [PubMed]
21. Harris, W.S.; Pottala, J.V.; Lacey, S.M.; Vasan, R.S.; Larson, M.G.; Robins, S.J. Clinical correlates and heritability of erythrocyte eicosapentaenoic and docosahexaenoic acid content in the framingham heart study. *Atherosclerosis* **2012**, *225*, 425–431. [CrossRef] [PubMed]
22. Marquardt, A.; Stohr, H.; White, K.; Weber, B.H. cDNA cloning, genomic structure, and chromosomal localization of three members of the human fatty acid desaturase family. *Genomics* **2000**, *66*, 175–183. [CrossRef] [PubMed]
23. NCBI. National Center for Biotechnology Information dbSNP Database. Available online: http://www.ncbi.nlm.nih.gov/SNP/ (accessed on 25 February 2016).
24. Schaeffer, L.; Gohlke, H.; Muller, M.; Heid, I.M.; Palmer, L.J.; Kompauer, I.; Demmelmair, H.; Illig, T.; Koletzko, B.; Heinrich, J. Common genetic variants of the *FADS*1 *FADS*2 gene cluster and their reconstructed haplotypes are associated with the fatty acid composition in phospholipids. *Hum. Mol. Genet.* **2006**, *15*, 1745–1756. [CrossRef] [PubMed]
25. Baylin, A.; Ruiz-Narvaez, E.; Kraft, P.; Campos, H. Alpha-linolenic acid, delta6-desaturase gene polymorphism, and the risk of nonfatal myocardial infarction. *Am. J. Clin. Nutr.* **2007**, *85*, 554–560. [PubMed]
26. Malerba, G.; Schaeffer, L.; Xumerle, L.; Klopp, N.; Trabetti, E.; Biscuola, M.; Cavallari, U.; Galavotti, R.; Martinelli, N.; Guarini, P.; *et al.* SNPS of the FADS gene cluster are associated with polyunsaturated fatty acids in a cohort of patients with cardiovascular disease. *Lipids* **2008**, *43*, 289–299. [CrossRef] [PubMed]
27. Martinelli, N.; Girelli, D.; Malerba, G.; Guarini, P.; Illig, T.; Trabetti, E.; Sandri, M.; Friso, S.; Pizzolo, F.; Schaeffer, L.; *et al.* Fads genotypes and desaturase activity estimated by the ratio of arachidonic acid to linoleic acid are associated with inflammation and coronary artery disease. *Am. J. Clin. Nutr.* **2008**, *88*, 941–949. [PubMed]
28. Rzehak, P.; Heinrich, J.; Klopp, N.; Schaeffer, L.; Hoff, S.; Wolfram, G.; Illig, T.; Linseisen, J. Evidence for an association between genetic variants of the fatty acid desaturase 1 fatty acid desaturase 2 (*FADS*1 *FADS*2) gene cluster and the fatty acid composition of erythrocyte membranes. *Br. J. Nutr.* **2009**, *101*, 20–26. [CrossRef] [PubMed]
29. Truong, H.; DiBello, J.R.; Ruiz-Narvaez, E.; Kraft, P.; Campos, H.; Baylin, A. Does genetic variation in the delta6-desaturase promoter modify the association between α-linolenic acid and the prevalence of metabolic syndrome? *Am. J. Clin. Nutr.* **2009**, *89*, 920–925. [CrossRef] [PubMed]
30. Xie, L.; Innis, S.M. Genetic variants of the fads1 fads2 gene cluster are associated with altered (*n*-6) and (*n*-3) essential fatty acids in plasma and erythrocyte phospholipids in women during pregnancy and in breast milk during lactation. *J. Nutr.* **2008**, *138*, 2222–2228. [CrossRef] [PubMed]
31. Hellstrand, S.; Ericson, U.; Gullberg, B.; Hedblad, B.; Orho-Melander, M.; Sonestedt, E. Genetic variation in fads1 has little effect on the association between dietary PUFA intake and cardiovascular disease. *J. Nutr.* **2014**, *144*, 1356–1363. [CrossRef] [PubMed]
32. Smith, C.E.; Follis, J.L.; Nettleton, J.A.; Foy, M.; Wu, J.H.; Ma, Y.; Tanaka, T.; Manichakul, A.W.; Wu, H.; Chu, A.Y.; *et al.* Dietary fatty acids modulate associations between genetic variants and circulating fatty acids in plasma and erythrocyte membranes: Meta-analysis of nine studies in the charge consortium. *Mol. Nutr. Food Res.* **2015**, *59*, 1373–1383. [CrossRef] [PubMed]

33. Harslof, L.B.; Larsen, L.H.; Ritz, C.; Hellgren, L.I.; Michaelsen, K.F.; Vogel, U.; Lauritzen, L. Fads genotype and diet are important determinants of DHA status: A cross-sectional study in danish infants. *Am. J. Clin. Nutr.* **2013**, *97*, 1403–1410. [CrossRef] [PubMed]
34. Molto-Puigmarti, C.; van Dongen, M.C.; Dagnelie, P.C.; Plat, J.; Mensink, R.P.; Tan, F.E.; Heinrich, J.; Thijs, C. Maternal but not fetal fads gene variants modify the association between maternal long-chain PUFA intake in pregnancy and birth weight. *J. Nutr.* **2014**, *144*, 1430–1437. [CrossRef] [PubMed]
35. Lemaitre, R.N.; Tanaka, T.; Tang, W.; Manichaikul, A.; Foy, M.; Kabagambe, E.K.; Nettleton, J.A.; King, I.B.; Weng, L.C.; Bhattacharya, S.; *et al.* Genetic loci associated with plasma phospholipid *n*-3 fatty acids: A meta-analysis of genome-wide association studies from the charge consortium. *PLoS Genet.* **2011**, *7*, e1002193. [CrossRef] [PubMed]
36. Tanaka, T.; Shen, J.; Abecasis, G.R.; Kisialiou, A.; Ordovas, J.M.; Guralnik, J.M.; Singleton, A.; Bandinelli, S.; Cherubini, A.; Arnett, D.; *et al.* Genome-wide association study of plasma polyunsaturated fatty acids in the inchianti study. *PLoS Genet.* **2009**, *5*, e1000338. [CrossRef] [PubMed]
37. Tintle, N.L.; Pottala, J.V.; Lacey, S.; Ramachandran, V.; Westra, J.; Rogers, A.; Clark, J.; Olthoff, B.; Larson, M.; Harris, W.; *et al.* A genome-wide association study of saturated, mono- and polyunsaturated red blood cell fatty acids in the Framingham heart offspring study. *Prostaglandins Leukot. Essent. Fat. Acids* **2015**, *94*, 65–72. [CrossRef] [PubMed]
38. Wang, L.; Athinarayanan, S.; Jiang, G.; Chalasani, N.; Zhang, M.; Liu, W. Fatty acid desaturase 1 gene polymorphisms control human hepatic lipid composition. *Hepatology* **2015**, *61*, 119–128. [CrossRef] [PubMed]
39. Gregory, M.K.; Gibson, R.A.; Cook-Johnson, R.J.; Cleland, L.G.; James, M.J. Elongase reactions as control points in long-chain polyunsaturated fatty acid synthesis. *PLoS ONE* **2011**, *6*, e29662. [CrossRef] [PubMed]
40. Molto-Puigmarti, C.; Plat, J.; Mensink, R.P.; Muller, A.; Jansen, E.; Zeegers, M.P.; Thijs, C. Fads1 fads2 gene variants modify the association between fish intake and the docosahexaenoic acid proportions in human milk. *Am. J. Clin. Nutr.* **2010**, *91*, 1368–1376. [CrossRef] [PubMed]
41. Aulchenko, Y.S.; Ripatti, S.; Lindqvist, I.; Boomsma, D.; Heid, I.M.; Pramstaller, P.P.; Penninx, B.W.; Janssens, A.C.; Wilson, J.F.; Spector, T.; *et al.* Loci influencing lipid levels and coronary heart disease risk in 16 european population cohorts. *Nat. Genet.* **2009**, *41*, 47–55. [CrossRef] [PubMed]
42. Sabatti, C.; Service, S.K.; Hartikainen, A.L.; Pouta, A.; Ripatti, S.; Brodsky, J.; Jones, C.G.; Zaitlen, N.A.; Varilo, T.; Kaakinen, M.; *et al.* Genome-wide association analysis of metabolic traits in a birth cohort from a founder population. *Nat. Genet.* **2009**, *41*, 35–46. [CrossRef] [PubMed]
43. Fumagalli, M.; Moltke, I.; Grarup, N.; Racimo, F.; Bjerregaard, P.; Jorgensen, M.E.; Korneliussen, T.S.; Gerbault, P.; Skotte, L.; Linneberg, A.; *et al.* Greenlandic inuit show genetic signatures of diet and climate adaptation. *Science* **2015**, *349*, 1343–1347. [CrossRef] [PubMed]
44. Al-Hilal, M.; Alsaleh, A.; Maniou, Z.; Lewis, F.J.; Hall, W.L.; Sanders, T.A.; O'Dell, S.D. Genetic variation at the fads1-fads2 gene locus influences delta-5 desaturase activity and LC-PUFA proportions after fish oil supplement. *J. Lipid Res.* **2013**, *54*, 542–551. [CrossRef] [PubMed]
45. Alsaleh, A.; Maniou, Z.; Lewis, F.J.; Hall, W.L.; Sanders, T.A.; O'Dell, S.D. ELOVL2 gene polymorphisms are associated with increases in plasma eicosapentaenoic and docosahexaenoic acid proportions after fish oil supplement. *Genes Nutr.* **2014**, *9*. [CrossRef] [PubMed]
46. Abdelmagid, S.A.; Clarke, S.E.; Roke, K.; Nielsen, D.E.; Badawi, A.; El-Sohemy, A.; Mutch, D.M.; Ma, D.W. Ethnicity, sex, fads genetic variation, and hormonal contraceptive use influence delta-5- and delta-6-desaturase indices and plasma docosahexaenoic acid concentration in young canadian adults: A cross-sectional study. *Nutr. Metab.* **2015**, *12*. [CrossRef] [PubMed]
47. Minihane, A.M.; Jofre-Monseny, L.; Olano-Martin, E.; Rimbach, G. Apoe genotype, cardiovascular risk and responsiveness to dietary fat manipulation. *Proc. Nutr. Soc.* **2007**, *66*, 183–197. [CrossRef] [PubMed]
48. Shore, V.G.; Shore, B. Heterogeneity of human plasma very low density lipoproteins. Separation of species differing in protein components. *Biochemistry* **1973**, *12*, 502–507. [CrossRef] [PubMed]
49. Zhong, N.; Weisgraber, K.H. Understanding the association of apolipoprotein e4 with alzheimer disease: Clues from its structure. *J. Biol. Chem.* **2009**, *284*, 6027–6031. [CrossRef] [PubMed]
50. Bennet, A.M.; Di Angelantonio, E.; Ye, Z.; Wensley, F.; Dahlin, A.; Ahlbom, A.; Keavney, B.; Collins, R.; Wiman, B.; de Faire, U.; *et al.* Association of apolipoprotein E genotypes with lipid levels and coronary risk. *JAMA* **2007**, *298*, 1300–1311. [CrossRef] [PubMed]

51. Khan, T.A.; Shah, T.; Prieto, D.; Zhang, W.; Price, J.; Fowkes, G.R.; Cooper, J.; Talmud, P.J.; Humphries, S.E.; Sundstrom, J.; *et al.* Apolipoprotein e genotype, cardiovascular biomarkers and risk of stroke: Systematic review and meta-analysis of 14,015 stroke cases and pooled analysis of primary biomarker data from up to 60,883 individuals. *Int. J. Epidemiol.* **2013**, *42*, 475–492. [CrossRef] [PubMed]
52. Masson, L.F.; McNeill, G.; Avenell, A. Genetic variation and the lipid response to dietary intervention: A systematic review. *Am. J. Clin. Nutr.* **2003**, *77*, 1098–1111. [PubMed]
53. Sarkkinen, E.; Korhonen, M.; Erkkila, A.; Ebeling, T.; Uusitupa, M. Effect of apolipoprotein e polymorphism on serum lipid response to the separate modification of dietary fat and dietary cholesterol. *Am. J. Clin. Nutr.* **1998**, *68*, 1215–1222. [PubMed]
54. Humphries, S.E.; Talmud, P.J.; Hawe, E.; Bolla, M.; Day, I.N.; Miller, G.J. Apolipoprotein e4 and coronary heart disease in middle-aged men who smoke: A prospective study. *Lancet* **2001**, *358*, 115–119. [CrossRef]
55. Beekman, M.; Blanche, H.; Perola, M.; Hervonen, A.; Bezrukov, V.; Sikora, E.; Flachsbart, F.; Christiansen, L.; De Craen, A.J.; Kirkwood, T.B.; *et al.* Genome-wide linkage analysis for human longevity: Genetics of healthy aging study. *Aging Cell* **2013**, *12*, 184–193. [CrossRef] [PubMed]
56. Broer, L.; Buchman, A.S.; Deelen, J.; Evans, D.S.; Faul, J.D.; Lunetta, K.L.; Sebastiani, P.; Smith, J.A.; Smith, A.V.; Tanaka, T.; *et al.* Gwas of longevity in charge consortium confirms APOE and FOXO3 candidacy. *J. Gerontol. Ser. A Biol. Sci. Med. Sci.* **2015**, *70*, 110–118. [CrossRef] [PubMed]
57. Bertram, L.; McQueen, M.B.; Mullin, K.; Blacker, D.; Tanzi, R.E. Systematic meta-analyses of alzheimer disease genetic association studies: The alzgene database. *Nat. Genet.* **2007**, *39*, 17–23. [CrossRef] [PubMed]
58. Huang, T.L.; Zandi, P.P.; Tucker, K.L.; Fitzpatrick, A.L.; Kuller, L.H.; Fried, L.P.; Burke, G.L.; Carlson, M.C. Benefits of fatty fish on dementia risk are stronger for those without Apoe ε4. *Neurology* **2005**, *65*, 1409–1414. [CrossRef] [PubMed]
59. Quinn, J.F.; Raman, R.; Thomas, R.G.; Yurko-Mauro, K.; Nelson, E.B.; Van Dyck, C.; Galvin, J.E.; Emond, J.; Jack, C.R., Jr.; Weiner, M.; *et al.* Docosahexaenoic acid supplementation and cognitive decline in Alzheimer disease: A randomized trial. *JAMA* **2010**, *304*, 1903–1911. [CrossRef] [PubMed]
60. Whalley, L.J.; Deary, I.J.; Starr, J.M.; Wahle, K.W.; Rance, K.A.; Bourne, V.J.; Fox, H.C. *n*-3 fatty acid erythrocyte membrane content, APOE ε4, and cognitive variation: An observational follow-up study in late adulthood. *Am. J. Clin. Nutr.* **2008**, *87*, 449–454. [PubMed]
61. Chouinard-Watkins, R.; Conway, V.; Minihane, A.M.; Jackson, K.G.; Lovegrove, J.A.; Plourde, M. Interaction between BMI and apoe genotype is associated with changes in the plasma long-chain-PUFA response to a fish-oil supplement in healthy participants. *Am. J. Clin. Nutr.* **2015**, *102*, 505–513. [CrossRef] [PubMed]
62. Gregg, R.E.; Zech, L.A.; Schaefer, E.J.; Stark, D.; Wilson, D.; Brewer, H.B., Jr. Abnormal *in vivo* metabolism of apolipoprotein e4 in humans. *J. Clin. Investig.* **1986**, *78*, 815–821. [CrossRef] [PubMed]
63. Chouinard-Watkins, R.; Rioux-Perreault, C.; Fortier, M.; Tremblay-Mercier, J.; Zhang, Y.; Lawrence, P.; Vohl, M.C.; Perron, P.; Lorrain, D.; Brenna, J.T.; *et al.* Disturbance in uniformly 13C-labelled DHA metabolism in elderly human subjects carrying the apoe ε4 allele. *Br. J. Nutr.* **2013**, *110*, 1751–1759. [CrossRef] [PubMed]
64. Vandal, M.; Alata, W.; Tremblay, C.; Rioux-Perreault, C.; Salem, N., Jr.; Calon, F.; Plourde, M. Reduction in DHA transport to the brain of mice expressing human apoe4 compared to apoe2. *J. Neurochem.* **2014**, *129*, 516–526. [CrossRef] [PubMed]
65. Bazinet, R.P.; Laye, S. Polyunsaturated fatty acids and their metabolites in brain function and disease. *Nat. Rev. Neurosci.* **2014**, *15*, 771–785. [CrossRef] [PubMed]
66. Nguyen, L.N.; Ma, D.; Shui, G.; Wong, P.; Cazenave-Gassiot, A.; Zhang, X.; Wenk, M.R.; Goh, E.L.; Silver, D.L. Mfsd2a is a transporter for the essential omega-3 fatty acid docosahexaenoic acid. *Nature* **2014**, *509*, 503–506. [CrossRef] [PubMed]
67. Carvalho-Wells, A.L.; Jackson, K.G.; Lockyer, S.; Lovegrove, J.A.; Minihane, A.M. Apoe genotype influences triglyceride and c-reactive protein responses to altered dietary fat intake in uk adults. *Am. J. Clin. Nutr.* **2012**, *96*, 1447–1453. [CrossRef] [PubMed]
68. Caslake, M.J.; Miles, E.A.; Kofler, B.M.; Lietz, G.; Curtis, P.; Armah, C.K.; Kimber, A.C.; Grew, J.P.; Farrell, L.; Stannard, J.; *et al.* Effect of sex and genotype on cardiovascular biomarker response to fish oils: The fingen study. *Am. J. Clin. Nutr.* **2008**, *88*, 618–629. [PubMed]
69. Harris, W.S.; Pottala, J.V.; Thiselton, D.L.; S, A.V.; Baedke, A.M.; Dayspring, T.D.; Warnick, G.R.; McConnell, J.P. Does apoe genotype modify the relations between serum lipid and erythrocyte omega-3 fatty acid levels? *J. Cardiovasc. Transl. Res.* **2014**, *7*, 526–532. [CrossRef] [PubMed]

70. Liang, S.; Steffen, L.M.; Steffen, B.T.; Guan, W.; Weir, N.L.; Rich, S.S.; Manichaikul, A.; Vargas, J.D.; Tsai, M.Y. Apoe genotype modifies the association between plasma omega-3 fatty acids and plasma lipids in the multi-ethnic study of atherosclerosis (MESA). *Atherosclerosis* **2013**, *228*, 181–187. [CrossRef] [PubMed]
71. Minihane, A.M.; Khan, S.; Leigh-Firbank, E.C.; Talmud, P.; Wright, J.W.; Murphy, M.C.; Griffin, B.A.; Williams, C.M. ApoE polymorphism and fish oil supplementation in subjects with an atherogenic lipoprotein phenotype. *Arterioscler. Thromb. Vasc. Biol.* **2000**, *20*, 1990–1997. [CrossRef] [PubMed]
72. Olano-Martin, E.; Anil, E.; Caslake, M.J.; Packard, C.J.; Bedford, D.; Stewart, G.; Peiris, D.; Williams, C.M.; Minihane, A.M. Contribution of apolipoprotein e genotype and docosahexaenoic acid to the ldl-cholesterol response to fish oil. *Atherosclerosis* **2010**, *209*, 104–110. [CrossRef] [PubMed]
73. Khan, S.; Minihane, A.M.; Talmud, P.J.; Wright, J.W.; Murphy, M.C.; Williams, C.M.; Griffin, B.A. Dietary long-chain *n*-3 PUFAs increase LPL gene expression in adipose tissue of subjects with an atherogenic lipoprotein phenotype. *J. Lipid Res.* **2002**, *43*, 979–985. [PubMed]
74. Jackson, K.G.; Poppitt, S.D.; Minihane, A.M. Postprandial lipemia and cardiovascular disease risk: Interrelationships between dietary, physiological and genetic determinants. *Atherosclerosis* **2012**, *220*, 22–33. [CrossRef] [PubMed]
75. Madden, J.; Williams, C.M.; Calder, P.C.; Lietz, G.; Miles, E.A.; Cordell, H.; Mathers, J.C.; Minihane, A.M. The impact of common gene variants on the response of biomarkers of cardiovascular disease (CVD) risk to increased fish oil fatty acids intakes. *Annu. Rev. Nutr.* **2011**, *31*, 203–234. [CrossRef]
76. Bouchard-Mercier, A.; Rudkowska, I.; Lemieux, S.; Couture, P.; Vohl, M.C. Polymorphisms, *de novo* lipogenesis, and plasma triglyceride response following fish oil supplementation. *J. Lipid Res.* **2013**, *54*, 2866–2873. [CrossRef] [PubMed]
77. Bouchard-Mercier, A.; Rudkowska, I.; Lemieux, S.; Couture, P.; Vohl, M.C. Polymorphisms in genes involved in fatty acid beta-oxidation interact with dietary fat intakes to modulate the plasma tg response to a fish oil supplementation. *Nutrients* **2014**, *6*, 1145–1163. [CrossRef] [PubMed]
78. Ouellette, C.; Cormier, H.; Rudkowska, I.; Guenard, F.; Lemieux, S.; Couture, P.; Vohl, M.C. Polymorphisms in genes involved in the triglyceride synthesis pathway and marine omega-3 polyunsaturated fatty acid supplementation modulate plasma triglyceride levels. *J. Nutrigenet. Nutrigenom.* **2013**, *6*, 268–280. [CrossRef] [PubMed]
79. Rudkowska, I.; Julien, P.; Couture, P.; Lemieux, S.; Tchernof, A.; Barbier, O.; Vohl, M.C. Cardiometabolic risk factors are influenced by Stearoyl-Coa Desaturase (SCD)-1 gene polymorphisms and *n*-3 polyunsaturated fatty acid supplementation. *Mol. Nutr. Food Res.* **2014**, *58*, 1079–1086. [CrossRef] [PubMed]
80. Tremblay, B.L.; Cormier, H.; Rudkowska, I.; Lemieux, S.; Couture, P.; Vohl, M.C. Association between polymorphisms in phospholipase A2 genes and the plasma triglyceride response to an *n*-3 PUFA supplementation: A clinical trial. *Lipids Health Dis.* **2015**, *14*. [CrossRef] [PubMed]
81. Rudkowska, I.; Guenard, F.; Julien, P.; Couture, P.; Lemieux, S.; Barbier, O.; Calder, P.C.; Minihane, A.M.; Vohl, M.C. Genome-wide association study of the plasma triglyceride response to an *n*-3 polyunsaturated fatty acid supplementation. *J. Lipid Res.* **2014**, *55*, 1245–1253. [CrossRef] [PubMed]
82. The Food and Agriculture Organization of the United Nations (FAO). *The State of World Fisheries and Aquaculture*; FAO: Rome, Italy, 2012.

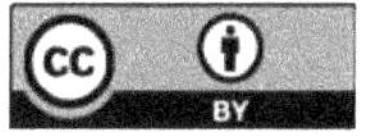

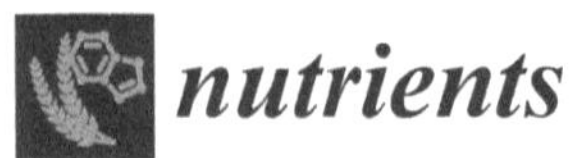
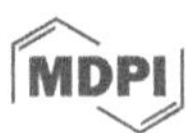

Article

A Correlation Study of DHA Dietary Intake and Plasma, Erythrocyte and Breast Milk DHA Concentrations in Lactating Women from Coastland, Lakeland, and Inland Areas of China

Meng-Jiao Liu [1,2,†], Hong-Tian Li [1,2,†], Li-Xia Yu [3], Gao-Sheng Xu [4], Hua Ge [5], Lin-Lin Wang [1,2], Ya-Li Zhang [1,2], Yu-Bo Zhou [1,2], You Li [1,2], Man-Xi Bai [6] and Jian-Meng Liu [1,2,*]

1 Institute of Reproductive and Child Health/Ministry of Health Key Laboratory of Reproductive Health, Peking University Health Science Center, 38 Xueyuan Rd., Beijing 100191, China; liumengjiao_bjmu@163.com (M.-J.L.); liht@bjmu.edu.cn (H.-T.L.); linlinwang@bjmu.edu.cn (L.-L.W.); zhangyl@bjmu.edu.cn (Y.-L.Z.); zhouyubo@yeah.net (Y.-B.Z.); liyou@pku.edu.cn (Y.L.)
2 Department of Epidemiology and Biostatistics, School of Public Health, Peking University Health Science Center, 38 Xueyuan Rd., Beijing 100191, China
3 Department of Obstetrics and Gynaecology, Weihai Maternal and Child Health Hospital, 51 Guangming Rd., Weihai 264200, China; Whyulixia@126.com
4 Department of Pediatrics, Yueyang Maternal and Child Health Hospital, 693 Baling Middle Rd., Yueyang 414000, China; xugaosheng0414@163.com
5 Department of Obstetrics and Gynecology, the First Affiliated Hospital of Baotou Medical School, 41 Linyin Rd., Baotou 014000, China; byyfygh2010@163.com
6 Wyeth Nutrition Science Center, 582 Wuzhong Rd., Shanghai 201103, China; Manxi.Bai@wyethnutrition.com
* Correspondence: liujm@pku.edu.cn; Tel.: +86-10-8280-1136
† These authors contributed equally to this work.

Received: 8 March 2016; Accepted: 18 May 2016; Published: 20 May 2016

Abstract: We aimed to assess the correlation between docosahexaenoic acid (DHA) dietary intake and the plasma, erythrocyte and breast milk DHA concentrations in lactating women residing in the coastland, lakeland and inland areas of China. A total of 408 healthy lactating women (42 ± 7 days postpartum) were recruited from four hospitals located in Weihai (coastland), Yueyang (lakeland) and Baotou (inland) city. The categories of food containing DHA, the average amount consumed per time and the frequency of consumption in the past month were assessed by a tailored DHA food frequency questionnaire, the DHA Intake Evaluation Tool (DIET). DHA dietary intake (mg/day) was calculated according to the Chinese Food Composition Table (Version 2009). In addition, fasting venous blood (5 mL) and breast milk (10 mL) were collected from lactating women. DHA concentrations in plasma, erythrocyte and breast milk were measured using capillary gas chromatography, and were reported as absolute concentration (μg/mL) and relative concentration (weight percent of total fatty acids, wt. %). Spearman correlation coefficients were used to assess the correlation between intakes of DHA and its concentrations in biological specimens. The study showed that the breast milk, plasma and erythrocyte DHA concentrations were positively correlated with DHA dietary intake; corresponding correlation coefficients were 0.36, 0.36 and 0.24 for relative concentration and 0.33, 0.32, and 0.18 for absolute concentration ($p < 0.05$). The median DHA dietary intake varied significantly across areas ($p < 0.05$), which was highest in the coastland (24.32 mg/day), followed by lakeland (13.69 mg/day), and lowest in the inland (8.84 mg/day). The overall relative and absolute DHA concentrations in breast milk were 0.36% ± 0.23% and 141.49 ± 107.41 μg/mL; the concentrations were significantly lower in inland women than those from coastland and lakeland. We conclude that DHA dietary intake is positively correlated with DHA concentrations in blood and breast milk in Chinese lactating women, suggesting that the tailored DHA food frequency questionnaire, DIET, is a valid tool for the assessment of DHA dietary intake.

Keywords: docosahexaenoic acid; lactating women; food frequency questionnaire; breast milk; plasma; erythrocyte; correlation

---

1. Introduction

Docosahexaenoic acid (DHA, 22:6*n*-3) plays an important role in infant growth and development, especially during early postnatal months, a period of rapid brain growth [1,2]. The accretion of DHA into brain during this period mainly depends on dietary sources [3]. Therefore, for breastfeeding infants, their nutritional status concerning DHA is largely determined by their mothers' DHA status [4,5]. Many professional organizations, including the Chinese Nutrition Society, recommend lactating women to consume a minimum of 200 mg DHA per day in order to meet their own needs and to achieve optimal growth of infants [6,7]. However, as noted by the European Commission with the International Society for the Study of Fatty Acids and Lipids, only 25% of women at 3 months postpartum met the recommendation [8]. In China, there is a scarcity of relevant data for lactating women [9], possibly because there is no valid tool for the assessment of DHA intake.

The food frequency questionnaire (FFQ) has been suggested as an optimal tool in estimating dietary intake of DHA as it cannot be synthesized *in vivo* and primarily comes from aquatic products [10,11]. Most FFQs available in the literature covered the whole diets and were originally designed to assess a wide range of nutrients, which were quite lengthy and not ideal for dietary assessment focusing specifically on DHA [12,13]. Given that DHA is contained in only a small range of foods, efforts have also been made to develop a tailored DHA specific FFQ [14,15], which demonstrated comparable validity (0.42–0.52) as compared with the whole diet-based FFQs (0.19–0.54) [16]. To our knowledge, previous studies were primarily conducted in the general populations but none in lactating women [16]. Due to the possibility of changed dietary patterns and different metabolic profile of fatty acid during lactation [17], the validity of FFQ in assessing dietary DHA intake of lactating women remains to be determined.

In this study, we aimed to evaluate the performance of a newly-developed DHA specific FFQ by assessing the correlation between dietary DHA intake and its concentration in plasma, erythrocyte and breast milk among Chinese lactating women residing in coastland, lakeland and inland areas of China.

2. Materials and Methods

2.1. Subjects

In this study, we recruited totally 408 healthy lactating women (42 $\pm$ 7 days postpartum) from four hospitals located in Weihai (coastland), Yueyang (lakeland) and Baotou (inland) city between May and July of 2014. The inclusion criteria were: (1) healthy women aged 18–35; (2) currently exclusive breastfeeding or partial breastfeeding (women who feed infants formula other than breast milk); (3) having had a singleton pregnancy; (4) local permanent residents. Women were considered not eligible if they had been diagnosed as having severe heart, liver, kidney or lung diseases, had serious mental illness, were allergic to fish, shrimp, shellfish or other DHA-rich food, or had participated in other research projects in the past 30 days. The Institutional Review Board/Human Subjects Committee at Peking University Health Science Center (IRB00001052-14012; date of approval: 22-04-2014) approved the study protocol, and all participating women signed informed consents.

2.2. Data Collection

The survey consisted of two parts. Firstly, we collected information about socio-demographic and maternal characteristics, including age, ethnicity, education level, annual family income per capita, height, breastfeeding patterns, pre-pregnancy and postpartum weight of mothers, as well as neonatal birth weight and gender. Then, we collected dietary information of the previous month by a newly designed electronic version DHA specific FFQ, the DHA Intake Evaluation Tool (DIET), where the pictures of various kinds of food and intake reference diagrams were provided. The DIET was designed to capture all food containing DHA listed in the China Food Composition Table (CFCT, Version 2009) [18], including three categories: seafood (75 kinds such as mackerel, lobster and crab), freshwater food (38 kinds such as carp, shrimp and river crab) and mutton. Totally, there were 12 food frequency options ranging from once per month to three times per day, and 9 food intake options ranging from 25 g to 250 g of edible portion. The survey was self-administered by lactating mothers and took approximately 10 min on average to complete. DHA dietary intake was calculated on the basis of the CFCT (Version 2009) [18].

To ensure the data quality, we trained all project staff intensively, standardized data collection procedures across sites, and designated an investigator at each site to supervise the study and reported the study process weekly.

2.3. *Sample Collection and Analysis*

For each participant, fasting venous blood (5 mL) and breast milk (10 mL) were collected. The detailed procedure for blood collection and processing has been described in our previous publication [19]. In brief, the blood samples were collected into an ethylenediaminetetraacetic acid (EDTA)-containing tube, and placed in the refrigerator at 5 °C for 30 min before centrifuging at 3000 rpm for 10 min to separate plasma and erythrocytes. Breast milk samples were collected into a sterile container in the morning (10 ± 2 a.m.) from the non-feeding breast manually or with a breast pump. In the study, mothers were allowed to breastfeed the baby using one side of the breast in the morning, and if a mother did breastfeed her baby, breast milk was collected from the non-feeding breast. If not, breast milk was collected from either side. It has been suggested by a study [20], that fat concentrations in the non-feeding breast are less likely to be influenced by the breastfeeding behavior using the other breast. Both blood and milk samples were stored at the local hospital at −20 °C for about 10 days before being transported on dry ice frozen to the central laboratory where samples were stored at −80 °C in a freezer.

Total lipids in blood and breast milk samples were extracted and derived following a modified method of Folch *et al.* [20], and were analyzed by capillary gas chromatography. The detailed analysis procedure for total lipids in the blood has been descried previously [21]. The same methods were used for breast milk analysis. Briefly, the internal standard solution with methyl ester (C11:0) was added to each sample, and mixed with boron trifluoride and methanol. The mixture was heated at 115 °C for 20 min and extracted with n-hexane after cooling down to room temperature. The n-hexane containing methyl esters of total lipids was analyzed by Agilent 6890N capillary gas chromatography (Agilent Technologies, Palo Alto, CA, USA) equipped with a capillary column (CP-Sil 88, 50 m, 0.25 mm ID, 0.20 μm film thickness). The fatty acids were separated by a programmed temperature ramping method, and the results were recorded via the Agilent Open LAB software (Agilent Technologies, Santa Clara, CA, USA). Both absolute (μg/mL) and relative (weight percent of total fatty acids, wt. %) concentrations of DHA were reported.

2.4. *Statistical Analysis*

The total dietary intake of DHA in the past month was calculated based on food consumption frequency, the average amount consumed per time, and the DHA content in the food. Of the 408 participants, 3 (1 lakeland, 2 inland) with obviously abnormal dietary intake and 9 (3 coastland, 5 lakeland, 1 inland) who had consumed DHA supplements in the past month were excluded; thus, 396 subjects were included in the analysis. There were no missing data on all socio-demographic and maternal characteristics, except that the information on education level and annual family income per capita was missing for 3% and 6% of subjects.

Data were presented as means ± SDs, median (interquartile range), or percentage (%) as appropriate. The statistical differences between regions in DHA dietary intake and the DHA concentrations in blood and breast milk were examined by one-way analysis of variance (ANOVA) and Kruskal-Wallis tests, followed by Tukey's HSD and Kruskal-Wallis one-way ANOVA by ranks for multiple comparisons, as appropriate. In addition, we explored whether DHA concentrations in breast milk varied across subgroups defined by maternal ethnicity, age (18.0–24.9, 25.0–29.9, and over 30.0 years), pre-pregnancy BMI (<18.5, 18.5–23.9, and 24.0 kg/m^2), annual family income per capita, education attainment (middle school or less, high school, and college or above), maternal dietary intake and feeding methods by using multiple linear regression with adjustment for region.

Spearman correlation analysis was used to assess the correlation between DHA dietary intake and its concentrations in biological specimens. To facilitate the description of dietary sources of DHA, we defined a category of food (seafood, freshwater food, and mutton) as the major DHA source for an individual if this food category comprised ⩾50% of total DHA intake. We compared the regional differences in major DHA sources by using the Chi-square test. Statistical analyses were performed by using SPSS version 20.0 (Chicago, IL, USA). *P* values were two-sided, and $p < 0.05$ was considered statistically significant.

3. Results

3.1. Maternal Characteristics

The mean age, height, pre-pregnancy BMI, postpartum BMI of the 396 lactating mothers and mean birth weight of their infants were 27.34 ± 2.97 years old, 162.04 ± 4.95 cm, 21.07 ± 3.31 kg/m^2, 23.61 ± 3.32 kg/m^2, 3.39 ± 0.46 kg, respectively. The mean annual family income per capita was 27,507 ± 18,789 Chinese Yuan. In total, 95.7% of the mothers were of Han ethnicity, and 36.8% had high school or above education; approximate 60% of mothers breastfed exclusively. Table 1 shows the characteristics of mothers and the infants by region. The overall tests showed that there were significant regional differences in all the characteristics except mothers' education, ethnics, feeding methods and infants' gender. Specifically, lakeland women were relatively younger, shorter in stature, and had lower pre-pregnancy BMI and postpartum BMI.

3.2. DHA Dietary Intake

Table 2 shows the DHA dietary intake of lactating women by region. The median intake varied significantly across the three areas ($p < 0.001$), which was highest in the coastland (24.32 mg/day), followed by the lakeland (13.69 mg/day), and lowest in the inland (8.84 mg/day). Totally, 126 women consumed mutton (19 in the coastland and 107 in the inland). The mean DHA dietary intake from mutton was 0.15 mg/day and 6.18 mg/day for women residing in coastland and inland.

The major DHA food sources differed significantly by region ($\chi^2 = 153.49$, $p < 0.001$) (Table 3). In coastland, seafood was the major food source for 48% of lactating mothers and for another 48% was freshwater food. In inland, the major food source for 40% of the mothers was freshwater food and 35% was mutton. In lakeland, the major food source for four fifths of women was freshwater food.

3.3. DHA Concentrations in Breast Milk and Multiple Regression Analyses

The overall mean DHA absolute and relative concentrations in breast milk were 141.49 μg/mL and 0.36%, respectively; the concentration was higher for coastland and lakeland than inland mothers in both absolute and relative DHA concentrations (Table 4). Plasma and erythrocyte DHA concentrations have been reported previously [19].

In multiple linear regression analyses, maternal dietary intake and geographical region were significantly associated with both absolute and relative DHA concentrations. Maternal feeding method was significantly associated with absolute DHA concentrations. As the results showed, none of the characteristics (including maternal ethnic, age, pre-pregnancy BMI, annual family income per capita, education attainment) have an impact on DHA concentrations in breast milk.

Table 1. Characteristics of the mothers and infants by region.

Characteristics	Total (n = 396)	Coastland (n = 133)	Lakeland (n = 130)	Inland (n = 133)	p Value
Mothers:					
Age (year)	27.34 ± 2.97	27.79 ± 2.69 [a]	26.61 ± 3.08 [b]	27.60 ± 3.00 [a]	<0.01
Ethnics (%)					>0.05
Han	95.7	97.0	97.7	92.5	
Others	4.3	3.0	2.3	7.5	
Education (%)					>0.05
College or above	36.8	38.6	32.5	39.2	
High school	52.5	51.5	53.2	52.8	
Middle school or less	10.7	9.9	14.3	8.0	
Annual family income per capita	27,507 ± 18,789	21,474 ± 11,291 [a]	30,298 ± 23,201 [b]	31,579 ± 18,524 [b]	<0.001
Height (cm)	162.04 ± 4.95	163.28 ± 5.05 [a]	159.75 ± 4.31 [b]	163.05 ± 4.68 [a]	<0.001
Pre-pregnancy BMI (kg/m^2)	21.07 ± 3.31	21.88 ± 3.52 [a]	20.12 ± 2.96 [b]	21.19 ± 3.22 [a]	<0.001
Postpartum BMI (kg/m^2)	23.61 ± 3.32	24.52 ± 3.52 [a]	22.54 ± 2.92 [b]	23.75 ± 3.20 [a]	<0.001
Feeding methods (%)					>0.05
Exclusively breastfeeding	58.8	54.1	63.8	58.6	
Partially breastfeeding	41.2	45.9	36.2	41.4	
Infants:					
Birth weight (kg)	3.39 ± 0.46	3.46 ± 0.43 [a]	3.28 ± 0.44 [b]	3.42 ± 0.48 [a]	<0.01
Gender, Male (%)	53.5	51.9	46.9	61.7	>0.05

Means ± SDs within a row with unlike superscript letters are significantly different ($p < 0.05$).

Table 2. Docosahexaenoic acid (DHA) dietary intake of lactating women by region (mg/day).

Dietary Sources of Foods	All (n = 396)	Coastland (n = 133)	Lakeland (n = 130)	Inland (n = 133)	p Value
Seafood					
Mean ± SDs	18.37 ± 33.23	27.89 ± 39.73 [a]	9.98 ± 25.07 [b]	13.43 ± 26.40 [b]	<0.001
Median (interquartile range)	3.28 (0.48, 20.72)	12.26 (1.65, 31.42) [a]	1.70 (0, 7.81) [b]	1.20 (0, 10.01) [b]	<0.001
Freshwater food					
Mean ± SDs	14.75 ± 24.42	19.76 ± 32.08 [a]	17.12 ± 22.50 [a]	7.56 ± 14.07 [b]	<0.001
Median (interquartile range)	5.97 (2.18, 15.63)	7.44 (2.79, 19.54) [a]	10.63 (4.42, 21.33) [a]	2.95 (0.76, 7.46) [b]	<0.001
Mutton					
Mean ± SDs	2.13 ± 8.55	0.15 ± 0.87 [a]	0 ± 0 [a]	6.18 ± 13.90 [b]	<0.001
Median (interquartile range)	0 (0, 0.43)	0 (0, 0) [a]	0 (0, 0) [a]	1.84 (0.22, 5.53) [b]	<0.001
Total food intake					
Mean ± SDs	30.00 ± 43.85	44.37 ± 56.77 [a]	24.20 ± 32.95 [b]	21.29 ± 33.95 [b]	<0.001
Median (interquartile range)	13.42 (5.54, 32.28)	24.32 (8.46, 57.49) [a]	13.69 (6.16, 25.47) [b]	8.84 (2.80, 21.96) [c]	<0.001

Means ± SDs or median (interquartile range) within a row with unlike superscript letters are significantly different ($p < 0.05$).

Table 3. Major food source [a] of DHA by region.

The Major DHA Source	Coastland		Lakeland		Inland	
	n	%	n	%	n	%
Seafood	64	48.12	23	17.69	22	16.54
Freshwater food	64	48.12	107	82.31	53	39.85
Mutton	2	1.50	-	-	47	35.34
None	3	2.26	-	-	11	8.27

[a] If a category of food (seafood, freshwater food, or mutton) contributed to ⩾50% of total DHA intake for an individual, this category of food was defined as the major food source of DHA for this individual. If all the three categories of food contributed to <50% of total DHA intake for an individual, we considered that there was no specific major food source of DHA for this individual.

Table 4. DHA concentrations in breast milk and multiple linear regression.

Variables	Breast Milk DHA (μg/mL)				Breast Milk DHA (wt. %)			
	Mean ± SDs	β	95% CI	*p*	Mean ± SDs	β	95% CI	*p*
Region								
Inland	113.09 ± 72.90	Ref.	Ref.	-	0.28 ± 0.19	Ref.	Ref.	-
Coastland	163.36 ± 133.82	29.69	8.61–48.01	<0.01	0.43 ± 0.28	0.09	0.05–0.13	<0.01
Lakeland	148.17 ± 100.98	−2.34	−27.85–20.95	0.85	0.38 ± 0.17	−0.03	−0.08–0.02	0.26
Age (year)								
<25.0	150.06 ± 121.28	Ref.	Ref.	-	0.36 ± 0.19	Ref.	Ref.	-
25.0–29.9	135.12 ± 90.72	−33.08	−66.81–1.96	0.06	0.36 ± 0.24	−0.02	−0.08–0.04	0.54
⩾30.0	161.98 ± 152.89	−16.75	−58.14–28.83	0.45	0.27 ± 0.19	−0.04	−0.11–0.04	0.34
Ethnicity								
Others	128.29 ± 117.84	Ref.	Ref.	-	0.38 ± 0.44	Ref.	Ref.	-
Han	142.08 ± 107.05	−3.50	−85.34–48.13	0.91	0.36 ± 0.21	−0.06	−0.33–0.10	0.64
Education								
Middle school or less	124.00 ± 92.11	Ref.	Ref.	-	0.34 ± 0.18	Ref.	Ref.	-
High school	138.18 ± 103.90	16.52	−12.85–44.42	0.27	0.36 ± 0.23	0.002	−0.05–0.05	0.94
College or above	153.61 ± 117.84	25.26	−5.58–56.55	0.10	0.38 ± 0.24	0.005	−0.048–0.06	0.86
Pre-pregnancy BMI								
<18.5	139.93 ± 95.16	Ref.	Ref.	-	0.38 ± 0.27	Ref.	Ref.	-
18.5–23.9	143.25 ± 111.83	9.29	−15.89–34.13	0.48	0.36 ± 0.20	−0.02	−0.08–0.04	0.62
⩾24.0	136.51 ± 105.04	−2.41	−34.60–32.78	0.86	0.25 ± 0.27	−0.04	−0.14–0.04	0.34
Annual family income per capita (ten thousand Yuan)		2.66	−4.59–9.70	0.50		0.01	−0.01–0.02	0.58
Feeding method								
Exclusive breastfeeding	131.20 ± 99.74	Ref.	Ref.	-	0.35 ± 0.24	Ref.	Ref.	-
Partial breastfeeding	156.20 ± 116.26	24.68	4.65–43.48	<0.05	0.38 ± 0.21	0.03	−0.01–0.07	0.12
Dietary DHA intake		0.75	0.44–1.15	<0.01		0.002	0.001–0.003	<0.01

β, regression coefficient; Ref., reference category.

3.4. Spearman Correlation Analysis

In overall analyses, the DHA dietary intake was significantly correlated with its relative concentrations in the breast milk, plasma and erythrocyte; corresponding spearman correlation coefficients were 0.36, 0.36 and 0.24, respectively ($p < 0.001$) (Table 5); similar but slightly lower correlation coefficients were observed for absolute concentrations in the three biomarkers. In stratified analyses by region, moderate correlations of DHA intake with both relative (0.18–0.45) and absolute (0.15–0.41) concentrations in plasma and breast milk were identified in the three regions, although some did not reach statistical significance. The correlations between DHA intake and erythrocyte DHA (relative: 0.05–0.30; absolute: 0.02–0.18) were relatively lower than those of plasma and breast milk DHA.

Table 5. Spearman correlation analysis between dietary DHA intake and DHA levels in biomarkers.

Biomarkers	All		Coastland (n = 133)		Lakeland (n = 130)		Inland (n = 133)	
	r (95%CI)	p	r (95%CI)	p	r (95%CI)	p	r (95%CI)	p
wt. %								
Breast milk	0.36 (0.26–0.45)	<0.001	0.45 (0.30–0.58)	<0.001	0.16 (−0.02–0.33)	0.06	0.23 (0.05–0.38)	<0.01
Plasma	0.36 (0.27–0.45)	<0.001	0.46 (0.31–0.60)	<0.001	0.21 (0.03–0.38)	<0.05	0.18 (0.01–0.34)	<0.05
Erythrocyte	0.24 (0.14–0.33)	<0.001	0.30 (0.14–0.44)	<0.01	0.05 (−0.13–0.23)	0.55	0.08 (−0.10–0.25)	0.38
μg/mL								
Breast milk	0.33 (0.23–0.42)	<0.001	0.39 (0.23–0.54)	<0.001	0.23 (0.06–0.41)	<0.01	0.25 (0.07–0.42)	<0.01
Plasma	0.32 (0.23–0.41)	<0.001	0.41 (0.26–0.55)	<0.001	0.21 (0.04–0.39)	<0.05	0.15 (−0.01–0.32)	0.08
Erythrocyte	0.18 (0.08–0.27)	<0.001	0.17 (0.01–0.32)	0.06	0.18 (−0.01–0.35)	0.05	0.02 (−0.16–0.20)	0.82

4. Discussion

In this large cross-sectional study conducted in the three typical urban areas of China, the DHA dietary intake was significantly and positively correlated with plasma, erythrocyte, and breast milk DHA concentrations, suggesting the possibility of using the DIET to assess DHA dietary intake. We also found that the DHA dietary intake of lactating women residing in the coastland, lakeland and inland areas of China was substantially lower than the adequate intake (200 mg/day) recommended by the Chinese Nutrition Society [7].

In our study, the breast milk, plasma and erythrocyte DHA concentrations were positively correlated with DHA dietary intake; corresponding correlation coefficients were 0.36, 0.36 and 0.24 for relative concentration and 0.33, 0.32, and 0.18 for absolute concentration. The magnitude of correlation in our study is slightly lower than that reported by a Canadian study and a Norwegian study, both of which also utilized DHA specific FFQ [14,15]. In the Canadian study, the correlation coefficient between DHA dietary intake and whole blood DHA was 0.42 [15], and in the Norwegian study, the correlation coefficient between DHA dietary intake and erythrocyte DHA was 0.52 [14]. The underlying reasons might be complex. Firstly, such difference may be a reflection of race differences in metabolic profile regarding DHA. Secondly, the relatively lower correlation in our study may suggest that our estimation of dietary intake might be less accurate than in aforementioned studies. If so, the reduced precision may be partially because we did not consider the variations in cooking methods of aquatic products. In China, the aquatic products could be cooked in a variety of ways, and it is unrealistic for us to accurately quantify the impacts of various cooking ways on fatty acids. Thirdly, both the Canadian and the Norwegian study were conducted in general population [14,15], whereas our study focused on lactating mothers whose fatty acid metabolic profile might be quite different from other populations [17]. In any case, the magnitude of our correlation for plasma and erythrocyte DHA was comparable to some other studies utilizing the FFQs covering the whole diet [16]. In addition to the correlation between dietary intake of DHA and its concentrations in plasma and erythrocytes, we also identified clear evidence of a positive correlation for breast milk, which further enhances the validity of our findings, suggesting that the DIET is suitable for the estimation of dietary intake of DHA. In the present study, the overall correlation coefficients were generally lower than those of coastland women, but higher than those of lakeland and inland women, which is in accordance with the variations of dietary DHA intake (*i.e.*, the overall interquartile range of intake was 5.54–32.28, the range for coastland women 8.46–57.49, for lakeland women 6.16–25.47, and for inland women 2.80–21.96), suggesting that it is quite important for future studies to validate FFQs in a population with diverse dietary patterns. Moreover, the correlation coefficients for plasma and breast milk were generally higher than those for erythrocytes, which corresponds to the fact that erythrocyte DHA is an indicator of longer term nutritional status [22], whereas plasma and breast milk DHA often reflect short term dietary intake [12,22,23].

In our study, the median DHA dietary intake was highest in lactating mothers residing in the coastland area (24.3 mg/day) and lowest in those from the inland area (8.8 mg/day), and the intake of lakeland mothers (13.7 mg/day) was intermediate between them. Compared to other studies carried out among Chinese population, the dietary intake of our population was relatively lower. On the basis of the whole diet FFQ, three cross-sectional studies reported the dietary intake of DHA of 54.7–93.9 mg/day, 35.4–51.7 mg/day, and 11.8–41.1 mg/day, in coastland, lakeland, and inland pregnant women of China, respectively [24–26]. In addition to the differences in study population, our study was carried out during the fish close season when the supply of aquatic products might reduce materially. Another reason might be due to the differences of the questionnaire [27]. Specifically, the food list of DIET was determined strictly following the CFCT (Version 2009) [18], and therefore only food containing DHA indicated by CFCT was included, enabling us to calculate the dietary intake of DHA based on standardized DHA content value for a specific food. However, foods like eggs which have been demonstrated by other studies as a non-negligible food source for DHA were not included in DIET as the CFCT states that DHA in eggs is not detectable [28].

It is noteworthy that the DHA dietary intake in our study as well as other studies conducted in China are much lower than reports from other countries. In developed countries like Spain, Japan and Korea, the dietary intake of the general population based on the whole diet FFQ was 400 mg/day, 290 mg/day and 174 mg/day, respectively [29–31]. In the USA, Australia, and Canada, the dietary intake of general population based on DHA specific FFQ were 206 mg/day, 201 mg/day, and 128 mg/day, respectively [21,27,32]; notably, only marine food was included in the FFQ of the USA study. Apparently, even in the coastland of China the DHA dietary intake was only one-fifth of that in Canada and one-tenth of that in USA [21,32]. The DHA intake differences between Chinese and other populations are rather consistent with the differences in aquatic food consumption patterns. Firstly, the intake of aquatic products per capita is substantially lower in China than other countries [33]. For example, the amount of aquatic products consumed by lactating women in China was only 7% of that in Sweden [34]. Secondly, most common seafood consumed in China were scallops and lean fish which contain less fatty acids, while people in other countries usually consumed fatty fish such as salmon and herring with higher content of DHA [26,35]. The Chinese Nutrition Society recommends the adequate intake of DHA as 200 mg/day for lactating women [7]. Obviously, even for women residing in the coastal area, their DHA dietary intake was only one eighth of the recommended value, indicating the necessity for lactating women to consume more fatty fish or take DHA supplements under the guidance of doctors [9].

Interestingly, despite substantially insufficient dietary intake relative to the recommendations, the mean breast milk DHA concentration in our study (0.36%) was slightly higher than the mean level of 65 studies worldwide (0.32%) [36], which is worth studying in the future. Except dietary intake and geographical location, we observed in multiple regression analyses that none of the common characteristics (including maternal ethnic, age, pre-pregnancy BMI, annual family income per capita, education attainment, and feeding methods) seemed to have an important impact on DHA concentrations in breast milk.

Our study has strengths. Firstly, we developed a user-friendly electronic version FFQ where food pictures and intake reference diagrams were provided, which could help the participants to recall more accurately. Secondly, our study was conducted in three areas of China, representing three typical areas with different dietary habits related to aquatic products. Thirdly, compared to other studies in the literature, our study had large sample size and simultaneously assessed the correlation between DHA dietary intake and its concentrations in plasma, erythrocytes, and breast milk.

Our study also has limitations. First, we did not include food that may contain DHA but was not listed in the CFCT (Version 2009). Second, this study is conducted in urban areas, which may limit the generalization of its findings to a broader population because the availability and consumption patterns of aquatic products between rural and urban China may be different. Third, we did not assay α-linolenic acid that can convert to DHA and therefore may be of importance with respect to the interpretation of the correlation between dietary intake of DHA and its concentrations. Additionally, erythrocyte DHA measurements may be lower than the true values because of the temporary storage of blood samples under −20 °C [37,38], and consequently, the correlation between dietary intake DHA and its concentrations in erythrocytes may be slightly compromised.

5. Conclusions

To summarize, this study is the first in China to assess the correlation between DHA dietary intake and its concentrations of biological specimens in lactating women. The DHA dietary intake is positively correlated with the three biomarkers, suggesting that the tailored FFQ can be used to assess the dietary intake of DHA. Consistent with the findings from other studies, the DHA dietary intake of lactating women in China is substantially inadequate. Given the importance of DHA nutritional status of lactating women on the health of both mothers and infants, it is of great significance to improve the maternal DHA nutritional status.

Acknowledgments: This study was supported by the grant from Wyeth Nutrition Science Center (Project Number: 14.10.CN.INF). We thank all participants for their cooperation. We thank all the physicians, nurses and other staff members from Weihai Maternal and Child Health Hospital, Yueyang Maternal and Child Health Hospital, the First Affiliated Hospital of Baotou Medical School, and the Third Hospital of Baogang Group for their supports in the field work.

Author Contributions: The authors' responsibilities were as follows—Jian-Meng Liu, Hong-Tian Li and Man-Xi Bai conceived and designed the study; Jian-Meng Liu, Hong-Tian Li, Meng-Jiao Liu, Hua Ge, Li-Xia Yu, Gao-Sheng Xu, Lin-Lin Wang, Ya-Li Zhang, Yu-Bo Zhou and You Li conducted the field work; Meng-Jiao Liu and Hong-Tian Li analyzed data; Meng-Jiao Liu and Hong-Tian Li drafted the manuscript. Jian-Meng Liu made critical reviews and revisions. All authors have reviewed and approved the final manuscript. Jian-Meng Liu had primary responsibility for final content.

Conflicts of Interest: Jian-Meng Liu has received a grant from Wyeth Nutrition Science Center and presented part of the results at a scientific workshop organized by Wyeth Nutrition Science Center. Man-Xi Bai is working for Wyeth Nutrition Science Center. All other authors declared no conflict of interest.

References

1. Innis, S.M. Impact of maternal diet on human milk composition and neurological development of infants. *Am. J. Clin. Nutr.* **2014**, *99*, 734S–741S. [CrossRef] [PubMed]
2. Lapillonne, A.; Clarke, S.D.; Heird, W.C. Plausible mechanisms for effects of long-chain polyunsaturated fatty acids on growth. *J. Pediatr.* **2003**, *143*, S9–S16. [CrossRef]
3. Salem, N., Jr.; Wegher, B.; Mena, P.; Uauy, R. Arachidonic and docosahexaenoic acids are biosynthesized from their 18-carbon precursors in human infants. *Proc. Natl. Acad. Sci. USA* **1996**, *93*, 49–54. [CrossRef] [PubMed]
4. Oh, R. Practical applications of fish oil (Omega-3 fatty acids) in primary care. *J. Am. Board Fam. Pract.* **2005**, *18*, 28–36. [CrossRef] [PubMed]
5. Hibbeln, J.R. Seafood consumption, the DHA content of mothers' milk and prevalence rates of postpartum depression: A cross-national, ecological analysis. *J. Affect. Disord.* **2002**, *69*, 15–29. [CrossRef]
6. Koletzko, B.; Lien, E.; Agostoni, C.; Bohles, H.; Campoy, C.; Cetin, I.; Decsi, T.; Dudenhausen, J.W.; Dupont, C.; Forsyth, S.; *et al.* The roles of long-chain polyunsaturated fatty acids in pregnancy, lactation and infancy: Review of current knowledge and consensus recommendations. *J. Perinat. Med.* **2008**, *36*, 5–14. [CrossRef] [PubMed]

7. Yiyong, C. The introduction of the Chinese resident meals nutrition DRIs (Version 2013). *Acta Nutr. Sin.* **2014**, *36*, 313–317.
8. Jia, X.; Pakseresht, M.; Wattar, N.; Wildgrube, J.; Sontag, S.; Andrews, M.; Subhan, F.B.; McCargar, L.; Field, C.J. Women who take *n*-3 long-chain polyunsaturated fatty acid supplements during pregnancy and lactation meet the recommended intake. *Appl. Physiol. Nutr. Metab.* **2015**, *40*, 474–481. [CrossRef] [PubMed]
9. Supplimentation CpoCmaiD. Experts consensus on China's maternal and infant DHA supplementation. *Chin. J. Reprod. Health* **2015**, *107*, 99–101. (In Chinese)
10. Pawlosky, R.J.; Hibbeln, J.R.; Novotny, J.A.; Salem, N., Jr. Physiological compartmental analysis of alpha-linolenic acid metabolism in adult humans. *J. Lipid Res.* **2001**, *42*, 1257–1265. [PubMed]
11. Plourde, M.; Cunnane, S.C. Extremely limited synthesis of long chain polyunsaturates in adults: Implications for their dietary essentiality and use as supplements. *Appl. Physiol. Nutr. Metab.* **2007**, *32*, 619–634. [CrossRef] [PubMed]
12. Sartorelli, D.S.; Nishimura, R.Y.; Castro, G.S.; Barbieri, P.; Jordao, A.A. Validation of a FFQ for estimating omega-3, omega-6 and trans fatty acid intake during pregnancy using mature breast milk and food recalls. *Eur. J. Clin. Nutr.* **2012**, *66*, 1259–1264. [CrossRef] [PubMed]
13. Iranpour, R.; Kelishadi, R.; Babaie, S.; Khosravi-Darani, K.; Farajian, S. Comparison of long chain polyunsaturated fatty acid content in human milk in preterm and term deliveries and its correlation with mothers' diet. *J. Res. Med. Sci.* **2013**, *18*, 1–5. [PubMed]
14. Dahl, L.; Maeland, C.A.; Bjorkkjaer, T. A short food frequency questionnaire to assess intake of seafood and *n*-3 supplements: Validation with biomarkers. *Nutr. J.* **2011**, *10*, 127. [CrossRef] [PubMed]
15. Patterson, A.C.; Hogg, R.C.; Kishi, D.M.; Stark, K.D. Biomarker and dietary validation of a Canadian food frequency questionnaire to measure eicosapentaenoic and docosahexaenoic acid intakes from whole food, functional food, and nutraceutical sources. *J. Acad. Nutr. Diet.* **2012**, *112*, 1005–1014. [CrossRef] [PubMed]
16. Serra-Majem, L.; Nissensohn, M.; Overby, N.C.; Fekete, K. Dietary methods and biomarkers of omega 3 fatty acids: A systematic review. *Br. J. Nutr.* **2012**, *107*, S64–S76. [CrossRef] [PubMed]
17. Butte, N.F.; Hopkinson, J.M.; Mehta, N.; Moon, J.K.; Smith, E.O. Adjustments in energy expenditure and substrate utilization during late pregnancy and lactation. *Am. J. Clin. Nutr.* **1999**, *69*, 299–307. [PubMed]
18. Yang, Y.X.; Wang, G.Y. *The China Food Composition Table*; Peking University Medical Press: Beijing, China, 2009. (In Chinese)
19. Li, Y.; Li, H.T.; Trasande, L.; Ge, H.; Yu, L.X.; Xu, G.S.; Bai, M.X.; Liu, J.M. DHA in Pregnant and Lactating Women from Coastland, Lakeland, and Inland Areas of China: Results of a DHA Evaluation in Women (DEW) Study. *Nutrients* **2015**, *7*, 8723–8732. [CrossRef] [PubMed]
20. Lucas, M.; Asselin, G.; Merette, C.; Poulin, M.J.; Dodin, S. Validation of an FFQ for evaluation of EPA and DHA intake. *Public Health Nutr.* **2009**, *12*, 1783–1790. [CrossRef] [PubMed]
21. Hassiotou, F.; Hepworth, A.R.; Williams, T.M.; Twigger, A.J.; Perrella, S.; Lai, C.T.; Filgueira, L.; Geddes, D.T.; Hartmann, P.E. Breastmilk cell and fat contents respond similarly to removal of breastmilk by the infant. *PLoS ONE* **2013**, *8*, e78232. [CrossRef] [PubMed]
22. Sullivan, B.L.; Williams, P.G.; Meyer, B.J. Biomarker validation of a long-chain omega-3 polyunsaturated fatty acid food frequency questionnaire. *Lipids* **2006**, *41*, 845–850. [CrossRef] [PubMed]
23. Hodge, A.M.; Simpson, J.A.; Gibson, R.A.; Sinclair, A.J.; Makrides, M.; O'Dea, K.; English, D.R.; Giles, G.G. Plasma phospholipid fatty acid composition as a biomarker of habitual dietary fat intake in an ethnically diverse cohort. *Nutr. Metab. Cardiovasc. Dis.* **2007**, *17*, 415–426. [CrossRef] [PubMed]
24. Meng, L.P.; Zhang, J.; Wang, Y.Q.; Wang, C.R.; Ghebremskel, K.; Zhao, W.H. Survey on the fatty acids intake in pregnant women in different auqatic product intake regions. *Acta Nutr. Sin.* **2008**, *30*, 249–252.
25. Zhang, J.; Wang, Y.; Meng, L.; Wang, C.; Zhao, W.; Chen, J.; Ghebremeskel, K.; Crawford, M.A. Maternal and neonatal plasma *n*-3 and *n*-6 fatty acids of pregnant women and neonates in three regions in China with contrasting dietary patterns. *Asia Pac. J. Clin. Nutr.* **2009**, *18*, 377–388. [PubMed]
26. Zhang, J.; Wang, C.; Gao, Y.; Li, L.; Man, Q.; Song, P.; Meng, L.; Du, Z.Y.; Miles, E.A.; Lie, O.; *et al.* Different intakes of *n*-3 fatty acids among pregnant women in 3 regions of China with contrasting dietary patterns are reflected in maternal but not in umbilical erythrocyte phosphatidylcholine fatty acid composition. *Nutr. Res.* **2013**, *33*, 613–621. [CrossRef] [PubMed]

27. Dickinson, K.M.; Delaney, C.L.; Allan, R.; Spark, I.; Miller, M.D. Validation of a Brief Dietary Assessment Tool for Estimating Dietary EPA and DHA Intake in Australian Adults at Risk of Cardiovascular Disease. *J. Am. Coll. Nutr.* **2015**, *34*, 333–339. [CrossRef] [PubMed]
28. Meyer, B.J.; Mann, N.J.; Lewis, J.L.; Milligan, G.C.; Sinclair, A.J.; Howe, P.R. Dietary intakes and food sources of omega-6 and omega-3 polyunsaturated fatty acids. *Lipids* **2003**, *38*, 391–398. [CrossRef] [PubMed]
29. Kim, J.; Lim, S.Y.; Shin, A.; Sung, M.K.; Ro, J.; Kang, H.S.; Lee, K.S.; Kim, S.W.; Lee, E.S. Fatty fish and fish omega-3 fatty acid intakes decrease the breast cancer risk: A case-control study. *BMC Cancer* **2009**, *9*, 216. [CrossRef] [PubMed]
30. Amiano, P.; Machon, M.; Dorronsoro, M.; Chirlaque, M.D.; Barricarte, A.; Sanchez, M.J.; Navarro, C.; Huerta, J.M.; Molina-Montes, E.; Sanchez-Cantalejo, E.; *et al.* Intake of total omega-3 fatty acids, eicosapentaenoic acid and docosahexaenoic acid and risk of coronary heart disease in the Spanish EPIC cohort study. *Nutr. Metab. Cardiovasc. Dis.* **2014**, *24*, 321–327. [CrossRef] [PubMed]
31. Miyake, Y.; Tanaka, K.; Okubo, H.; Sasaki, S.; Arakawa, M. Maternal fat intake during pregnancy and wheeze and eczema in Japanese infants: The Kyushu Okinawa Maternal and Child Health Study. *Ann. Epidemiol.* **2013**, *23*, 674–680. [CrossRef] [PubMed]
32. Arsenault, L.N.; Matthan, N.; Scott, T.M.; Dallal, G.; Lichtenstein, A.H.; Folstein, M.F.; Rosenberg, I.; Tucker, K.L. Validity of estimated dietary eicosapentaenoic acid and docosahexaenoic acid intakes determined by interviewer-administered food frequency questionnaire among older adults with mild-to-moderate cognitive impairment or dementia. *Am. J. Epidemiol.* **2009**, *170*, 95–103. [CrossRef] [PubMed]
33. Zhai, F.Y.; He, Y.N.; Ma, G.S.; Li, Y.P.; Wang, Z.H.; Hu, Y.S.; Zhao, L.Y.; Cui, Z.H.; Li, Y.; Yang, X.G. Study on the current status and trend of food consumption among Chinese population. *Chin. J. Epidemiol.* **2005**, *26*, 485–488.
34. Xiang, M.; Harbige, L.S.; Zetterstrom, R. Long-chain polyunsaturated fatty acids in Chinese and Swedish mothers: Diet, breast milk and infant growth. *Acta Paediatr.* **2005**, *94*, 1543–1549. [CrossRef] [PubMed]
35. Jeppesen, C.; Jorgensen, M.E.; Bjerregaard, P. Assessment of consumption of marine food in Greenland by a food frequency questionnaire and biomarkers. *Int. J. Circumpolar Health* **2012**, *71*, 18361. [CrossRef] [PubMed]
36. Turcot, V.; Brunet, J.; Daneault, C.; Tardif, J.C.; Des Rosiers, C.; Lettre, G. Validation of fatty acid intakes estimated by a food frequency questionnaire using erythrocyte fatty acid profiling in the Montreal Heart Institute Biobank. *J. Hum. Nutr. Diet.* **2015**, *28*, 646–658. [CrossRef] [PubMed]
37. Metherel, A.H.; Stark, K.D. Cryopreservation prevents iron-initiated highly unsaturated fatty acid loss during storage of human blood on chromatography paper at −20 °C. *J. Nutr.* **2015**, *145*, 654–660. [CrossRef] [PubMed]
38. Metherel, A.H.; Aristizabal Henao, J.J.; Stark, K.D. EPA and DHA levels in whole blood decrease more rapidly when stored at −20 °C as compared with room temperature, 4 and −75 °C. *Lipids* **2013**, *48*, 1079–1091. [CrossRef] [PubMed]

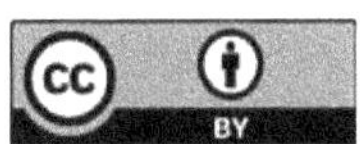

MDPI
St. Alban-Anlage 66
4052 Basel, Switzerland
Tel. +41 61 683 77 34
Fax +41 61 302 89 18
http://www.mdpi.com

Nutrients Editorial Office
E-mail: nutrients@mdpi.com
http://www.mdpi.com/journal/nutrients

www.ingramcontent.com/pod-product-compliance
Lightning Source LLC
Chambersburg PA
CBHW051724210326
41597CB00032B/5591
* 9 7 8 3 0 3 8 4 2 9 7 1 5 *